Stanfield's Introduction to

Health Professions

Eighth Edition

Nanna Cross, PhD

Dana C. McWay, JD, RHIA, FAHIMA

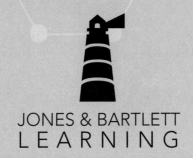

JONES & BARTLETT
LEARNING

World Headquarters
Jones & Bartlett Learning
25 Mall Road
Burlington, MA 01803
978-443-5000
info@jblearning.com
www.jblearning.com

Jones & Bartlett Learning books and products are available through most bookstores and online booksellers. To contact Jones & Bartlett Learning directly, call 800-832-0034, fax 978-443-8000, or visit our website, www.jblearning.com.

> Substantial discounts on bulk quantities of Jones & Bartlett Learning publications are available to corporations, professional associations, and other qualified organizations. For details and specific discount information, contact the special sales department at Jones & Bartlett Learning via the above contact information or send an email to specialsales@jblearning.com.

29377-7

Production Credits

Vice President, Product Management: Marisa R. Urbano
Vice President, Product Operations: Christine Emerton
Director of Product Management: Matthew Kane
Product Manager: Bill Lawrensen
Director, Content Management: Donna Gridley
Manager, Content Strategy: Carolyn Pershouse
Content Strategist: Ashley Malone
Content Coordinator: Elena Sorrentino
Director, Project Management and Content Services: Karen Scott
Project Manager: Kristen Rogers
Project Specialist: Belinda Thresher
Senior Digital Project Specialist: Angela Dooley
Director of Marketing: Andrea DeFronzo
Marketing Manager: Dana Burford

Marketing Specialist: Emma Limperis
Vice President, International Sales, Public Safety Group: Matthew Maniscalco
Director of Sales, Public Safety Group: Brian Hendrickson
Content Services Manager: Colleen Lamy
Vice President, Manufacturing and Inventory Control: Therese Connell
Composition: Straive
Project Management: Straive
Cover Design: Briana Yates
Media Development Editor: Faith Brosnan
Rights & Permissions Manager: John Rusk
Rights Specialist: Rebecca Damon
Cover Image (Title Page, Part Opener, Chapter Opener):
    © kanetmark/Shutterstock.
Printing and Binding: LSC Communications

Library of Congress Cataloging-in-Publication Data
Names: Cross, Nanna, author. | McWay, Dana C., author.
Title: Stanfield's introduction to health professions / Nanna Cross, Dana C. McWay.
Other titles: Introduction to health professions
Description: Eighth edition. | Burlington, Massachusetts : Jones & Bartlett Learning, [2023] | Includes bibliographical references and index.
Identifiers: LCCN 2021034318 | ISBN 9781284219456 (paperback)
Subjects: LCSH: Medicine—Vocational guidance. | Allied health personnel—Vocational guidance.
Classification: LCC R690 .S727 2023 | DDC 610.69—dc23
LC record available at https://lccn.loc.gov/2021034318

6048

Printed in the United States of America
26 25 24 23 22   10 9 8 7 6 5 4 3 2 1

BRIEF CONTENTS

CONTENTS

NOTE FROM THE AUTHORS

Careers in the healthcare field are growing more rapidly than other careers because of longevity and greater numbers of the elderly needing health care as well as advanced technology with more treatment options. Within health care, there is a career for nearly everyone—from entry-level positions as home health or personal care aides, which require no prior training, to being employed as a physician, which requires 7 to 8 years of college plus an internship to enter a career.

Although the COVID-19 pandemic dramatically impacted the demand for many healthcare professionals, the authors did not attempt to predict how the pandemic might change future job opportunities for individual health professions. The pandemic increased the demand and appreciation for respiratory therapists—the health professional who manages patients on ventilators—and critical care physicians and nurses. The high number of residents in nursing homes ill from the virus demonstrated the importance of infection control in healthcare settings and the need for skilled nursing assistants. The virus also demonstrated the value of public health workers who monitored the pandemic on the local, state, and federal levels and communicated changing recommendations to prevent the public from becoming ill from the virus. It is hoped that living through the pandemic has expanded our knowledge and appreciation for the many healthcare workers who have the responsibility for protecting our health.

This text is designed so that the instructor can select individual chapters for a course. Most college texts are organized to be followed from the beginning of the book through the last chapter. By contrast, instructors using this text can select certain chapters based on their course objectives since each chapter is written to be understandable and comprehensive as a standalone. Key terms unique to health care are defined in the glossary at the end of the text and are listed at the beginning of each chapter so students can refer to the glossary as needed.

WHAT ARE THE LATEST TRENDS IN THIS MARKET?

The current trend is to require more education for entry-level health professionals. Educational programs for registered nurses are moving to a bachelor's degree, while programs for dietitians and occupational therapists are moving to a master's degree. The profession of physical therapy now requires a Doctor of Physical Therapy to practice. Educational requirements for support personnel are typically an associate's degree—for example, occupational therapy assistants and physical therapy assistants.

The health inequities in the United States were exacerbated by the COVID-19 pandemic. The health system was not prepared, and disparities in access to health care became more evident with the pandemic. Advances in healthcare treatment are not readily available to low-income communities and minorities. Historically, our healthcare system has not addressed social needs and social determinants of health (SDOH). The future of health care for all requires that the system address SDOH (safe and affordable education, housing, transportation, food, and mental health services). Unless these needs are addressed, there will continue to be disparities in access to health care and health outcomes. The entire health community—hospitals and primary care providers—will be expected to address these unmet needs of the population.

Information technology is changing the way health care is delivered as well as the way consumers manage their health. Electronic health records that are accessible by professionals regardless of physical location are cost-effective and improve the quality and safety of health care. Many patients now have access to lab values and other text results through a patient portal within the electronic health record. Technology also makes it possible for patients to do more self-monitoring and to communicate results back to their physician, nurse, or caseworker. For example, blood glucose and blood pressure can be monitored by the patient and the results transmitted to the healthcare provider.

Nanna Cross, PhD
Dana C. McWay, JD, RHIA, FAHIMA

PREFACE

The eighth edition of *Stanfield's Introduction to Health Professions* provides comprehensive coverage of all the major health professions. This product is designed for students who are interested in pursuing a health-related career but are still exploring and have not yet decided on a specific career. The eighth edition outlines more than 75 careers and touches on every major facet of the field, including a description of the profession and typical work settings; educational, licensure, and certification requirements; salary and growth projections; and internet resources on educational programs and state requirements for licensure and/or certification. In addition, this resource provides a thorough review of the U.S. healthcare delivery system, managed care, healthcare financing, reimbursement, insurance coverage, Medicare, Medicaid, and the impact of new technology on healthcare services. Information on career preparation and development is also included. All chapters are updated to reflect current demographics and new policies.

HOW IS THIS BOOK ORGANIZED?

The new edition of this text has been reorganized into five sections.

- **Part I—The Healthcare System in the United States**. This section provides an overview of the healthcare system in the United States, with separate chapters on categories of health services, financing health care, the impact of aging on demands for healthcare providers, healthcare reform, and medical and information technology.
- **Part II—Jobs and Careers**. This section focuses on career planning and career development.
- **Parts III through V** contain chapters on individual careers that are organized so that students will be able to quickly identify a particular career of interest. Each chapter is organized to follow the same general format, making it easy for students to explore many different health careers. Each chapter follows the same format with a description of the profession and typical work setting; educational, licensure and certification requirements; salary and growth projections; and internet resources on educational programs and requirements for licensure and/or certification. For example, in the chapter on dentistry, the career is described based on the education and training requirements from most education—dentist—to least education—dental assistant. For each career within the dentistry profession, the student has access to the usual responsibilities, work setting, salary, and expected demand for that career. Each chapter lists internet resources to explore educational programs as well as state requirements for licensure and certification options for advancing in the profession.
- **Part III—Health Practitioners and Technicians**. This section is the core of the product and contains 21 chapters directed at health careers that involve direct patient contact and care, ranging from diagnosis to treatment to education and counseling and medical or surgical interventions.
- **Part IV—Healthcare Support Personnel**. This section contains five chapters directed at health careers that support or supplement other health professionals in providing ongoing care for patients—medical and nursing assistants; personal, home, and psychiatric aides; medical information technology; and alternative therapies including massage, recreation, art, dance, and music therapists.
- **Part V—Health-Related Professions**. This section focuses on health-related professionals who usually do not have direct contact with human patients but often have an impact on human health—veterinary medicine and occupational health and environmental sciences.

ABOUT THE AUTHORS

Nanna Cross, PhD, has worked as a faculty member in dietetic and physician education programs teaching clinical nutrition courses and supervising dietetic interns in clinical practicums. Dr. Cross worked as a clinical dietitian at the University of Missouri Hospitals and Clinics and as a consulting dietitian for Home Care, Hospice, Head Start, and Long-Term Care facilities.

Dana C. McWay, JD, RHIA, FAHIMA, is both a lawyer and a health information management professional. She works as an adjunct faculty member at Saint Louis University in the Health Informatics and Pre-Law Studies programs. She serves as the Clerk of Court for the U.S. Bankruptcy Court for the Eastern District of Missouri, an executive position responsible for all operational, administrative, financial, and technological matters of the court. She has worked as both a director and assistant director of medical records in a large teaching hospital and a for-profit psychiatric and substance abuse facility. She is a past Director on the Board of Directors of the American Health Information Management Association and serves as a voting member of the Institutional Review Board at Washington University School of Medicine, from 1992 to the present.

NEW FEATURES

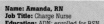

Professional Profiles

Interviews with professionals, including frequently asked questions and answer sections.

Learning Portfolio

At the end of each chapter, this review section includes Study Points, Issues for Discussion, Enrichment Activities, and Case Studies.

All sections are thoroughly updated to reflect current training requirements, responsibilities, and salaries, as established in the *Occupational Outlook Handbook 2020–2021 Edition.*

© kanetmark/Shutterstock.

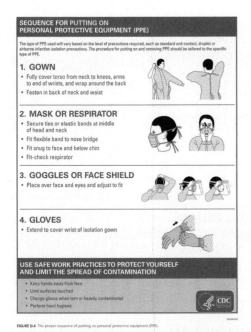

FIGURE D.4 The proper sequence of putting on personal protective equipment (PPE).

New Appendix

Appendix D, "Infection Control," has been added. This appendix reviews standard precautions for all patient care to prevent the spread of infectious diseases in healthcare settings. Included is a brief overview of the key elements needed for the transmission of infections: a source of the infectious organism, a susceptible person, and a method of transmitting the infection to the susceptible person. There is a review of the proper use of personal protective equipment (PPE), hand washing, sources of viruses and bacteria in a healthcare setting, and a glossary. The appendix also includes posters and infographics that illustrate the concepts of infection control in a way that is easy to understand.

New Careers

Includes seven new careers!

- Dietary Manager (Chapter 13)
- Speech-Language Pathology and Audiology Assistants (Chapter 16)
- Kinesiotherapists (Chapter 19)
- Chiropractor (Chapter 20)
- Art Therapists (Chapter 31)
- Dance Therapists (Chapter 31)
- Music Therapists (Chapter 31)

THE LEARNING AND TEACHING PACKAGE
The Learning Package for the Student

Students can review the Learning Portfolios at the end of each chapter. For the first eight chapters of the text, the Learning Portfolio includes Study Points and a brief summary of the chapter content. All chapters also include Issues for Discussion, Enrichment Activities, and Case Studies designed to be used by the student for self-study and exploration.

The Teaching Package for the Instructor

Teacher resources include the Learning Portfolios at the end of each chapter, which are designed to be used by both the student and instructor. In addition, the following items are part of the Instructor's Teaching Package:

- Test Bank for each chapter
- Slides in PowerPoint format for each chapter
- Instructor's Manual
- Lecture Outline

Bloom's Taxonomy

The Learning Package for the student and the Teaching Package for the instructor are designed to incorporate Bloom's levels of learning from the lowest level of knowledge to the highest level of evaluation. The learning and teaching packages that accompany the text encourage going beyond the content of the text. The text is expected to be a starting point.

REVIEWERS

Seventh Edition

Jennifer M. Hatfield, MHS
Clinical Assistant Professor
Indiana University South Bend

Rebecca Manriquez
Health Science Technology Instructor
El Paso Center for Career and Technology

Sixth Edition

Karen Bakuzonis, PhD, MSHA, RHIA
Chair Health Informatics Department
Ashford University

William Ballard, MA, MEd
Academic Advisor College of Business
Florida Atlantic University

Dr. Barry Brock
Academic Coordinator/Health Services Administration
Barry University School of PACE

Dr. Kenneth L. Campbell, MPH, MBA, MA
Adjunct Professor
Department of Health Sciences at Chicago State University
Adjunct Professor and Interim Community Health Worker
(CHW) Program Director at City Colleges of Chicago
Cook County System Operations Analyst
Cook County Health and Hospitals System (CCHHS) and
Cook County Department of Public Health (CCDPH)

Karen Collins Gibson, MSA, RHIA, FAHIMA
Delaware County Community College

Nicole L. Hatcher, PH.Sc, MPAS, PA-C
Assistant Professor
Howard University

Andrea Koepke, PhD, RN
Dean—College of Health Professions
The University of Findlay

Barbara Marchelletta, CMA (AAMA), CPC, RHIT, CPT
Program Director—Allied Health Beal College

Darlene Martin, MEd, ATC
Liberty University

Kristen L. McHenry, MS, RRT-ACCS
Director of Cardiopulmonary Science Program Assistants
Professor—Department of Allied Health Sciences
College of Clinical and Rehabilitative Health Sciences
East Tennessee State University

Jahangir Moini, MD, MPH
Professor of Science and Health
Eastern Florida State College

Cindy Mulder, MSN
Instructor
University of South Dakota

Amy Nelson, MS OTR/L, MT(ASCP)
University of South Dakota

Dr. Dennis Palkon, PhD, MPH, MSW
Professor and Director of Management Programs/Health
Administration/Business
Florida Atlantic University

Bonita Sasnett, EdD
East Carolina University

Erin Sayer, PhD
Chief Academic Advisor—School of Biological Sciences
University of Nebraska—Lincoln

PART ONE

The Healthcare System in the United States

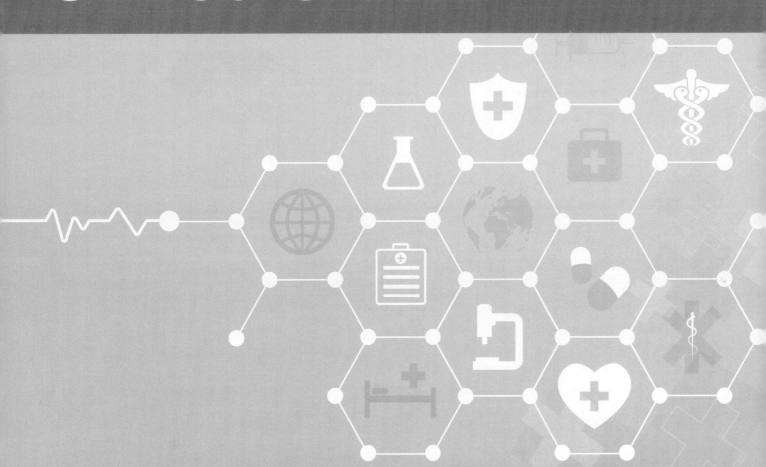

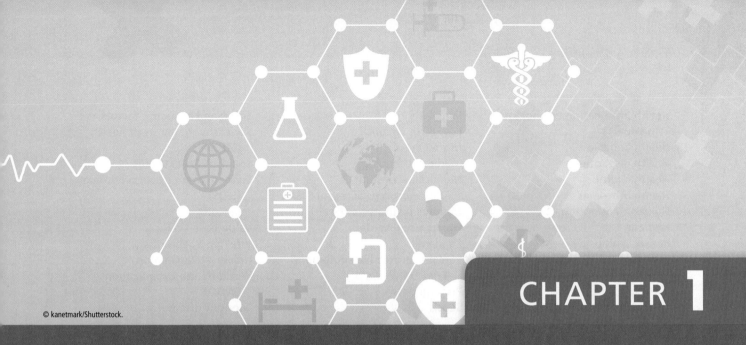

© kanetmark/Shutterstock.

CHAPTER **1**

U.S. Health Care

After studying this chapter, the student should be able to:

- Discuss the changes in health problems of the population in the United States over the past 150 years.
- Discuss some of the reasons for changes in the causes of mortality and life expectancy between 2010 and 2020.
- Explain the role of social determinants of health in health outcomes.
- Identify expected future changes in the health of the population that will influence healthcare needs and career opportunities in health care.
- Explain the role of the government in the expansion of health care.

KEY TERMS

Acute infectious disease
Affordable Care Act (ACA)
American Academy of Family Physicians
American Hospital Association (AHA)
Applied behavior analysis (ABA)
Artificial intelligence (AI)
Autism spectrum disorders (ASD)
Avian (bird) influenza

Birth defects
Centers for Disease Control and Prevention (CDC)
Centers for Medicare and Medicaid (CMS) Innovation programs
Chronic disease
Clinical care
Clinical preventive services
Congenital malformation
Coronavirus (COVID-19)

Discrimination
Disparities
Doulas
Ebola virus
Electronic health records (EHRs)
Epidemics
Equality
Equity
Federal Poverty Level (FPL)
Foodborne illness
Globalization

3

Health information technology (health IT)	Longevity	Social and economic factors
Health behaviors	Low birth weight	Social determinants of health (SDOH)
Health disparities	Mortality	Spanish Flu (1918 Flu)
Health equity	Medical technology	Sudden infant death syndrome (SIDS)
Health outcomes	Methicillin-resistant *Staphylococcus aureus* (MRSA)	Telehealth
Human Genome Project	National Institutes of Health (NIH)	Value-based care
Hygiene	Opioid use disorder	Viral gastroenteritis
Immunizations	Pandemic	Universal vaccination
Infant mortality	Personal protective equipment (PPE)	World Health Organization (WHO)
Infectious disease	Preterm birth	Zoonotic diseases
Life expectancy	Sepsis	
Lifestyle		

Introduction

This chapter will review historical, current, and emerging trends that have impacted the health status of individuals and health delivery systems in the United States. Information added since the seventh edition includes the current approach of healthcare systems to address social needs as part of delivering health care and public health efforts to respond to the COVID-19 pandemic. The chapter will introduce topics that will be discussed in more detail in later chapters.

HISTORICAL EVENTS IMPACTING HEALTH CARE

Controlling healthcare costs and increasing access to health care were policy priorities for President Barack Obama with the passage of the **Affordable Care Act (ACA)** signed into law on March 23, 2010.[1] Some of the reasons for the rising costs of health care are the use of expensive **medical technology** and prescription drugs, reimbursement systems that reward the volume of medical services instead of outcomes, inadequate preventive services, the aging of the population, and the increased prevalence of **chronic disease** as well as high administrative costs.[2] Healthcare costs have been a concern of the government because growth in healthcare costs exceeded growth of the U.S. economy beginning in the 1970s with a high of 14% in 1980 followed by a decrease equal to that of inflation at 3% in 2018.[3]

Another critical issue that needs to be addressed is the inefficiencies and **disparities** in the current system. Comparisons with other countries and across states show large variations in spending without commensurate differences in **health outcomes**.[4]

The most significant change in health care in the United States in the past 10 years is the number of individuals who have gained access to health care with the implementation of the ACA. In 2008, 46.5 million individuals (17% of the population) were uninsured; by 2017, the number of uninsured dropped to 26.7 million or 10%. As a result of the ACA, Medicaid expanded health coverage to nearly all adults with incomes at or below 138% of poverty in states that adopted the expansion, and tax credits are available for people with incomes up to 400% of poverty who purchased coverage through a health insurance marketplace.[4] The ACA has narrowed racial and ethnic disparities in access to health insurance with increased access for Blacks and Hispanics primarily in states that expanded Medicaid.[5] Those who remain uninsured after the ACA are non-elderly adults with income below 200% of the **Federal Poverty Level (FPL)** who work for an employer who doesn't provide health insurance and those who are unable to buy insurance because of the cost of the premiums. Hispanic, American Indians/Alaskan Natives, and those living in the South and West—in states that did not expand Medicaid—are more likely to be uninsured.[6]

Greater access to health care increased demand for providers (physicians, nurses, and other healthcare workers), hospitals, outpatient clinics, and home-care services. The healthcare environment has become more competitive, in large part because of the requirements for hospitals to improve both the quality of care and efficiency as a result of the ACA.

The United States will need to continue to improve the efficiency and quality of health care and reduce disparities in access to health care for all Americans. With that premise, we begin this chapter with a look back at healthcare issues and treatments developed in the past 150 years. Much of the material from the seventh edition of this text is still relevant.

The succeeding chapters have been updated to reflect the anticipated changes and demographics of the twenty-first century and the changing nature of health care and opportunities for health careers.

A LOOK BACK

Since the dawn of recorded history (and undoubtedly before), human beings have suffered sudden and devastating epidemics and diseases. In the United States in the second half of the nineteenth century, the most critical health problems were related to industrialization and crowded living conditions in cities. Improper sewage disposal resulted in contaminated water, and lack of refrigeration resulted in contaminated food. Illness caused by infectious agents—pneumonia, tuberculosis, diarrhea, and diphtheria—accounted for one-third of all deaths with children under five years of age accounting for 40% of all deaths.[7]

By 1900, infectious disease **epidemics** had been brought under control as a result of the discovery of microbes as the cause for **infectious diseases** and the development of antibiotics that were effective in treating bacterial infections such as pneumonia and tuberculosis. However, the most important factor in the decline in mortality in the twentieth century was improvements in sanitation and **hygiene**, supported by home and workplace improvements and attempts to improve the environment. Cities developed systems for safeguarding the milk, food, and water supply, and health departments began to grow, applying case findings and quarantines with good results. Better personal hygiene (for example, handwashing) accounted for approximately one-fifth of the reduction in mortality or death. The major epidemics that had caused deaths had been eliminated in the United States, and the pendulum swung away from acute infectious diseases and toward chronic conditions.[7]

Another reason for the falling death rate was the improvement of nutrition, which led to an increase in the resistance to diseases. Once sanitation improved, lack of food and the resulting malnutrition were largely responsible for infectious diseases. Nutritional status is a critical factor in a person's response to infectious diseases, especially young children. According to the **World Health Organization (WHO),** the best "vaccine" against common diseases is an adequate diet.

With epidemics behind them, the scientific community began working on better surgical techniques, new treatment methods, new tests to facilitate accurate diagnoses, and the treatment of individual diseases. The number of hospitals grew rapidly, and medical schools flourished. Within a few years, medical care and patterns of disease had totally changed. The arrival of antibiotics in the 1940s and the implementation of childhood **universal vaccination** in the 1950s for measles, mumps, rubella, and polio signaled the end of the dominance of **acute infectious disease** (FIGURE 1.1).[7]

By the late 1940s, chronic illnesses such as heart disease and cancer accounted for nearly half of the deaths in the United States. By the twenty-first century, the development of

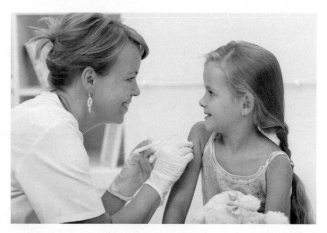

FIGURE 1.1 Universal child immunization beginning in the 1950s dramatically reduced death from infectious disease in the United States.
© Ilike/Shutterstock.

new drugs to control risk factors for heart disease—for example, drugs to control hypertension, cholesterol, and diabetes—reduced death from heart disease by 16% between 2007 and 2017. During this same time, deaths from cancer decreased to a greater extent (29%) due to fewer people smoking and advances in early detection and treatment.[8] The introduction of antiviral therapy in the 1990s reduced the death rate from the human immunodeficiency virus (HIV) by 80%.[9] Death rates continue to be highest for heart disease and cancer; however, rates for unintentional injuries (accidental death) and Alzheimer's disease are on the rise.[8] **FIGURE 1.2** shows death rates for men and women in 2017.

RECENT TRENDS

Although the United States has made great strides in improving the health of the nation and improving access to health care, recent changes in the cause of death and **longevity** are cause for concern. Monitoring of **mortality**—the causes and rates of death—along with **life expectancy** at birth is used to describe the health of a population. Changes in mortality or life expectancy are used to evaluate and develop health policy and allocate resources. After decades of gains in longevity, life expectancy at birth plateaued at 78 years between 2013 and 2017.[8] Between 2000 and 2016, increases in mortality from four causes of death—unintentional injuries, Alzheimer's disease, suicide, and chronic liver disease—contributed to the recent decline in life expectancy.[10]

Death rates for unintentional drug overdoses—a subset of unintentional injuries—in particular—contributed to the negative change in life expectancy observed in recent years. Most unintentional drug overdoses were because of **opioid use disorders**. An increase in suicides was also seen between 2006 and 2016 with suicide being among the top five leading causes of death for persons from 1 to 44 years of age. Chronic liver disease—caused by excessive alcohol intake—also increased in men.[10] Deaths from these three causes—drug overdose, suicide, and chronic liver disease—are often described as

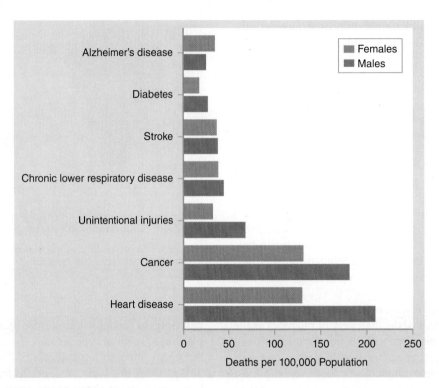

FIGURE 1.2 Causes of death by sex: United States, 2017.
Data from National Center for Health Statistics. *Health, United States, 2018.* Accessed March 2, 2021. https://www.cdc.gov/nchs/data/hus/hus18.pdf

"deaths of despair," or markers for complex socioeconomic problems manifested in behavioral health problems such as excessive use of alcohol or addiction to opioids. Communities with limited opportunities for employment and the ready availability of synthetic opioids to treat pain contributed to opioid addiction. States most impacted by the opioid crisis were West Virginia, Pennsylvania, and Ohio.[11]

The rise in opioid use disorders and overdose has been fueled by inappropriate opioid prescribing as well as aggressive trafficking of heroin, often laced with fentanyl, a highly potent synthetic opioid. Sales of prescription opioid painkillers nearly quadrupled from 1999 to 2014 in response to efforts of health professionals to treat patients more effectively with pain. States are addressing the opioid crisis by educating healthcare providers on appropriately prescribing opioids for treatment of pain and educating patients on proper disposal of unused opioids. Other strategies are increasing patient access to medication-assisted treatment (e.g., methadone treatment programs) and behavioral health treatment programs. The medication naloxone (Narcan) is now available to reverse opioid overdose and is being used by emergency medical technicians and emergency room staff to prevent death.

Reversing the upward trend in deaths from suicide, alcohol, and drug overdose will require greater cooperation across sectors, at both the state and federal level, including the public health, healthcare delivery, and criminal justice systems.[11] Health professionals who treat mental and behavioral health conditions—psychologists, clinical social workers, and behavioral disorder counselors—are needed to treat those with alcohol and opioid addictions.

Infant mortality—the death of a baby before their first birthday—is an indicator of maternal health and the availability and use of appropriate health care by pregnant women and their infants. The overall infant mortality rate in the United States has decreased over the past seven decades, yet there are disparities in infant mortality by race, geography, and socioeconomic status. For example, in 2017, infants of non-Hispanic Black mothers and American Indians/Alaskan Natives had the highest infant mortality rate, nearly twice the rate of Asians. The death rates for Hispanic and White infants were similar between 2007 and 2017 (**FIGURE 1.3**).[8]

Leading causes of infant deaths in 2017 were **congenital malformations**, **preterm birth** and **low birth weight**, **sudden infant death syndrome (SIDS)**, maternal complications of pregnancy, and unintentional injuries or accidents.[8] Many causes of preterm birth and low birth weight are preventable with appropriate prenatal care. The disparities in infant death by race suggest disparities in access to health care (health insurance, primary care providers) and lack of opportunities to obtain necessary resources such as healthy food, prenatal vitamins, and safe housing (**FIGURE 1.4**).[8]

Living in a rural area limits access to health care because of the growing shortage of providers in rural communities. Many rural hospitals are closing, and fewer than half of all rural counties have physicians that specialize in pregnancy and postpartum care. This lack of prenatal care increases the likelihood that women will die a pregnancy-related death and contributes to higher rates of infant mortality.[13] Data indicate that the first 100 days after delivery are critical for follow-up by healthcare personnel to identify and treat complications. Women who are on Medicaid during pregnancy

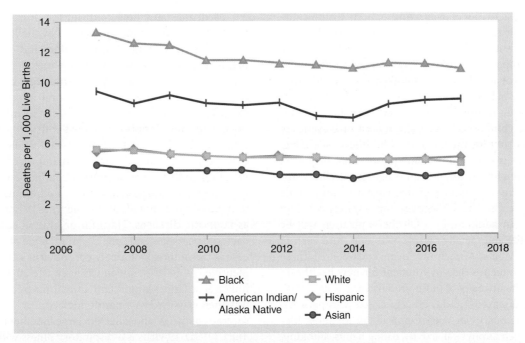

FIGURE 1.3 Infant mortality rates by race: United States, 2007–2017.
Data from National Center for Health Statistics. *Health, United States, 2018*. Accessed March 2, 2021. https://www.cdc.gov/nchs/data/hus/hus18.pdf

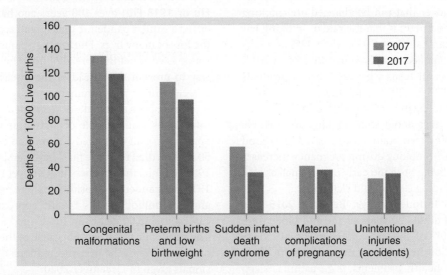

FIGURE 1.4 Leading causes of infant deaths: United States, 2007 and 2017.
Modified from National Center for Health Statistics. *Health, United States, 2018*. Accessed March 2, 2021. https://www.cdc.gov/nchs/data/hus/hus18.pdf

often lose their benefits six months after delivery of the baby. Current recommendations are a follow-up visit at 12 weeks postpartum to improve the mortality rate for both infants and mothers.[14]

Programs that provide prenatal support that address racial, socioeconomic, and structural barriers to optimum care improve health outcomes. Examples are programs that utilize **doulas** to support the mother and programs that offer classes on possible medical complications during pregnancy as well as what to expect during labor and delivery. Addressing structural barriers to care—lack of health insurance, child care, and transportation—is needed to reduce disparities for low-income and other marginalized groups. Women often need assistance with transportation and child

care in order to keep clinic appointments.[15] Many health professionals—nurse-midwives, advanced practice nurses, community health workers, and social workers—can support women and their babies to reduce infant and maternal mortality. Nurse-midwives and advanced practice nurses can serve as primary care providers in communities that lack primary care physicians.

A LOOK FORWARD

Longevity and greater numbers of the elderly have increased the prevalence of chronic and degenerative diseases associated with aging. Chronic diseases are defined as conditions that last one year or more and require ongoing medical attention, limit activities of daily living, or both. Chronic diseases such as heart disease, cancer, and diabetes are the leading causes of death and disability in the United States. The downside to improved health care and longevity is that those above 65 years of age often have multiple chronic conditions. In 2016, nearly half of people above 65 years of age had two to three chronic health conditions, and 15% had four or more chronic conditions.[16] Also, the frailest or chronically ill patients account for the majority of healthcare spending, both by the government and by individuals in out-of-pocket spending. In the future, physical and cognitive decline associated with aging will require personal assistance from family or paid caregivers and health services from a variety of health professionals. In addition, by 2050 the population will be more ethnically and racially diverse, with one-third each of Hispanic non-White, African American, and White.[17] These changes will influence the environment for new healthcare workers and the diversity of those needing care.

Chronic diseases of today are associated with personal **lifestyle**. Individuals can take responsibility for most lifestyle factors such as physical activity, eating habits, smoking, drinking alcoholic beverages, using illicit drugs, and personal hygiene. Two lifestyle factors associated with a high risk for heart disease and cancer that can be changed are smoking and obesity.[18] The good news is that the rate of smoking has dropped by more than half since 1965, when 42% of adults over 18 years of age smoked compared to only 14% in 2017. However, the number of teens who use tobacco products remained high at 27% in 2018, with the majority using electronic cigarettes (e-cigarettes) introduced in the United States in 2007. Concerns about teen smoking are possible harm to the developing teen brain and increased likelihood of lifelong addiction.[18] Smoking during pregnancy increases the risk of an infant being born too early or too small as well as **birth defects** including cleft lip and cleft palate.[19]

Obesity rates continue to rise. Between 2015 and 2016, nearly 40% of adults 20 years of age and older were obese, and nearly 20% of children and teens 2 to 19 years of age were obese. Children who are obese are more likely to develop chronic health problems (e.g., asthma, sleep apnea, joint problems, and type 2 diabetes). These conditions often continue through adulthood with greater risk for heart disease.[8]

As a result of requirements to include preventive services by insurance plans purchased through health exchanges under the ACA and coverage by Medicare, **clinical preventive services** are being utilized by more Americans. For example, **immunizations** and cancer screening—mammography and colonoscopy—are the most common preventive services. However, utilization remains suboptimal for some services. In 2016, only 70% of children 19 to 35 months of age received a combined vaccination series protecting them against seven infectious diseases. Also, only 42% of adults 18 years and older received the influenza vaccine, and only 67% of adults over 65 years of age received a vaccine against pneumonia.[10]

Medicine must now confront the diseases and health problems that are greatly influenced by the local and international environment. **Globalization** and ease in international travel increase the risk for infectious diseases. In the United States, **viral gastroenteritis**—caused by the norovirus—is the most common viral infection, and salmonellosis is the most common bacterial infection—both organisms cause **foodborne illness** with symptoms of vomiting and diarrhea.[20] Although most infectious diseases are now prevented with vaccines and improved methods of infection control, new organisms continue to appear from mutations and transmission from wild animals or insects to domesticated animals and sometimes to humans, known as **zoonotic diseases**. Harmful organisms can be viruses, bacteria, parasites, and fungi.[21] An example of zoonotic disease is the outbreak of a new **coronavirus (COVID-19)** first identified as an epidemic in China in late 2019 and initially linked to a large seafood and animal market.[22] The disease was then classified as a **pandemic** because it spread across several countries and affected large numbers of people.[23] The COVID-19 virus is a respiratory illness with symptoms similar to the flu; however, the virus is different than viruses that cause the flu. Not since the flu pandemic (the **Spanish Flu** or **1918 Flu**) over 100 years ago has the world experienced a similar pandemic that spread around the world with the loss of many lives. During the Spanish Flu outbreak, less was known about the spread of infectious diseases. The only way to prevent the spread of the disease was for everyone to wear a mask and to remain socially isolated.[24] Since then there have been outbreaks of viral infections. However, none infected as many people or caused as many deaths as the Spanish Flu; an estimated 500 million became infected and 50 million died from the flu.[25] In the first year of the COVID-19 pandemic, the numbers had not yet reached those of the 1918 Flu pandemic. Worldwide there were 82 million cases and 1.8 million deaths,[26] with approximately 20 million cases and 345,00 deaths in the United States during 2020.[27] The pandemic was slowed because of the rapid development of vaccines with the first vaccinations of healthcare professionals given in December 2020.[28]

Although scientists had predicted the possibility of a pandemic similar to the Spanish Flu as early as 2000, the world was unprepared to respond to COVID-19. The coronavirus of 2020 was deadly because the virus is easily transmitted from person to person through aerosol droplets spread by coughing, sneezing, and talking and because the virus is unlike other influenza viruses for which there are vaccines. By the time the United States acknowledged the presence of the virus, there were already thousands of people infected, and many had died. Ways that the country was unprepared for the pandemic were the lack of needed **personal protective equipment (PPE)** masks, gloves, and gowns for healthcare workers and the lack of a quick and reliable test to identify those infected with the virus. One of the reasons for the slow response to the pandemic was growing public skepticism of science and scientists at the

National Institutes of Health (NIH) and the **Centers for Disease Control and Prevention (CDC).** Politics interfered with a rapid response to the pandemic because even though infectious disease experts were aware of the impending pandemic, they had difficulty being heard by those in government, and there was a lack of a centralized coordinated response from the federal government.[29] The impact of the COVID-19 pandemic on the world and the economy resulted in closed businesses, schools, and colleges; unemployment; and restricted local and international travel. The response and recovery times in some countries were much quicker than in the United States, and the numbers of cases and deaths were also lower. Scientists around the world worked quickly to develop a vaccine for COVID-19 to prevent the rapid spread of the virus. Without a vaccine, precautions to control the disease were to wear protective masks, self-isolation, proper handwashing, and sanitizing common areas in public buildings, for example, the insides of elevators and doors. **Telehealth** became a common way to deliver health care during this period of social isolation to prevent spread of the virus.

Other examples of zoonotic diseases caused by viruses are the **Ebola** and avian viruses. Between 2014 and 2016, Ebola, a deadly viral infection, was localized primarily to West Africa. Ebola can be transmitted to humans by an infected animal (bat or nonhuman primate) or a sick or dead person infected with the virus. The 2014 Ebola epidemic in West Africa was spread to the United States by healthcare workers employed in West Africa.[30] The CDC—the U.S. government agency that monitors infectious diseases—developed infection-control measures for hospitals treating infected patients in the United States. WHO and the CDC also deployed teams of experts to West Africa to implement infection-control measures to prevent further spread of the disease in Africa.[31]

In 2015, cases of the **avian (bird) influenza** were identified in Europe and China; in the United States, entire commercial poultry flocks required culling or removal of infected turkeys and chickens—and sometimes an entire flock was destroyed to prevent further spread of the disease, at great financial cost to the poultry business.[32] The avian virus occurs naturally in wild aquatic birds and is easily transmitted to domestic birds; however, transmission from birds to humans is rare.

A particularly virulent or antibiotic-resistant bacterial strain—**methicillin-resistant *Staphylococcus aureus* (MRSA)**—is present in hospitals and nursing homes but also in the community: in child-care facilities, schools, and athletic programs.[33] MSRA can cause skin infections after a cut or abrasion and increases the risk for surgical infections, pneumonia, and **sepsis** in hospitalized patients. Preventing MSRA infection requires stringent infection-control measures to prevent spread of the bacteria causing the infection from patient to patient and among healthcare workers because the *Staphylococcus aureus* organism has become resistant to antibiotic treatment (**FIGURE 1.5**).[33]

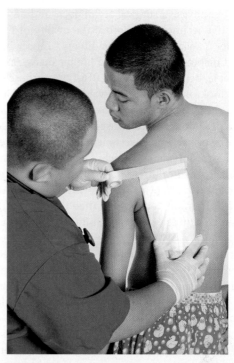

FIGURE 1.5 Methicillin-resistant *Staphylococcus aureus* (MRSA) is a common cause of skin infection.
© Joseph Dilag/Shutterstock.

Preventing the spread of infectious disease requires a team of public health experts to track and contain diseases to prevent epidemics in both humans and animals. Physicians, nurses, veterinarians, medical laboratory technologists, epidemiologists, and public health officials at the local, state, and federal level are examples of healthcare workers involved in preventing the spread of infectious disease. Pandemics require cooperation and ongoing communication among scientists, epidemiologists, and healthcare workers in countries around the world to control the spread of the infectious agent causing the infection. The CDC is responsible for coordinating the team of healthcare workers at the city and state levels across the United States during an epidemic. WHO is the international governmental agency responsible for coordination of this effort. One of the important components of public health work is communication with the public about the disease—how it is transmitted and treated and recommendations for preventing the spread of disease (e.g., proper handwashing and self-isolation for those who are infected). All healthcare workers need to be knowledgeable about the transmission of infectious diseases and the proper procedures for preventing the spread of the disease.

IMPACT OF TECHNOLOGY ON HEALTHCARE SERVICES

Technology has made many new procedures and methods of diagnosis and treatment possible. Advances in medical technology have improved the survival rates of trauma victims and the severely ill. Clinical developments, such as infection control, less invasive surgical techniques, and advances in reproductive technology, improve the quality of life. Drug therapy for managing chronic conditions—cancer, heart disease, and diabetes—has extended life for many Americans. For example, between 2015 and 2016, 40% of those 65 years or older took one or more prescription drugs.[8] More prescription drugs are being used because of the development of new drugs to treat chronic disease and the growth of drug coverage by private and government health insurance.[9]

Two forms of computer technology that have improved the efficiency of health care are augmented intelligence—sometimes referred to as **artificial intelligence (AI)**—and **health information technology (health IT)**. AI is the use of computers and technology to simulate intelligent behavior and critical thinking comparable to a human being. AI can sort through data in public health settings to predict the spread of infectious diseases or to assist a healthcare provider in making decisions about the best medication to use for a specific patient based on symptoms, chronic health problems, and other medications.

Health IT is the use of computers to store health data to support health information management across computerized systems and the secure exchange of health information among providers, consumers, and payers. AI in medicine can be separated into two subtypes: virtual and physical. Virtual AI applications are **electronic health record (EHR)** systems or computer-assisted analysis used by radiologists to identify abnormal X-rays or magnetic resonance images. An example of physical AI is the use of robots to assist in performing surgeries using 3D images and magnification. Other examples of physical AI are the use of multiple sensors to track the movements of patients in smart intensive care units (ICUs) and monitoring movements of an elderly person who lives alone. Remote monitoring of patient clinical data—for example, blood pressure, blood glucose, or heart monitoring—allows healthcare workers to provide care after the patient returns home.[34]

EHRs make it possible for multiple team members to schedule a patient-team conference regardless of physical location. Sharing of EHRs among different providers for the same patient—hospital, emergency room, and outpatient clinic—has the potential to improve patient safety by preventing drug interactions and reducing costs by avoiding duplicate laboratory tests.[22] Patients are able to access their EHR to review lab results, schedule appointments, and receive appointment reminders. Hospitals use EHR to monitor hospital-acquired infections. The federal government uses data to monitor outcomes such as hospital readmission rates and surgical complications as well as healthcare costs.

The continuing surge of technological advances is not without problems. Medical technology can also prolong life for the critically ill, unresponsive patient who has little or no chance of recovery. Services such as mechanical ventilation, kidney dialysis, parenteral (tube) feeding, and other means can keep even comatose patients alive. For the healthcare system, dying can be extremely expensive. The use of EHR by hospitals, clinics, and providers raises ethical concerns for patient privacy and security to prevent data breaches. Issues yet to be

addressed with the use of AI are meeting state and federal regulatory laws and determining policies related to payment and coverage of AI services.[35] The use of technology can increase the efficiency of health delivery; however, start-up costs may be prohibitive for small group practices. The high cost of technology affects the financial structure of the entire healthcare system. These increased costs are visible in the form of higher health insurance costs, higher costs for hospital stays, government payments to the system, and total medical bills. This advanced technology has not only increased medical costs but also created a social and ethical problem. Because of limits in funding, advanced treatment is not available to all people. The poor, who may need it desperately, have no access to it.

The incredible growth of technology has affected all the health professions. Students entering the health field today recognize that they must excel academically and master technical skills. Less time is spent learning personal, non-technical aspects of care. This value system is reinforced by professionals, peers, and administrators and by the public as well. Excellent technical performance has become a standard at the cost of the personal, human touch.

The federal government plays an increasingly powerful role in the direction of health care. It dominates the healthcare system by virtue of its expanding monetary support of technology and services and because it sets the rules for the provision of health care. As health services enter the twenty-first century, it becomes apparent that the social philosophy of the twentieth century is obsolete and is moving toward a philosophy that holds society, through the government, responsible for organizing and maintaining adequate health care for all people. Health care was once considered an individual matter, but it is now considered a right to which everyone should have access.

TRENDS THAT WILL IMPACT HEALTH SERVICES AND HEALTH CAREERS

Changes in disease patterns and methods of diagnosis and treatment impact the demand for health services and healthcare workers. The **Human Genome Project** has identified gene mutations that increase the risk for disease and modify response to drugs used to treat disease. The lower cost of genetic testing and coverage by health insurance have made it possible for this technology to be available for more people. This new information allows a physician to ask patients for a family disease history and order DNA testing to target preventive measures specific to the disease. Genetic counselors play an important role in counseling patients about DNA testing to identify risk for disease as well as treatment interventions.[36]

Public health research shows that more and more children are being diagnosed with **autism spectrum disorders (ASD)**, with 1 in 59 children in the United States receiving this diagnosis. Children with ASD are often treated by a team of health professionals, including occupational therapists, speech therapists, and **applied behavior analysis (ABA)** therapists[37] (**FIGURE 1.6**).

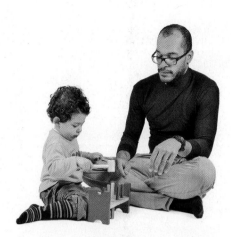

FIGURE 1.6 Autism spectrum disorders (ASD) affects 1 in 59 children in the United States.
© JGA/Shutterstock.

Many diseases of the brain cause disabilities that impact productivity and quality of life and contribute to high health-care costs. New technology makes it possible to identify genes for these brain diseases—Alzheimer's disease, Parkinson's disease, epilepsy, ASD, and psychiatric disorders such as schizophrenia and depression—and to capture images of the brain to develop treatment for such diseases.[38] Awareness of the need for pain control and freedom to make choices about treatment for those with life-limiting illnesses is beginning to shift the focus of both patients and physicians from curative therapy to quality of life and greater use of palliative and hospice services.[39]

As hospitals and health systems work to improve health outcomes and reduce healthcare costs, they are recognizing the necessity of addressing nonmedical factors that affect health. An individual's ability to achieve good health is influenced by more than access to high-quality medical services. Historically, identifying and addressing patients' social needs has not been part of medical practice in the United States. However, tying health outcomes of patients to reimbursement payments to hospitals has demonstrated that high-quality medical care alone cannot ensure optimal health outcomes. Though many other industrialized nations spend less on medical services for each person than the United States, they spend more on social services relative to medical services, and their residents have better health and lead longer lives. For example, as a nation the United States spends about 16% on medical services but only 9% on social services; this compares to equal amounts (10%) for each in Canada.[40]

There is increasing interest in the role of the healthcare sector in addressing adverse **social determinants of health (SDOH)**—the conditions in which people are born, grow, work, live, and age.[41] Examples of SDOH are a lack of access to stable housing, nutritious food, employment, education, personal safety, or reliable transportation. Considering SDOH is critical to improving both primary prevention and the treatment of acute and chronic illness because SDOH influence the delivery and outcome of health care as well as the cost of health care.

A model that describes factors that contribute to health outcomes is the County Health Rankings and Roadmaps Model. The model is helpful in examining the health of a community and the impact of the community on the health of individuals living in the community (**FIGURE 1.7**).[42]

When evaluating health care, we often think of the care provided by a primary care provider, hospital, or clinic to be the most important factor. However, as shown by the model in Figure 1.7, only 20% of health outcomes—length of life and quality of life—are determined by **clinical care** or access to high-quality health care. **Health behaviors** account for 30% of health outcomes—for example, individual behaviors that contribute to risk for disease: tobacco use, diet and exercise, alcohol use, and sexual activity. The greatest influence—40% of health outcomes—is attributed to **social and economic factors**: lack of access to stable housing, nutritious food, employment, education, personal safety, or personal and family support. The physical environment—air and water quality and housing and transportation—accounts for 10% of health outcomes.[42]

The need to address unmet social determinants of health became evident with the implementation of the **Centers for Medicare and Medicaid (CMS) Innovation programs** designed to improve the quality of health care while controlling costs. Payment to hospitals is based on **value-based care**—paying for the quality of care rather than quantity (number of procedures) for Medicare patients. Medicare reduces payments to hospitals if the readmission rate of these patients is excessive.[43] Often the reasons for high hospital readmission rates are unmet social needs (social determinants)—for example, homelessness, food insecurity, or access to transportation. Data collected by the **American Hospital Association (AHA)** has demonstrated that patients with the following characteristics had higher readmission rates: racial and ethnic minority, limited English proficiency, low health literacy, disability, and lack of primary care provider. Hospitals are identifying unmet needs of patients before hospitalization and using a team approach to address unmet needs before hospital discharge to prevent frequent readmissions to the hospital.[44] In 2016, the Innovation Center at CMS introduced the Accountable Health Communities model to support communities in addressing health-related social needs of patients obtaining health care through Medicare and Medicaid by connecting clinical and community service providers. Medicaid funds the cost of some social needs—for example, money for transportation or food.[45]

Hospitals have developed strategies to reduce hospital readmission rates. A strategy used by a hospital in Camden, New Jersey, was to identify barriers that prevented patients from making clinic appointments as well as providing financial incentives for the hospital staff to schedule follow-up clinic visits. Patients were provided transportation to clinic visits and a $20 gift card after the visit while the hospital was reimbursed an additional $150 for each follow-up clinic visit made within seven days of hospital discharge.[46] The University of Illinois Hospital in Chicago was able to reduce emergency department (ED) utilization by 57% and reduce

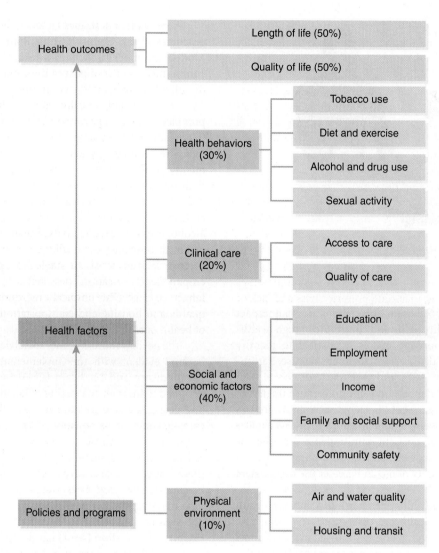

FIGURE 1.7 The County Health Rankings Model for Health Outcomes.
Reproduced from The University of Wisconsin Population Health Institute. *County Health Rankings & Roadmaps, 2021.* www.countyhealthrankings.org

healthcare costs by 21% through the Better Health Through Housing program that provided supportive housing for chronically homeless patients that frequented the ED. The program was successful because the hospital partnered with community organizations and patients were assigned to a housing caseworker who worked with them to find permanent housing.[47]

The American Hospital Association (AHA) and the **American Academy of Family Physicians** have developed screening programs to assess patients for unmet social needs. Both programs include documentation of social needs in the patients' medical records as well as referring patients to community resources for needed services such as emergency food or permanent housing. Both groups have developed materials to assist in developing a screening program and training hospital and clinic staff to carry out the screening. Patients are screened for core social needs: housing, food, transportation, child care, employment, education, finances, utilities, and personal safety. Many different health professionals can be used for screening patients to identify unmet social

needs. For example, receptionists and medical assistants can administer the screening tool; nurses, physician assistants, or health educators can review the completed screening tool to determine patient needs, identify community resources, and develop an action plan; the primary care provider can review the action plan and refer the patient to other team members for education or follow-up; social workers or community health workers can identify community resources and make necessary referrals and provide ongoing case management; and administrators can ensure adequate human and financial resources and provide training on the screening program.[48,49]

Unmet social needs result in **health disparities** or differences in health outcomes. For example, there are disparities in infant mortality in the United States with greater numbers of Black and American Indian/Alaskan Native infant deaths during the first year of life compared to White, Hispanic, and Asian infants. These statistics prompt us to ask why there are differences in health outcomes based on race even when women give birth in the same hospital and receive prenatal care from the same healthcare provider. In this example of disparities in infant mortality, we assume that the women and their infants received equal healthcare services. However, those living in Black and American Indian/Alaskan Native communities often have unmet social needs and experience **discrimination** that impacts their ability to obtain safe housing, healthy food, good-paying jobs, and health care. Others who experience discrimination include marginalized groups from different cultural or socioeconomic backgrounds, ethnicities, or gender identities or sexual orientations and those with physical or mental disabilities.[50]

Equality and **equity** are terms used to describe opportunities for best health outcomes. Equality means treating everyone the same even though not everyone starts at the same place. The Robert Wood Johnson Foundation's definition states, "**Health equity** means that everyone has a fair and just opportunity to be as healthy as possible. This requires removing obstacles to health such as poverty, discrimination, and their consequences, including powerlessness and lack of access to good jobs with fair pay, quality education and housing, safe environments, and health care."[50] Fairness or equity aims to overcome such obstacles so that everyone has the same opportunities.[50]

Equality is giving everyone the same opportunities or the same bicycle. However, not everyone is able to ride the same bicycle because of their size or physical ability. Equity is when people are given a bicycle based on their needs. The same is true for achieving health outcomes. **FIGURE 1.8** illustrates the difference between equality and equity.[51]

Addressing inequities in health care requires that each community examine the underlying causes and barriers to equal opportunity for all citizens, including poverty, high unemployment, low educational achievement, high crime rates, and availability of affordable health care. Policies at the national and state levels can remove some of these barriers. For example, CMS has allowed Medicaid health plans to cover the cost of nonmedical services such as food or transportation. The County Health Rankings and Roadmap model includes resources to examine communities and develop action plans for changing the local environment to reduce barriers. Structural changes will require legislation and policies at the local, state, and national levels that provide economic opportunities for all.

SUMMARY

To improve the health of all Americans, it is critical to continue collecting data on all components of health; documenting trends in risk factors, health status, and access to and utilization of healthcare services; and disseminating reliable and accurate information about the health of our population. Equally important is gaining an understanding of the healthcare needs and utilization patterns of population subgroups. Such insights will enable policy makers to set program priorities and allocate target resources most effectively. Healthcare and population trends and healthcare reform will affect all health professionals in every career and will change the practice of medicine as we know it.

Because there is no single "U.S. healthcare system," the many ways in which health care is delivered can be puzzling. This should not be surprising, given the historical perspective of health services, the diverse subsystems in operation in the United States, and the dynamics of social and technological changes.

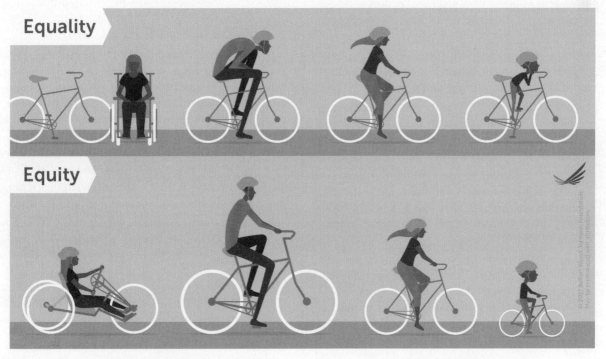

FIGURE 1.8 Visualizing health equity: One size does not fit all.
Data from Robert Wood Johnson Foundation. Visualizing Health Equity: One Size Does Not Fit All Infographic. June 30, 2017. www.rwjf.org/en/library/infographics/visualizing-health-equity.html

LEARNING PORTFOLIO

Study Points

1. As a result of the 2010 Affordable Care Act (ACA), more Americans have access to health insurance. The percentage of the uninsured dropped from 17% to 10% between 2008 and 2017. Those who remained uninsured were non-elderly adults with incomes below 200% of the federal poverty level living in states that did not expand Medicaid.

2. In the second half of the nineteenth century, the most critical health problems were related to poor sanitation resulting in contaminated water and food.

3. Diseases caused by infectious agents—pneumonia, tuberculosis, diarrhea, and diphtheria—accounted for one-third of all deaths in the 1900s with 40% of the deaths in children under five years of age.

4. By the 1950s, with the use of antibiotics and universal childhood immunizations, the causes of death changed from acute infectious diseases to chronic diseases of heart disease and cancer.

5. Life expectancy at birth plateaued between 2014 and 2017; the plateau is attributed to increases in death from unintentional injuries (including unintentional drug overdose), Alzheimer's disease, suicide, and chronic liver disease.

6. Deaths from drug overdose, suicide, and chronic liver disease have been labeled "deaths of despair," attributed to living in a community with limited opportunities for employment and a readily available source of opioids.

7. Factors contributing to drug (opioid) addiction and overdose are inappropriate prescribing of synthetic opioids for treatment of pain and aggressive trafficking of heroin laced with synthetic opioids.

8. Even though infant mortality rates continue to decrease, there are disparities by race, geography, and socioeconomic status with higher infant mortality rates from non-Hispanic Black and American Indian/Native Alaskan women.

9. Leading causes of infant mortality are congenital malformations, preterm birth and low birth weight, sudden infant death syndrome, and maternal complications of birth.

10. Programs that improve pregnancy outcomes and prevent infant mortality are classes on normal pregnancy and childbirth and possible complications of pregnancy, addressing structural barriers to making prenatal visits, and using doulas to support women during pregnancy and childbirth.

11. Chronic diseases are conditions that last one year or more and require ongoing medical attention, limit activities of daily living, or both; chronic diseases that are leading causes of death and disability are heart disease, diabetes, and cancer.

12. By age 65, half of seniors will have two to three chronic diseases, and with increasing age many will become frail and require personal assistance from family or paid caregivers.

13. Lifestyle factors related to the development of chronic diseases are physical activity, eating habits, smoking, drinking alcoholic beverages, using illicit drugs, and personal hygiene.

14. Smoking for those 18 years of age and older has declined, but it has increased for teens.

15. The obesity rate for adults is twice as high (40%) as for children (20%).

16. Vaccines to prevent infectious diseases are not utilized by everyone; about 70% of infants receive vaccines against childhood diseases, about two-thirds of adults receive the pneumonia vaccine, and fewer than half of children and adults receive the vaccine for influenza.

17. Gastroenteritis is a common foodborne illness caused by the norovirus and the salmonella bacteria with symptoms of vomiting and diarrhea.

18. Zoonotic diseases are infectious diseases that are transmitted from wild animals or insects to domesticated animals and humans.

19. The coronavirus COVID-19 originated in China and spread throughout the world in 2020 causing a pandemic similar to the 1918 influenza (Spanish Flu); methods used to stop the spread of the disease were for individuals to wear face masks, practice social distancing, and wash hands frequently.

20. The Centers for Disease Control and Prevention (CDC) in the United States and the World Health Organization (WHO) are the governmental organizations that monitor infectious and chronic diseases.

21. Augmented or artificial intelligence (AI) and health information technology (health IT) are used to improve the efficiency of health care. AI is used to follow infectious disease epidemics, use robots to perform surgery, and monitor patient movements in the hospital and at home. Health IT uses computers to document and share health information among healthcare workers in different locations.

LEARNING PORTFOLIO

22. The Human Genome Project will increase understanding and treatment of diseases that have a genetic basis.

23. The healthcare system is recognizing the importance of considering nonmedical factors (social needs or social determinants of health [SDOH]) that impact health outcomes such as hospital readmission rates, compliance with scheduled clinic visits, and taking prescribed medications.

24. SDOH are socioeconomic factors: housing, food, education, employment, personal safety, personal and family support; SDOH account for 40% of health outcomes.

25. There continue to be disparities in health outcomes based on socioeconomic factors, race, ethnicity, gender and gender identity, sexual orientation, and physical or mental disability.

26. Equality and equity are terms used to describe opportunities for best health outcomes; equality is treating everyone the same even though their needs are different, while equity is removing obstacles that interfere with achieving the best health outcomes.

Issues for Discussion

1. Discuss changes in access to health care in the United States as a result of the Affordable Care Act of 2010.

2. Discuss how the causes of death have changed since 1900 in the United States. Discuss three major factors that have contributed to these changes.

3. Go to the *2020 County Health Rankings & Roadmaps* website to review the health of the county in which you live. Review all of the components of the model shown in Figure 1.7, "The County Health Rankings Model for Health Outcomes." Link to trend tables and percentages according to race (for example, low birth weight). Compare the rankings of the county with the ranking of the state in which you live and the entire United States. www.countyhealthrankings.org /explore-health-rankings

4. Review the one-minute video "Equity vs. Equality" from the Robert Wood Johnson Foundation. Explain the difference between equity and equality as it relates to health care. https://youtu.be/MlXZyNtaoDM. August 6, 2018.

5. Discuss the role of government in providing access to health care through legislation and financial support of health care and technology.

6. Review the social needs screening tool "The Every-ONE Project," developed by the American Academy of Family Physicians. Select one social need—for example, housing—and describe how health outcomes are impacted by insecure housing. www.aafp .org/dam/AAFP/documents/patient_care/everyone _project/hops19-physician-guide-sdoh.pdf

Enrichment Activities

1. Methicillin-resistant *Staphylococcus aureus* (MRSA) is a cause of skin infection in the community—for example, in high schools and day care centers. Review information from the CDC to learn how MRSA can be transmitted in the community setting. www.cdc .gov/mrsa/community/index.html

2. Explore CDC Vital Signs to learn more about differences in cigarette smoking across states and different groups within the United States. Learn more about the health risks of smoking and secondhand smoke. www.cdc.gov/vitalsigns/TobaccoUse/Smoking /index.html

3. Learn more about the role of genomics from the CDC's *Healthy People 2020* website. Which diseases have a strong relationship to genomics, and how can this information be used by consumers and physicians to prevent disease? www.healthypeople.gov/2020 /topics-objectives/topic/genomics

4. Review the five-minute video clip "The Cliff of Good Health" by Dr. Camara Jones, who explains the structural causes of health inequity. List ways that structural barriers limit health equity. https://youtu.be /to7Yrl50iHI7

5. Review the CDC website that summarizes past pandemics. How were past pandemics similar to and different from the coronavirus pandemic of 2020? www.cdc.gov/flu/pandemic-resources/basics/past -pandemics.html

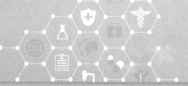

LEARNING PORTFOLIO

CASE STUDY: U.S. HEALTH CARE

Will is a 20-year-old male who is attending a community college and is enrolled in a physical therapy assistant program with an ultimate goal of applying for a physical therapy program. He also works part time as an emergency medical technician (EMT) in the college town where he lives. He has been smoking since he was 15 years old and has recently tried to quit because his father had a heart attack several months ago and his mother has diabetes and is overweight.

While working as an EMT, Will makes many trips to nursing homes to pick up residents and take them to the hospital. He has concerns about contracting the flu because his younger brother's school was shut down because of a flu epidemic. Although his brother didn't contract the flu, Will is concerned that he could become exposed since he often examines patients that are very ill.

Based on the information in this chapter, answer these questions related to this case study.

1. If Will is able to quit smoking, what are his risks for developing the same health problems as his parents?
   A. Increased health risk for heart disease
   B. Risk will be the same because of genetics
   C. Decreased risk for heart disease
   D. Increased risk for lung cancer
2. What recommendations do you have for Will to prevent becoming ill with the flu?
   A. Getting the annual flu vaccine
   B. Getting tested for the coronavirus
   C. Getting the pneumococcal vaccine
   D. Getting a booster shot to protect against childhood infections
3. What percentage of health outcomes (length of life and quality of life) can be attributed to social and economic factors?
   A. 10%
   B. 20%
   C. 30%
   D. 40%
4. _____ is the causes and rates of death.
5. _____ is the death of a baby before one year of age.

References

1. Office of the Legislative Counsel, U.S. House of Representatives. *Compilation of Patient Protection and Affordable Care Act*. 111th Congress, 2d Session. May 10, 2010. http://housedocs.house.gov/energycommerce/ppacacon.pdf

2. Goodman DC, Brownlee S, Chang C-H, Fisher E. *Regional and Racial Variation in Primary Care and the Quality of Care Among Medicare Beneficiaries. A Report of the Dartmouth Atlas Project* . Hanover, NH: Dartmouth Institute for Health Policy and Clinical Practice Center for Health Policy Research; 2010. Accessed February 9, 2021.

3. Kamal R, McDermott D, Cox C. *How Has Health Spending Changed Over Time?* Menlo Park, CA: Kaiser Family Foundation. December 20, 2019. www.healthsystemtracker.org/chart-collection/u-s-spending-healthcare-changed-time/#item-start Accessed February 9, 2021.

4. Garfield, R, Orgera, K, Damico, A. *The Uninsured and the ACA: A Primer—Key Facts about Health Insurance and the Uninsured amidst Changes to the Affordable Care Act*. Kaiser Family Foundation, January 2019. www.kff.org/uninsured/report/the-uninsured-and-the-aca-a-primer-key-facts-about-health-insurance-and-the-uninsured-amidst-changes-to-the-affordable-care-act/ Accessed February 9, 2021.

5. Baumgartner, JC, Collins SR, Radley, DC, Hayes, SL. How the Affordable Care Act Has Narrowed Racial and Ethnic Disparities in Access to Health Care. *Data Brief*. The Commonwealth Fund. January 2020. www.commonwealthfund.org /press-release/2020/new-report-affordable-care Accessed February 9, 2021.

6. Tolbert J, Orgera K, Singer N, Damico A. *Key Facts about the Uninsured Population*. Kaiser Family Foundation, December 2019. https://www.kff.org/uninsured/issue-brief/key-facts-about-the-uninsured-population/ Accessed February 9, 2021.

7. National Center for Environmental Health; National Center for Health Statistics; National Center for Infectious Diseases, CDC. Achievements in Public Health, 1900–1999: Control of Infectious Diseases. *MMWR* 1999; 48:621–629.

8. National Center for Health Statistics. *Health, United States, 2018*. Hyattsville, MD. 2019. www.cdc.gov/nchs/data/hus/hus18.pdf Accessed February 9, 2021.

9. National Center for Health Statistics. *Health, United States, 2013. With Special Features on Prescription Drugs*. Hyattsville, MD. 2014. www.cdc.gov/nchs/data/hus/hus13.pdf Accessed February 9, 2021.

10. National Center for Health Statistics. *Health, United States, 2017: With Special Feature on Mortality*. Hyattsville, MD. 2018. www.cdc.gov/nchs/data/hus/hus17.pdf Accessed February 9, 2021.

11. Radley DC, Collins SR, Hayes SL. *2019 Scorecard on State Health System Performance*. The Commonwealth Fund, June 2019. www.commonwealthfund.org/publications/fund-reports/2019/jun/2019-scorecard-state-health-system-performance-deaths-suicide Accessed February 9, 2021.

LEARNING PORTFOLIO

12. Murphy K, Becker M, Locke J, Kelleher C, McLeod J, Isasi F. *Finding Solutions to the Prescription Opioid and Heroin Crisis: A Road Map for States*. Washington, DC: National Governors Association Center for Best Practices, July 2016. www.nga.org/wp-content/uploads/2019/08/1607NGAOpio idRoadMap.pdf Accessed February 9, 2021.

13. Lewis C, Paxton I, Zephyrin I. The Rural Maternity Care Crisis. [Blog] *To the Point*. https://doi.org/10.26099 /j0nn-ap16 Accessed 14 March 2020.

14. Zephyrin L, Coleman A, Nuzum R, Getachew Y. Increasing Postpartum Medicaid Coverage Could Reduce Maternal Deaths and Improve Outcomes. [Blog] *To the Point*. https:// doi.org/10.26099/ejtb-tw04 Accessed February 9, 2021.

15. Novoa C. *Ensuring Healthy Births through Prenatal Support. Innovations from Three Models*. Center for American Progress, January 11, 2020. www.americanprogress.org/issues /early-childhood/reports/2020/01/31/479930/ensuring -healthy-births-prenatal-support/ Accessed February 9, 2021.

16. Administration for Community Living. *2018 Profile of Older Americans*. Administration on Aging (AOA), Administration for Community Living, April, 2018.

17. Centers for Disease Control and Prevention. *The State of Aging and Health in America 2013*. Atlanta, GA: Centers for Disease Control and Prevention, 2013

18. Ortman JM, Velkoff VA. An Aging Nation: The Older Population in the United States. *Current Population Reports*. P25-1149. Washington, DC: U.S. Census Bureau. May 2014. www.census.gov/prod/2014pubs/p25-1140.pdf

19. Centers for Disease Control and Prevention. *Smoking, Pregnancy, and Babies*. Office on Smoking and Health, National Center for Chronic Disease Prevention and Health Promotion, www.cdc.gov/tobacco/campaign/tips/diseases/pregnancy .html Reviewed March 23, 2020. Accessed February 9, 2021.

20. Smith KF, Goldberg M, Rosenthal S, et al. Rise in Human Infectious Disease Outbreaks. *J R Soc Interface*. 2014; *11*(101): 20140950. https://doi.org/10.1098/rsif.2014.0950

21. Centers for Disease Control and Prevention. *Zoonotic Diseases*. Centers for Disease Control and Prevention. National Center for Emerging and Zoonotic Infectious Diseases (NCEZID). www.cdc.gov/onehealth/basics/zoonotic-diseases .html Reviewed July 14, 2017. Accessed February 9, 2021.

22. Centers for Disease Control and Prevention. *COVID-19*. National Center for Immunization and Respiratory Diseases (NCIRD), Division of Viral Diseases, February 5, 2020. www.cdc.gov/coronavirus/2019-ncov/about/index .html Accessed February 9, 2021.

23. WHO Director-General's opening remarks at the media briefing on COVID-19. March 11, 2020. www.who.int/dg /speeches/detail/who-director-general-s-opening-remarks -at-the-media-briefing-on-covid-19—11-march-2020 Accessed February 9, 2021.

24. Centers for Disease Control and Prevention. *1918 Pandemic Influenza Historic Timeline*. www.cdc.gov/flu/pandemic -resources/1918-commemoration/pandemic-timeline-1918 .htm Reviewed March 20, 2018.

25. Centers for Disease Control and Prevention. *1918 Pandemic (H1N1virus)*. www.cdc.gov/flu/pandemic-resources/1918 -pandemic-h1n1.html Reviewed March 20, 2019. Accessed February 9, 2021.

26. World Health Organization. *WHO Coronavirus Disease (COVID-19) Dashboard*. https://covid19.who.int/ Updated February 9, 2021.

27. Centers for Disease Control and Prevention. *COVID Data Tracker*. https://covid.cdc.gov/covid-data-tracker/#global -counts-rates Accessed February 9, 2021.

28. Loftus P, Grayer West, M. First Covid-19 Vaccine Given to U.S. Public. *Wall Street Journal*. December 14, 2020. www .wsj.com/articles/covid-19-vaccinations-in-the-u-s-slated -to-begin-monday-11607941806

29. Lewis W. Disaster Response Expert Explains why the U.S. wasn't more Prepared for the Pandemic. *USC Dornsife*. March 24, 2020. University of Southern California. https:// dornsife.usc.edu/news/stories/3182/why-u-s-wasn't-better -prepared-for-the-coronavirus/ Accessed February 9, 2021.

30. Centers for Disease Control and Prevention. *Ebola Virus Disease*. National Center for Emerging and Zoonotic Infectious Diseases (NCEZID), Division of High-Consequence Pathogens and Pathology (DHCPP), Viral Special Pathogens Branch (VSPB). www.cdc.gov/vhf/ebola/index.html Reviewed November 18, 2020. Accessed February 9, 2021.

31. Centers for Disease Control and Prevention. *2014-2016 Ebola Outbreak in West Africa*. Centers for Disease Control and Prevention, National Center for Emerging and Zoonotic Infectious Diseases (NCEZID), Division of High-Consequence Pathogens and Pathology (DHCPP), Viral Special Pathogens Branch (VSPB). Reviewed March 8, 2019. www.cdc.gov/vhf/ebola/outbreaks/2014-west-africa/index .html Accessed February 9, 2021.

32. Centers for Disease Control and Prevention. *Avian Influenza in Birds*. Centers for Disease Control and Prevention, National Center for Immunization and Respiratory Diseases (NCIRD). www.cdc.gov/flu/avianflu/avian-in-birds .htm Reviewed February 6, 2017. Accessed February 9, 2021.

33. Centers for Disease Control and Prevention. *Methicillin-resistant Staphylococcus aureus (MRSA)*. National Center for Emerging and Zoonotic Infectious Diseases (NCEZID), Division of Healthcare Quality Promotion (DHQP). www .cdc.gov/mrsa/community/index.html Reviewed June 26, 2019. Accessed February 9, 2021.

34. Amisha MP, Pathania M, Rathaur VK. Overview of Artificial Intelligence in Medicine. *J Family Med Prim Care*. 2019; 8(7):2328–2331. doi:10.4103/jfmpc.jfmpc_440_19

35. Gerke S, Minssen T, Cohen G. Ethical and Legal Challenges of Artificial Intelligence-Driven Healthcare. *Artificial Intelligence in Healthcare*. 2020;295–336. doi:10.1016/B978-0 -12-818438-7.00012-5

36. National Human Genome Research Institute. *JHU/NIH Genetic Counseling Training Program (GCTP).* Updated October 8, 2020. Accessed February 9, 2021. www.genome.gov/careers-training/Professional-Development-Programs/Genetic-Counseling-Training

37. Maenner MJ, Shaw KA, Baio J, et al. Prevalence of Autism Spectrum Disorder among Children Aged 8 Years—Autism and Developmental Disabilities Monitoring Network, 11 Sites, United States, 2016. *MMWR Surveill Summ* 2020;69 (No. SS-4):1–12. DOI: http://dx.doi.org/10.15585/mmwr.ss6904a1external icon

38. National Institutes of Health. *What is the Brain Initiative?* The Brain Initiative. U.S. Department of Health and Human Services. https://braininitiative.nih.gov/ Accessed February 9, 2021.

39. National Hospice and Palliative Care Organization. *2020 Edition: Hospice Facts and Figures.* Alexandria, VA: National Hospice and Palliative Care Organization. August 20, 2020. www.nhpco.org/factsfigures

40. National Academies of Sciences, Engineering, and Medicine. Introduction. In: *Integrating Social Care into the Delivery of Health Care: Moving Upstream to Improve the Nation's Health.* Washington, DC: The National Academies Press; 2019: 19-31. https://doi.org/10.17226/25467

41. World Health Organization. *Social Determinants of Health.* www.who.int/social_determinants/en/ Accessed August 1, 2020.

42. The University of Wisconsin Population Health Institute. *2020 County Health Rankings & Roadmaps.* www.countyhealthrankings.org. Accessed February 9, 2021.

43. Centers for Medicare and Medicaid. *Hospital Readmissions Reduction Program (HRRP).* www.cms.gov/Medicare/Medicare-Fee-for-Service-Payment/AcuteInpatientPPS/Readmissions-Reduction-Program Modified August 24, 2020. Accessed February 9, 2021.

44. Centers for Medicare and Medicaid. *Guide to Reducing Disparities in Readmissions.* August 2018. http://cms.gov/about-cms/agency-information/omh/downloads/omh_readmissions_guide.pdf Accessed February 9, 2021.

45. Centers for Medicare and Medicaid Services. *Accountable Health Communities Model.* https://innovation.cms.gov/innovation-models/ahcm. Updated May 19, 2020. Accessed February 9, 2021.

46. West D, Yang Q, Wilson C, Dravid N. Outcomes of a City-wide Campaign to Reduce Medicaid Hospital Readmissions with Connection to Primary Care within 7 Days of Hospital Discharge. *JAMA Network Open.* 2019; 2(1):e187369. doi:10.1001/jamanetworkopen.2018.7369.

47. Castrucci B, Auerbach J. Meeting Individual Social Needs Falls Short of Addressing Social Determinants of Health. *Health Affairs* Blog. January 16, 2019. DOI: 10.1377/hblog20190115.234942

48. American Academy of Family Physicians. *Social Determinants of Health. Guide to Social Needs Screening.* The Every-ONE Project. 2019. www.aafp.org/dam/AAFP/documents/patient_care/everyone_project/hops19-physician-guide-sdoh.pdf Accessed February 9, 2021.

49. American Hospital Association. *Screening for Social Needs: Guiding Care Teams to Engage Patients.* 2019. www.aha.org/toolkitsmethodology/2019-06-05-screening-social-needs-guiding-care-teams-engage-patients Accessed February 9, 2021.

50. Braverman P, Arkin F, Orleans T, Proctor D, Plough A. *What Is Health Equity?* Princeton, NJ: Robert Wood Johnson Foundation. 2017. https://www.rwjf.org/en/search-results.html?at=Proctor+D Accessed February 9, 2021.

51. Robert Wood Johnson Foundation. *Visualizing Health Equity: One Size Does Not Fit All Infographic.* June 30, 2017. www.rwjf.org/en/library/infographics/visualizing-health-equity.html Accessed February 9, 2021.

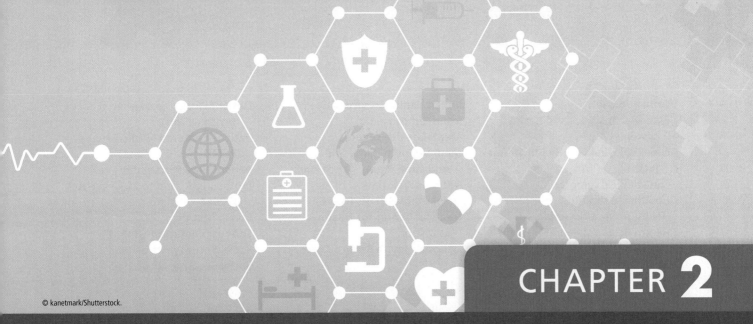

© kanetmark/Shutterstock.

CHAPTER 2

Categories of Health Services

OBJECTIVES

After studying this chapter, the student should be able to:

- List direct health services provided by the federal government.
- Compare financing and governing of private, public, and volunteer healthcare facilities.
- Identify the five broad types of health services in the United States.
- Compare the population served by federally funded primary care health centers and free clinics.
- Name health agencies within the U.S. Department of Health and Human Services (HHS).
- Summarize the six major points of the Patient Care Partnership.
- Describe public health and mental health services in the United States.

KEY TERMS

Affordable Care Act (ACA)
Almshouse
Ambulatory care
Behavioral Risk Factor
  Surveillance System (BRFSS)
Centers for Disease Control and
  Prevention (CDC)

Certified Community Behavioral
  Health Clinics (CCBHCs)
Chronic care
Civilian Health and Medical
  Program of the Department of
  Veterans Affairs (CHAMPVA)
Commissioned Corps

Community hospital
Community Mental Health Act
Community Mental Health
  Centers (CMHC)
Diagnosis and treatment of
  illness
Disease prevention services

Drug addiction
Essential hospitals and health
    systems
Federally Qualified Health Center
    (FQHC)
Free medical clinic (FMC)
Healthcare facilities
Health promotion services
Health Resources and Services
    Administration (HRSA)
Hospital system

Indian Health Service (IHS)
Informed consent
Mental health services
Mental Health Parity and
    Addiction Equity Act of 2008
National Association of Free &
    Charitable Clinics (NAFC)
National Center for Health
    Statistics
National Health Service Corps

National Institute of Mental
    Health (NIMH)
Patient-Centered Medical Home
    (PCMH)
Patient Care Partnership
Protecting Access to Medicare Act
    of 2014
Rehabilitation
Serious mental illness (SMI)
Social Security Act of 1935
Social Security Act of 1965

OVERVIEW OF THE U.S. HEALTHCARE SYSTEM

The healthcare industry is a complex system of diagnostic, therapeutic, and preventive services. Hospitals, clinics, government and volunteer agencies, pharmaceutical and medical equipment manufacturers, and private insurance companies provide these services. In terms of jobs in the healthcare industry, hospitals employ the largest percentage (39%), followed by offices of health practitioners (26%) and nursing and other residential facilities (20%). Home health services and outpatient, laboratory, and other ambulatory care settings make up the remaining healthcare jobs, at 8% each.[1]

The focus of this chapter is hospitals and outpatient or ambulatory care provided by both private and government institutions as well as the federal agencies responsible for ensuring the health and safety of all Americans under the U.S. Department of Health and Human Services (HHS) through research and financial support. Chapter 4 includes long-term care—nursing home care and other supportive living facilities.

Unlike most developed countries, the United States does not have a centralized healthcare delivery system in which individuals automatically receive health care. Instead, consumers obtain healthcare services—choosing their doctor, clinic, or hospital—from a variety of locations and providers funded by private insurance or government-subsidized insurance. Consumers often are left to coordinate their own care; thus, the quality of health care can vary.

Two countries similar to the United States, Canada and the United Kingdom (UK), have national health insurance systems. Canada implemented a national health insurance system in 1966, and each province or territory has its own unique health insurance plan. The health insurance program is funded by provincial taxes as well as a fixed amount from the federal government. The UK health delivery system—the National Health Service (NHS)—is funded primarily through general taxation. The system emphasizes preventive community services and coordination of primary and acute care. All patients insured through this system are required to register with a local general practitioner or physician who coordinates their care. The federal government owns and operates the hospitals and clinics, and most of the healthcare workers are employed by the government.[2]

In contrast, the U.S. federal government provides very few direct health services, preferring to support new or improved services by providing money to fund expanded services—for example, through the **Affordable Care Act (ACA)**. The exceptions are the health services of TRICARE, through the U.S. Department of Defense (DoD), the Civilian Health and Medical Program of the Department of Veterans Affairs (CHAMPVA), and the **Indian Health Service (IHS)**. The federal government has no authority to provide direct services; this is a function of the private sector and the states. The federal government is involved, however, in financing research through the National Institutes of Health (NIH) and individual health care for the elderly through Medicare as well as health care for the low-income uninsured through Medicaid. The federal government also funds loans and scholarships for students in the health professions through the **Health Resources and Services Administration (HRSA)**. The most important federal agency concerned with health affairs is the HHS, with 11 operating divisions, including eight agencies in the U.S. Public Health Service and three human services agencies.[3] Congress plays a key role in this federal activity by making laws, allocating funds, and doing investigative work through committees.

CATEGORIES OF HEALTHCARE SERVICES

The healthcare system offers five broad types of services: health promotion, disease prevention, diagnosis and treatment, rehabilitation, and chronic care.

Health promotion services help clients reduce the risk of illness, maintain optimal function, and follow healthy lifestyles. These services are provided in a variety of ways and settings. Examples include hospitals that offer prenatal nutrition classes and local health departments that offer selected recipients prenatal nutrition classes plus a food package that meets their nutritional requirements (the Women, Infants, and Children [WIC] program). Classes at both locations promote the general health of women and children. Exercise and aerobic classes offered by city recreation departments, adult education programs, and private or nonprofit gymnasiums encourage consumers to exercise and maintain cardiovascular fitness, thus promoting better health through lifestyle changes.

Disease prevention services offer a wide variety of assistance and activities. Educational efforts aimed at involving consumers in their own care include attention to and recognition of risk factors, environmental changes to reduce the threat of illness, occupational safety measures, and public health education programs and legislation. Examples of public health programs are a smoking cessation class offered through the hospital or the local department of public health or a lead abatement program for older homes offered to homeowners by the city health department. An example on the individual level is women participating in screening for breast and cervical cancer. It is evident that preventive measures such as these can reduce the overall costs of health care.

Diagnosis and treatment of illness have been the most used of the healthcare services, most often provided in the hospital or **ambulatory care** setting. Diagnosis of illness involves physician visits and, if necessary, laboratory tests, X-rays, and other technology to make a diagnosis; examples of treatment are surgery, physical and speech therapy, and medications. Recent advances in technology and early diagnostic techniques have greatly improved the diagnosis and treatment capacity of the healthcare delivery system, but the advances have also increased the complexity and price of health care (**FIGURE 2.1**).

Rehabilitation involves the restoration of a person to normal or near-normal function after a physical or mental illness, including chemical addiction. These programs take place in many settings: homes, community centers, rehabilitation centers, hospitals, outpatient clinics, and long-term care facilities. Rehabilitation is a long process, and both the client and family require extra assistance in adjusting to a chronic disability. Common conditions requiring rehabilitation are physical injuries such as strokes and head injuries, hip and knee replacement surgery, and substance use disorders such as alcohol or drug addiction.

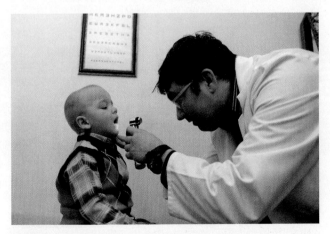

FIGURE 2.1 Diagnosis and treatment are the most used healthcare services.
© thomas koch/Shutterstock.

Chronic care is ongoing care for a chronic health condition such as diabetes, which requires long-term monitoring with adjustments in diet, medication, and physical activity to maintain blood glucose levels and the prevention of complications. Most individuals with diabetes have a primary physician or a specialist physician, an endocrinologist, who coordinates care. Nurses, dietitians, and other healthcare professionals who specialize in diabetes care provide patient education. The primary care provider refers patients to other physician specialists when complications of the disease develop—for example, an ophthalmologist for eye health and a nephrologist to monitor kidney function.

HEALTHCARE FACILITIES

A wide variety of **healthcare facilities** are available. These facilities—the places where people involved in the healthcare industry work—are broadly summarized in this chapter but are individually detailed elsewhere. This discussion of numerous healthcare settings should assist students in selecting a health career and becoming knowledgeable about their chosen field.

Expansion of the healthcare system and professional specialization have broadened the range and types of healthcare settings. Medical care settings include offices of health practitioners, nursing and residential facilities, home health services, and outpatient clinics, laboratories, and ambulatory services as well as the primary inpatient setting, hospitals. Public health settings are usually community-based and may be voluntary organizations, such as the American Cancer Society, or government-supported entities, such as the city, county, or state public health department.

Clients requiring diagnosis and treatment can find health care in physicians' offices, ambulatory care centers, and outpatient clinics. In addition, there are freestanding immediate-care clinics staffed by physicians or located inside a pharmacy and staffed by nurse practitioners or physician assistants who provide immunizations and treat minor, acute illnesses such as colds, cuts, or sprains. Although physicians in office practice focus mainly on the diagnosis and treatment of specific diseases, many clinics and ambulatory centers offer health education and rehabilitation as well. For example, outpatient cardiac rehabilitation centers provide classes on nutrition and stress management and the use of exercise equipment to increase strength and endurance while monitoring heart function. Other health professionals who provide rehabilitation services are physical therapists for physical rehabilitation and psychologists, social workers, and behavioral counselors, who provide therapy for chemical addiction and mental illness.

Community-based agencies provide health care within defined neighborhoods. Such diverse facilities include federally supported health centers, adult day care centers, home health agencies, crisis intervention and drug rehabilitation centers, halfway houses, and various support groups. All work in a wide variety of ways to maintain the integrity of the community.

Federally funded primary care health centers—**Federally Qualified Health Centers (FQHC)**—are the largest comprehensive safety net of primary and preventive care in the country with nearly 1,400 centers in the United States. The health centers are supported by the HRSA within the HHS and are public and private nonprofit healthcare organizations governed by a board, most of whose members are from the community being served by the health center. The centers provide a medical home for medically underserved populations—for example, the homeless, veterans, residents of public housing, and the uninsured—or special, medically underserved populations, such as migrant and seasonal farmworkers. The health centers receive assistance in recruiting and staffing primary care providers through the **National Health Service Corps**, also funded by HRSA.[4] The FQHC manage patients with multiple healthcare needs and use key quality improvement practices, including health information technology—nearly 97% of the centers use electronic health records.[5] The majority of the operating funds come from Medicaid, Medicare, private insurance, and patient fees; services are provided regardless of ability to pay. The quality of care is comparable to private primary care centers.[4]

Comprehensive medical, prenatal, dental, pharmacy, and behavioral health services are available at the health centers. A multidisciplinary team of physicians, physician assistants, nurses and nurse practitioners, midwives, social workers, health educators, behavioral health counselors, and other providers staff the health centers.[5] Supportive services—health education, language translation, and transportation—increase language access and reduce barriers to keeping scheduled appointments because of limited public transportation.[4]

The health centers use the **Patient-Centered Medical Home (PCMH)** model, whereby patient care is coordinated by a primary care provider to ensure that patients receive culturally appropriate care when and where they need it. The centers are able to achieve strong patient outcomes even though the patients are often sicker than the general population. Because of the care received in the clinics, patients have fewer emergency room or hospital visits, resulting in a cost savings to the government.[6]

The first federally funded health centers were established in 1962 for migrant and seasonal farmworkers, and by 1964, two neighborhood health centers were opened in the Boston area. As of 2019, centers provided care to over 28 million patients in all states within the United States, the District of Columbia, Puerto Rico, the U.S. Virgin Islands, and the Pacific Basin.[6] The ACA provided funds to expand the number of health centers and increased access to health care for many low-income individuals. In 2019, one in every 12 Americans received health care through one of the health centers[6]; over 60% of those receiving services were members of an ethnic or minority group, and 23% had no health insurance.[5]

The FQHC network addresses public health priorities—for example, the opioid crisis and the HIV epidemic. For example, in 2018, health centers screened and identified over 1 million people for substance use disorder and provided medication-assisted treatment—naloxone, used to prevent death from an overdose—to nearly 95,000 patients. These health centers serve the HIV community with testing and diagnosis of HIV and in 2018 provided testing for over 2 million patients and treated one in six individuals diagnosed with HIV from across the United States.[6]

Privately funded **free medical clinics (FMCs)** are nonprofit, community-based or faith-based organizations that provide health care at little or no charge to low-income individuals—at or below 200% of the federal poverty level—who are uninsured or underinsured and are residents of the county in which the clinic is located. The **National Association of Free & Charitable Clinics (NAFC)** was established in 2001; in 2019, 2 million people received health care at 1,400 clinics and pharmacies.[7] A nationwide survey reported that those who used a free clinic were homeless (42%) and immigrants (40%) and had substance use disorders (18%) or HIV/AIDs (10%). When the ACA was implemented, more people were eligible for health insurance through Medicaid or the Marketplace. However, barriers to health care access persisted for individuals not eligible for government-subsidized health insurance—for example, the undocumented and those who live in states that have not expanded Medicaid programs. Also, FMCs provide services less readily available elsewhere, free or low-cost medications and eyeglasses, and health education (**FIGURE 2.2**).[8]

In contrast to the FQHC, the free clinics receive little or no state or federal funds. FMCs are financially supported by a variety of individuals or organizations such as hospitals, medical associations, secular community organizations, faith-based entities, and foundations as well as fund-raising events. Pharmaceutical companies and other organizations donate low-cost or free medications and medical supplies. Clinics may be housed in temporary physical facilities similar to those used for humanitarian relief in response to disasters such as a hurricane or tornado.[9] For example, from 2009 through 2016, large-scale free clinics were held in several cities including Kansas City, MO; Dallas, TX; New Orleans, LA; Charlotte, NC; Madison, WI; and Tacoma, WA. Permanent clinics are housed in existing physical spaces such as

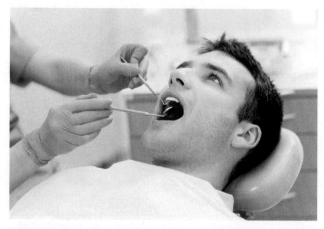

FIGURE 2.2 Free clinics provide dental services to the uninsured.
© pikselstock/Shutterstock.

churches.[10] Most FMCs provide medical, dental, pharmaceutical, behavioral health, vision, and health education services to ensure that the uninsured and underinsured have a medical home. Clinics are staffed by a variety of volunteer health professionals: doctors, dentists, nurses, nurse practitioners, social workers, psychologists, optometrists, pharmacists, and non-licensed medical personnel or lay volunteers. Board-certified physicians typically devote one to four half-days per month. Some clinics develop networks with local physician specialists such as cardiologists or endocrinologists or with hospitals to pool resources to enable the uninsured or undocumented to receive specialty care.[9]

There is a popular misconception that free clinics are no longer necessary after the implementation of the ACA. However, an estimated 29 million (11%) of those living in the United States were uninsured in 2019. Nearly half of the uninsured were not eligible for insurance because they lived in a state that did not expand Medicaid, were restricted because of immigration status, or were not eligible for subsidized health insurance premiums because their income was too high. Those without health insurance included noncitizens (23%); undocumented immigrants are not eligible for federally funded health insurance through Medicaid, the Marketplace, or the FQHC.[11] Immigrants are more likely to be uninsured because most work in low-paying jobs that do not include a health insurance benefit. In addition, documented immigrants must have lived in the United States for at least five years to be eligible for federally funded insurance; however, immigrants granted refugee status are eligible.[11]

Individuals who are unemployed or working in low-paying jobs and living in the 12 states that have not expanded Medicaid often are unable to pay for the premiums for health insurance policies through the Marketplace because of the cost. They fall into a coverage gap because they earn too much to be eligible for Medicaid and don't earn enough to be able to pay for health insurance premiums, even when the premiums are subsidized. However, they would be able to receive care in federally supported health centers. Undocumented immigrants often rely on free clinics for health care since they are not eligible for government programs, either Medicaid or services through the FQHC.

HOSPITALS: DEVELOPMENT AND SERVICES

Hospitals are the major agency in the healthcare system and vary greatly in size, depending on the location. A rural hospital may have two dozen beds; a hospital in a large city may have more than a thousand. The hospital is the key resource and center of the U.S. healthcare system. Hospitals not only deliver primary patient care, but some also train health personnel, conduct research, and disseminate information to consumers. Since the turn of the century, hospitals have gradually become the professional heart of all medical practice. Accelerating technological advances and changing societal factors have thrust hospitals into the grasp of big business.

Hospitals are the second-largest business in the United States. They employ approximately 40% of healthcare personnel, with a collective payroll that accounts for at least one-third of the nation's health expenditures. Approximately 41% of federal health spending goes to hospitals as reimbursement for patients who are enrolled in Medicare or Medicaid.

American hospitals started around the time of the Civil War in response to urbanization and economic expansion during the Second Industrial Revolution as well as the arrival of large numbers of immigrants. When the country was first settled, most Americans lived in rural areas and received health care in the home. Hospitals emerged from **almshouses**, institutions that cared for the poor who were chronically ill or disabled. The first two hospitals in the United States were originally almshouses; a six-bed almshouse founded in 1736 in New York City later became Bellevue Hospital, and an almshouse founded in the same year in New Orleans later became Charity Hospital. Before the 1920s, the doctors donated their services, and the nurses and other staff received low pay; however, as healthcare staff became more professional, funds were required to operate the hospitals. From these first hospitals developed public hospitals established by cities, counties, or states that were committed to serving all people but especially the poor. The passage of the **Social Security Act of 1965** created the Medicare and Medicaid programs that funded health care for those over 65 years of age through Medicare and for the indigent through Medicaid. These programs provided federal funds to alleviate poverty; Medicare and Medicaid provided a source of funds to hospitals.[12]

The major forces affecting the development of hospitals include the following: (1) advances in medical science, most notably the discovery of antiseptic techniques and sterilization processes and the use of anesthesia; (2) advances in medical education, with predominant use of scientific theory and standardization of academic training for physicians; and (3) transformation of nursing into a profession by requiring training in caring for the wounded and ill, cleanliness and sanitation procedures, dietary instruction, and simple organized care. These effective, although simple, procedures were a great boon to the growth of hospitals, as the public began to see hospitals as a safe, effective place to go when they were ill. The fourth major force was the development of specialized technology such as X-rays, blood typing, and electrocardiograms, which all came into being early in the twentieth century.[13]

The growth of health insurance (which is discussed in Chapter 3) and of the role of government in the hospital industry has had a substantial impact on hospitals. The federal government has financed hospital construction, regulated the type of construction, financed the provision of care, and set policy for the ways in which hospitals are operated.

The complex hospital industry is usually categorized by three methods: function or type of service provided (from those treating a single disease such as cancer to those with multiple specialties, usually teaching hospitals); length of stay (many short-term, with five days being the average length of stay, and fewer long-term, such as psychiatric or chronic disease hospitals, where the average stay is several weeks to months); and owner-ship or source of financial support—for example, government (or public), proprietary (private for-profit), or voluntary and religious (private nonprofit) ownership.[13] The majority of hospitals (5,141) in the United States are **community hospitals**, with nearly 3,000 of community hospitals being nonprofit (TABLE 2.1).

Hospitals are either private or public. Private hospitals are owned and operated by groups such as churches, businesses, corporations, and physicians. This type of facility is operated in such a way as to make a profit for the owners. A public hospital is financed and operated by a government agency—for example, by the city, county, or state. Such facilities are termed nonprofit facilities, and they admit many patients who cannot afford to pay for medical care. Patients in private hospitals have insurance, private funds, or medical assistance to pay for their care. Voluntary hospitals are usually nonprofit and often are owned and operated by religious organizations. Community hospitals are independent, non-profit corporations consisting of local citizens interested in providing hospital care for their community.[13]

Proprietary hospitals or for-profit hospitals are operated for the financial benefit of the persons, partnerships, or corporations that own them. The current trend is toward a buyout of substantial numbers of these smaller hospitals by large investment firms, creating large, for-profit hospital systems. Management contracts are also on the rise, not only in for-profit hospitals but also in community hospitals. Both trends are expected to continue, as will adverse reaction to them, especially in regard to management corporations taking over community-based hospitals. Philosophy, policies, and operations change drastically under management systems—sometimes for the better and at other times with dubious benefit. However, the proliferation of multisystem hospitals (corporation owned, leased, or managed) will probably persist.[13]

Community hospitals are defined as short-term general and specialty hospitals designed to treat specific health problems, which may include obstetrics and gynecology; ear,

nose, and throat; rehabilitation; and orthopedic conditions. These may include academic medical centers and teaching hospitals. A **hospital system** is defined as either more than one hospital managed by one organization or a single hospital that includes other healthcare organizations—for example, a single hospital that has ownership in a pre-acute outpatient clinic and/or in a post-acute rehabilitation center. A network is a group of hospitals, physicians, and other providers such as physical therapists or mental health workers, insurers, and other community agencies that work together to coordinate and deliver a broad spectrum of services within a town or geographic region.[14]

Public hospitals are owned by local, state, or federal agencies. Federally owned hospitals are generally reserved for the military, veterans, American Indians and Alaska Natives, or other special groups. State governments usually operate long-term hospitals treating chronic illnesses, such as mental institutions. Local governments have city, county, or district hospitals that are primarily short term and staffed by physicians who also have private practices. These types of hospitals in small cities and towns are generally small and function as community healthcare facilities. Public hospitals in major urban areas are large and are staffed by salaried physicians and resident physicians. They take care of the economically deprived and furnish all types of services—from drug abuse treatment to family planning.[13] Another term used to describe public hospitals is **essential hospitals and health systems** that provide significant levels of care to vulnerable populations with limited or no access to health care because of financial circumstances, insurance status, or health condition.[15]

Every state operates hospitals that provide long-term care (if necessary) for the treatment of the mentally ill or developmentally disabled persons; for example, Lincoln Regional Center is a hospital that provides care for Nebraskans who are mentally ill. These state hospitals are run by state administrative agencies; at the local level, district hospitals are supported by taxes from those who live in the district. These hospitals are not involved with the governments of cities, states, or counties. County and city hospitals provide services for the poor and for private patients. Municipal and county governments usually control city hospitals. An example of a locally governed public hospital is Cook County Hospital in Chicago, IL (now Stroger Hospital), which provided uncompensated care for residents without health insurance for years at a cost to taxpayers.

The federal government operates hospitals and clinics for three agencies—the VA, the DoD, and the IHS. The **Civilian Health and Medical Program of the Department of Veterans Affairs (CHAMPVA)** is a comprehensive healthcare program in which the VA shares the cost of covered healthcare services with eligible veterans of the armed services. VA services are organized into regional centers that include hospitals and clinics. TRICARE is a managed healthcare program for active-duty and retired members of the armed services, their families, and survivors. Military retirees and spouses of

TABLE 2.1 Number of Hospitals in the United States by Type of Hospital, 2021[14]

Type of hospital	Number
Community	5,141
Nonprofit	2,946
For-profit	1,233
State and local	962
Federal government	208
Non-federal psychiatric	625

Data from American Hospital Association. *Fast Facts on U.S. Hospitals*, 2021. Accessed August 16, 2021. https://www.aha.org/system/files/media/file/2021/01/Fast-Facts-Hospitals-Infographic-2021-jan21.pdf

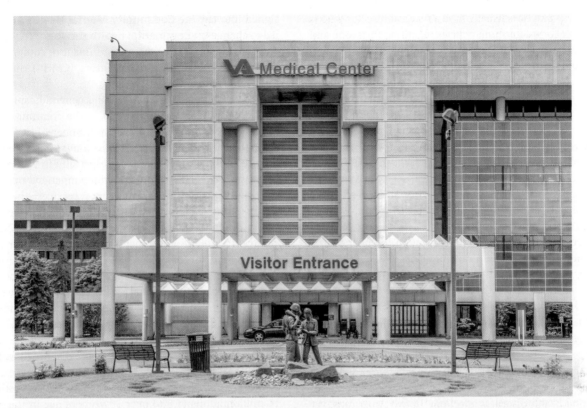

FIGURE 2.3 The federal government operates hospitals for the military and VA.
© Ken Wolter/Shutterstock.

veterans killed in action are also eligible for health services through TRICARE. Walter Reed National Military Medical Center in Bethesda, MD, is one of the largest military hospitals in the United States and provides care for military personnel who are injured or need medical care (**FIGURE 2.3**).[16]

The IHS provides health services to 2.2 million American Indians (AI) and Alaska Natives (AN) who are members of 566 federally recognized tribes. IHS is administered through a system of 12 area offices and 170 IHS and tribally managed service units that include both hospitals and clinics. In addition, there are 33 urban health service programs to meet the needs of AI/AN who live off the reservation.[17]

AMBULATORY HEALTHCARE SERVICES

Care that is provided outside institutional settings is considered ambulatory care and is the most frequent contact that most people have with the healthcare system. Ambulatory care can be any type of care, from simple and routine to complex and specialized. Probably the most familiar kind of ambulatory care, and the one that most people receive, is in the office of either a single practitioner or a group practice or in a non-institutional clinic. The type of service is primary or secondary care, and the principal health practitioners are physicians, dentists, nurses, medical lab technicians, physical therapists, and medical and nursing assistants. If the community can afford an emergency transportation and immediate care system, paramedics and

emergency medical technicians are also part of the ambulatory care network. Emergency advice is furnished from community hotlines and poison control centers.

Primary and secondary care is given at neighborhood health centers and migrant health centers as previously discussed in this chapter. Psychologists and social workers staff community mental health centers. Nurses staff home health and school health services and give both primary and preventive care. Public health services include targeted programs such as family planning, immunizations, screening, maternal and child nutrition, and health education. The health practitioners in these settings are physicians, nurses, dietitians, clinical assistants, and aides. The roster may also include environmental health specialists and health inspectors who do inspections of factories, hospitals, and food establishments to ensure the safety of workers and the public. Pharmacies are ambulatory care facilities staffed by registered pharmacists who dispense drugs and health education. Optical shops with optometrists and opticians provide vision care, while medical technicians provide specialized services in medical laboratories. The federal health system, previously detailed, furnishes all types of ambulatory care, as do prison services.

Many of the ambulatory care services evolve into large, highly complex organizations. For example, an executive committee may be elected to administer the service's business and operations functions. Designated group members may form a credentials committee to screen prospective members, or a building committee may be established.

Large group practices usually have a medical director who is responsible for establishing policies regarding the scope and quality of care as well as personnel practices.[13]

Hospitals are expanding their role to include ambulatory services. They have established fully staffed outpatient facilities and clinics. Hospital outpatient clinics include not only primary care but also specialties such as cardiology, neurology, and endocrinology. Teaching hospitals operate many specialty ambulatory clinics that expose medical students and residents to more extensive experiences. Ambulatory surgery centers and emergency medical services have both expanded, with emergency medicine becoming a specialty for physicians, and regional, hospital-based trauma centers have sprung up in many communities. Forces are at work within communities throughout the nation to enhance primary and specialized health care for all citizens.[13]

BEHAVIORAL HEALTH SERVICES

Behavioral health disorders include mental illness and substance use disorders. Mental illnesses are specific, diagnosable disorders characterized by intense alterations in thinking, mood, and/or behavior. Substance use disorders are conditions resulting from the inappropriate use of alcohol and drugs. Behavioral health disorders affect one in five Americans, yet finding affordable services can be a challenge for many.[18] In 2016, only 43% of nearly 45 million adults with any mental health disorder received treatment, and fewer than 11% of those with substance use disorder received treatment.[19]

Behavioral health personnel involved in the delivery of services include psychiatrists, who are physicians who make a diagnosis, prescribe medications, and may provide psychotherapy. Other health professionals include psychologists, clinical social workers, behavioral disorder counselors, and psychiatric nurses who have advanced degrees and who provide case management and/or psychotherapy. Primary care providers—physicians, nurse practitioners, and physician assistants—screen patients for mental health and substance use disorders and frequently prescribe psychotherapeutic medications. A number of allied health fields have developed in response to the growing needs of the community and the availability of funding. These include school counselors, special education teachers, and others such as art, music, and recreational therapists.

Mental health facilities in the United States were developed in the nineteenth century (as was the American Psychiatric Association), but they were little more than warehouses for large numbers of poor, homeless, alcoholics, drug addicts, and social misfits. They were state hospitals in which the primary purpose, instead of treating the patient, was to protect the public. The creation of the **National Institute of Mental Health (NIMH)** in 1946 and the development of psychopharmaceuticals in the 1950s were the major breakthroughs that led to the real treatment of mental illnesses. Psychotropic drugs enabled thousands of people to return to their communities and to be treated on an outpatient basis.[20] On October 31, 1963, President John F. Kennedy

signed into law the **Community Mental Health Act,** which led to changes in how **mental health services** were delivered and provided funds for the establishment of comprehensive **Community Mental Health Centers (CMHC)** throughout the United States.[21]

By 1964, over 1,600 CMHC and general hospitals were providing mental health services in the community. General hospitals designated a certain number of beds as psychiatric beds for short-term stays. Grants were provided to finance staffing and conversion, especially in economically depressed areas. The centers provided inpatient, outpatient, and day care as well as emergency services; the centers were required to provide specialized services for the mental health of children and the elderly and offered special preventive, treatment, and rehabilitation programs for behavioral health disorders.[22]

Deinstitutionalization appeared to be an acceptable approach for treating mental illness; most patients who had been living in institutions could be treated in community facilities if a comprehensive program was available. Unfortunately, the government failed to adequately fund the CMHC needed for addressing the needs of those diagnosed with **serious mental illness (SMI)**—schizophrenia and severe bipolar disorder—with serious consequences. In 2017, an estimated 11 million adults (4.5%) over 18 years of age in the United States suffered from SMI, yet nearly half of those needing treatment were not getting it because (1) they could not afford the cost of treatment, (2) they didn't know where to go for treatment, or (3) they thought they could handle the problem on their own.[19] The publicly funded psychiatric system that was originally created to protect both the patients and the public no longer exists. Those with SMI are more likely to be homeless or incarcerated or attempt suicide. The psychiatric care they receive is fragmented and uncoordinated, coming at great cost to taxpayers, often with poor outcomes.[23]

Drug addiction became a public health crisis beginning in 2001 when deaths from drug overdoses needed to be addressed. In 2014, nearly 2 million people in the United States suffered from substance use disorders fueled by addiction to prescription opioids and heroin, with a 200% increase in death from overdose between 2001 and 2014. States addressed the opioid crisis by increasing patient access to medication-assisted treatment (e.g., methadone treatment and naloxone [Narcan]) and behavioral health treatment programs. Naloxone was made available to emergency medical technicians and emergency room staff to reverse an opioid overdose and prevent death.[24]

In response to the opioid crisis and decades of declining federal funding for both mental health and addiction treatment services, the bipartisan **Protecting Access to Medicare Act of 2014** funded **Certified Community Behavioral Health Clinics (CCBHC)** to expand access to comprehensive mental health and substance use disorder services. States applied for grants for Medicaid demonstration projects and were required to meet specific criteria including 24-hour crisis services and rapid response non-crisis services, tailored services for active duty military and veterans, and access for all regardless of ability to pay. In 2017, eight states received funding for 66 CCBHC, and by 2020, 13 additional states were funded for a total of 113 clinics in 21 states. Other states can use Medicaid waivers to fund CCBHC. The clinics partner with primary care providers, hospitals, and other healthcare providers to coordinate care, integrate mental and physical health, and reduce hospital readmission; clinics also partner with local law enforcement to prevent recidivism.[25]

Hospitals can become "safety nets" for behavioral health care especially when there is a shortage of CMHC and CCBHC in the community. As a way to identify settings more appropriate for providing behavioral health services, hospitals are now partnering with CMHC, CCBHC, FQHC, academic medical centers, churches, community advocacy groups, and other social service agencies to connect those suffering from behavioral health disorders with care and resources. Hospitals are also working with healthcare workers in primary care settings to integrate assessment and treatment for behavioral health disorders.[18] Approximately one in eight emergency department (ED) visits involves a behavioral health condition, the most common being suicide ideation. This occurs in communities where access to behavioral health care is limited. To avoid repeat visits to the ED, hospitals are involving community resources for care.[18]

Many problems exist within the behavioral health system, including a society that stigmatizes mental illness and substance use disorders. One in 5 Americans suffers from mental illness or substance use disorders every year, yet only half of those seek treatment. Mental illness and substance use disorders are leading causes of disability and death. Adequate and appropriate treatment for mental illness has been difficult, especially for long-term treatment, because of lack of public funding. Historically, most private health insurance policies limited the number of days in the hospital and the number of outpatient visits for treating mental illness and substance use disorders. It has only been since 2008 that services began to be covered by health insurance policies as a result of the **Mental Health Parity and Addiction Equity Act of 2008**.[26] In addition, the ACA requires that all health insurance policies include mental and behavioral health services (see Chapter 5). These requirements are expected to increase access to mental health services for Americans. Unfortunately, those with SMI often are unable to seek treatment, including follow-up care, because of the disabling effects of mental illness. The consequences of untreated mental illness too often are unemployment, homelessness, and incarceration. Treatment requires an integrated system of social and medical services and greater awareness of mental health and mental illness, prevention, and early intervention. There are also disparities in behavioral healthcare access for various populations, including racial and ethnic minority groups, the LGBTQ community, military service members and veterans, and rural residents. These disparities continue to result in poorer health outcomes and increased costs across the healthcare system.[27] The CCBHC model addresses these issues, but not all states have these clinics, and as in the past, the federal government may reduce funding for these clinics, leaving those most vulnerable to a behavioral health crisis without the needed services.

THE CONSUMER'S RIGHTS

In 1973, the American Hospital Association (AHA) developed a Patient's Bill of Rights. The bill, although not a legally binding document, stated the responsibilities of the hospital and staff toward the patient and the patient's family. In 1997, President Bill Clinton appointed an advisory commission on consumer protection and quality in the healthcare industry that further refined the Patient's Bill of Rights. In 2003, the AHA developed the **Patient Care Partnership** to replace the Patient's Bill of Rights, which has six expectations for patients during hospitalization: (1) high-quality hospital care, (2) a clean and safe environment, (3) patient involvement in their own care, (4) protection of patient privacy, (5) help when leaving the hospital, and (6) help with billing claims. A brochure is available in several languages in addition to English and is posted on the AHA webpage.[28]

One of the patient's most important legal rights is **informed consent**; that is, the physician must obtain permission from the patient to perform certain actions or procedures. Informed consent must be obtained before beginning any invasive procedure, administering an experimental drug, or entering the patient into any research project. Specific criteria must be adhered to for informed consent to be valid. Important factors are that the client must be rational and competent or be represented by someone (an advocate) and that the document must be written in a language the client can understand, delineate all the risks involved, state that participation is voluntary, and list the benefits of the procedure and alternatives to the procedure. The client's right to informed consent affects how the healthcare system delivers care. It usually results in increased costs from extra paperwork, but it is necessary for the consumer's protection (and may reduce the care provider's vulnerability to malpractice suits).

Healthcare professionals working in such a wide variety of facilities find challenges and diversity that require them to become knowledgeable in specialized areas and to expand their range of services. The healthcare professional who prefers research may choose to work in primary research institutions, such as the NIH and agencies that administer health and welfare programs. Two major agencies are the VA hospitals and clinics and the U.S. Public Health Service (PHS). If you choose to practice in Canada, the Canada Health Care System covers medical care for all residents of Canada.

PUBLIC HEALTH SERVICES

The mission of HHS is to enhance and protect the health and well-being of all Americans by providing for effective health and human services and fostering advances in medicine, public health, and social services. The Secretary, Operating

Divisions, and Regional Offices administer HHS programs including the ACA. Many HHS-funded services are provided at the local level by state or county agencies or through private-sector grantees (**TABLE 2.2**).[2]

HHS is responsible for Medicare, Medicaid, public health, biomedical research, food and drug safety, disease control and prevention, Indian health services, and mental health services. HHS works closely with state and local governments and provides leadership in public health emergency preparedness in the event of severe weather, infectious disease epidemics, or biological terrorism.[2]

The focus of public health is the community instead of the individual. The community may be limited to a city or may include an entire state, country, or the world. The recent outbreaks of infectious diseases such the coronavirus and Ebola demonstrate the importance of global disease surveillance, pooling of research efforts to help identify pathogens, and international cooperation to develop diagnostic tests, prevention measures, and treatments.

The emphasis in public health is on prevention in contrast to medical care, in which the emphasis is treatment of disease. Public health practitioners are represented by a variety of disciplines such as nursing, medicine, veterinary medicine, dentistry, health education, and nutrition.

Practitioners in public health, including epidemiologists and statisticians, study the nature of new threats and organize public measures to combat them. Because the government is usually involved in the financing and policy-making procedures, the term "public health" has come to include research, assessment, and control measures.

The threats to health change over time. As one set of diseases, epidemics, and conditions is brought under control or eliminated, new diseases appear. The past focus of services, as previously discussed, was to prevent or mitigate the effects of acute infectious diseases such as smallpox, bubonic plague, typhoid fever, childhood infectious diseases, and the 1918 flu pandemic. With the changes in living conditions in the twentieth century, degenerative, debilitative diseases such

TABLE 2.2 Operating Divisions and Functions within the U.S. Department of Health and Human Services (HHS)[2]

Administration for Children and Families (ACF)	Promotes economic and social well-being of families, children, individuals, and communities through educational and supportive programs in partnership with states, tribes, and community organizations.
Administration for Community Living (ACL)	Ensures access to community support and resources to meet needs of older Americans and people with disabilities.
Agency for Healthcare Research and Quality (AHRQ)	Supports research designed to improve quality and patient safety, reduce healthcare costs and medical errors, and broaden access to essential services.
Agency for Toxic Substances and Disease Registry (ATSDR)	Prevents exposure to toxic substances and the adverse health effects and diminished quality of life associated with exposure from waste sites, unplanned releases, and other sources of environmental pollution.
Centers for Disease Control and Prevention (CDC)	Protects the public health of the nation by providing leadership and direction in the prevention and control of diseases and other preventable conditions, and responding to public health emergencies.
Centers for Medicare and Medicaid Services (CMS)	Combines oversight of the Medicare program, the federal portion of the Medicaid program and State Children's Health Insurance Program, the Health Insurance Marketplace, and related quality-assurance activities.
Food and Drug Administration (FDA)	Ensures that food is safe, pure, and wholesome; human and animal drugs, biological products, and medical devices are safe and effective; and electronic products that emit radiation are safe.
Health Resources and Services Administration (HRSA)	Improves access to healthcare services for people who are uninsured, isolated, or medically vulnerable.
Indian Health Service (IHS)	Provides American Indians and Alaska Natives with comprehensive health services by developing and managing programs to meet their health needs.
National Institutes of Health (NIH)	Supports biomedical and behavioral research in the United States and abroad, conducts research in its own laboratories and clinics, trains promising young researchers, and promotes collecting and sharing medical knowledge.
Substance Abuse and Mental Health Services Administration (SAMHSA)	Improves access and reduces barriers to high-quality, effective programs and services for individuals who suffer from or are at risk for addictive and mental disorders as well as for their families and communities.

Reproduced from Department of Health and Human Services, HHS Agencies & Offices. https://www.hhs.gov/about/agencies/hhs-agencies-and-offices/index.html[3]

as chronic obstructive pulmonary disease (COPD), cancer, arthritis, strokes, and coronary heart disease have replaced infectious diseases. That is, until 2020, when the pandemic caused by COVID-19 caught the world unprepared to manage a public health crisis. The virus caused many hospitalizations and deaths comparable to the worldwide 1918 influenza.

The public health system requires cooperation among federal, state, and local governments. Great changes in the roles played by government agencies have occurred over time, with the most important one being the **Social Security Act of 1935**. This act established annual grants-in-aid from the federal government to the states, part of the purpose of which was to fund full-time local health departments. These grants provided for maternal and child health services and extended the services of local public health departments according to the needs of their communities. They were matching-fund grants, in which the states matched federal money on a dollar-for-dollar basis.

Public health at the city and state level now includes such functions as licensing and accrediting health professionals and health facilities, setting standards for automobile

safety devices, and supervising the quality of medical payment programs such as Medicaid.

The establishment of public health and social services in the United States has evolved over time. TABLE 2.3 is a timeline of the HHS beginning in 1798 with an act to provide health care for sick and disabled seamen.[9]

Six basic functions were established for the Public Health Service between 1935 and 1946, and with few revisions they remain the foundation for public health agencies. These are (1) collecting and reporting vital statistics such as birth, death, and incidence of diseases; (2) controlling communicable diseases such as influenza and measles; (3) maintaining a sanitary and safe supply of food and water; (4) ensuring maternal and child health by providing prenatal care; (5) improving health education on common diseases through publications and state and local outreach; and (6) providing laboratory services to track communicable diseases such as HIV/AIDS, COVID-19, influenza, and outbreaks of foodborne illnesses. States conduct annual telephone surveys of residents as part of the **Behavioral Risk Factor Surveillance System (BRFSS)** to evaluate behaviors that increase risk for

TABLE 2.3 Historical Highlights of Health and Human Services in the United States[29]

Year	Event
1798	Passage of an act for the relief of sick and disabled seamen, which established a federal network of hospitals for the care of merchant seamen, the forerunner of today's U.S. Public Health Service.
1862	President Lincoln appointed a chemist, Charles M. Wetherill, to serve in the new Department of Agriculture. This was the beginning of the Bureau of Chemistry, the forerunner to the Food and Drug Administration.
1871	Appointment of the first Supervising Surgeon (later called Surgeon General) for the Marine Hospital Service, which was organized the previous year.
1878	Passage of the National Quarantine Act began the transfer of quarantine functions from the states to the federal Marine Hospital Service.
1887	The federal government opened a one-room laboratory on Staten Island for research on disease, thereby planting the seed that was to grow into the National Institutes of Health.
1891	Passage of immigration legislation, assigning to the Marine Hospital Service the responsibility for the medical examination of arriving immigrants.
1902	Conversion of the Marine Hospital Service into the Public Health and Marine Hospital Service in recognition of its expanding activities in the field of public health. In 1912, the name was shortened to the Public Health Service (PHS).
1906	Congress passed the Pure Food and Drugs Act, authorizing the government to monitor the purity of foods and the safety of medicines, which is now a responsibility of the Food and Drug Administration (FDA).
1912	President Theodore Roosevelt's first White House Conference urged the creation of the Children's Bureau to combat the exploitation of children.
1921	The Bureau of Indian Affairs Health Division was created, the forerunner to the Indian Health Service.
1930	Creation of the National Institute (later Institutes) of Health, out of the Public Health Service's Hygienic Laboratory.
1935	Passage of the Social Security Act.
1938	Passage of the Federal Food, Drug, and Cosmetic Act.
1939	The Federal Security Agency was created, bringing together related federal activities in the fields of health, education, and social insurance.
1946	The Communicable Disease Center was established, forerunner of the Centers for Disease Control and Prevention (CDC).

(Continued)

TABLE 2.3 Historical Highlights of Health and Human Services in the United States[29] *(Continued)*

1955	Licensing of the Salk polio vaccine. The Indian Health Service was transferred to the U.S. Department of Health and Human Services from the Department of the Interior.
1961	First White House Conference on Aging.
1962	Passage of the Migrant Health Act, providing support for clinics serving agricultural workers.
1964	Release of the first Surgeon General's Report on Smoking and Health.
1965	Creation of the Medicare and Medicaid programs, making comprehensive health care available to millions of Americans. The Older Americans Act created nutrition and social programs administered by the HHS's Administration on Aging. Head Start program was created.
1966	International Smallpox Eradication program was established; led by the U.S. Public Health Service, the worldwide eradication of smallpox was accomplished in 1977. The Community Health Center and Migrant Health Center programs were launched.
1970	Creation of the National Health Service Corps.
1971	National Cancer Act signed into law.
1975	Child Support Enforcement program was established.
1977	Creation of the Health Care Financing Administration (HCFA) to manage Medicare and Medicaid separately from the Social Security Administration.
1980	Federal funding provided to states for foster care and adoption assistance.
1981	Identification of AIDS. In 1984, the Public Health Service and French scientists identified HIV. In 1985, a blood test to detect HIV was licensed.
1984	National Organ Transplantation Act signed into law.
1988	Creation of the JOBS program and federal support for child care. Passage of the McKinney Act to provide health care to the homeless.
1989	Creation of the Agency for Health Care Policy and Research (now the Agency for Healthcare Research and Quality).
1990	Human Genome Project established. Passage of the Nutrition Labeling and Education Act, authorizing the food label. Ryan White Comprehensive AIDS Resource Emergency (CARE) Act began providing support for people with AIDS.
1993	The Vaccines for Children Program was established, providing free immunizations to all children in low-income families.
1995	The Social Security Administration became an independent agency.
1996	Enactment of welfare reform under the Personal Responsibility and Work Opportunity Reconciliation Act. Enactment of the Health Insurance Portability and Accountability Act (HIPAA).
1997	Creation of the State Children's Health Insurance Program (CHIP), enabling states to extend health coverage to more uninsured children.
1999	The Ticket to Work and Work Incentives Improvement Act of 1999 made it possible for millions of Americans with disabilities to join the workforce without fear of losing their Medicaid and Medicare coverage. Initiative on combating bioterrorism was launched.
2000	Publication of human genome sequencing.
2002	Office of Public Health Emergency Preparedness was created to coordinate efforts against bioterrorism and other emergency health threats.
2003	Enactment of the Medicare Prescription Drug Improvement and Modernization Act of 2003, the most significant expansion of Medicare since its enactment, including a prescription drug benefit.
2010	The Affordable Care Act was signed into law, putting in place comprehensive U.S. health insurance reforms.

Modified from U.S. Department of Health and Human Services. *HHS Historical Highlights*, 2017. http://www.hhs.gov/about/historical-highlights/[29]

chronic disease, including diet, physical activity, smoking, and drug and alcohol use. Individual states report health statistics to the **National Center for Health Statistics**, and the **Centers for Disease Control and Prevention (CDC)** compiles, analyzes, and reports data on disease prevalence. The CDC works in cooperation with infectious disease specialists around the world to track outbreaks of infectious diseases and to develop vaccines and other treatment protocols. In addition, the CDC monitors air and water quality and provides support in emergencies, such as severe weather conditions that impact health and safety (**FIGURE 2.4**).

In the United States, career opportunities in public health exist in the **Commissioned Corps**, an essential component of the largest public health program in the world. Corps officers are eligible for a variety of positions throughout the HHS and certain non-HHS federal agencies and programs in the areas of disease control and prevention; biomedical research; regulation of food, drugs, and medical devices; mental health and drug abuse; healthcare delivery; and international health. Opportunities are also available at the community level in public health departments and professional organizations—for example, the American Heart Association.

The student desiring to go into public health must be aware of the political battles that are being waged over the structure of the system as well as a lack of financial support. New and changed roles for local, state, and federal public health agencies are apparent. The nation will continue to need public health services and leaders who keep abreast of new research and who have a grasp of modern health problems and solving problems from both a preventive and curative standpoint. Also needed is an understanding of the political system and societal expectations and demands. The student who chooses a public health service career will be in a role with changing dynamics while still fulfilling fundamental, long-accepted functions. Table 2.3 lists achievements in public health in the United States.

HEALTH CARE IN THE TWENTY-FIRST CENTURY

From its humble, unscientific, and often haphazard beginnings to the present multibillion-dollar industry, the private U.S. healthcare system has undergone broad and often drastic changes. Its present visibility and highly technical orientation have led to thousands of jobs, created new professions, and provided care to millions of people. It is not without the attendant problems of a giant industry, however, and in the twenty-first century, the system must face and solve yet more problems. Preventive health care will play an important role

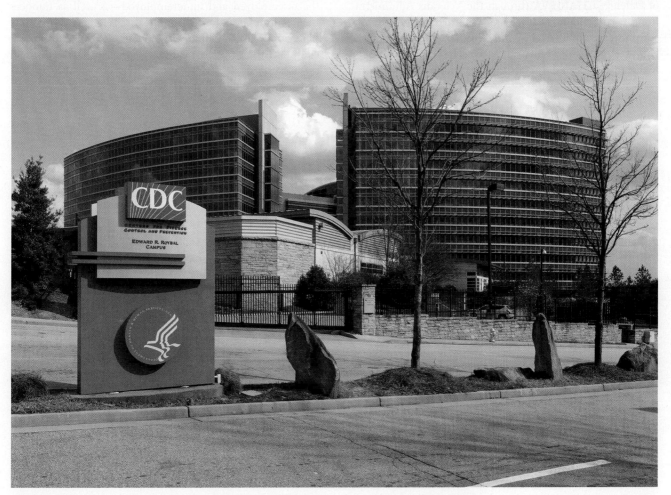

FIGURE 2.4 The CDC monitors air and water quality and provides support in weather emergencies.
© Katherine Welles/Shutterstock.

in achieving health care for all through recently expanded federally funded primary care clinics and behavioral health clinics in response to the opioid crisis and high rates of incarceration of those with serious mental illness. Although many infectious diseases have been nearly eliminated through vaccination programs, new infectious threats can reappear, as happened in 2019–2020 with COVID-19. American ingenuity will face a difficult challenge in formulating a workable, affordable system for all people.

SUMMARY

Unlike most developed countries the United States does not have a centralized health care delivery system (national health system) in which individuals automatically receive health care. Instead, the majority of Americans obtain health care services from a variety of locations and providers; services are employer-funded private insurance or government-subsidized Medicare or Medicaid. Five broad categories of healthcare services are health promotion, disease prevention, diagnosis and treatment, rehabilitation, and chronic care.

The only direct health services provided by the federal government are TRICARE, through the Department of Defense, CHAMPVA through the Veterans Administration, and the Indian Health Service. The federal government administers public health programs through 11 agencies within Health and Human Services (HHS) responsible for Medicare, Medicaid, public health, biomedical research, food and drug safety, disease control and prevention, Indian health services, and mental health services. HHS works closely with state and local governments and provides leadership in public health emergency preparedness. The role of the U.S. Congress is making laws, allocating funds, and doing investigative work through committees.

Hospitals are the second-largest industry in the United States and the largest employer of healthcare workers. Public hospitals are financed by the government, while private hospitals are financed by businesses, churches, physicians, and others. Hospitals provide patient care, train health professionals, conduct research, and provide public education for consumers and members of the community. The American Hospital Association's Patient Care Partnership informs patients of their rights and responsibilities during hospitalization and after hospital discharge.

Ambulatory healthcare is delivered outside of a hospital setting and employs the second-highest number of healthcare workers to provide care for simple to complex health conditions. Federally Qualified Health Centers are funded by Medicare, Medicaid, and private insurance, and serve high-need and medically underserved people including those with substance use disorders and HIV. Free Medical Clinics are privately funded and serve those who are uninsured—the unemployed and underemployed—as well as undocumented immigrants and the homeless. Certified Community Behavioral Health Clinics are federally funded and provide comprehensive mental health and substance use disorder services.

Learning Portfolio   **33**

LEARNING PORTFOLIO

Study Points

1. The healthcare industry is a complex system of hospitals, ambulatory care, laboratories, pharmaceutical and medical equipment manufacturers, and private and government-funded programs. However, the United States does not have a centralized healthcare delivery system common in other countries including Canada and the United Kingdom.

2. Hospitals are the second-largest industry and the largest employer of healthcare workers in the United States.

3. Direct healthcare services provided by the federal government are limited to the U.S. Department of Defense, the U.S. Veterans Administration, and Indian Health Services.

4. Most health care is delivered in ambulatory care settings by a variety of health professionals.

5. Five broad categories of health care are health promotion, disease prevention, diagnosis and treatment, rehabilitation, and chronic care.

6. Nearly 1,400 Federally Qualified Health Centers (FQHC) are funded by Medicare, Medicaid, private insurance, and patient fees. FQHC serve high-need and medically underserved people living in urban and rural areas, including large populations with substance abuse disorders and HIV.

7. About 1,400 privately funded free medical clinics (FMCs) serve those who are uninsured—the unemployed and underemployed as well as undocumented immigrants and the homeless.

8. Inadequate public funding for treating serious mental illness (SMI) has had serious consequences for those with SMI: unemployment, homelessness, and incarceration.

9. In response to deaths from the opioid crisis and homelessness and incarceration of those with serious mental illness, federal legislators funded Certified Community Behavioral Health Clinics (CCBHC) beginning in 2017.

10. Hospitals provide patient care, train health professionals, conduct research, and provide public education for consumers and members of the community.

11. Four major forces responsible for the development of hospitals in the United States are (1) aseptic techniques, (2) advances in medical education, (3) professional development of nurses, and (4) specialized technology.

12. Hospitals are categorized by function, length of stay, and financial support or ownership. Public hospitals are financed by the government, while private hospitals are financed by businesses, churches, physicians, and others. There are more community, nonprofit hospitals than all other categories of hospitals.

13. Most health care is delivered in ambulatory care settings by a variety of health professionals.

14. The American Hospital Association developed the Patient Care Partnership as a guide for hospital personnel in providing care to patients and to inform hospital patients of their rights and responsibilities.

15. The coronavirus, COVID-19, caught the world unprepared for an infectious disease pandemic resulting in the infection and death of thousands around the world.

16. The most important federal agency responsible for the health of the United States is the U.S. Department of Health and Human Services, which administers 11 operating divisions responsible for Medicare, Medicaid, public health, biomedical research, food and drug safety, disease control and prevention, mental health services, and Indian Health Services.

Issues for Discussion

1. View the 5½-minute video "American's Health Centers: An Enduring Legacy, Value for Today & Tomorrow," March 21, 2015. National Association of Community Health Centers. Discuss the history of federally funded national health centers. Discuss the medical services provided at these centers and the medical and economic benefits for local communities. https://www.youtube.com/watch?v=aV9jJpX0PZI

2. View the 2-minute cartoon video "My Hospital—Advancing Health in America" from the American Hospital Association. Discuss community outreach programs of the hospital and how health care is coordinated with other health service facilities in the wider community that make up health care in the entire community. https://www.youtube.com/watch?v=NFiLJksGOxA

3. Go to the Centers for Disease Control and Prevention (CDC) webpage, link to *Emergency Preparedness and Response,* and select one disaster to review what to do before, during, and after the event, especially regarding food and water safety.

    Which weather-related disasters are common in your area? What can you do to be prepared to prevent injury or illness? Which agencies in your community provide support during emergencies? https://www.cdc.gov/disasters/alldisasters.html

LEARNING PORTFOLIO

4. Review the infographic titled "Multicultural Mental Health Infographic" from the National Alliance for Mental Illness.

   At what age does chronic mental illness appear? Which ethnic group has the highest incidence of mental illness? Which other minority groups have a high incidence of mental illness? https://www.nami.org/NAMI/media/NAMI-Media/Infographics/MulticulturalMHFacts10-23-15.pdf

Enrichment Activities

1. Access the website for the National Association of Free and Charitable Clinics; enter the zip code where you live to find out if there are any free clinics where you live. https://www.nafcclinics.org/find-clinic

2. Go to the Indian Health Services' website to find out what healthcare services are provided and how the quality of the health services are monitored. http://www.ihs.gov/forpatients/healthcare/

3. Go to the Centers for Disease Control and Prevention website and review information about the 1918 Pandemic Flu (H1N1 virus). What are the similarities with the COVID-19 pandemic in 2020? What are the differences? https://www.cdc.gov/flu/pandemic-resources/1918-pandemic-h1n1.html

CASE STUDY: CATEGORIES OF HEALTH CARE

Jenny was enlisted in the United States Navy and was on active duty as a hospital corpsman serving as an operating room technician during surgery. Jenny was able to begin taking basic college courses while in the Navy with a goal of becoming a registered nurse. She has been admitted to a community college in a suburb of Chicago to begin an associate's degree that will enable her to complete the requirements to take the national licensing exam required to become a registered nurse. Jenny plans to work part time as a waitress; however, she will have no health benefits through her job. Jenny is a single mother of a 5-year-old daughter and is concerned about obtaining health care for herself and her daughter while she attends college.

Based on the information about healthcare systems, answer the following questions.

1. Jenny has found it challenging to follow a routine of regular physical activity since leaving the military. Which of the following category of health services would assist Jenny in meeting her goal of becoming physically fit?
   A. Diagnosis
   B. Health promotion
   C. Disease prevention
   D. Treatment

2. Which category of health services are immunizations?
   A. Diagnosis
   B. Health promotion
   C. Disease prevention
   D. Treatment

3. Jenny's boyfriend Joe is also a veteran. He is a construction worker and injured his back several months ago. Joe's doctor prescribed a pain medication, and Joe was able to continue to work because the medication stopped the pain. Joe has tried to stop taking the pain medication but experienced withdrawal symptoms. Where would you recommend that Joe not go for treatment of his addiction?
   A. VA clinic
   B. Primary doctor
   C. Certified Community Behavioral Health Clinic
   D. Emergency room

References

1. Torpey E. Healthcare: Millions of Jobs Now and in the Future. *Occup Outlook Q.* Spring 2014. https://www.bls.gov/careeroutlook/2014/spring/art03.pdf Accessed July 2, 2020.

2. Shi L, Singh DA. *Delivering Health Care in America. A Systems Approach.* 7th ed. Burlington, MA: Jones & Bartlett Learning; 2019.

3. HHS.gov. *HHS Agencies and Offices.* January 2015. U.S. Department of Health and Human Services. https://www.hhs.gov/about/agencies/hhs-agencies-and-offices/index.html Accessed July 2, 2020.

4. Bureau of Primary Health Care. Health Resources and Service Administration. *What Is a Health Center?* U.S. Department of Health and Human Services, November 2018. http://bphc.hrsa.gov/about/what-is-a-health-center/index.html Accessed July 2, 2020.

5. Bureau of Primary Health Care. Health Resources and Services Administration. *2018 National Health Center Data.* U.S. Department of Health and Human Services. https://bphc.hrsa.gov/uds/datacenter.aspx Accessed July 2, 2020.

6. Bureau of Primary Health Care. Health Resources and Service Administration. *Health Center Program Fact Sheet,*

LEARNING PORTFOLIO

2018. https://bphc.hrsa.gov/sites/default/files/bphc/about/healthcenterfactsheet.pdf Accessed July 2, 2020.

7.   The National Association of Free & Charitable Clinics (NAFC). *2019 Public Policy Objectives*. https://www.nafcclinics.org/sites/default/files/NAFC%202019%20Federal%20Policy%20Objectives%20FINAL%20.pdf Accessed July 2, 2020.

8.   Darnell JS. Free Clinics in the United States. A Nationwide Survey. *Arch Int Med*. 2010; 946–953.

9.   American Health Lawyers Association/American Medical Association Foundation. *The Free Medical Clinic: A Practical Handbook for Health Care Providers*, 2016. https://www.ama-assn.org/sites/ama-assn.org/files/corp/media-browser/public/ama-foundation/free-medical-clinic-handbook.pdf Accessed July 2, 2020.

10.   National Association of Free and Charitable Clinics. *NAFC History*. https://www.nafcclinics.org/content/nafc-history Accessed July 2, 2020.

11.   Tolbert J, Orgera K, Singer N, Damico A. *Key Facts about the Uninsured Population*, December 2019. Kaiser Family Foundation. http://files.kff.org/attachment/Issue-Brief-Key-Facts-about-the-Uninsured-Population Accessed July 2, 2020.

12.   America's Essential Hospitals. *History of Public Hospitals in the United States*. http://essentialhospitals.org/about-americas-essential-hospitals/history-of-public-hospitals-in-the-united-states/ Accessed July 2, 2020.

13.   Bernstein AB, Hing E, Moss AJ, Allen KF, Siller AB, Riggle RB. *Health Care in America. Trends in Utilization*. Hyattsville, MD. National Center for Health Statistics; 2003.

14.   American Hospital Association. *Fast Facts on U.S. Hospitals*, March, 2020. https://www.aha.org/system/files/media/file/2020/01/2020-aha-hospital-fast-facts-new-Jan-2020.pdf Accessed July 2, 2020.

15.   America's Essential Hospitals. *Frequently Asked Questions*. http://essentialhospitals.org/about-americas-essential-hospitals/frequently-asked-questions/ Accessed July 2, 2020.

16.   U.S. Department of Veteran's Affairs. *CHAMPVA*. https://www.va.gov/communitycare/programs/dependents/champva/index.asp#resources Accessed July 2, 2020.

17.   Indian Health Services. *Trends in Indian Health, 2014 Edition*, March 2015. U.S. Department of Health and Human Services. https://www.ihs.gov/sites/dps/themes/responsive2017/display_objects/documents/Trends2014Book508.pdf Accessed August 16, 2021.

18.   American Hospital Association. Increasing Access to Behavioral Health Care Advances Value for Patients, Providers and Communities. *TrendWatch*, May 2019. https://www.aha.org/system/files/media/file/2019/05/aha-trendwatch-behavioral-health-2019.pdf Accessed July 2, 2020.

19.   Substance Abuse and Mental Health Services Administration. *Key substance use and Mental Health Indicators in the United States: Results from the 2017 National Survey on Drug Use and Health, 2018*. HHS Publication No. SMA 18-5068, NSDUH Series H-53. Rockville, MD: Center for Behavioral Health Statistics and Quality, Substance Abuse and Mental Health.

20.   Satcher DS, Executive Summary: A Report of the Surgeon General on Mental Health. *Public Health Rep*. 2000; 115:89–101.

21.   National Council for Behavioral Health. *Community Mental Health Act*. https://www.thenationalcouncil.org/about/national-mental-health association/overview/community-mental-health-act/ Accessed July 2, 2020.

22.   Ornstein G. *Community Mental Health Centers*, 1967. Chicago: American Society of Planning Officials. https://planning-org-uploaded-media.s3.amazonaws.com/document/PAS-Report-223.pdf Accessed July 2, 2020.

23.   Treatment Advocacy Center. *Consequences of Non-Treatment*. https://www.treatmentadvocacycenter.org/key-issues/consequences-of-non-treatment Accessed May 19, 2020.

24.   Murphy K, Becker M, Locke J, Kelleher C, McLeod J, Isasi F. *Finding Solutions to the Prescription Opioid and Heroin Crisis: A Road Map for States*. Washington, DC: National Governors Association Center for Best Practices, July 2016.

25.   National Council for Behavioral Health. *Hope for the Future. CCBHCs Expanding Mental Health and Addiction Treatment. An Impact Report*, 2020.

26.   Federal Register. *Final Rules Under the Paul Wellstone and Pete Domenici Mental Health Parity and Addiction Equity Act of 2008; Technical Amendment to External Review for Multi-State Plan Program. November 2013*. https://www.federalregister.gov/documents/2013/11/13/2013-27086/final-rules-under-the-paul-wellstone-and-pete-domenici-mental-health-parity-and-addiction-equity-act Accessed August 16, 2021.

27.   National Conference for State Legislature (NCSL). *The Costs and Consequences of Disparities in Behavioral Health Care*, 2018. http://www.ncsl.org/Portals/1/HTML_LargeReports/DisparitiesBehHealth_Final.htm Accessed July 2, 2020.

28.   American Hospital Association. *The Patient Care Partnership*. 2003. https://www.aha.org/system/files/2018-01/aha-patient-care-partnership.pdf Accessed August 16, 2021.

29.   HHS.gov. *HHS Historical Highlights*. 2017. U.S. Department of Health and Human Services. http://www.hhs.gov/about/historical-highlights/ Accessed July 2, 2020.

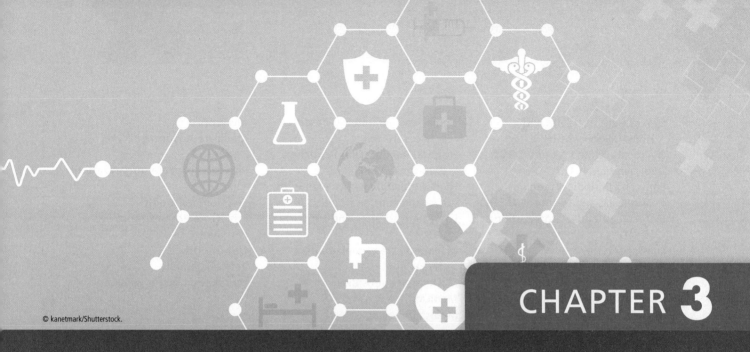

© kanetmark/Shutterstock.

CHAPTER 3

Paying for Health Services

OBJECTIVES

After studying this chapter, the student should be able to:

- Explain how public healthcare systems are financed.
- Characterize the populations served by Medicare, Medicaid, and the Children's Health Insurance Program (CHIP).
- Estimate the percentage of the total federal budget expended for government-funded healthcare programs.
- Compare traditional and contemporary methods of reimbursement for healthcare services.
- Describe the similarities and differences of managed care organizations used by private insurance.
- Identify the role of the government in the expansion of health care.

KEY TERMS

Accountable care organization (ACO)	Capitation	Initiative
Affordable Care Act (ACA)	Centers for Medicare and Medicaid Services (CMS)	Copayment
American Medical Association (AMA)	Children's Health Insurance Program (CHIP)	Coinsurance
Bundled payment	Community Engagement	Cost-sharing subsidy
		Deductible

Department of Health and Human Services (HHS)	Home- and community-based services (HCBS)	Medicare
Diagnosis-related groups (DRGs)	Hospital Readmission Reduction Program (HRRP)	Medicare Advantage Plan
Dual-eligible		Network
Early and Periodic Screening, Diagnostic, and Treatment (EPSDT)	High-deductible health plan with a savings option (HDHP/SO)	Preferred provider organizations (PPOs)
Exclusive provider organization (EPO)	Long-term services and supports (LTSS)	Premium tax credit
		Private health insurance
Fee-for-service	Managed care organizations (MCOs)	Premium
Federal poverty level (FPL)		Out-of-pocket
Health Insurance Marketplace	Marketplace subsidies	Reimbursement
Health maintenance organization (HMO)	Medicaid	Work requirement waiver
	Medicaid waiver	

HEALTHCARE FINANCING

Health care in the United States is funded through a variety of private payers and public programs. Public spending represents expenditures by federal, state, and local governments. Private funding is primarily through private health insurance. In addition to private insurance, privately funded health care includes out-of-pocket expenditures, philanthropy, and non-patient revenues (such as revenue from hospital gift shops and parking lots) as well as health services that are provided at employers' establishments, immediate care clinics, or clinics within pharmacies.[1]

A significant portion of public health spending can be attributed to the programs administered by the **Centers for Medicare and Medicaid Services (CMS)**—Medicare, Medicaid, the **Children's Health Insurance Program (CHIP)**, and the **Health Insurance Marketplace**. In 2019, three budget items accounted for the largest expenditures for the federal budget; government-funded health care programs—Medicare, Medicaid, CHIP, and Marketplace subsidies—accounted for 25%, Social Security for 23%, and defense for 16% **(FIGURE 3.1)**[2]

The sources of federal revenue to cover the costs of the national budget are income tax (50%); payroll tax (36%); excise, estate, and other taxes (7%); and corporate income tax (7%) **(FIGURE 3.2)**. Payroll taxes are assessed on the wage or salary paychecks of almost all workers and split between the employer and employee. Payroll taxes are used to fund Social Security, Medicare Hospital Insurance, and unemployment insurance. Excise taxes are collected on the sale of such items as fuel, alcohol, and tobacco. Estate tax is a tax on assets transferred to the deceased heirs on items such as cash, real estate, or stock (Figure 3.2).[3]

PAYMENT TO PROVIDERS

The traditional method of **reimbursement** for health services before passage of the **Affordable Care Act (ACA)** was **fee-for-service**; that is, paying the provider at the time of service. Under fee-for-service, the provider—doctor, hospital, or clinic—is financially rewarded for the volume of services

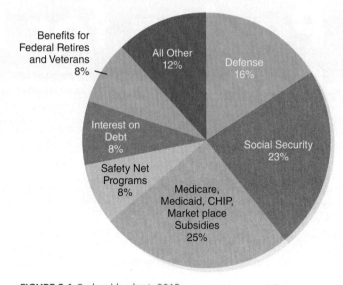

FIGURE 3.1 Federal budget, 2019.

Data from Center on Budget and Policy Priorities. *Where Do Our Federal Tax Dollars Go?* April 9, 2020. https://www.cbpp.org/sites/default/files/atoms/files/4-14-08tax.pdf

performed—for example, the number of laboratory tests, number of surgeries, and number of days in the hospital—rather than for the quality and cost control (value) of those services. In an effort to control rising healthcare costs, both public and private health insurance programs have moved to **capitation**, defined as paying the practitioner or hospital a fixed amount for a specific service. In capitation, the insurance pays a set fee to cover all the services; fee-for-service pays only for the particular service(s) rendered (itemized) at a given time.[4]

An example of capitation for private insurance is **health maintenance organizations (HMOs)**, which limit consumer choice to health professionals and hospitals that contract with the HMO. Both Medicare and Medicaid use long-term contracts with providers for a population or group of patients. An example of long-term contracts is **managed care organizations (MCOs)**, a healthcare delivery system designed to manage cost, utilization, and quality. State Medicaid agencies contract with MCOs that accept payment for a specific dollar

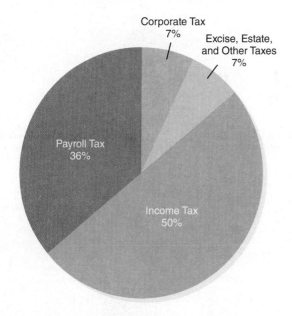

FIGURE 3.2 Sources of federal tax revenue, 2019.

Modified from Center on Budget and Policy Priorities. *Where Do Federal Tax Revenues Come From?* June 2019. https://www.cbpp.org/sites/default/files/atoms/files/PolicyBasics_WhereDoFederalTaxRevsComeFrom_08-20-12.pdf

amount per member per month (capitation) regardless of the services delivered. **Medicare Advantage Plans** are a form of MCO; Medicare pays a fixed dollar amount per enrollee per month to the insurance company offering Medicare Advantage Plans. Providers are motivated to give quality care rather than increase the number of procedures or hospitalizations when patients are enrolled in an MCO.

Shifting away from fee-for-service to improve quality while reducing costs requires changed expectations for both consumers and providers. Under fee-for-service, there were few limits on the length of hospital stay or number of doctor visits; however, MCOs often require preapproval for surgery and other costly treatments.[4] The consequence for consumers is that scheduling non-emergency surgery and other procedures will involve a waiting period. Consumers will need to be knowledgeable about their insurance requirements for treatment.

In an effort to reduce costs and improve quality, the CMS set a goal of reducing Medicare fee-for-service payments to providers (doctors, hospitals) over a period of several years. One of the changes CMS made to reward quality of care instead of volume is the **Hospital Readmission Reduction Program (HRRP)**, in which hospitals receive lower reimbursement rates for all patients on Medicare if hospital readmission occurs sooner than 30 days after discharge.[5] Other CMS programs designed to improve quality and reduce costs are **bundled payments** and **accountable care organizations (ACOs)**; both are examples of capitation. Bundled payments are made for an episode of care; for example, hospital and homecare services, including physical therapy for a patient receiving hip-replacement surgery. ACOs address quality and costs for a population—for example, payment for comprehensive care for end-stage renal disease for patients receiving regular dialysis.[4]

GOVERNMENT-FUNDED HEALTH INSURANCE

Medicare and Medicaid are government or public health insurance programs that benefit one in three Americans. The **Medicare** program is a federal health program for people aged 65 years and older, certain disabled people younger than 65, and any adult with permanent kidney failure (end-stage renal disease) or amyotrophic lateral sclerosis (ALS, or Lou Gehrig's disease). Patients on Medicare are entitled to the same benefits and care as those with private insurance. The main difference is that the government pays the healthcare bills instead of the individual or private insurance. Medicare pays for many healthcare services—hospitalizations, doctor visits, and prescription drugs. It also covers the cost of short-term stays in a skilled nursing facility, home health care, hospice, and preventive services such as immunizations (flu shots and pneumococcal shots) and cancer screenings.[6] In 2019, Medicare provided health insurance for 61.5 million people—8.5 million with permanent disabilities under age 65 (14%) and 53 million 65 years of age and older (86%).[7]

Medicaid is the federal–state cooperative health insurance plan for those who are not eligible for health insurance through an employer and cannot afford to buy health insurance through the Marketplace. Title XIX of the Social Security Act and other federal regulations govern Medicaid by defining federal requirements and state options.[8] The CMS within the **Department of Health and Human Services (HHS)** is responsible for implementing Medicaid. The program is jointly funded by the federal and state governments and is administered by individual states. People with incomes below the poverty level established by a state can use this government-sponsored health insurance program. Until Medicaid was expanded as a result of the ACA, only certain low-income individuals were eligible: U.S. citizens or legal immigrants, pregnant women, children, parents of low-income children, seniors, and those with disabilities.[9] The ACA set new guidelines requiring states to cover all children and pregnant women living in households with incomes up to at least 138% of the **federal poverty level (FPL)**; however, about half of the states cover children from households with higher incomes—above 250% of the FPL.[9] Since implementation of the ACA, states that chose to expand Medicaid cover adults at 133% of the FPL.[9]

Medicaid as an entitlement is based on two guarantees: (1) All Americans who meet Medicaid eligibility requirements are guaranteed coverage, and (2) states are guaranteed matching funds from the federal government to help pay for Medicaid coverage. The matching rate ranges from 50% to 75% depending on a state's per-capita income and changes from year to year; wealthier states receive lower federal matches, and poorer states receive higher matches. Some Medicaid services are funded at even higher levels; family planning is funded at 90%, while home health and Indian Health Services are funded at 100%.[10] Matching funds from states are generated through local and state sales tax, state income taxes, or assessments on health

TABLE 3.1 Mandatory Health Services Required by Medicaid Programs	
Inpatient hospital services	Laboratory and X-ray services
Outpatient hospital services	Family planning services
Early and periodic screening, diagnostic, and treatment services	Certified pediatric and family nurse practitioner services
Nursing facility services	Nurse-midwife services
Home health services	Freestanding birth center services
Physician services	Transportation to medical care
Rural health clinic services	Tobacco cessation counseling for pregnant women
Federally qualified health centers (FQHC)	

Data from Centers for Medicare & Medicaid Services. *Mandatory & Optional Medicaid Benefits.* https://www.medicaid.gov/medicaid/benefits/mandatory-optional-medicaid-benefits/index.html

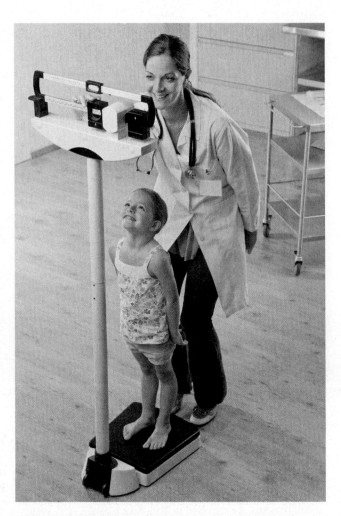

FIGURE 3.3 A mandatory requirement for Medicaid is early and periodic screening of children.
© AVAVA/Shutterstock.

plans and providers. A temporary source of funding at the state level came as a result of the ACA. A provision of the ACA was that the federal government paid state governments the costs of expanding Medicaid at the level of 100% from 2014 through 2016, with a gradual decrease to 90% by 2020. To date, 38 states and Washington, D.C., have adopted Medicaid expansion, while 12 states have not adopted the expansion. The majority of states that chose not to expand through the ACA are states in the South and Southeast except for South Dakota, Wisconsin, and Wyoming.[11]

States administer Medicaid programs and have the flexibility to determine eligibility, which services will be provided, and a specific healthcare delivery and payment model.[9] The majority of Medicaid programs use a managed care model, while others use a fee-for-service model. Medicaid beneficiaries receive care through community clinics, public hospitals, and academic health centers. A limitation for those enrolled in Medicaid is that not all providers (specialty physicians such as cardiologists and dentists) accept patients because of the low reimbursement rate, which can limit access to care. State Medicaid programs can establish cost-sharing in the form of **copayments** for outpatient visits, hospitalizations, and other care; fees are based on income and are nominal.[8] Some health services for those on Medicaid are considered mandatory by the federal government, while others are considered optional. Many states cover additional optional benefits such as dental care, vision care, prescription drugs, physical and occupational therapy, and others (**TABLE 3.1**).[12] See **FIGURE 3.3** for mandatory care.

In 2019, Medicaid provided coverage to one in five Americans, which makes it the nation's largest public health insurance program. Medicaid covers the lowest-income and most medically complex children and adults. For example, Medicaid is the largest source of funding for mental health and substance use disorders, maternal health, and long-term care services in nursing homes and **home- and community-based services (HCBS)**.[8] Medicaid covered more than one-third of all children, more than three-fourths of children living in households below 100% of the (FPL), and nearly half of all births.[8] In addition, Medicaid covered 45% of non-elderly adults with disabilities (physical disabilities such as cerebral palsy and developmental disabilities such as autism), serious mental illness, traumatic brain injury, and Alzheimer's disease.[8] Examples of health services provided by Medicaid are listed in **TABLE 3.2**.[8]

Medicaid spends a larger portion of money on beneficiaries with physical or mental disabilities who have high medical needs. **FIGURES 3.4** and **3.5** show the distribution of different populations enrolled in Medicaid and the average annual federal spending for the same population groups. For example, even though 43% of the total Medicaid enrollees are children, less money is spent on children than all other

TABLE 3.2 Medicaid Benefits for Families, Individuals, and the Elderly

Population	Medicaid Benefits
Low-Income Families	• **Pregnant women**: Prenatal care and delivery • **Children**: Routine and specialized care (immunizations, dental, vision, speech therapy) • **Families**: Affordable coverage for the unexpected (emergency dental, hospitalization)
Individuals with Disabilities	• **Child with autism**: In-home speech/occupational therapy • **Cerebral palsy**: Assistance to gain independence (personal care, case management, assistive technology) • **HIV/AIDS**: Physician services, prescription drugs • **Mental illness**: Physician services, prescription drugs
Elderly Individuals	• **Medicare beneficiary**: Pays for Medicare premiums; cost sharing • **Community waiver participant**: Community-based and personal care • **Nursing home resident**: Costs paid by Medicaid since Medicare does not cover institutional care

Modified from Rudowitz R, Garfield R, Hinton E. *10 Things To Know About Medicaid: Setting The Facts Straight.* San Francisco, CA: Kaiser Family Foundation. March 2019. https://www.kff.org/medicaid/issue-brief/10-things-to-know-about-medicaid-setting-the-facts-straight/

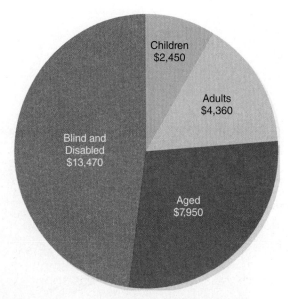

FIGURE 3.5 Average annual federal spending per Medicaid enrollee, 2019.

Data from *Medicaid: Congressional Budget Office's May 2019 Baseline.* https://www.cbo.gov/system/files/2019-05/51301-2019-05-medicaid.pdf

groups ($2,450 per enrollee per year). The smallest group—the blind and disabled—is only 12% of the total Medicaid enrollment, yet the total amount of money spent on the blind and disabled was $13,470 per enrollee per year.[13]

Infants, children, and adolescents under age 21 who are enrolled in Medicaid receive **Early and Periodic Screening, Diagnostic, and Treatment (EPSDT)** to identify and treat physical and developmental conditions and mental illness. Individual states arrange for children to receive physicals, mental health, vision, hearing, and dental services as needed by a physician, dentist, nurse practitioner, speech/language therapist, occupational therapist, or other professionals.[14]

Those enrolled in both Medicare and Medicaid are **dual-eligibles**. Medicaid covers one in five Medicare beneficiaries and almost two-thirds of all nursing home residents. Medicaid also covers additional services beyond those provided under Medicare—for example, health insurance premiums, prescription drugs, eye glasses, and hearing aids. Services covered by both programs are paid first by Medicare, with Medicaid filling in the difference up to the state's payment limit (**FIGURE 3.6**).[15]

Medicaid uses a mechanism that allows individual states to use **Medicaid waivers** to test new or existing ways to deliver and pay for healthcare services in Medicaid and CHIP. In 2017, CMS responded to the opioid addiction problem in the United States by allowing states to apply for funds for demonstration projects to improve access to treatment programs for opioid use disorder and other substance use disorders.[16] Medicaid also allows states to use waivers for HCBS to allow individuals with intellectual or developmental disabilities, physical disabilities, and/or mental illnesses to receive care in their home instead of an institution or nursing home.[17] In 2018, CMS under the **Community Engagement Initiative**, Medicaid established a waiver to allow states to use **work requirement waivers** among non-elderly,

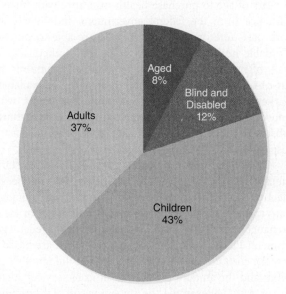

FIGURE 3.4 Average monthly Medicaid enrollment, 2019.

Data from *Medicaid: Congressional Budget Office's May 2019 Baseline.* https://www.cbo.gov/system/files/2019-05/51301-2019-05-medicaid.pdf

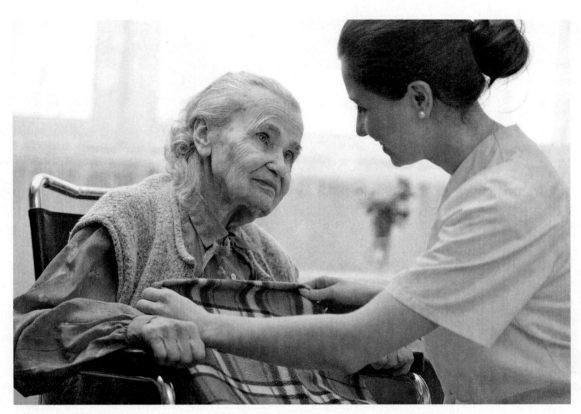

FIGURE 3.6 Medicaid covers the cost of nearly two-thirds of nursing home residents.
© Alexander Raths/Shutterstock.

nonpregnant adult Medicaid beneficiaries as a requirement for continued Medicaid eligibility. Medicaid beneficiaries were required to verify employment and other work-related activities such as job training and the job search to continue to receive Medicaid benefits.[18] Several states either applied or received work requirement waivers; however, in February 2021, President Biden directed CMS to withdraw all work requirement waivers because adding a work requirement for those enrolling in Medicaid would prevent low-income people from obtaining health coverage.[19]

CHIP was signed into law in 1997 to provide federal matching funds to states to provide healthcare coverage to children in families with incomes too high to qualify for Medicaid but unable to afford private insurance. All states have expanded children's coverage significantly through their CHIP programs, with nearly every state providing coverage for children up to at least 200% of the FPL. Federal and state governments jointly finance CHIP similar to the way Medicaid is funded. States may elect to provide coverage to qualifying children by expanding their Medicaid programs or through a state program separate from Medicaid. A number of states have also been granted waivers to cover parents of children enrolled in CHIP. As of January 2021, a total of 38 million children were enrolled in both Medicaid and CHIP with 6.7 million enrolled in CHIP.[20] In order to be eligible for CHIP, a child must be:

- Under 19 years of age,
- Uninsured (not eligible for Medicaid and not covered by private insurance),
- A citizen or meet immigration requirements,
- A resident of the state, and
- Eligible within the state's CHIP income range based on family income and any other state specified rules in the CHIP state plan[21]

Marketplace subsidies were implemented as part of the ACA as a way for low- and middle-income adults under 65 years of age to purchase health insurance with financial assistance from the federal government. Individuals who work part-time or are self-employed are able to purchase affordable health insurance through the Marketplace. The ACA offers subsidies to reduce monthly **premiums** and **out-of-pocket** costs. The two types of subsidies available to Marketplace enrollees are the **premium tax credit**, which reduces the cost of monthly premiums, and the **cost-sharing subsidy** to minimize out-of-pocket costs for doctor visits or hospital stays.[22]

One of the most important parts of the ACA started January 1, 2014, when health insurance coverage became effective for those purchasing insurance from nongroup plans through the Health Insurance Marketplace (or Health Exchange) established by individual states or the federal government. Plans in the Marketplace categories are based on how the costs are split between the cost of the monthly premium and the amount paid for healthcare services such as doctor visits. For example, the higher the cost of the premium for the health insurance policy, the lower the amount paid to healthcare providers at the time of service, and the lower the amount paid for premiums when buying the insurance, the higher the cost for health care at the time of service.[22]

The number of individuals who have health insurance through the Marketplace is lower than the number enrolled in Medicare, Medicaid, or CHIP, and federal expenditures for Marketplace subsidies are lower than for other public programs. An estimated 8 million adults obtained health insurance through the Marketplace in 2019, costing a total cost of $43 billion.[23] Eligibility requirements are citizenship or legal immigration status; ineligibility for coverage through an employer or through any federal government programs such as Medicaid, Medicare, Veterans Health Programs, or TRICARE; and an income between 100% and 400% of the FPL.[22]

HISTORY OF HEALTH INSURANCE IN THE UNITED STATES

Health insurance coverage has been a hotly debated topic in the United States since the early 1900s. From the beginning, the main issue has been whether health insurance should be publicly or privately financed. Government-sponsored healthcare efforts were initiated between 1915 and 1920 at the state level and in the 1930s at the federal level. However, the only outcome of these efforts was limited financial support for public health and healthcare services for mothers and children. Congress enacted legislation to improve access to medical care for those on public assistance in the 1950s and for the needy elderly in the 1960s.[1]

The most significant change in government healthcare financing was when Congress approved Medicare and Medicaid with the passage of Title XVIII and Title XIX, respectively, of the Social Security Act of 1965 signed into law by President Lyndon B. Johnson. Medicare funded health care for all elderly regardless of income, and Medicaid was established for those on public aid. In 1973, Medicare was expanded to include those with certain disabilities, chronic kidney disease, and ALS. Congress has expanded Medicaid for those living at or near the poverty level, including working and jobless families, individuals with diverse physical and mental conditions, and low-income seniors. Further expansion of health care for children—CHIP—came with the passage of Title XXI of the Social Security Act, a program initiated by the Balanced Budget Act of 1997.[1]

Private health insurance started with hospital coverage in the 1920s because of increased consumer demand and increased costs for hospital care. The first private hospital insurance plan was developed in 1929, when a group of Dallas teachers contracted with Baylor University Hospital to provide 21 days of hospitalization for a fixed $6.00 payment. The contract ensured that teachers had access to hospital care and that the hospital was paid. Community hospitals later joined together to develop prepaid hospital plans to avoid competition among hospitals. These plans eventually combined under the name Blue Cross and allowed subscribers a free choice of physician and hospital. Expanding medical

services became a reality after World War II when the federal government began subsidizing hospital construction and medical research.[24]

Physicians were concerned that Blue Cross hospital plans would underwrite physician services, interfere with the physician–patient relationship, and lower their incomes, so by the 1930s, physicians began to organize to develop prepaid plans that covered physician services to protect themselves from competition with Blue Cross.[24] In 1939 the California Physicians' Service began the first prepayment plan to cover physicians' services. Employees with incomes less than $3,000 annually were eligible for a fee of $1.70 per month. Later, the **American Medical Association (AMA)** encouraged state and local medical societies to form their own prepayment plans. In 1946, these physician-sponsored plans affiliated and became known as Blue Shield. These plans offered medical and surgical benefits for hospitalized members, and some plans covered outpatient doctors' visits. Doctors charged patients the difference between their actual charges and the amount for which they were reimbursed by Blue Shield. This allowed doctors to maintain control and to price discriminate by charging different prices to different patients.[24]

Other private insurance companies began offering health insurance after Blue Shield demonstrated that financial loss could be prevented by offering health insurance only to the young and healthy who were employed. The government aided the expansion of private insurance companies by excluding employers' contributions to health insurance from taxable income. During World War II, private health insurance coverage grew rapidly as an employee fringe benefit because the government limited direct wage increases. Demand for health insurance increased as medical technology advanced.[24]

The first managed care insurance programs were started with HMOs—Kaiser Permanente in California and Group Health Cooperative in Washington state. Kaiser Permanente started in California during the Depression of the 1930s and expanded to mostly the Western states of Washington, Oregon, Hawaii, and Colorado.[25] Group Health Cooperative began in Washington in 1947 and was purchased by Kaiser Permanente in 2017.[26] Kaiser evolved from healthcare programs to cover on-the-job injuries of workers (now known as workers' compensation) constructing the Los Angeles Aqueduct and the Grand Coulee Dam. The HMO started with one physician, Stanley Garfield, MD, in the small town of Desert Center, as an effort to receive payment for treating sick and injured workers during the building of the aqueduct. Later, Dr. Garfield established health care for workers of the Kaiser Shipyards in the San Francisco Bay area during World War II. Thereafter, the HMO expanded through efforts of unions, and the Kaiser HMO became available to the public on October 1, 1945.[25]

By the mid-1970s, the United States entered a new stage in the history of health insurance. Fee-for-service payment was no longer appropriate or sufficient for managing medical expenses. As one of the four most inflationary sectors of the economy (energy, food, and housing being the top three), medical care logically became a target of anti-inflationary measures. Attempts to slow the increasing costs of health care included industry-wide wage and price controls initiated in 1971, followed by Medicare policies to slow price increases by doctors and hospitals and to decrease the unnecessary use of hospital services. During the 1980s, there was another radical change in the way health care was financed. The term *managed care* came into common usage and remains a significant aspect of the sector's current evolution.[27]

In 1983, Congress passed a prospective payment bill, under which hospitals are paid a set amount for each patient in any of the established disease categories and **diagnosis-related groups (DRGs)**. This means that Medicare would not pay beyond the set fees for the identified type of illness, no matter how long the patient was hospitalized or what services he or she received. As a result, Medicare hospital admissions dropped, and the lengths of stay became shorter—but Medicare payments continued to rise. In 1985, Congress began to regulate direct Medicare payments to physicians by a resource-based relative-value scale for payment and established the Physician Payment Review Commission. In 1988, the commission replaced the "customary, prevailing, and reasonable" system with a fee schedule that was implemented in 1992 in an effort to control healthcare costs.[27]

A shift in the balance of power between unions and management is another dramatic change that has radically altered health care. The 1980s saw a weakening of union bargaining power and a high unemployment rate. These two factors enabled management to decrease employee benefits. Prior to this time, fringe benefits, especially in the areas of health care, had been escalating with the same intensity as healthcare costs. Employees had come to expect more free health benefits with each ensuing contract. Now employers were able to restrain costs by requiring the employee to pay higher **deductibles** and copayments. Many companies went to managed care health plans, which direct patients to the most cost-effective sources of care.[27]

The oversupply of physicians led to competition, the reorganization of medical practice, advertising for clients, and increased medical costs. The government directly intervened in medical education more than 30 years ago to ensure that there would be enough physicians to keep up with the demands of Medicare. This was accomplished with grants, scholarships, low-interest or no-interest loans, and other incentives, making access to a medical education easy for qualified individuals.[27]

Medical care has shifted from the hospital into the community because revolutionary advances in medical technology created a new dimension in healthcare delivery. Examples of recent advances are portable, mobile units for diagnosing almost every known disease without hospital admission; magnetic resonance imaging (MRI), mammography, ultrasound, telemedicine, and other technological advances are available in doctors' offices and outpatient clinics and can even be taken into homes. Freestanding surgical centers and outpatient surgery are thriving, facilitated especially by advances made in fiber optics and lasers. These factors have led to what is called distributive health care, which is changing the healthcare system as well as creating different ways of paying for health care.[28]

MANAGED CARE: HMOs, PPOs, AND EPOs

MCOs are divided primarily into HMOs, **preferred provider organizations (PPOs),** and **exclusive provider organizations (EPOs)**. The term *managed care* means a system in which employers and health insurers channel patients to the most cost-effective site of care. The umbrella label *health maintenance organization* was coined in the 1970s to describe independent plans that offer benefits to an enrolled group of subscribers. HMOs are a form of prepaid health insurance that only covers care provided by providers and healthcare facilities inside the HMO **network**. Patients must have a referral from a primary care provider to see a specialist. The consumer's cost is generally less than that in other facilities. Physicians and other providers agree to provide certain services for a specified cost, often with a cap on total patient visits or procedures during a benefit period. An HMO provides basic and supplemental health maintenance and treatment services to enrollees who pay a fixed fee. The range of health services delivered depends on the voluntary contractual agreement between the enrollee and the plan. The greatest drawback of the HMO lies in the fact that the enrollee must find a physician within the HMO group for services. This often creates problems for those who live in rural areas because HMO group physicians tend to practice in large, metropolitan medical centers. If enrollees go outside the HMO for health care, no benefits are available to them.

PPOs are another option open to the consumer for the delivery of health care. PPOs cover care provided both inside and outside the plan's provider network. However, consumers typically pay a higher percentage of the cost for out-of-network care. PPOs are made up of groups of physicians or a hospital that provides employers with comprehensive health services for their employees at a discount. The majority of Americans with **private health insurance** receive their care through a PPO. The benefits of a PPO are choice of provider and hospital and cost control. PPOs are either a group of providers who have voluntarily joined together to render health care on a contractual basis or a group of providers who have been organized by a payer through contractual arrangement for a particular delivery system. The providers can be hospitals, physicians, other healthcare services, or any combination of these. PPOs are fee-for-service systems, as opposed to HMOs, which are capitated (that is, insurance pays providers a set fee in advance to cover all required services that the insured person needs). Patients subscribing to a PPO have the freedom to go wherever they want, including outside the PPO system. From an economic standpoint, however, the incentive to use PPO contract providers is that they are less expensive. Under a PPO contract, standard fee-for-service charges are generally discounted. These discounts range from 10% to 20% for hospital services performed by a physician in a hospital environment. The essential elements of a PPO, then, are as follows: fee-for-service, contractual arrangements, organization of providers, discounts, free choice, and economic incentives. EPOs are similar to HMOs since services outside the network are not covered. The primary difference between an

HMO and EPOs is that an EPO usually doesn't require that the primary care provider make referrals to specialists.

The biggest impact on healthcare delivery by the managed care explosion is a substantial reduction in hospital use. As more and more people are covered by managed care plans, incentives to cut hospital use will continue to bring the number of hospital days down. As this trend continues, it is probable that marginal providers will leave the market and the remainder will compete based on convenience, price, and quality.

PRIVATE HEALTH INSURANCE COVERAGE IN THE UNITED STATES

Most Americans with private health insurance belong to a group plan financed through their employer; 60% of adults ages 18 to 64 in the United States had coverage through an employer or union in 2018.[29] The larger the firm—1,000 employees compared to nine employees—the more likely health insurance will be offered by the employer. Of those with employer-based health insurance, the majority are enrolled in a PPO (44%), HMO (19%), or **high-deductible health plan with a savings option (HDHP/SO)** (30%). Although the majority of workers are employed by firms that offer health benefits, many who are part-time or temporary workers either are not eligible or choose not to enroll because of the cost of the premiums; thus, only 61% who are offered health insurance through their employer actually enroll.[30]

In 2019, the annual premium for employer-based health insurance for family coverage was $20,576; for single-person coverage of the worker alone, the cost was $7,188. Workers and employers share in the cost of the premiums, with single workers contributing 18% of the cost ($1,293 per year) and workers with families contributing 30% of the cost ($6,172 per year). Workers share in other costs as well. Eighty-two percent of plans required an annual deductible before services were paid by the plan; the average annual yearly deductible for single coverage was $1,655. The average premium for family coverage increased 22% between 2014 and 2019 and 54% between 2009 and 2019, significantly more than either workers' wages or inflation. Most plans require copayments (a fixed dollar amount) or **coinsurance** (a percentage of the covered amount) for office visits, hospitalizations, outpatient surgery, and prescription drugs. However, some health insurance policies have an annual out-of-pocket maximum that ranges from $2,000 to $6,000 or more.[30]

HEALTHCARE EXPENDITURES

In 2019, total healthcare spending was $3.8 trillion, or $11,582 per person and representing 17.7% of the gross domestic product (GDP).[31] This compares with costs in 2010 with a total healthcare spending of $2.6 trillion, or $8,402 per person and 17.9% of the GDP.[32] In 2019, the cost of hospital care represented the largest amount of the total cost (31%), followed by the cost of physician and clinical services (20%), retail prescription drugs (10%) and nursing care facilities/continuing care communities (5%) (**FIGURE 3.7**).[33]

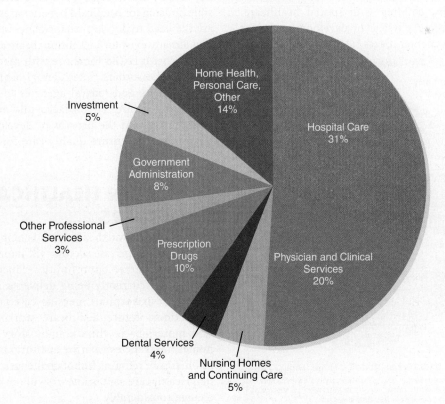

FIGURE 3.7 The nation's health dollar. Where did it go, 2019?

Date from Centers for Medicare & Medicaid Services, Office of the Actuary, National Health Statistics Group. *The Nation's Health Dollar (3.8 Trillion), Calendar Year 2019, Where It Went.* https://www.cms.gov/files/document/nations-health-dollar-where-it-came-where-it-went.pdf

Nearly 73% of the funds came from public and private health insurance; with 31% from private or employer-based health insurance and 41% from government-sponsored insurance. The percentages for government-sponsored insurance were Medicare 21% and Medicaid 16%; while CHIP, the Department of Defense, and the Veterans Administration accounted for, 4%. A significant 11% of the money came from out-of-pocket expenses paid by individuals to cover the cost of **deductibles, copayments**, prescription drugs, and services not covered by Medicare such as vision care, dental care, and hearing aids. The remaining 17% came from other third-party payers, public health activities, and investments (**FIGURE 3.8**).[33]

Total spending for Medicare in 2019 was $799 billion, which accounted for 21% of total national health spending.[31] The average annual growth in Medicare spending was only 1.7% between 2010 and 2018, down from 7.3% between 2000 and 2010. The slower growth is attributed to the ACA, which reduced payments to providers and plans, as well as an influx of relatively younger and healthier Baby Boomer enrollees in Medicare.[35]

Medicaid financed nearly a fifth of all personal healthcare spending and provided significant financial support for hospitals, community health centers, and nursing homes. In 2019, total Medicaid expenditures were $613 billion.[31] In 2018, about one-third of Medicaid expenditures were for **long-term services and supports (LTSS)** for the disabled and those over 65 years of age. About half received LTSS in nursing homes; the other half received care through HCBS.[36] Medicaid paid for nearly 50% of these services: births, children with special healthcare needs, adults with either physical or developmental disabilities, and serious mental illness.[8] Also, Medicaid paid

Medicare premiums (for Plan B, outpatient services) for 20% of those on Medicare.[8]

LTSS help seniors and people with disabilities with self-care, such as bathing and dressing, and household activities, such as preparing meals and managing medication. LTSS needs arise from a range of conditions, such as cognitive disabilities, like dementia or Down syndrome; physical disabilities, like multiple sclerosis or spinal cord injury; mental health disabilities, like depression or schizophrenia; and disabling chronic conditions, like cancer or HIV/AIDS.[36] CMS has been working with individual states, consumers, and providers to develop LTSS in the community instead of in institutions for people with disabilities and chronic conditions. Goals are to offer consumers greater choice and control with access to quality services, resulting in optimal outcomes including health, quality of life, and independence.[37]

One of the significant changes over the past decade is that all states have expanded HCBS and have been able to reduce the number residing in institutions as well as the cost for providing LTSS. Other evidence that HCBS is less costly than institutionalization is that in 2008, yearly costs in California for HCBS for an individual was $9,129 compared to $32,406 for institutional care.[37] One of the challenges of providing HCBS is that the cost of room and board is not reimbursed by Medicaid for people with intellectual or developmental disabilities in home-based settings, whereas room and board costs are reimbursed for residents living in institutions. A barrier for expanding HCBS, therefore, is providing affordable and accessible housing for Medicaid beneficiaries. Other challenges are the need to develop performance standards for HCBS that already exist for institutional care and to link housing services with HCBS for those with mental illness or substance use disorders.[37] Residential facilities are regulated by both state and federal agencies for compliance with standards of care. HCBS lacks this oversight, although CMS has started the process of developing policies and mechanisms to ensure quality care for those who live in the community.[37]

EFFECT ON HEALTHCARE PROVIDERS

Changes in the way health care is being paid for in both the public and private sectors will impact healthcare personnel and career opportunities. Since more healthcare services are currently being delivered in the community instead of in hospitals, nursing care facilities, and other institutions, future healthcare workers can expect to find more jobs in clinics, ambulatory care centers, and homecare agencies than in institutions. The health field of the future remains full of challenges for health personnel. Health care as it is known will not disappear but may change considerably.

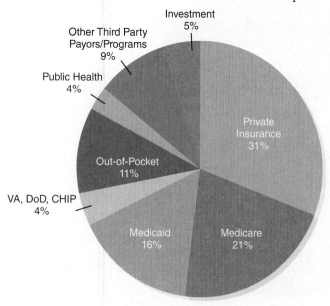

FIGURE 3.8 Where the nation's health dollar came from, 2019.

Data from Centers for Medicare & Medicaid Services, Office of the Actuary, National Health Statistics Group. *The Nation's Health Dollar ($3.8 Trillion), Calendar Year 2019: Where It Came From.* https://www.cms.gov/files/document/nations-health-dollar-where-it-came-where-it-went.pdf

SUMMARY

Health care in the United States is funded through a combination of private and government funds. Private spending is primarily through private health insurance jointly funded by premiums paid by both the employee and the employer while government-sponsored health insurance is funded by federal, state, and local governments. The sources of government-funded health care are Medicaid, Medicare, the Children's Health Insurance Program (CHIP), and the Health Insurance Marketplace. Individuals share in the cost of government funded health care through premiums or copayments. Medicaid was designed for low-income children and pregnant women, however, after the Affordable Care Act (ACA), adults with incomes at 133% of the federal poverty level were eligible for Medicaid. CHIP provides healthcare coverage to children in families with incomes too high to qualify for Medicaid but too low to afford the cost of the premiums for private insurance. Medicare was designed for those over 65 years of age but has been expanded to provide coverage for the disabled under 65 years of age. Medicaid and CHIP are jointly funded by federal and state governments and administered by individual states, while Medicare is funded and administered by the federal government. As a result of the ACA, individuals without access to private insurance through an employer can purchase health insurance through an exchange and receive government subsidies to share in the cost of the premiums. Managed care organizations are used to manage healthcare utilization, cost, and quality through contracts in both the private and government-funded sectors.

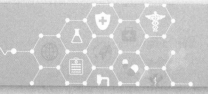

LEARNING PORTFOLIO

Study Points

1. Congress approved legislation for the public health programs Medicare and Medicaid in 1965. Medicare is a federal health program for those 65 years and older and for the disabled under 65 years of age. Medicaid was designed primarily for low-income children and pregnant women but was expanded to include low-income adults with introduction of the Affordable Care Act in 2010.

2. The Centers for Medicare and Medicaid (CMS) administers public health programs—Medicare, Medicaid, the Children's Health Insurance Program (CHIP), and the Marketplace.

3. Medicaid and CHIP are jointly funded by the federal government and individual state governments for those not eligible for insurance through an employer and for those who cannot afford to purchase health insurance through the Marketplace.

4. Adults who are not eligible for employer-based health insurance, Medicare, or Medicaid can purchase affordable health insurance through the Marketplace.

5. Medicaid funds health care for one in five Americans and is the largest public health insurance program in the United States. Medicaid covers the cost of health care for the lowest-income and the most medically complex individuals. Medicaid pays for nearly 50% of these services: births, children with special health care needs, adults with either physical or developmental disabilities, and serious mental illness.

6. Individuals enrolled in both Medicare and Medicaid are designated as dual-eligibles; Medicaid covers one in five low-income Medicare patients.

7. In 2019, expenditures for Medicare, Medicaid, CHIP, and Marketplace subsidies represented 25%, or about one-fourth, of the total federal budget.

8. The traditional method of paying providers for health services is fee-for-service or payment for the volume of services—for example, number of procedures, surgeries, or lab tests. Capitation is a defined payment for a designated set of healthcare services to control costs while providing high-quality health care.

9. Managed care organizations (MCOs) are health insurance programs that control healthcare costs by agreeing to provide health services in exchange for a set dollar amount received from Medicare or Medicaid for each enrollee; MCOs use capitation to control healthcare costs.

10. Private health insurance started in the 1920s to cover the cost of hospital care. Prepaid private health insurance for physician services started in the 1930s with the development of Blue Cross and Blue Shield.

11. The federal government has supported medical education with grants, scholarships, and low-interest loans for students to ensure an adequate supply of trained physicians.

12. MCOs in the private health insurance industry include health maintenance organizations (HMOs), preferred provider organizations (PPOs), and exclusive provider organizations (EPOs).

13. HMOs are a capitation system that only covers the cost of health services to providers and facilities within a network and requires specialty referrals from a primary care provider. PPOs use fee-for-service to pay for health services, but payment is less for providers and facilities out of the network. EPOs are similar to HMOs except that specialty referrals from a primary care provider are not required.

14. All MCOs contract with providers (hospitals, physicians, laboratories, and other services) and agree to provide all healthcare services for a set price for each enrollee in exchange for premiums paid by individuals and/or the employer. Medicare and Medicaid primarily use MCOs to contract for healthcare services for enrollees.

15. In 2018, only 61% of employees eligible for employer-sponsored health insurance actually enrolled because of the cost of the premiums to the employee. The majority of employees are enrolled in PPOs (44%) or high-deductible health plans with a savings option (30%).

16. For those who obtain health insurance through their employer, the employee's share of the cost of yearly premiums was $1,293 for an individual and $6,172 for families in 2019. The cost of premiums increased by 54% over the 10 year period from 2009 to 2019.

17. About one-fourth of Medicare payments in 2019 were for hospital services and one-fifth for physician and clinical services.

18. Medicaid is the largest source of funding for long-term services and supports (LTSS) in nursing homes and home- and community-based care (HCBC). In 2018, 34% of Medicaid expenditures were for LTSS for those over 65 years of age.

19. Individual states use Medicaid waivers to test new or existing ways to deliver and pay for healthcare services in Medicaid and CHIP. In 2018, work requirement waivers were used to require non-elderly, nonpregnant adult Medicaid beneficiaries to verify employment as a requirement for continued Medicaid eligibility.

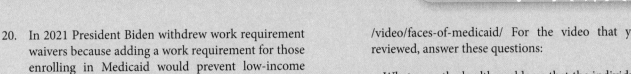

LEARNING PORTFOLIO

20. In 2021 President Biden withdrew work requirement waivers because adding a work requirement for those enrolling in Medicaid would prevent low-income people from obtaining health coverage.

Issues for Discussion

1. View the video "Health Insurance Explained," from Kaiser Family Foundation which explains health insurance. After viewing the video, define these terms: *premium, deductible, copay, out-of-pocket,* and *provider network.* https://www.kff.org/health-reform /video/health-insurance-explained-youtoons/

2. Take the self-study "Health Insurance Quiz" from the Kaiser Family Foundation. After taking the quiz, explain these terms: *annual health insurance deductible, out-of-pocket limit, health insurance formulary,* and *provider network.* http://kff.org/quiz/health-insurance-quiz/

3. Describe your source of health insurance: private health insurance or employer-sponsored insurance, Medicare, Medicaid, or Marketplace. Review the policy to determine if the policy is a preferred provider organization (PPO), health maintenance organization (HMO), or high-deductible health plan with a savings option (HDHP/SO). If you are responsible for paying the premiums for the insurance, share the monthly cost of the premium. What factors determine the cost of the premiums?

4. View one of the 10 videos of personal stories of those receiving Medicaid benefits from Kaiser Family Foundation. *Faces of Medicaid.* http://kff.org/medicaid /video/faces-of-medicaid/ For the video that you reviewed, answer these questions:

- What were the health problems that the individual or family experienced that required treatment?
- Did the individual or family have other health insurance?
- What services did Medicaid provide?

Enrichment Activities

1. Go to the website InsureKidsNow.gov and search for a dentist who would be close enough for your child to obtain care by either driving or taking public transportation. How many dentists are available? InsureKidsNow. gov. *Find Coverage for Your Family.* https://www.insu rekidsnow.gov/coverage/index.html

2. View the 17-minute video "Medicine and Medicaid at 50" from the Kaiser Family Foundation, https://www.kff .org/medicare/video/medicare-and-medicaid-at-50/ As you view the video, answer these questions:

- Which U.S. president was the first to propose Medicare?
- Which president signed the Medicare and Medicaid legislation, and in which year?
- In what year did Medicaid begin coverage of the permanently disabled?
- In what year was Part D for Medicare added, and which president signed the bill into law?

CASE STUDY: PAYING FOR HEALTH SERVICES

Mary Ann is a 67-year-old woman who recently retired from her job as a college professor at a small community college. She is a widow; her husband of 50 years passed away less than one year ago. Fortunately, she has enough money in her retirement fund to live comfortably for the rest of her life. She is doing some research to find healthcare plans for which she may be eligible. She does have a medical history that includes some significant health problems.

Based on the information you have read about paying for health services, answer the following questions.

1. Is Mary Ann eligible for Medicaid?
2. Does Mary Ann meet the age requirements for eligibility for Medicare?

3. Based on her health history, which of the following conditions/diseases would allow her eligibility for Medicare?
   A. End-stage renal disease
   B. Lou Gehrig's disease (ALS)
   C. Both A and B
   D. None of these are correct.
4. Mary Ann is very concerned about being able to afford expensive prescription drugs in her retirement. Will Medicare help pay for these expensive prescription drugs?
5. Mary Ann is concerned about the quality of care and the benefits she will be eligible for compared to those she had with her private insurance plan. How does Medicare compare to private insurance plans?

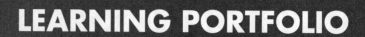

LEARNING PORTFOLIO

References

1. Klees BS, Wolfe CJ, Curtis CA. *Medicare & Medicaid. Title XVIII and Title XIX of the Social Security Act.* Baltimore, MD: Office of the Actuary Centers for Medicare and Medicaid Services, DHHS; 2009.

2. Center on Budget and Policy Priorities. *Where Do Our Federal Tax Dollars Go?* April 9, 2020. https://www.cbpp.org/sites/default/files/atoms/files/4-14-08tax.pdf Accessed August 31, 2021.

3. Center on Budget and Policy Priorities. *Where Do Federal Tax Revenues Come From?* August 2020. https://www.cbpp.org/sites/default/files/atoms/files/PolicyBasics_WhereDoFederalTaxRevsComeFrom_08-20-12.pdf Accessed August 20, 2021.

4. Centers for Medicare and Medicaid Services. Fact Sheet: *Better Care. Smarter Spending. Healthier People: Paying Providers for Value, Not Volume.* January 26, 2015. https://www.cms.gov/newsroom/fact-sheets/better-care-smarter-spending-healthier-people-paying-providers-value-not-volume Accessed July 2, 2020.

5. Centers for Medicare and Medicaid Services. *Readmissions Reduction Program.* http://cms.gov/Medicare/Medicare-Fee-for-Service-Payment/AcuteInpatientPPS/Readmissions-Reduction-Program.html/ Accessed January 25, 2021.

6. Cubanski J, Swoope C, Boccuti C, et al. A *Primer on Medicare: Key Facts about the Medicare Program and the People It Covers.* Kaiser Family Foundation. March 20, 2015. http://kff.org/medicare/report/a-primer-on-medicare-key-facts-about-the-medicare-program-and-the-people-it-covers/ Accessed July 2, 2020.

7. Data.CMS.gov. *Total Medicare Enrolled 2019.* https://data.cms.gov/beta/search?keywords=Total%20Medicare%20enrolled%202019&sort=Relevancy Accessed July 23, 2021.

8. Rudowitz R, Garfield R, Hinton E. *10 Things to Know about Medicaid: Setting the Facts Straight,* March 2019. Kaiser Family Foundation. https://www.kff.org/medicaid/issue-brief/10-things-to-know-about-medicaid-setting-the-facts-straight Accessed July 2, 2020.

9. Medicaid.Gov. *Eligibility.* https://www.medicaid.gov/medicaid/eligibility/index.html Accessed July 12, 2021.

10. Manatt, Phelps & Phillips, LLP. *Medicaid: The Basics.* February 2019. Robert Wood Johnson Foundation. https://www.rwjf.org/en/library/research/2019/02/medicaid-the-basics.html Accessed July 2, 2020.

11. *Status of State Medicaid Expansion Decisions: Interactive Map.* Kaiser Family Foundation. https://www.kff.org/medicaid/issue-brief/status-of-state-medicaid-expansion-decisions-interactive-map/ Accessed July 23, 2021.

12. Medicaid.Gov. *Mandatory & Optional Medicaid Benefits.* https://www.medicaid.gov/medicaid/benefits/mandatory-optional-medicaid-benefits/index.html Accessed July 2, 2020.

13. Congressional Budget Office. *Medicaid- Congressional Budget Office's May 2019 Baseline.* https://www.cbo.gov/system/files/2019-05/51301-2019-05-medicaid.pdf Accessed July 2, 2020.

14. Medicaid.gov. *Early and Periodic Screening, Diagnostic and Treatment (EPSDT),* July 2014. https://www.medicaid.gov/sites/default/files/2019-12/epsdt_coverage_guide.pdf Accessed July 2, 2020.

15. Centers for Medicare and Medicaid Services. *Seniors & Medicare and Medicaid Enrollees.* https://www.medicaid.gov/medicaid/eligibility/seniors-medicare-and-medicaid-enrollees/index.html Accessed July 2, 2020.

16. Medicaid.gov. *Section 1115 Demonstrations: Substance Use Disorders, Serious Mental Illness, and Serious Emotional Disturbance.* https://www.medicaid.gov/medicaid/section-1115-demonstrations/1115-substance-use-disorder-demonstrations/section-1115-demonstrations-substance-use-disorders-serious-mental-illness-and-serious-emotional-disturbance/index.html Accessed July 2, 2020.

17. Medicaid.gov. *Home & Community Based Services.* https://www.medicaid.gov/medicaid/home-community-based-services/index.html Accessed July 2, 2020.

18. Centers for Medicare and Medicaid Services. *CMS Announces New Policy Guidance for States to Test Community Engagement for Able-Bodied Adults* https://www.cms.gov/newsroom/press-releases/cms-announces-new-policy-guidance-states-test-community-engagement-able-bodied-adults Accessed August 19, 2021.

19. Kaiser Family Foundation. *Medicaid Waiver Tracker: Approved and Pending. Section 1115 Waivers by State.* June 28, 2021. https://www.kff.org/medicaid/issue-brief/medicaid-waiver-tracker-approved-and-pending-section-1115-waivers-by-state/ Accessed July 12, 2021.

20. Medicaid.gov. *December 2020 and January 2021 Medicaid and CHIP Enrollment Trends Snapshot.* https://www.medicaid.gov/medicaid/national-medicaid-chip-program-information/downloads/december-2020-january-2021-medicaid-chip-enrollment-trend-snapshot.pdf Accessed July 12, 2021.

21. Medicaid.gov. *Eligibility.* https://www.medicaid.gov/chip/eligibility/index.html

22. *Explaining Health Care Reform: Questions about Health Insurance Subsidies.* January 2020. Kaiser Family Foundation. https://www.kff.org/health-reform/issue-brief/explaining-health-care-reform-questions-about-health/ Accessed July 2, 2020.

23. Congressional Budget Office. *Federal Subsidies for Health Insurance Coverage for People under Age 65: Tables from CBO's May 2019 Projections,* May 2019. https://www.cbo.gov/system/files/2019-05/51298-2019-05-healthinsurance.pdf Accessed July 2, 2020.

24. Thomasson M. *Health Insurance in the United States.* Economic History Association. 2010. https://eh.net/encyclopedia/health-insurance-in-the-united-states/ Accessed August 19, 2021.

LEARNING PORTFOLIO

25. Kaiser Permanente. *A History of Leading the Way.* https://about.kaiserpermanente.org/our-story/our-history/a-history-of-leading-the-way Accessed August 23, 2021.

26. Kaiser Permanente. *Acquisition of Group Health Cooperative in Washington State Complete.* February 1, 2017. https://about.kaiserpermanente.org/our-story/news/announcements/kaiser-permanente-a-national-leader-in-integrated-health-care-an Accessed August 19, 2021.

27. Oliver TR. Analysis, Advice and Congressional Leadership: The Physician Payment Review Commission and the Politics of Medicare. *Journal of Health Politics, Policy and Law.* 1993; 18:113–174.

28. National Center for Health Statistics/Centers for Disease Control and Prevention. *Health, United States, 2009: With Special Feature on Technology.* Hyattsville, MD: NCHS; 2010.

29. Hamel L, Muñana C, Brody M. *Kaiser Family Foundation/LA Times Survey of Adults with Employer-Sponsored Health Insurance.* May 2019. Kaiser Family Foundation. https://www.kff.org/private-insurance/report/kaiser-family-foundation-la-times-survey-of-adults-with-employer-sponsored-insurance/ Accessed July 2, 2020.

30. *Employer Health Benefits. 2019 Summary of Benefits.* Kaiser Family Foundation. http://files.kff.org/attachment/Summary-of-Findings-Employer-Health-Benefits-2019 Accessed July 2, 2020.

31. Centers for Medicare and Medicaid. *National Health Expenditures 2019 Highlights.* National Health Expenditure Data. https://www.cms.gov/files/document/highlights.pdf Accessed July 14, 2020.

32. The Henry J. Kaiser Family Foundation. *Health Care Costs: A Primer. Key Information on Health Care Costs and Their Impact.* Publication no. 7670-03. May 2012. http://kff.org/health-costs/issue-brief/health-care-costs-a-primer/ Accessed July 2, 2020.

33. Centers for Medicare & Medicaid Services, Office of the Actuary, National Health Statistics Group. *The Nation's Health Dollar ($3.8 Trillion), Calendar Year 2019: Where It Went.* https://www.cms.gov/files/document/nations-health-dollar-where-it-came-where-it-went.pdf Accessed July 14, 2021.

34. Centers for Medicare & Medicaid Services, Office of the Actuary, National Health Statistics Group. *The Nation's Health Dollar ($3.8 Trillion), Calendar Year 2019: Where It Came From.* https://www.cms.gov/files/document/nations-health-dollar-where-it-came-where-it-went.pdf Accessed July 14, 2021.

35. Cubanski J, Neuman T, Freed M. The Facts on Medicare Spending and Financing. *Issue Brief.* August 2019. https://www.kff.org/medicare/issue-brief/the-facts-on-medicare-spending-and-financing/ Accessed July 2, 2020.

36. O'Malley Watts M, Musumeci MB, Chidambaram P. Medicaid Home and Community-Based Services Enrollment and Spending. *Issue Brief,* February 2020. Kaiser Family Foundation. https://files.kff.org/attachment/Issue-Brief-Medicaid-Home-and-Community-Based-Services-Enrollment-and-Spending Accessed August 19, 2021.

37. Ryan J, Edwards B. Health Policy Brief: Rebalancing Medicaid Long-Term Services and Supports. *Health Affairs.* September 17, 2015. https://www.healthaffairs.org/do/10.1377/hpb20150917.439553/full/ Accessed July 23, 2021.

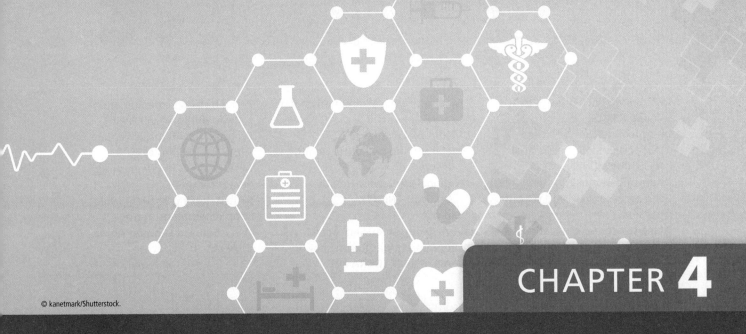

CHAPTER **4**

Aging, Health, and Long-Term Care

OBJECTIVES

After studying this chapter, the student should be able to:

- Describe projected changes in demographics in the United States—age, ethnicity, and race—through 2050.
- Discuss how aging and disease impact the ability to complete instrumental activities of daily living (IADLs) and basic activities of daily living (ADLs).
- Compare options for long-term care for the physically and intellectually disabled and older adults.
- Summarize Medicaid benefits for low-income older people.
- Explain how shifts in demographics will impact the skills and training needs of healthcare workers.
- Define the role of health literacy in delivering quality health care.

KEY TERMS

Activities of daily living (ADLs)	Caregiving	Demographic
Adult day care services	Centers for Medicare and	Frail elderly
Aging Network	Medicaid Services (CMS)	Geriatricians
Alzheimer's disease	Chronic diseases	Health literacy
Area Agencies on Aging (AAAs)	Continuing care community	Healthy People 2020
Assisted living facilities	Dementia	Home health agencies (HHAs)

Instrumental activities of daily living (IADLs)

Intermediate care facilities for people with intellectual disability (ICF/ID)

Interprofessional Education (IPE)

Long-term services and support (LTSS)

Managed care organization (MCO)

Medicaid spousal impoverishment provisions

Medicare Advantage

Medicare Supplemental Health Insurance

National Center for Health Statistics (NCHS)

Old-old

1973 Older Americans Act (OAA)

Omnibus Budget Reconciliation Act of 1987 (OBRA 87)

Preadmission Screening and Resident Review (PASRR)

Program for All-Inclusive Care for the Elderly (PACE)

Residential Care Communities

Senior centers

Skilled nursing facility (SNF)

Supplemental insurance

U.S. Administration on Aging (AOA)

THE IMPACT OF FUTURE DEMOGRAPHIC CHANGES ON HEALTHCARE NEEDS

In Chapter 1, we summarized trends that will impact healthcare services and health careers. This chapter briefly explores the role of **demographic** changes in determining the nation's future healthcare needs. The size of the older population is projected to grow by almost 50% from 2016 to 2030 will likely change demands for health care, social services, and caregiving in the United States.[1] Growth in the number of people over 65 is expected to increase dramatically as a result of the aging of "Baby Boomers" (those born between 1946 and 1964) that began in 2011 with growth projected through 2030.[2] As the older segment of the population increases, more services will be required for the treatment and management of chronic and acute health conditions and disabilities. In addition, Medicare beneficiaries with multiple chronic conditions, especially the **frail elderly** with functional or cognitive impairments in addition to chronic disease, will need care coordination.[3]

In 2016, 49 million people living in the United States were age 65 and older; more than half (58%) were ages 65 to 74, 29% were ages 75 to 84, and 13% were age 85 and older.[4] By 2034, those 65 years of age and older are projected to outnumber children under the age of 18, and by 2060, nearly one in four Americans will be at least 65 years old. The overall aging of the population is the result of increasing life expectancy and decreasing fertility; this trend follows that of other developed countries.[5] The **old-old** (those over age 85) have been the fastest-growing segment of the population and are projected to grow rapidly after 2030 as the Baby Boomers move into this age group. In contrast, the percentage of those 65 years and older is projected to grow at a much slower rate after 2030.[2] Also, those over 65 years of age are projected to become more racially and ethnically diverse, with about 53% being non-White in 2050 compared to 21% non-White in 2014.[2]

COMMON HEALTH PROBLEMS IN AN AGING POPULATION

Chronic diseases are defined as conditions that last 1 year or more and require ongoing medical attention, limit activities of daily living, or both.[6] Chronic diseases arising from both emotional and physical causes will be the most important of the future disabilities. Conditions range from relatively minor to very severe. The minor problems require little care from others, but the severe ones require increasing amounts of care and professional help. Chronic conditions tend to be cumulative, so older adults, especially the old-old, often experience multiple problems and require a substantial number of services.

Americans continue to live longer because of more effective diagnosis and treatment for heart disease and cancer, the two leading causes of death in those 65 years and older. As a consequence, the numbers of older Americans above both 65 and 85 years of age continue to increase. Common chronic diseases in older adults are arthritis, stroke, diabetes, chronic lower respiratory diseases, and dementia, including Alzheimer's disease. In addition, those with chronic diseases may have preexisting health problems such as alcoholism or substance abuse, mental illness, or developmental disabilities.

Also, with aging there is a loss of functional ability including limitations in vision, hearing, mobility, communication, cognition, and self-care. All affect the well-being of the older population and the ability to live independently. Early in the aging process there is a loss of the ability to perform activities that require more complex thinking and organizational skills: **instrumental activities of daily living (IADLs)**. Examples are managing money, shopping, preparing meals, and taking prescribed medications. **Activities of daily living (ADLs)** is a term used to describe basic skills required to independently care for oneself, such as eating, bathing, dressing, maintaining personal hygiene, and mobility. With further mental and physical decline, there is a loss of ability to carry out basic tasks or ADLs such as bathing, toileting, getting dressed, and self-feeding.[7] A combination of chronic disease and a loss of ability to complete IADLs and ADLs in older adults often leads to the need for long-term care services or support from either family members or professional caregivers.[7] Refer to **TABLE 4.1.**

In a 2016 survey of those living independently, about 69% of those age 85 and older had at least one type of disability, compared with just 9% of the population under the age of 65. The most common disability was mobility impairment, the ability to walk or climb stairs, at 25% for those 75 to 84 years of age and nearly 50% for those age 85 and older. Often mobility impairment limits the ability to complete ADLs without assistance from others and limits the ability to drive or use public transportation. Lack of mobility limits contact with family and friends and can lead to social isolation and depression.[7] For those ages 65 to 74, difficulty hearing was the second most common disability (9%), followed by difficulties with IADLs (8%). It was the opposite for those 85 and older, with 43% having difficulty with IADLs, the second most common, and difficulty hearing, the third most common (35%).[2] Although normal vision and hearing are not listed as either ADLs or IADLs, being visually impaired limits the ability to complete many IADLs, and loss of hearing can impair the ability to safely use public transportation and result in social isolation and depression.

The most debilitating conditions accompanied by functional impairments among older adults are stroke and dementia, with the most common cause of dementia being **Alzheimer's disease**. Stroke ranks fifth and Alzheimer's disease ranks sixth among all causes for death after diseases of the heart, cancer, chronic lower respiratory disease, and accidents. Stroke is more common in women, Asians and Pacific Islanders, African Americans, and Hispanics and in those over 85 years of age.[8] Stroke is also a leading cause of long-term disability, since a stroke can cause either left- or right-sided paralysis that impairs mobility and the ability to swallow and speak. Functional ability may improve with rehabilitation; however, permanent disability can cause a loss of independence and require long-term institutional care.

Dementia is a decline in cognitive function that affects memory, language, and problem-solving skills. Moderate decline impairs the ability to complete IADLs without assistance—for example, paying bills or managing medications. In contrast, someone with mild dementia would be able to carry out IADLs, but with great effort. Dementia is characteristic of Parkinson's disease, cardiovascular disease of the brain, and Alzheimer's disease, with 60% to 80% of those with Alzheimer's disease showing symptoms of dementia. The early symptoms of Alzheimer's disease are difficulty remembering names or events. Later symptoms are disorientation and confusion as well as personality and behavior changes (e.g., suspicion and agitation). In the later stages, symptoms are an inability to complete ADLs and eventually difficulty in speaking, swallowing, and mobility, requiring total bed care 24 hours a day.[9] Alzheimer's dementia is one of the most devastating diseases in older adults because there are no known treatments to prevent or slow progression of the disease. According to the Alzheimer's Association, one in 10 people age 65 and older and one in three of those age 85 and older have the disease, and at the time of death, one in three Americans will have dementia. Women, African Americans, and Hispanics are more likely to develop the disease. Those diagnosed with the disease at age 65 can expect to live an additional 4 to 8 years, though some live 20 years after the initial diagnosis, and most will require nursing home care. Among adults age 80 years and older, living in nursing homes, 75% will have Alzheimer's disease. However, many with the disease live in their home, and family members, friends, or others assume the responsibility as unpaid caregivers. **Caregiving** refers to attending to another person's health needs and well-being and often includes assistance with one or more ADLs such as bathing and dressing as well as multiple IADLs such as paying bills, shopping, and providing transportation.[9]

MEDICARE FOR OLDER ADULTS

The **Centers for Medicare and Medicaid Services (CMS)** administers the Medicare program. Medicare-covered benefits apply mostly to the treatment of patients with acute illnesses who require hospitalization, short-term skilled nursing care in rehabilitation centers or nursing homes, or home health care. Medicare is divided into four parts. All have deductibles and copayments.[10] Review **TABLE 4.2** for more detailed information about benefits and premium requirements.

Part A is hospital insurance, and all elderly beneficiaries are automatically enrolled. Part B is supplemental medical insurance and is voluntary, although over 90% of older adults purchase Part B. Most older adults also purchase a **Medicare Supplemental Health Insurance** (often called Medigap insurance) from a private company to cover deductibles and copayments for Parts A and B. Part C is supplemental hospital and medical insurance, and Part D is medication insurance, and both are optional.

Under Part A, Medicare pays for hospital expenses minus a deductible for the first 60 days of each benefit period.

TABLE 4.1 Basic and Complex Activities of Daily Living	
Basic Activities of Daily Living (ADLs)	**Complex (Instrumental) Activities of Daily Living (IADLs)**
Bathing	Doing laundry
Continence	Housekeeping
Dressing	Managing finances
Eating	Preparing meals
Toileting	Shopping
Mobility	Using the telephone
	Using transportation

Data from Centers for Disease Control and Prevention. *The State of Aging and Health in America 2013.* Atlanta, GA: Centers for Disease Control and Prevention; 2013. https://www.cdc.gov/aging/pdf/state-aging-health-in-america-2013.pdf

TABLE 4.2 Medicare Programs for Those 65 Years of Age and Older or Under 65 and Disabled

Part A Hospital Insurance	Citizens and permanent residents are automatically eligible. Annual deductible. Covered benefits: • Inpatient hospital care • Skilled nursing facility care • Hospice care • Home health care
Part B Medical Insurance	Citizens and permanent residents are automatically eligible. Requires payment of monthly premium. Covered benefits at 80%: • Services from doctors and other healthcare providers • Outpatient care • Home health care • Durable medical equipment • Some preventive services Most beneficiaries purchase supplementary private insurance to cover the cost of copayments.
Part C Medicare Advantage	Optional. Requires payment of monthly premium (for Medicare Part B). Medicare-approved private insurance managed care plan. Replaces benefits and services under Parts A, B, and usually D. Requires using doctors who are in the network. May need a referral to see a physician specialist. May include additional services such as dental, hearing, or vision care.
Part D Prescription Drug Coverage	Optional. Requires payment of monthly premium (except for some Medicare Advantage plans). Covers the cost of prescription drugs.

Data from Centers for Medicare & Medicaid Services. *Medicare & You 2020*. CMS Product no. 10050-23. September 2019. https://www.medicare.gov/Pubs/pdf/10050-Medicare-and-You.

Part B pays 80% of the cost of the outpatient services of doctors, physical, occupational and speech therapy, diagnostic and laboratory tests, and durable medical equipment such as wheelchairs or oxygen tanks as well as preventive screening for diabetes, cardiovascular disease, and cancer. Many older adults purchase Part C, also called **Medicare Advantage**, and Part D, Prescription Medications, from private insurance companies. Medicare Advantage Plans provide all of Part A (hospital insurance) and Part B (medical insurance) coverage and may offer extra coverage such as vision, hearing, dental, and/or health and wellness programs. Most also include Part D, the Medicare prescription drug coverage. Medicare pays a fixed amount to the private insurance company offering Medicare Advantage Plans to cover the cost of Medicare Part B premiums and additional services.

The structure of Medicare Advantage Plans follows that of a **managed care organization (MCO)** designed to manage costs and often requires preapproval for surgery and other procedures. In addition, care must be provided by healthcare workers and facilities that are in the MCO network to prevent additional costs.[10] (Refer to Chapter 3.)

MEDICAID FOR OLDER ADULTS

Other than both being administered by the Centers for Medicare and Medicaid (CMS), Medicaid and Medicare structures have little in common. Medicaid covers a broad range of services not covered by Medicare, acting as a **supplemental insurance** for older adults and the disabled. It also pays their Medicare premiums, includes cost-sharing requirements, and covers prescription drugs. However, a large number of older adults do not take advantage of Medicaid coverage because of the inability to navigate the publicly run system.

The Medicaid program is the primary payer and the only safety-net program for **long-term services and supports (LTSS)** for many low- and middle-income families. Long-term care in a nursing home in the United States can cost $7,500 to $8,500 per month or $90,000 to $102,000 per year.[11] Under the **Medicaid Spousal Impoverishment provisions**, a certain amount of the couple's combined resources is protected for the spouse living in the community since the cost of long-term care can rapidly deplete the lifetime savings of elderly couples. These provisions help ensure that this situation will not occur and that spouses of individuals in nursing homes are able to live out their lives with independence and dignity.[12]

Even though Medicaid pays for the largest share of long-term services, beneficiaries must meet certain requirements, including having income and assets that do not exceed levels defined by the state of residence. Most states use a specific number of basic care (ADLs) and other service needs to qualify for nursing home or community-based services. Costs for long-term care vary depending on the services provided and the geographic location.[11]

LONG-TERM SERVICES AND SUPPORTS (LTSS)

Long-term health care is defined as the help needed by people of any age who are unable to complete ADLs because of physical and/or mental impairment. As the term implies, this care is for extended periods, ranging from months to years to a lifetime. Long-term care is provided in institutions or the community, or it can be home-based.

Although families, friends, and neighbors may be able to help the disabled, family units have become smaller over the years, and most able people are working. Frequently, no one is available to take care of the disabled or older adults who cannot manage the tasks of daily living. For some, community-based services are an alternative to institutional care, but for many others, such services are not enough. These individuals include the vast numbers of mentally ill, the intellectually and developmentally disabled, the frail elderly, and the permanently disabled.

Long-term care facilities funded by the federal government include more than just nursing homes. Institutional services refer to specific benefits authorized under the Social Security Act. These are **intermediate care facilities for people with intellectual disability (ICF/ID)**, inpatient psychiatric services for individuals under age 21, and services for individuals age 65 or older in an institution for mental disease. Another federal requirement is the **Preadmission Screening and Resident Review (PASRR)**, designed to ensure that individuals are not inappropriately placed in a nursing home for long-term care. All applicants to a Medicaid-certified nursing home are required to be evaluated for mental illness and/or intellectual disability and be placed in the appropriate long-term care setting based on their needs.[13]

Intermediate Care Facilities for People with Intellectual Disability (ICF/ID)

ICF/ID are available only for individuals in need of and receiving active treatment, which consists of a program of specialized and generic training, treatment, and health services. The emphasis in an ICF is on personal care and social services, and most participants attend workshops during the day. Independent clients who are able to function with little supervision and do not require a continuous program of habilitation services are not eligible for ICF.[13]

Inpatient Psychiatric Services for Individuals under Age 21

This program provides comprehensive mental health treatment for children and adolescents who, due to acute mental illness, substance abuse, or severe emotional disturbance, are in need of treatment that can most effectively be provided in a residential treatment facility.[13]

Services for Individuals Age 65 or Older in an Institution for Mental Diseases

The services of an institution for mental diseases (IMD) meet federal and state requirements of a hospital or nursing facility but are also considered an IMD for older adults with mental or intellectual disabilities who require ongoing long-term care.[13]

Nursing Facilities (NF)

Nursing facility services are provided by Medicaid-certified nursing homes, which primarily provide three types of services:

- Skilled nursing or medical care and related services
- Rehabilitation needed due to injury, disability, or illness
- Long-term care—health-related care and services (above the level of room and board) not available in the community, needed regularly due to a mental or physical condition

A **skilled nursing facility (SNF)** is a nursing home that provides the level of care closest to hospital care. Twenty-four-hour nursing services, medical supervision, rehabilitation, pharmacy and dietetic services, and physical, occupational, and recreational therapy are provided in accordance with federal guidelines. Medicare covers the cost of short-term skilled nursing and rehabilitation after surgery or disease—for example, for hip replacement surgery or after a stroke. Long-term care is required for those requiring care 24 hours a day for assistance with ADLs. The cost of long-term care is funded either through private payment or by Medicaid for those who are eligible based on income and assets.[13]

History of Nursing Homes

Nursing homes originated with county poorhouses (almshouses). They were first established in the nineteenth century to care for the poor and provide food, shelter, and clothing. Over time, they became community dumps for castoff unfortunates. The conditions in these places were atrocious. The mentally ill and developmentally disabled were placed in nursing homes because there were few other options. However, this population did not need skilled nursing care or supervision 24 hours a day. Before Medicare and Medicaid were established in 1965, states were responsible for monitoring nursing homes. The poor conditions in the nursing homes prompted states to set up regulations governing nursing home care, but most states were unwilling to close the proprietary or voluntary nursing homes because they would then be responsible for the occupants. Instead, they chose to look the other way if conditions violated regulations.[14] The **Omnibus Budget Reconciliation Act of 1987 (OBRA 87)** was enacted in response to concerns about the poor quality of care and inadequate regulation in nursing homes in the United States. A change brought about by OBRA 87 required Medicare and Medicaid standards and certification procedures regarding long-term care facilities to merge, and ICF/ID standards were upgraded to correspond to those for skilled care facilities.[15] The federal government, through the Center for Medicare and Medicaid Services (CMS), is responsible for nursing home standards, while individual states are responsible for monitoring facilities to ensure that standards are met. The OBRA 87 created minimum standards of care, including staffing requirements and rights for residents. These standards emphasized quality-of-life issues and the prevention of abuse, neglect, and mistreatment, including the use of physical and chemical restraints.[15]

COMMUNITY LONG-TERM CARE SERVICES

Privately funded long-term care providers that are regulated by federal and/or state governments in addition to nursing homes are adult day care facilities, residential care communities, home health agencies, and hospice. The **National Center for Health Statistics (NCHS)** conducted the first portion of the National Study of Long-Term Care Providers in 2012. The survey is conducted biennially and used for planning long-term care needs of the aging population.[16] The 2016 survey results are shown in **TABLE 4.3**.[16]

A survey was conducted in 2016 by the National Center for Health Statistics to determine data on long-term care services in the U.S.[16] There were a total of 65,000 regulated

TABLE 4.3 Long-Term Care Providers in the United States, 2016

Long-Term Care Services	Number	Percent
Residential care communities	28,900	44%
Nursing homes	15,600	24%
Home health agencies	12,200	19%
Adult day care services	4,600	7%
Hospice	4,300	7%

Data from Harris-Kojetin L, Sengupta M, Lendon JP, Rome V, Valverde R, Caffrey C. Long-term care providers and services users in the United States, 2015–2016. National Center for Health Statistics. *Vital Health* Stat;2019;3(43).

long-term care service providers serving over 8.3 million people annually. The majority (about two-thirds) were residential care communities and nursing homes, and about one-fifth were home health agencies. Both adult day care and hospice represented less than 10% each. The majority of the providers were for-profit except for adult day care, where the majority were nonprofit. Clients in adult day care and home health were younger than clients in other settings. Adult day care clients were also more racially diverse, with 23% Hispanic and 15% non-Hispanic black. The diagnosis of Alzheimer's and depression was highest in nursing home residents, at 48% for those with Alzheimer's and 46% for those with depression. Clients receiving home care services were being managed for chronic diseases of arthritis, diabetes, and heart disease (**FIGURE 4.1**).[16]

An evaluation of the ADLs—bathing, dressing, toileting, and eating—was used to measure physical and cognitive function for users of long-term services. Nearly half of those receiving long term support services needed assistance with at least one ADL. A need for assistance with bathing was most common (39% to 97%), while needing assistance with eating was least common (19% to 61%). Assistance with all ADLs was highest for residents in nursing homes and clients of home health agencies. Clients of adult day care services needed less assistance with ADLs than all other long-term services, except for assistance with eating, which was lower for those living in residential care communities. For those using adult day services, assistance with physical mobility was the most common (46%) (refer to **FIGURE 4.2**).[16]

The cost for long-term care services varies based on needed assistance with IADLs and ADLs. Based on a survey conducted in 2019, the median yearly cost was least expensive for **adult day care** at $19,500, followed by assisted living at $48,612 for a one-bedroom apartment and $90,155 for a semi-private room in a nursing home. The cost of the services of a homemaker or health care aide varied depending on the number of hours required; however, for homemaking services, the cost was $22.50 per hour, and it was $23 per hour for home health aide services.[11]

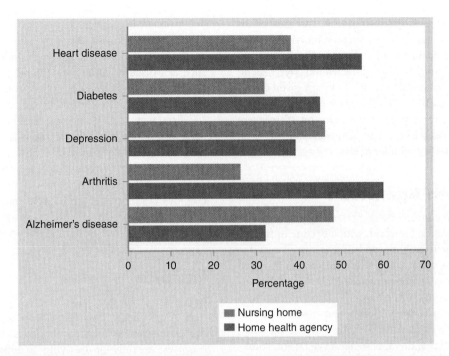

FIGURE 4.1 Comparison of most common diagnoses by type of long-term care services, 2015–2016.

Data from Harris-Kojetin L, Sengupta M, Lendon JP, Rome V, Valverde R, Caffrey C. Long-term care providers and services users in the United States, 2015–2016. National Center for Health Statistics. *Vital Health Stat* 2019;3(43). https://www.cdc.gov/nchs/data/series/sr_03/sr03_43-508.pdf

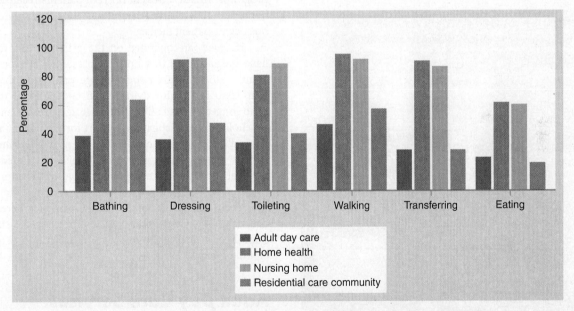

FIGURE 4.2 Percentage of those using long-term care services needing assistance with ADLs, 2015–2016.

Modified from Harris-Kojetin L, Sengupta M, Lendon JP, Rome V, Valverde R, Caffrey C. Long-term care providers and services users in the United States, 2015–2016. National Center for Health Statistics. *Vital Health Stat* 2019;3(43).

Residential Care Communities/ Assisted-Living Facilities

Residential care communities or **assisted-living facilities** are nonmedical facilities that provide a room or apartment, meals, housekeeping, medication management, assistance with ADLs as needed, and recreational activities. Some also provide transportation for shopping or doctor visits. These facilities may be part of a retirement community, nursing home, or senior housing complex or a stand-alone facility. Some facilities are part of a retirement community, known as a **continuing care community**, that allows residents to move from independent living to assisted living to a skilled nursing facility on the same campus as their needs change. Licensing requirements vary by state, and the facilities are known by numerous different names, such as residential care, board and care, congregate care, supported care, sheltered care, and personal care. Financing arrangements include private pay or coverage through long-term care insurance. Some states cover the cost for low-income individuals who qualify through Medicaid waiver programs. These facilities are regulated by the states instead of the federal government, and standards vary from state to state.[17] On any given day in 2015–2016, there were 811,500 residents living in these communities. About half were 85 years and older, one-third were between 75 and 84 years of age, and 11% were 65 to 74 years of age. The remainder were under 65 years of age.[16]

Home Health Agencies

"Aging in place" is a concept that is preferred by many older adults and their families. However, with a decline in health, outside assistance is usually needed. Home health services are often ordered by a physician after a hip fracture or hip replacement. Others need ongoing assistance with ADLs or need supervision because of dementia. **Home health agencies (HHA)** provide part-time nursing and medical care in patients' homes as well as other services such as physical, speech, and occupational therapy; social services; and sometimes medical supplies and equipment such as wheelchairs, walkers, and so forth (**FIGURE 4.3**).

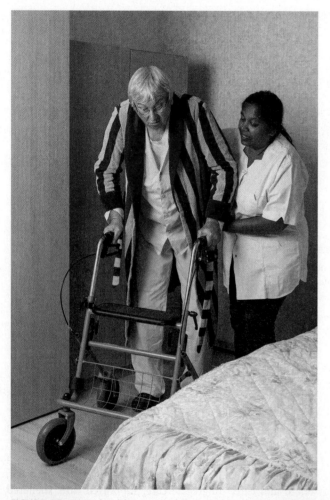

FIGURE 4.3 Home health care services include physical therapy.
© Anneka/Shutterstock.

Homemaker services may also be part of the package. Physicians, physician assistants, and nurse practitioners provide medical care at home. Ongoing custodial or supportive care such as assistance with ADLs (bathing, dressing, eating) and IADLs (shopping, meal preparation, housekeeping) is provided by home health aides, homemakers, or personal assistants.[17]

The agency may be independently operated or managed by a public health department or hospital. Patient fees, government grants, private insurance, or Medicare and Medicaid may finance agency services. Variations include the well-known Visiting Nurse Association, which most often employs U.S. Public Health Service nurses. These nurses go to patients' homes and change dressings, give injections, and perform other types of services as needed.[18]

Hospice

In 1967, the hospice movement was resurrected from its beginnings during the medieval era in England. Whereas the first hospices cared for the wounded, sick, and dying, modern hospices care only for the dying. In 1986, the Medicare Hospice Benefit was made permanent by Congress, and states were given the option of including hospice in their Medicaid programs. In 2017, 56% of hospice patients received care at home and 42% received care in a nursing facility including a hospice in-patient facility.[19]

Hospices are operated on the principle that the dying have special needs that hospital personnel are too busy to handle. Hospice care helps manage pain and other symptoms associated with dying when conventional treatment is no longer of value. Other hospice services are emotional, psychological, and spiritual support for the patient and family and bereavement counseling for surviving family and friends. Medical care may include necessary medications, medical supplies, and equipment. Health professionals who work in hospice are physicians who serve as the medical directors, registered nurses, social workers, bereavement counselors, spiritual counselors, and personal assistants and home health aides. Hospice programs function as a multidisciplinary team.[19]

Adult Day Care Services

Adult day care services are provided in a community-based group setting, usually in a freestanding facility. Some centers may be affiliated with other health facilities or organizations including hospitals, nursing homes, residential care facilities, or senior centers. Adult day care is used to supplement home care services or as a less costly alternative to a residential care facility or a nursing care facility.[17] Adult day care centers are usually open during the day, five days a week, to allow the family to continue to work or to offer a respite from caregiving. However, some centers may offer evening or weekend hours. Participants in adult day care centers usually require some supervision because of dementia or assistance with ADLs. Others receive therapeutic treatment to maintain physical or cognitive functioning. Social and recreational activities and meals and snacks are offered as well as some medical services. Most also include transportation services.[17] The majority of adult day care centers employ registered nurses (62%), licensed practical nurses (46%), health aides (67%), social workers (40%), and activity directors (85%).[16]

OTHER COMMUNITY PROGRAMS FOR OLDER ADULTS AND DISABLED PERSONS
Program of All-Inclusive Care for the Elderly (PACE)

The **Program of All-Inclusive Care for the Elderly (PACE)** is a form of integrated care supported by CMS, one of several programs that encourage states to provide the full array of Medicaid and Medicare benefits through a single delivery system in order to provide quality care for dual-eligible enrollees, improve care coordination, and reduce administrative burdens. PACE provides comprehensive preventive, primary, acute, and long-term care services so older individuals with chronic care needs can continue living in the community.[20] The PACE model of care began in the 1970s in the Chinatown–North Beach area of San Francisco to meet the long-term care needs of elderly immigrants.[21] By 2015, PACE had expanded to 116 sites in urban and rural areas in 32 states across the United States. Services include adult day care at a PACE center, which has an on-site primary care provider—either a physician or nurse practitioner—and a multidisciplinary team of physical, occupational, and recreational therapists; dietitians; social workers; nurses; aides; and van drivers. Most participants attend the PACE center three days a week, and transportation services are covered by the program. As needs change, participants may receive home, hospital, or nursing home care. PACE programs receive Medicare and Medicaid capitation payments.

PACE is available to individuals 55 years of age or older who are certified by their state as needing home care but unable to otherwise live safely in the community. A typical PACE participant is very similar to the average nursing home resident: a woman, 80 years old, with eight medical conditions, who is limited in three ADLs and has nearly a 50% chance of having dementia. Even though PACE participants require high levels of care, more than 90% are able to continue living in the community.[23]

The Aging Network

The **Aging Network** is a system of federal, state, and local entities committed to supporting older Americans in living independently in their homes and communities. The network consists of the **U.S. Administration on Aging (AOA)**, 56 state Aging units, 622 **Area Agencies on Aging (AAAs),** and

more than 250 Title VI Native American aging programs. The network of agencies has successfully delivered aging services in communities across the United States for 47 years. Most AAAs service rural areas (41%) or a mix of rural, urban, and suburban communities (26%).[24] AAAs were established as part of the **1973 Older Americans Act (OAA)** and Title VI.

Native American aging programs were added to the 1978 amendment to the OAA. The federal government funds the Aging Network through individual states, which then distribute money to AAAs to fund direct services in local communities. Additional funding sources are general revenue from individual states, local funding and fund-raising, Medicaid waivers, and consumer cost-sharing. The organizational structure of AAAs varies; local AAAs are part of city, county, or council governments or are independent nonprofit organizations. All AAAs offer five core services: nutrition, health and wellness, elder rights, caregiver support, and supportive services including transportation (**FIGURE 4.4**).[25]

Senior centers are the focal point where 60% of services are delivered. Most centers offer a noon meal as well as social, wellness, educational, and recreational programs Monday through Friday. Senior centers serve as referral centers for other services and offer public benefit counseling.[25]

BOX 4.1 demonstrates how a senior center delivers nutrition services.[26]

Approximately 11,400 senior centers serve more than 1 million older adults every day. The majority of participants are women (70%); ethnicity is primarily Caucasian followed by African American, Latino, and Asian, and the average age is 75 years. An estimated 75% of participants visit their senior center one to three times a week.[25]

Most local agencies also offer case management, information and referral, and counseling on health insurance benefits. AAAs were designed for vulnerable adults 60 years and older; however, many agencies now offer services to adults younger than 60 years who have disabilities and chronic disease as well as to veterans.[26] The Aging Network continues to expand programming to serve consumers—for example, integration of acute care with home- and community-based care and chronic disease self-management. Local AAAs partner with other agencies to provide services.[27] Some of these partnerships and the percentage of AAAs with these partnerships are listed in **TABLE 4.4**.[26]

DEMOGRAPHIC TRENDS AND PROJECTIONS

Changes in the racial and ethnic composition of the U.S. population have important consequences for the nation's health because many of the measures of disease and disability differ significantly by race and ethnicity. Shifts in the U.S. population are expected to occur, with a decrease in the percentage of Caucasians and an increase in all other racial groups. Racial and ethnic minority populations have increased from 19% of the older adult population in 2007 to 23% in 2017 and are projected to increase to 34% in 2040. Between 2017 and 2040,

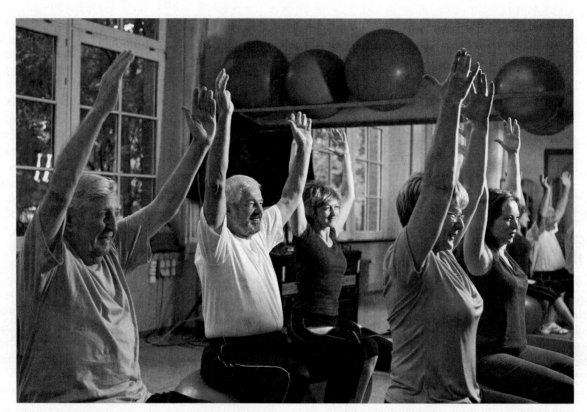

FIGURE 4.4 Area Agency on Aging (AAA) programming includes health and wellness.
© Robert Kneschke/Shutterstock.

BOX 4.1 AAA Profile: Nutrition

The Chautauqua County Office for the Aging in Mayville, NY, serves a rural area in western New York state. It provides services to 8,000 seniors, disabled adults, and caregivers each year. The aging office has close partnerships with three Meals on Wheels organizations and two hospital kitchens that serve meals at the senior center and to the homebound. The AAA is the central intake for all home-delivered meal requests and oversees congregate meals and home-delivered meals in the county. These partnerships are cost-effective but also ensure that frail seniors and disabled adults have access to good nutrition essential for recovery after discharge from the hospital.

Modified from Area Agencies on Aging. *Trends and New Directions. Area Agencies on Aging Survey 2014.* https://www.n4a.org/files/AAA%20 2014%20Survey.pdf

TABLE 4.4 Area Agency on Aging Partnerships, 2013

Partnership	Percent
Adult protective services	85
Transportation agencies	84
Medicaid agencies	83
Advocacy organizations	82
Hospitals	79
Emergency preparedness agencies	79
Mental health organizations	77
Disability service organizations	75
Public housing authority	75
Faith-based organizations	66
Community health providers	60
Businesses	46
Managed care/HMO networks	42

Data from Area Agencies on Aging. *Trends and New Directions. Area Agencies on Aging Survey 2014.* https://www.n4a.org/files/AAA%202014%20Survey.pdf

the Caucasians age 65 and older are projected to increase by 36% compared with 135% for older racial and ethnic minority populations, including Hispanics (188%), African Americans (96%), American Indians and Alaskan Natives (85%), and Asians (123%).[28] These shifts in the racial and ethnic makeup of the United States require health professionals and organizations to achieve cultural competence and to ensure that they utilize appropriate and tailored approaches in working with specific population groups. A **Healthy People 2020** recommendation is to increase the proportion of all degrees awarded to members of underrepresented racial and ethnic groups among the health professions to meet the needs of all patients, regardless of their background.[29]

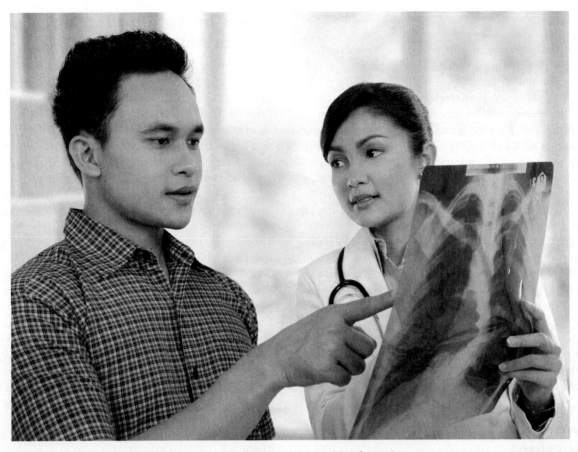

FIGURE 4.5 Health literacy is the ability to process and understand basic health information.
© Odua Images/Shutterstock.

Health Literacy

Limited **health literacy** affects people of all ages, races, incomes, and education levels, but the impact of limited health literacy disproportionately affects lower socioeconomic and minority groups, those with low English proficiency, and older adults. Nearly one-third of adults in the United States have low literacy skills. The impact on the individual with low literacy skills includes more frequent medical errors, illness and disability, and loss of wages. The impact on the larger economy is billions of dollars per year (**FIGURE 4.5**).[30]

Research over the past two decades has shown that health information is often presented in a way that is not usable to the majority of Americans. Health literacy is the degree to which individuals have the capacity to obtain, process, and understand basic health information and services needed to make appropriate health decisions. Examples of health literacy are the ability to understand instructions on prescription drug bottles, appointment slips, medical education brochures, doctors' directions, and consent forms and the ability to negotiate complex healthcare systems. Health literacy is not simply the ability to read. It requires a complex group of reading, listening, analytical, and decision-making skills and the ability to apply these skills to health situations. It affects people's ability to search for and use health

information, adopt healthy behaviors, and act on important public health alerts. Limited health literacy is also associated with worse health outcomes and higher costs.[31,32] An example of how the lack of health literacy impacts health delivery is shown in **BOX 4.2**.[33]

PERSONNEL NEEDS

Healthcare practitioners will routinely serve older people in the future as part of their regular duties. This care will make up approximately one-third to two-thirds of the workload of healthcare personnel. Although attention to aging and geriatrics has expanded in recent years, most health education programs give little emphasis to these issues. Greatly expanded training programs are required to prepare personnel to provide services in homes, hospice, nursing homes, and other community settings.

Requirements for personnel specifically prepared to serve older people will greatly exceed the current supply. This is especially true for nursing assistants or home health and personal care aides who provide direct care to patients receiving LTSS and make up the largest percentage of employees in these settings. For example, a 2016 survey reported the percentage of full-time aides working in different settings to be higher than any other health professional: residential care communities (83%), nursing homes (64%), and adult day care services (57%).[16] Retaining aides is challenging because of the low pay and high physical and emotional demands of the job.[34] There is also a shortage of physician specialists—**geriatricians** and neurologists—being trained to care for older patients with a primary diagnosis of Alzheimer's disease. Because there are not enough physicians specialized to diagnose and treat those with Alzheimer's disease, there is a need for training primary care physicians to become more knowledgeable about the disease.[9]

Future Education for the Health Professions

The healthcare personnel of tomorrow need to begin now to develop some special skills to deal with future changes. First, curricula must include the requirements and care of the older adult population. A second requisite is the need to assume an active role in developing acceptable health policies. Interdisciplinary respect and understanding will be critical for future health professionals. Students seeking a career in the health professions can expect to experience **interprofessional education (IPE)** in which students in different programs learn the roles and functions of other health professions and work together as a team to contribute to the assessment and treatment of individual patients. An ideal mechanism to achieve this would be shared educational experiences, with a health science core of studies and laboratories that allow students from many disciplines to interact and jointly provide care. Would-be healthcare professionals must learn to establish strong, effective, collegial relationships with practitioners of all healthcare disciplines. In this way, the student of today can prepare for a leadership role in clinical care, the political process, and national healthcare planning and research.

Shifts in Training Health Personnel

Health personnel in the coming years will need to develop a broader understanding and competence in geriatrics. An extended curriculum to encompass these goals should be established. It likely will include a variety of clinical settings and short-term, intensive courses to bring practitioners up to current knowledge levels. All physicians should receive education and training in geriatric medicine as part of their professional preparation. Care of chronically ill, frail elderly persons should be emphasized. Special attention should be focused on clinical pharmacology, especially for patients on multiple medications, and on the impact of sensory loss and dental health on nutritional status. Dentists, dental hygienists, and dental assistants will be serving substantially larger numbers of older adults. Like nurses, they should receive education concerning the special needs and conditions of older adults as part of their basic preparation. Innovative educational preparation with a focus on the needs and care of older adults must be emphasized. Nursing personnel need expanded knowledge and skills, with stress on health promotion and nutrition for older adults. They should be encouraged to go into geriatric nursing or to specialize in advanced gerontology education. Social work personnel must be prepared to meet the diverse social services needs of older adults. They will require a specialized knowledge of the aging process and the interpersonal dynamics of the aging and their families.

Health professionals need to be knowledgeable about the health problems of different ethnic, racial, and socioeconomic groups, including recent immigrants. Training in factors related to health literacy and approaches to simplify patient education are needed. Health literacy is critical in ensuring the delivery of quality health care and reducing hospital and emergency room admissions and healthcare costs.

Parts three to five of this book describes the work of many health professionals and supporting personnel in great detail. Each of the professions will need expanded personnel to take care of the aging population. Students considering a career in the health field are encouraged to continue—their services will be greatly needed.

SUMMARY

The future of health services will be concentrated among older and very old persons. This fact has important implications for the education and training of all healthcare personnel. The impact of these changes will have an increasing role in the delivery of health care and on the economy of the United States.

LEARNING PORTFOLIO

Study Points

1. Demographic shifts are projected in the population with an increase in those over 65 years until 2030 when the percentage of those over age 85 will increase. The population over age 65 will also be more racially and ethnically diverse with non-Whites being in the majority by 2050.

2. Those over 85 years of age are likely to have one or more chronic diseases and need assistance in performing complex activities—IADLs (e.g., preparing food, shopping, managing finances and medications, and using transportation); they are also more likely to have impaired mobility.

3. Stroke and Alzheimer's disease are the two most common causes of functional impairment requiring assistance with basic activities of daily living (ADLs): bathing, dressing, eating, and toileting.

4. Early symptoms of Alzheimer's disease are dementia or a loss of memory and problem-solving ability; in the later stages, there is a loss of ability to complete basic activities of daily living (ADLs) requiring total care 24 hours a day. An estimated 75% of nursing home residents over age 85 have a diagnosis of Alzheimer's disease.

5. There are four parts to Medicare: Part A, hospital and short-term skilled nursing home care; Part B, outpatient, home, and hospice care; Part C, supplemental insurance that replaces Parts A and B; and Part D, medication insurance. All parts have deductibles and copayments.

6. Medicaid covers the costs of long-term care for those who require assistance with ADLs and are either low-income and disabled or low-income and older than 65 years of age.

7. The federal government funds institutional care as specified by the Social Security Act: skilled nursing and rehabilitation; intermediate care for people with intellectual disability (ICF/ID); inpatient psychiatric services for individuals under age 21; and services for individuals age 65 or older in an institution for mental disease.

8. The Centers for Medicare and Medicaid (CMS) are responsible for nursing home standards, while individual states are responsible for monitoring facilities to ensure that standards are met.

9. In 2016, about two-thirds of those requiring long-term care services were residents of nursing homes or residential care communities, one-fifth received home health care, and fewer than 10% received either adult day care or hospice services.

10. Residents of nursing homes and those receiving home care usually require more assistance with ADLs than those using adult day care services or living in residential care communities.

11. Home health care provides both medical care and personal care after an acute illness or surgery plus medical, nursing, and therapy services.

12. Hospice services manage pain and other symptoms of dying and emotional, psychological, and spiritual support for patients and their families and grief support for survivors.

13. Adult day care services supplement home care services or provide a less costly alternative to nursing home care.

14. The Program of All-Inclusive Care for the Elderly (PACE) coordinates Medicare and Medicaid services for those eligible who are 55 years and older and need nursing home care but who can live safely in the community with supportive services offered through PACE.

15. The Aging Network is a system of the U.S. Administration on Aging, area and state aging units, and Title VI Native American aging programs that delivers services for those 60 years and older, veterans, and disabled persons under 60 years of age. The local senior center is the center for delivering services in nutrition, health and wellness, elder rights, caregiver support, transportation, and referrals for other services.

16. Health literacy is the ability to obtain, process, and understand basic health information and services needed to make appropriate health decisions; those more likely to have low health literacy are of lower socioeconomic status, those with low English proficiency, and older adults.

17. Based on projected demographics indicating greater diversity in ethnic and racial diversity and greater numbers older than age 65, future health professionals will need to be knowledgeable about cultural differences and the health conditions and needs of older adults.

Issues for Discussion

1. Use the interactive tool to estimate the cost of various long-term services such as homemaker services, adult day care, assisted living facility, or nursing home for the state in which you live. What are the costs of care in your state? Which service costs the least? Which service costs the most? https://www.genworth.com /aging-and-you/finances/cost-of-care.html

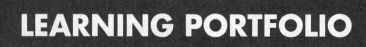

LEARNING PORTFOLIO

Enrichment Activities

1. Go to the Genworth website to the section on *Aging & You*. View the simulations to experience vision, mobility, and hearing impairments. Imagine how either a visual or hearing impairment could impact your ability to complete IADLs and ADLs. https://www.genworth.com/aging-and-you/health.html

2. Go to the website *Center for Health Care Strategies* and review fact sheets on health literacy. Choose one of the six fact sheets and provide two to three tips that you would use as a student in the health professionals to provide improved communication with clients who may have low literacy skills. https://www.chcs.org/resource/health-literacy-fact-sheets/

CASE STUDY: HEALTH INSURANCE BENEFITS FOR SENIORS

Sam is a 73-year-old man who currently has healthcare coverage through Medicare. Sam knows that Medicare programs are divided into four parts and that each covers different areas of health care. He is reviewing his plan to be sure he has adequate coverage. Based on the information you have read about aging, health, and long-term care, answer the following questions.

1. If Sam is admitted to the hospital, is there any type of coverage that will help pay the bill?

2. Is there any type of coverage available for prescription drugs?

3. Sam needs to wear glasses and realizes how expensive they can be. What coverage may include vision benefits?

4. Sam is happy that he has all his natural teeth—no dentures, implants, or partial plates. He is concerned, though, that he needs to have expensive dental exams and cleanings on a regular basis. Is there any type of Medicare coverage that may help with dental bills?

5. Sam is a widower. Although his children live close by, he wants to be sure he can afford home health services

if he needs them. What coverage would help pay for these services?

6. Some of the healthcare services paid for through Medicare are only paid at the rate of 80%. What can Sam do to be prepared in case he is financially responsible for 20% of a healthcare bill?

7. If Sam decides to have a knee replacement and spend part of his rehabilitation time in a skilled nursing facility to recuperate, will there be any coverage for this through Medicare?

8. Sam sees three different doctors on a regular basis. Is there Medicare coverage available to help pay for office visits?

9. Sam is concerned about the possibility of having a terminal illness in the future. Is there any coverage for such an eventuality available under any of the Medicare plans?

10. What if Sam is unable to pay his Medicare premiums? Is there help available through any government healthcare plans to pay those premiums? Do you have any other advice you can offer Sam regarding help with his healthcare needs? Please explain your answer.

References

1. Medina LD, Sabo S, Vespa J. Living Longer: Historical and Projected Life Expectancy in the United States, 1960 to 2060. *Current Population Reports*, P25-1145, U.S. Census Bureau, Washington, DC, 2020.

2. Federal Interagency Forum on Aging-Related Statistics. *Older Americans 2016: Key Indicators of Well-Being*. Washington, DC: U.S. Government Printing Office. August 2016.

3. Berenson R, Howell J. *Structuring, Financing and Paying for Effective Chronic Care Coordination*. A Report Commissioned by the National Coalition on Care Coordination (N3C); 2009. http://www.urban.org/research/publication/structuring-financing-and-paying-effective-chronic-care-coordination Accessed on June 27, 2020.

4. Roberts AW, Ogunwole SU, Blakeslee L, Rabe MA. The Population 65 Years and Older in the United States: 2016. *American Community Survey Reports*, ACS-38, U.S. Census Bureau, Washington, DC, 2018.

5. Medina LD, Sabo S, Vespa J. Living Longer: Historical and Projected Life Expectancy in the United States, 1960 to 2060. *Current Population Reports*, P25-1145, U.S. Census Bureau, Washington, DC, 2020.

6. Centers for Disease Control and Prevention. *About Chronic Diseases*, 2019. National Center for Chronic Disease Prevention and Health Promotion (NCCDPHP). https://www.cdc.gov/chronicdisease/about/index.htm Accessed June 27, 2020.

7. Centers for Disease Control and Prevention. *The State of Aging and Health in America 2013*. Atlanta, GA: Centers for Disease Control and Prevention; 2013.

8. Heron M. Death: Leading Causes for 2017. *National Vital Statistics Reports*; 68(6): Hyattsville, MD: National Center for Health Statistics. 2019.

9. Alzheimer's Association. 2020 Alzheimer's Disease Facts and Figures. *Alzheimers Dement* 2020;16(3):1–94.

LEARNING PORTFOLIO

10. Centers for Medicare and Medicaid Services. *Medicare & You, 2021.* CMS Product No. 10050 December 2020. https://www.medicare.gov/sites/default/files/2020-12/10050-Medicare-and-You_0.pdf Accessed August 20, 2021.

11. Genworth Financial, Inc. *Cost of Care Survey. Summary and Methodology.* December 2020. https://pro.genworth.com/riiproweb/productinfo/pdf/131168.pdf Accessed August 20, 2021.

12. Centers for Medicare and Medicaid Services. *Spousal Impoverishment.* https://www.medicaid.gov/medicaid/eligibility/spousal-impoverishment/index.html Accessed June 27, 2020.

13. Centers for Medicare and Medicaid Services. *Long-Term Services and Supports.* https://www.medicaid.gov/medicaid/long-term-services-supports/index.html Accessed August 20, 2021.

14. Watson SD. From Almshouses to Nursing Homes and Community Care: Lessons from Medicaid's History. *GSU Law Rev* 2009; 26:1–34.

15. Walshe K. Regulating U.S. Nursing Homes: Are We Learning from Experience? *Health Aff* 2001; 20:128–144.

16. Harris-Kojetin L, Sengupta M, Lendon JP, Rome V, Valverde R, Caffrey C. Long-Term Care Providers and Services Users in the United States, 2015–2016. National Center for Health Statistics. *Vital Health Stat* 3(43); 2019.

17. MetLife Mature Market Institute. *Market Survey of Long-Term Care Costs. The 2012 MetLife Market Survey of Nursing Homes, Assisted Living, Adult Day Services, and Home Care Cost.* November 2012. https://eadscares.files.wordpress.com/2012/12/metlife-ltc-cost-study.pdf Accessed August 20, 2021

18. VNA Foundation. *History.* http://vnafoundation.net/history-misson/. Accessed June 27, 2020.

19. *National Hospice and Palliative Care Organization (NHPCO) NHPCO's Facts and Figures. 2018 Edition.* Alexandria, VA: National Hospice and Palliative Care Organization; July 2019.

20. Centers for Medicare and Medicaid Services. *Program of All-Inclusive Care for the Elderly (PACE).* https://www.medicaid.gov/medicaid/long-term-services-supports/program-all-inclusive-care-elderly/index.html. Accessed June 27, 2020.

21. On Lok Pace Partners. *Our History.* On Lok, Inc. 2020. https://pacepartners.net/who-we-are/our-history/. Accessed June 27, 2020.

22. National PACE Association. *Understanding PACE.* https://www.npaonline.org/sites/default/files/PDFs/Profile%20of%20PACE_rev031621_v2.pdf Accessed August 20, 2021.

23. National PACE Association. *Eligibility Requirements for Programs of All-Inclusive Care for the Elderly. PACE.* https://www.npaonline.org/pace-you/eligibility-require

ments-programs-all-inclusive-care-elderly-pace%C2%AE Accessed August 20, 2021.

24. National Association of Area Agencies on Aging. *National Survey of Area Agencies on Aging 2017 Report Serving America's Older Adults.* https://www.n4a.org/Files/2017%20AAA%20Survey%20Report/AAANationalSurvey_web.pdf Accessed August 20, 2021.

25. National Council on Aging. *Senior Centers.* Fact Sheet. 2015. https://assets-us-01.kc-usercontent.com/ffacfe7d-10b6-0083-2632-604077fd4eca/d62574a5-2604-4454-8df8-461e7fbe7622/FactSheet_SeniorCenters.pdf Accessed August 20, 2021.

26. Area Agencies on Aging. *Trends and New Directions. Area Agencies on Aging Survey 2014.* https://www.n4a.org/files/AAA%202014%20Survey.pdf Accessed August 20, 2021.

27. National Association of Area Agencies on Aging. *2020 Policy Priorities.* March 2020. https://www.n4a.org/files/n4a_2020PolicyPriorities_Web%20(1).pdf Accessed August 20, 2021.

28. *A Profile of Older Americans: 2018.* U.S. Administration on Aging (AoA). Administration for Community Living, U.S. Department of Health and Human Services. April, 2018. https://acl.gov/sites/default/files/Aging%20and%20Disability%20in%20America/2018OlderAmericansProfile.pdf Accessed August 20, 2021.

29. *Healthy People 2020: Language and Literacy.* Centers for Disease Control and Prevention. U.S. Department of Health and Human Services. https://www.healthypeople.gov/2020/topics-objectives/topic/social-determinants-health/interventions-resources/language-and-literacy Accessed August 20, 2021.

30. Vernon J, Trujillo A, Rosenbaum S, DeBuono B. *Low Health Literacy: Implications for National Health Policy.* Washington, DC: Department of Health Policy, School of Public Health and Health Services, George Washington University; 2007.

31. U.S. Department of Health and Human Services. Office of Disease Prevention and Health Promotion. *National Action Plan to Improve Health Literacy.* Washington, DC: DHHS; 2010.

32. National Academies of Sciences, Engineering, and Medicine. 2018. *Building the case for health literacy: Proceedings of a workshop.* Washington, DC: The National Academies Press. doi: https://doi.org/10.17226/25068 Accessed August 20, 2021.

33. Mahadevan R. Improving *Oral Communication to Promote Health Literacy.* Fact Sheet #5. October 2013. Center for Health Care Strategies, Inc. https://www.chcs.org/media/Improving_Oral_Communication.pdf. Accessed June 27, 2020.

34. Bureau of Labor Statistics, U.S. Department of Labor, *Occupational Outlook Handbook,* Home Health Aides and Personal Care Aides. https://www.bls.gov/ooh/healthcare/home-health-aides-and-personal-care-aides.htm Accessed July 1, 2020.

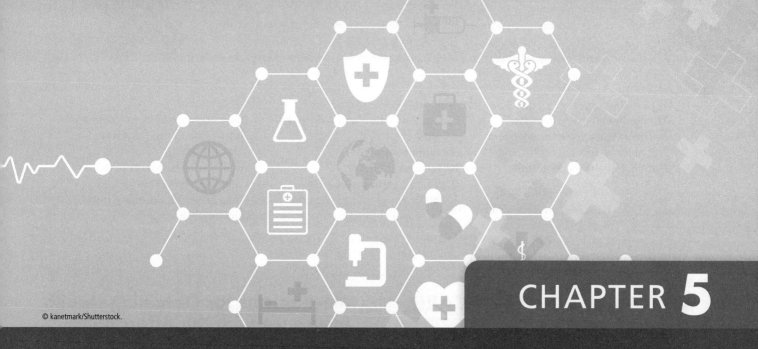
© kanetmark/Shutterstock.

CHAPTER 5

Healthcare Reform

OBJECTIVES

After studying this chapter, the student should be able to:

- Summarize the process of applying for health insurance through the HealthCare.gov website.
- Describe the impact of the Affordable Care Act (ACA) on insurance coverage and access to care.
- Explain modifications in the Affordable Care Act (ACA) of 2010 as a result of the U.S. Supreme Court decisions, underfunding of the navigator program, legislation, and executive action.
- Compare insurance coverage and access to care in states with and without expanded Medicaid.

KEY TERMS

Accountable care organizations (ACOs)
Advance premium tax credit
Affordable Care Act (ACA)
Bundling payments
Burwell v. Hobby Lobby, Inc.
Center for Medicare and Medicaid Innovation
Clinical preventive services
Closely held corporations
Cost sharing reduction
Coverage gap

Data Service Hub
Diagnosis-related group
Employer shared responsibility payment
Essential health benefits
Executive order
Expansion of Medicaid
Federally Facilitated Marketplace (FFM)
Federal poverty level (FPL)
Federally Qualified Health Center (FQHC)

FFM-P
Gross domestic product (GDP)
Health Care and Education Reconciliation Act of 2010
HealthCare.gov
Health Exchange (Marketplace)
Hospital Readmission Reduction Program (HRRP)
Individual mandate
King v. Burwell
Little Sisters of the Poor v. Pennsylvania

Minimum essential coverage
National Federation of Independent
  Business v. Sebelius
National health expenditures
  (NHE)
Navigator
Obamacare

Patient Protection and Affordable
  Care Act
Premium subsidies
Preexisting conditions
Qualified health plan (QHP)
Religious Freedom Restoration
  Act of 1993

Shared responsibility for coverage
Short-term, limited-duration
  health policy
Small Business Health Options
  Program (SHOP)
State-Based Marketplace (SBM)
Uncompensated care

OVERVIEW OF HEALTHCARE REFORM

President Barack Obama signed healthcare reform legislation into law in March 2010. The **Patient Protection and Affordable Care Act** (H.R. 3590) was modified by the **Health Care and Education Reconciliation Act of 2010** (H.R. 4872); the two are collectively called the **Affordable Care Act (ACA)**.[1] A more commonly used term is **Obamacare**, named for the president.

The ACA of 2010 was the most significant healthcare reform legislation in the United States since 1965, when Medicare and Medicaid legislation was passed by President Lyndon B. Johnson. The unique political circumstances made it possible for President Obama, a Democrat, to pass the ACA since the Democratic party had a solid majority in both the U.S. House and the Senate.[2] However, the public has had widely divided views on the ACA along partisan lines. A decade after the ACA was passed, the majority of Democrats (86%) had a favorable opinion of the law, while the majority of Republicans had an unfavorable opinion (71%).[3] Various components of the ACA have been modified, and with the election of a Republican president in 2016 the law was threatened with being overturned. The U.S. Supreme Court held initial hearings on the fate of the ACA on November 10, 2020 and on June 17, 2021, the court turned back the challenge to overturn the ACA; thus, the ACA remains a part of the U.S. healthcare system.[4] Concerns about rising healthcare costs and the large numbers of uninsured Americans led to passage of the ACA. The cost of health care has increased dramatically over the past 50 years. In 1970 the average cost of health care per person in the United States was $355 compared to $8,402 in 2010 and $11,172 in 2018, and it was nearly 18% of the **gross domestic product (GDP)** for both 2010 and 2018 compared to 7% in 1970.[5]

Three goals of the Affordable Care Act (ACA) of 2010 were to decrease the number of uninsured, slow the rising costs of health care, and increase the quality and efficiency of health care. This chapter will review the components of the ACA, compare the outcomes with the goals, and summarize changes made in the law since 2010.

Mechanisms for Obtaining Health Insurance with the Affordable Care Act

After implementation of the ACA, the primary source of health insurance continued to be the employer for most Americans (55%),[6] and the self-employed could continue to purchase a health plan from a private carrier. Three new sources of health insurance with the ACA were an **expansion of Medicaid**, the newly established Marketplace or Health Exchanges, and allowing young adults to remain on their parents' health insurance policy until age 26. With the passage of the ACA, individuals had more options for obtaining health insurance (**TABLE 5.1**).[7]

TABLE 5.1 Mechanisms for Obtaining Health Insurance Coverage after the Affordable Care Act (ACA)

Mechanism	Description
Employer	Most large companies offer health benefits, the same as before ACA. For new small-business markets, Small Business Health Options Program (SHOP) offers insurance for businesses with up to 100 employees.
Direct Enrollment	Consumers buy coverage directly from private insurers with new consumer protections.
Parents	Young adults can remain on their parents' health plan until age 26.
Marketplace	Consumers shop for private plans with different cost sharing through a State-Based Marketplace or the Federally Facilitated Marketplace. Based on income, consumers can also apply for Medicaid or the Children's Health Insurance Program (CHIP).
Medicaid	Medicaid coverage expanded in 38 states and Washington, DC.

Data from Blumenthal D, Collins SR. Health care coverage under the Affordable Care Act: a progress report. *N Engl J Med.* 2014;371(3):275-281. doi:10.1056/NEJMhpr1405667

Beginning in 2010, the ACA required that all states expand Medicaid to include nonpregnant adults younger than 65 with incomes 138% of the **federal poverty level (FPL).** The ACA stipulated that the federal government fund 100% of the cost of **Medicaid expansion** for years 2014, 2015, and 2016 with a gradual decrease in funding to 90% in 2020 and thereafter. As originally written, the ACA stipulated that if a state failed to comply with the requirement to expand Medicaid, the state could lose all federal Medicaid funding.[1] Medicaid coverage before the ACA varied by state, and most states did not cover adults without children. Even with the federal government covering much of the cost of Medicaid expansion, many states were reluctant to add the costs to struggling state budgets.[8]

Part-time and self-employed workers and those buying insurance from non-group plans were able to purchase insurance through the new **Health Exchange** (also known as the **Marketplace**) established by individual states or the federal government. States had the option to establish their own **State-Based Marketplace (SBM),** default to a **Federally Facilitated Marketplace (FFM)**, or operate in partnership with the federal government **(FFM-P).**[9] The **HealthCare.gov** site was established as a one-stop shopping site for purchasing a non-group health plan as well as determining eligibility for Medicaid and the Children's Health Insurance Program (CHIP). In addition, the site provides resources for small businesses to offer insurance to their employees through the **Small Business Health Options Program (SHOP).**[7] All marketplaces were required to have **navigators**, individuals employed and trained to assist consumers in selecting and enrolling in a **qualified health plan (QHP)** offered through either a SBM or FFM **(FIGURE 5.1).**[10]

The ACA's **premium subsidies** allowed consumers to purchase affordable health insurance through an **advance premium tax credit** for those with incomes between 100% and 400% of the **federal poverty level (FPL)** or **cost sharing reduction** for those with incomes between 100% and 250%

of the FPL. Employers with 50 or more employees were required to provide health insurance for employees. A fine, the **employer shared responsibility payment**, was triggered if a full-time employee was receiving a Marketplace premium subsidy since the employer is required to provide health insurance for employees. The Internal Revenue Service (IRS) allowed premium subsidies to be purchased through any Marketplace: SBM, FFM, or FFM-P.[11]

The Internet Technology (IT) systems for the Health Exchanges were designed to be streamlined, simple, and coordinated to determine eligibility and enroll consumers in all health subsidy programs and to be integrated with state Medicaid programs to allow consumers to switch from private insurance to Medicaid and CHIP with changes in eligibility status—for example, job changes or marriage. In addition, the process was designed to allow individuals to enroll online, by mail or telephone, or in person. The ACA created the federal **Data Service Hub** to connect the Marketplace with Medicaid and CHIP and common federal data sources (Homeland Security, Social Security Administration, and the Internal Revenue Service) for easy electronic verification of income, immigration, and citizenship status.[12] However, there were several sources of breakdown in the system, as shown by the red burst symbol **(FIGURE 5.2).**

Timeline for Implementing the Affordable Care Act

Parts of the ACA started in 2010, and each successive year additional parts of the ACA were implemented, with all parts of the ACA completed by 2018.[13] Different parts addressed the three major goals of the ACA: (1) to increase access to health care for more Americans: (2) to control healthcare costs; and (3) improve the quality of healthcare delivery **(TABLE 5.2).**

Americans with **preexisting conditions** previously denied health insurance were eligible for health insurance in the first year of implementation. For example, those with the preexisting diagnoses of diabetes or heart disease were often denied health insurance before ACA **(FIGURE 5.3).**

The most important parts of the law started January 1, 2014, when health insurance coverage became effective for those purchasing insurance through the Marketplace. Many Americans were able to purchase health insurance for the first time through the Health Exchanges with federal subsidies **(shared responsibility for coverage)** to pay part of the premium. Another source of health coverage for low-income Americans was Medicaid expansion for those living in states that expanded Medicaid.[13]

Other ways that access to health care were expanded include (1) expansion of the primary care workforce—physicians, nurse practitioners, and physician assistants—through scholarships and loan repayment programs and (2) expanding the **Federally Qualified Health Centers (FQHC)** designed to serve low-income individuals.[13]

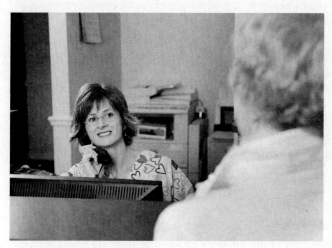

FIGURE 5.1 Navigators work for Health Exchanges to assist consumers in selecting and enrolling in health plans.

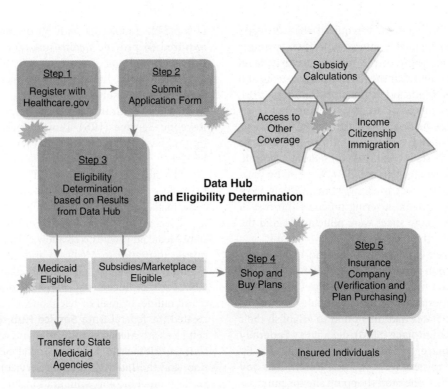

FIGURE 5.2 Federally Facilitated Marketplace eligibility and enrollment.

Modified from Courtot B, Coughlin TA, Upadhayay DK. *The Launch of the Affordable Care Act in Selected States: Building ACA-Compliant Eligibility and Enrollment Systems.* ACA Implementation–Monitoring and Tracking. The Urban Institute. March 2014. https://www.urban.org/sites/default/files/publication/22336/413038-The-Launch-of-the-Affordable-Care-Act-in-Selected-States-Building-ACA-Compliant-Eligibility-and-Enrollment-Systems.PDF

TABLE 5.2 Timeline for Implementing the Affordable Care Act

Year	
2010	• Adult children under 26 years of age are covered by parents' health insurance policy.
	• **Preexisting conditions** could no longer be **used** to exclude applicants from obtaining health insurance (for example, those with type 1 diabetes are able to obtain health insurance when changing jobs and insurance policies).
	• **Clinical preventive services** were required by all health insurance policies (for example, contraceptives, immunizations, and cancer screening).
	• **Scholarship and loan repayment** program for student training: physicians, nurses, and physician assistants.
	• **Federally qualified health centers** were expanded.
2011	• **Limits on nonmedical spending** by private health insurance plans to 15% of the cost of health insurance premiums.
	• The **Center for Medicare and Medicaid Innovation** was established to develop and evaluate new payment and delivery service models.
	• **Pharmaceutical fees** levied on drug manufacturers.
2012	• **Hospital Readmission Reduction Program**: Lowered Medicare payments to hospitals failing to meet the standard for readmission for three diagnoses: heart attack, stroke, and pneumonia.
	• **Accountable Care Organizations**: Incentives for healthcare providers (physicians, hospitals, clinics) to coordinate care to reduce costs and improve quality of care.
2013	• **Electronic health records** required by private health insurers.
	• **Payment reform**: Pilot programs that **bundle** services (for example, surgery plus home care after surgery).
2014	• **Health Exchanges** established by individual states and the federal government for individuals with incomes between 100% and 400% of the federal poverty level (FPL).
	• **Medicaid expansion** for individuals with incomes at 138% of the FPL living in states that chose to expand Medicaid.
	• **Essential health benefits** required by all health insurance policies sold through Health Exchanges.
	• **Shared responsibility for coverage**: Individuals must have health insurance or pay a penalty; employers with at least 100 employees must offer health insurance to employees.

Data from Institute of Medicine. *The Impacts of the Affordable Care Act on Preparedness Resources and Programs: Workshop Summary.* Washington, DC: The National Academies Press; 2014:135–146. Appendix F: Key Features of the Affordable Care Act by Year. https://doi.org/10.17226/18755.

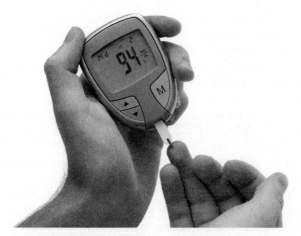

FIGURE 5.3 The Affordable Care Act removed restrictions for those with preexisting diseases such as diabetes from purchasing health insurance.
© gajdamak/Shutterstock.

Programs were established by the **Center for Medicare and Medicaid Innovation** to control costs while improving the quality of health care. The ACA included incentives for healthcare providers—hospitals, clinics, and physicians—to improve outcomes (for example, lower hospital readmissions and lower costs). **Accountable care organizations (ACO),** offered through Medicare, were rewarded for lowering healthcare costs and providing quality care. New payment reforms such as **bundling payments** for surgery and follow-up home health care were part of the ACA.[1]

A program established by the ACA, the **Hospital Readmission Reduction Program (HRRP),** includes incentives for healthcare providers to improve the quality and efficiency of health care. The HRRP used incentives for hospitals to avoid readmission rates for three conditions: heart attack, heart failure, and pneumonia. CMS data showed that one in five Medicare patients receiving hospital care was being readmitted within 30 days of discharge, at an estimated cost of $26 million.[14] Under the HRRP, the amount of money that hospitals receive from Medicare reimbursement is based on the readmission rate. The criteria for readmission is an unplanned hospital admission within 30 days of discharge from the same or another hospital. Conditions evaluated for hospital readmission were heart attack, heart failure, and pneumonia. For patients readmitted to the hospital for any of these three conditions, Medicare determined if the hospital met the criteria for readmission based on a formula adjusted for wages and the base amount paid per each **diagnosis-related group**—for example, pneumonia.[14] If the readmission rate failed to meet the standard, Medicare reimbursements were reduced for hospital admissions for Medicare patients admitted for any condition, not just the three conditions used to establish the hospital readmission rate.

TABLE 5.3 Essential Health Benefits Required by All Qualified Health Plans
Ambulatory patient services
Emergency services
Hospitalization
Maternity and newborn care
Mental health and substance use disorder services including behavioral health treatment
Prescription drugs
Rehabilitative services and devices
Laboratory services
Preventive and wellness services and chronic disease management
Pediatric services, including oral and vision care

Data from How the ACA Will Change the Health Care Delivery System. In Institute of Medicine. *The Impacts of the Affordable Care Act on Preparedness Resources and Programs: Workshop Summary.* Washington, DC: The National Academies Press; 2014:15–21.

ACOs are networks of physicians, hospitals, and other providers that agree to participate for at least three years. As part of the ACA, ACOs create incentives for hospitals and healthcare workers to coordinate patient care across all settings—physicians' offices, hospitals, and long-term care. These programs reward ACOs that reduce the rate of growth in healthcare spending while providing quality care—for example, reducing duplication of services and preventing medical errors. The ACO is eligible for additional Medicare payments or bonuses for improving quality and reducing costs of patient care. ACOs that failed to meet the standard for quality and cost savings were financially responsible for the healthcare costs of patients instead of Medicare. CMS monitors quality and financial data from each ACO to determine if goals are being met.[15]

Essential Health Benefits

Requiring **essential health benefits** in all health plans ensured the same benefits for all Americans regardless of the source of insurance coverage. All health plans, both private and government-sponsored plans—Medicare, Medicaid, and state and federal exchanges—were required to include essential health benefits beginning in 2014. **Clinical preventive services**—contraceptive services, cancer screening, and immunizations—were also required as a part of all health policies obtained through the Health Exchanges, Medicare, and Medicaid **(TABLE 5.3).**[16] Preventive services are less costly than treating a serious disease; for example, cancer diagnosed in the early stages is easier and less costly to treat than cancer that has spread throughout the body, and immunizations prevent costly illnesses requiring hospitalization.

MODIFICATION OF THE AFFORDABLE CARE ACT

Republicans threatened to repeal and replace the ACA during the presidency of Donald Trump beginning in 2016; instead, different parts of the ACA were weakened through various mechanisms including executive order, tax laws, underfunding components of the ACA, and lawsuits. Between 2016 and 2018, the Centers for Medicare and Medicaid Services (CMS) slashed funding by 80% for the navigator program in 34 states with Marketplaces facilitated by the federal government.[17] Navigators are needed to provide outreach and enrollment assistance to ensure that those who are eligible are able to purchase health insurance through the Marketplace.

In 2017, the Tax Cuts and Jobs Act of 2017 eliminated the **individual mandate** for everyone to have health insurance coverage and removed the tax penalty for those who did not purchase health insurance and were not eligible for public health insurance (Medicare, Medicaid, or Marketplace).[18] However, a few states implemented laws mandating that everyone have insurance for fear that young healthy adults would not purchase insurance through the Marketplace; the expectation was that the premiums would increase in price, causing health insurance to be unaffordable for many. In an effort to keep premiums affordable, these states have a mandate as of 2020: California, Massachusetts, New Jersey, Delaware, Rhode Island, and Vermont as well as the District of Columbia.[19]

In 2018, President Trump signed an **executive order**, "Promoting Healthcare Choice and Competition across the United States," that allowed states to offer **short-term, limited-duration** health insurance policies.[20] These policies are not required to comply with requirements of the ACA: covering preexisting conditions or providing minimal essential benefits, maternity care, mental health services, or prescription drugs. The costs of the premiums are usually lower than insurance policies that meet ACA requirements. However, short-term, limited-duration policies limit benefits by limiting the number of doctor visits or the dollar amount covered per day during hospitalizations; those with preexisting conditions are not eligible for these policies.[21]

Individual Mandate and Medicaid Expansion

The two most unpopular parts of the ACA were the requirements for individuals without access to employer-covered insurance to purchase insurance through the Marketplace (individual mandate) and for states to expand Medicaid. Beginning in 2014, all American citizens and permanent residents were required to have **minimum essential coverage** (health insurance) or pay a tax penalty. The Internal Revenue Service (IRS) monitored compliance to minimum essential coverage.[22]

Because of the unpopularity of the ACA, a lawsuit was filed in Federal District Court in 2011 to challenge the constitutionality of both the individual mandate and Medicaid expansion by the National Federation of Independent Business, 26 states, and several individuals (*National Federation of Independent Business v. Sebelius*). The Federal District Court upheld Medicaid expansion but not the individual mandate. When the case was brought to the Supreme Court in 2012, however, the individual mandate was upheld, but Medicaid expansion was ruled to be a violation of the Constitution, since states were threatened with loss of their existing Medicaid funding (an estimated 10% of state budgets) for failing to comply with the expansion. Therefore, the Supreme Court ruled that expansion of Medicaid by individual states was optional.[23] **TABLE 5.4** lists some of the modifications and methods used to change the ACA.

The interpretation of the IRS was that the cost of premiums purchased through any Marketplace—SBM, FFM, or FFM-P—ensured eligibility for tax credits by individuals.[11] However, the IRS ruling was challenged in the federal courts based on the wording of the ACA that specified that the Marketplace be established by the state. Lawsuits brought to federal appeals court disputed both the ACA language about Marketplace premium subsidies and the authority of the IRS to grant premium subsidies for those who purchased plans through the FFM. Because of the conflicting rulings on premium subsidies, the case moved to the Supreme Court to be resolved. In *King v. Burwell*, the Supreme Court ruled in favor of the U.S. government on June 25, 2015, allowing an estimated 6.4 million Americans who had purchased health plans through the federal marketplace to continue to receive premium subsidies.[28]

Contraceptive Coverage

The ACA requires that all health insurance policies cover women's preventive health services including Food and Drug Administration– (FDA-) approved prescription contraceptives and counseling on birth control methods. However, some employers with religious objections to contraceptives challenged this requirement. Women had contraceptive coverage if they had insurance through an employer that did not object to contraceptives based on religious grounds. Women who worked for nonprofit healthcare institutions or universities affiliated with religious organizations that objected to contraceptives usually had access to contraceptives; however, the employer was not required to pay for the coverage. Instead, women could obtain coverage directly through their insurance plans.[29]

The Supreme Court heard two cases with conflicting outcomes in lower courts involving for-profit employers that were opposed to contraceptive coverage on the grounds that requiring coverage interfered with religious freedom under the **Religious Freedom Restoration Act of 1993**. The two employers were Hobby Lobby, a chain of craft stores owned by a Christian family; and Conestoga Wood Specialties, a manufacturer of wooden cabinets owned by Mennonites. The lower courts ruled in favor of Hobby Lobby but not Conestoga Wood Specialties. On June 30, 2014, the Supreme Court in *Burwell v. Hobby Lobby, Inc.* ruled in favor of Hobby Lobby and Conestoga, both

TABLE 5.4 Changes in the Affordable Care Act (ACA) since 2010		
Modification of Affordable Care Act	**Law or Lawsuit**	**Impact of Change**
Medicaid Expansion	**Supreme Court Decision** *National Federation of Independent Business v. Sibelius,* June 28, 2012.[23]	Individual states not required to expand Medicaid.
Marketplace Premium Subsidies	**Supreme Court Decision** *King v. Burwell,* June 25, 2015.[24]	Individuals eligible for premium subsidies can purchase health insurance from either a state or federal exchange.
Navigators	**Centers for Medicare and Medicaid, 2018.**[17]	Reduced funding for outreach and enrollment assistance programs.
Contraceptives	**Supreme Court Decisions** *Burwell v. Hobby Lobby Stores, Inc.,* June 30, 2014.[25] *Little Sisters of the Poor v. Pennsylvania,* July 8, 2020.[26]	Religiously affiliated or closely affiliated corporations opposed to contraceptives are exempt Employers with moral or religious opposition to contraceptives are exempt.
Individual Mandate	Tax Cuts and Jobs Act of 2017, January 1, 2019.[18]	Individuals not required to have health insurance or pay a tax penalty.
Essential Benefits	**Executive Order** "Promoting Healthcare Choice and Competition across the United States," October 2, 2018.[19]	ACA requirements do not apply to short-term, limited-duration health insurance plans.

Data from Supreme Court of the United States of America. *National Federation of Independent Business v. Sebelius.* June 28, 2012.
Supreme Court of the United States of American. *King v. Burwell.* March 25, 2015. Center on Budget and Policy Priorities. Sabotage Watch: Tracking Efforts to Undermine the ACA.
January 4, 2021. https://www.cbpp.org/sabotage-watch-tracking-efforts-to-undermine-the-aca.
Supreme Court of the United States of America. *Burwell v. Hobby Lobby Stores, Inc.* June 30, 2014.
Supreme Court of the United States. 19–431. *Little Sisters of the Poor v. Pennsylvania.* July 8, 2020.
H.R. 1. (115th) Public Law 115–97, December 22, 2017. *Elimination of Shared Responsibility Payment for Individuals Failing to Maintain Minimum Essential Coverage.* Congressional Record, Vol 163 (2017).
Short-Term, Limited-Duration Insurance; Final Rule. 83 *Federal Register* 150. August 3, 2018. Garfield R, Oregera K, Damico A, *The Uninsured and the ACA: A Primer.* Kaiser Family Foundation. January 2019.

closely held corporations (50% or more of ownership held by a small number of family members), on grounds that requiring coverage of contraceptive drugs or devices would violate their religion beliefs.[25]

As a result of this ruling, female employees had no or limited coverage for contraceptives depending on the religious beliefs of their employer. Houses of worship are exempt from providing contraceptive coverage. Religiously affiliated employers or for-profit closely held corporations are required to request an accommodation—the insurance provider must pay for contraceptive coverage for female employees (instead of the employer). The *Burwell v. Hobby Lobby* ruling did not apply to other employers that were mandated to provide contraceptive coverage for female employees. An employer that qualifies for an accommodation must submit an application through the insurance provider or write a letter to the Secretary of Health and Human Services to request an accommodation.[25]

Another lawsuit challenged the mandatory contraceptive benefit by employers as well as the insurance provider. Little Sisters of the Poor, an organization of nuns that provides services for the elderly, were opposed to the contraceptive benefit of female employees on religious and moral grounds. In 2020, ***Little Sisters of the Poor v. Pennsylvania***, the U.S. Supreme Court ruled in favor of the Little Sisters of the Poor, which allowed an exemption from contraceptives, an essential benefit of the ACA.[26]

IMPACT OF THE AFFORDABLE CARE ACT

The most significant impact of the ACA was the number of people who had health insurance after 2010 when ACA was implemented. Health care costs as measured by the **national health expenditure (NHE)** slowed to 3.8% between 2010 and 2016 and increased to 4.6% in 2019. Programs through the Center for Medicare and Medicaid Innovation that showed the most success were ACOs, which saved in Medicare costs while improving the quality of care.

Increased Numbers of Individuals with Health Insurance

As a result of the ACA, an estimated 20 million individuals gained health coverage between 2010 and 2016, lowering the percentage of the uninsured from nearly 18% to 10%.[27] By 2018 the percentage of the uninsured had dropped to 8.5%, and only 5.5% of children under age 19 were uninsured (**FIGURE 5.4**).[6]

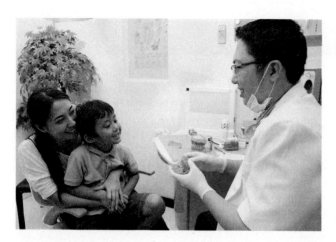

FIGURE 5.4 As a result of the Affordable Care Act, low-income adults and children were able to enroll in either Medicaid or the Children's Health Insurance Program.
© Creativa Images/Shutterstock.

The majority of the newly insured were Latinos as well as low- and middle-income adults who lived in states that expanded Medicaid.[30] As of August 2020, Medicaid expansion had been adopted in 38 states and Washington, DC, with expansion yet to be implemented in two of the states and 12 states that were not expected to expand Medicaid.[31] An estimated 2 million individuals were not able to obtain government-sponsored health care in states that didn't expand Medicaid because of income guidelines for both Medicaid and premium subsidies for those purchasing health insurance through Health Exchanges. Those who fell into the **coverage gap** had incomes that were too high to qualify for Medicaid and too low to qualify for premium subsidies through the Marketplace. The majority of individuals in the coverage gap were adults without dependent children who lived in the Southern states of Texas, Florida, Georgia, and North Carolina.[32]

The ACA could cause an unintended disparity in healthcare coverage and access, especially in the South where many states chose to not expand Medicaid. One-third of the U.S. population lives in the South, and nearly half of Southerners live in three states—Texas, Florida, and Georgia—none of which expanded Medicaid.[33] Southerners are also more likely to be uninsured than those living in the Midwest or Northeast primarily because of the type of work available in blue-collar industries and small businesses. Employers in these settings typically don't offer health coverage, and private insurance is unaffordable.[33] Although Medicaid expansion in the South would increase health coverage, 11 states in the South opted out of expansion.

Indicators of Healthcare Costs

One indicator of healthcare costs is the NHE, which slowed between 2010 and 2014 with an average annual rate of 3.8%, the lowest since tracking began in 1960.[34] These changes in the NHE parallel the period of time when the ACA was implemented. Then there was a gradual rise in the NHE beginning in 2017 (4.7% NHE) followed by a slight decrease in 2019 (4.6% NHE).[35]

Another indicator of healthcare cost is **uncompensated care**—also described as charity care—nonreimbursed hospital care for the uninsured or underinsured. Estimates are that uncompensated care costs were lowered by $5.7 billion in 2014 with $4.2 billion savings coming from Medicaid expansion states and $1.5 billion coming from non-expansion states.[36] The percentage of hospitals reporting uncompensated care was less in states that expanded Medicaid (2.8%) compared to non-expansion states (7.2%) before October 1, 2017.[37] Reduction in costs came primarily from fewer uncompensated hospital admissions and emergency room visits because the newly insured were able to obtain health care from a primary provider, which costs much less than going to the emergency room.[36] The estimated cost for each uninsured individual in 2013 was $1,005, and a total of $49 billion was spent for all uncompensated care in the United States.[38] Data analysis from eight states that expanded Medicaid reported a savings by replacing state general funds with federal funds received by expanding Medicaid. These states reported a drop in uncompensated hospital care.[39]

Programs to Control Healthcare Costs and Improve Quality of Care

Implementation of the ACA programs that were designed to reduce health care costs and improve the quality of care have shown mixed results. Ten years of data are now available to evaluate these programs and make modifications to continue to improve outcomes. Evaluations of the Hospital Readmission Reduction Program for the years 2010 through 2013 showed promising results with lower readmission rates; however, in the third year of the program, a record number of 2,610 hospitals received reduced payments for Medicare patients.[40] Penalties for excessive rates of hospital readmissions were expected to save the federal government $428 million as a result of lower reimbursement rates for these hospitals.[41] In 2019, 83% of eligible hospitals were penalized, with 2,583 hospitals charged a total of $563 million for readmissions. Over the 10 years of the program, a similar number of hospitals have paid a penalty for high readmission rates without a significant reduction in readmission rates.[42]

The ACOs were more successful in achieving the goals of saving costs while maintaining or improving the quality of care. Both the Medicare Shared Savings Program ACOs and the Pioneer ACOs showed improvements over time in the quality of care and a reduced cost of medical care. In 2018 there were 548 Medicare Shared Savings Program ACOs with a total of 10.1 million Medicare beneficiaries.[42]

Pioneer ACOs were able to demonstrate a net savings to Medicare of $314 million in 2012 and $99 million in 2013, while the Medicare Shared Savings Program ACOs showed a net savings to Medicare of nearly $740 million in 2018. The Pioneer ACOs also demonstrated a reduction in visits to the emergency department. Medicare Shared Savings Program ACOs led by physicians showed more improvement than those led by hospitals. Both ACO programs received high ratings for the quality of care.[42]

SUMMARY

The Affordable Care Act (ACA) of 2010 was designed to increase access to health insurance, reduce health care costs, and improve the efficiency and quality of health care. The ACA added two new ways to increase access to health insurance for those not covered by employer health insurance: expansion of Medicaid and the Marketplace.

Certain provisions of the ACA were opposed by the states and certain businesses. Opposition by states to expand Medicaid because of concerns about the long-term financial burden of state governments led to the U.S. Supreme Court modifying the ACA to make Medicaid expansion by states optional rather than mandatory. Controversy about the requirement of the law to cover prescriptions for contraceptives led to the Supreme Court decision to support religiously affiliated businesses, closely held corporations, or other employers that oppose contraceptives for female employees for religious or moral reasons to opt out of contraceptive coverage. The Supreme Court ruled in favor of the U.S. government in allowing premium subsidies for individuals buying policies through the Federal Facilitated Marketplace.

Other changes to the ACA were (1) elimination of the individual mandate and penalty for not having health insurance beginning in 2019, (2) underfunding the navigator program that provided outreach and assistance with enrolling in health insurance in 2018, and (3) introduction of short-term, limited-duration health insurance plans in 2018 that are not required to meet ACA requirements such as essential benefits.

The most significant impact of the ACA was the number of people who had health insurance after 2010 when the ACA was implemented. Healthcare costs as measured by the national health expenditure (NHE) slowed to 3.8% between 2010 and 2016 and increased to 4.6% in 2019. Programs through the Center for Medicare and Medicaid Innovation that showed the most success in improving efficiency and quality of care were ACOs, which saved in Medicare costs while improving the quality of care.

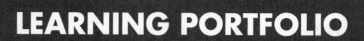

LEARNING PORTFOLIO

Study Points

1. Concerns about nearly one-fifth of the gross domestic product (GDP) being spent on health care and large numbers of individuals being uninsured led to passage of the Affordable Care Act (ACA) in 2010. The ACA, also known as Obamacare, became law in March 2010 with goals of increasing access to health care for the uninsured while at the same time improving healthcare quality and controlling healthcare costs.

2. As a result of the ACA, individuals were able to obtain health insurance in two new ways: Medicaid expansion to include those with incomes at 138% of the FPL and the Marketplace for individuals with income between 100% and 400% of the FPL. The federal government subsidizes plans purchased through the Marketplace, thus lowering the costs of premiums.

3. The ACA was implemented in phases beginning in 2010 and ending in 2018. The federal and state governments established the Marketplace between 2010 and 2012, and uninsured people were able to obtain health insurance through expanded Medicaid and the Marketplace beginning in January 2014.

4. The ACA requires all health insurance policies to include minimum essential benefits for all applicants, and individuals with preexisting health conditions such as diabetes were no longer denied access to health insurance.

5. The Data Service Hub was designed to determine eligibility for enrolling in Medicaid, CHIP, or subsidized Marketplace policies based on citizenship and income.

6. Supreme Court rulings modified three parts of the ACA that had been contested by lower courts. The outcomes of the rulings were that (1) expanding Medicaid became optional for individual states, (2) premium subsidies were allowed for individuals enrolling through a Federally Facilitated Marketplace, and (3) contraceptive coverage was exempted for female employees of religiously affiliated, closely affiliated corporations, or employers with moral or religious opposition to contraceptives.

7. Many Southern states opted out of Medicaid expansion, which resulted in a disparity in access to health insurance and health care for those living in the South compared to other regions of the United States where Medicaid was expanded.

8. Changes to the ACA beginning in 2017 were (1) elimination of the individual mandate and the penalty for individuals without health insurance, (2) underfunding the navigator program, and (3) introduction of short-term, limited duration health insurance policies that were exempt from ACA requirements.

9. National health expenditures (NHE) slowed between 2010 and 2014 to 3.8% and rose to 4.6% in 2019. Uncompensated care reported by hospitals was higher in states that did not expand Medicaid (7.2%) compared to states that expanded Medicaid (2.8%).

10. Accountable care organizations (ACOs) established by the ACA to reduce healthcare costs while improving quality were successful in achieving these goals with significant cost savings to Medicare while maintaining or improving the quality of care.

11. During the Republican administration of 2016–2020 a lawsuit was filed to overturn the ACA; however, the U.S. Supreme Court ruled against overturning the ACA on June 17, 2021, and the ACA remains a part of the U.S. healthcare system.

Issues for Discussion

1. Go to the HealthCare.gov website and find out if the state where you live has a State-Based Marketplace. Go through the steps of applying and enrolling in a healthcare plan for the state where you live. Was the website easy to use? If not, why not?

2. A video developed by the Henry J. Kaiser Family Foundation is a quick and understandable overview of the different mechanisms for obtaining healthcare coverage as a result of the ACA. What are four ways that individuals can obtain health insurance as a result of the ACA? Explain preexisting conditions. Define the individual mandate; which states have the individual mandate? *Note:* This video was developed before ACA was implemented; the individual mandate (as described in the video) is no longer required by the federal government, although some states have the individual mandate. https://www.youtube.com/watch?v=JZkk6ueZt-U

3. Go to the Kaiser Family Foundation website to the section *FAQs: Health Insurance Marketplace and the ACA*. Review one of the following sections and report during class discussion:

   - Cost Sharing Reduction
   - Employer-Sponsored Health Coverage
   - Help Paying Marketplace Premiums
   - Immigrants
   - Short-Term and Other Policies Sold outside of the Marketplace

   https://www.kff.org/faqs/faqs-health-insurance-marketplace-and-the-aca/?view=1

LEARNING PORTFOLIO

Enrichment Activities

1. Determine your eligibility for health insurance through the Marketplace or Medicaid.

   - Compare your income with the federal poverty level (FPL) by checking the U.S. Department of Health and Human Services website.
   - Compare your income with the FPL. What percent of the FPL is your income?

Use the Health Insurance Marketplace Calculator to determine your eligibility for insurance through the Marketplace or Medicaid.

U.S. Health and Human Services website: https://aspe.hhs .gov/poverty-guidelines

Health Insurance Marketplace Calculator: Kaiser Family Foundation website: https://www.kff.org/interactive/subsidy -calculator/

CASE STUDY: HEALTHCARE REFORM

Becky lives in Austin, TX, with her husband and their 10-year-old daughter. She plans to open a small bakery and coffee shop in her neighborhood and expects to hire several part-time college students to work 10 to 15 hours per week. Her husband works as a firefighter, and the family has health insurance through his employer. Becky is evaluating her options for health insurance for her employees.

The following questions are based on this case study.

1. True or false? All of Becky's employees are required to have health insurance, or they will be required to pay a penalty.

2. What option would not be available for health insurance for Becky's employees?
   A. Remain on their parent's health plan if younger than 26
   B. Enroll in Medicaid
   C. Purchase insurance through the Marketplace
   D. Purchase a health plan through the college or university

References

1. United States Congress (111th). *Health Care and Education Reconciliation Act of 2010*. H.R. 4872. https://www.hhs.gov /sites/default/files/reconciliation-law.pdf Accessed August 16, 2021.

2. Shi L, Singh DA. *Delivering Health Care in America. A Systems Approach.* 7th ed., Burlington, MA: Jones & Bartlett Learning; 2019:548–549.

3. Kaiser Family Foundation. *KFF Health Tracking Poll: The Public's Views on the ACA.* December 18, 2020. https://www.kff .org/interactive/kff-health-tracking-poll-the-publics-views -on-the-aca/. Accessed January 25, 2021.

4. Keith K. 2021. Supreme Court Rejects ACA Challenge; Law Remains Fully Intact. June 17, 2021. *Health Affairs Blog,* https://www.healthaffairs.org/do/10.1377/hblog20210617 .665248/full/ Accessed July 7, 2021.

5. Kamal R. Cox C, McDermott D, Kurani N. *COVID-19 Repercussions May Outweigh Recent Gains in U.S. Health System Performance.* Peterson-Kaiser FF Health Systems Tracker. July 23, 2020. https://www.healthsystemtracker .org/brief/covid-19-repercussions-may-outweigh-recent -gains-in-u-s-health-system-performance/. Accessed September 4, 2020.

6. Berchick ER, Barnett JC, Upton RD. *Current Population Reports,* P60-267(RV), Health Insurance Coverage in the United States: 2018, U.S. Government Printing Office, Washington, DC, 2019.

7. Blumenthal D, Collins SR. Health Care Coverage under the Affordable Care Act—A Progress Report. *N Engl J Med.* 2014; *371*:275–281.

8. Baron S. *10 Frequently Asked Questions about Medicaid Expansion.* Center for American Progress. April 2, 2013. https://www.americanprogress.org/issues/healthcare /news/2013/04/02/58922/10-frequently-asked-questions -about-medicaid-expansion/. Accessed September 14, 2020.

9. Centers for Medicare and Medicaid Services. The Center for Consumer Information and Insurance Oversight (CCIIO). *State-Based Exchanges.* https://www.cms.gov/CCIIO/Resources /Fact-Sheets-and-FAQs/state-marketplaces Accessed August 16, 2021.

10. Hill F, Courtot B, Wilkerson M. *Reaching and Enrolling the Uninsured: Early Efforts to Implement the Affordable Care Act.* The Urban Institute. October 2013. http://www.urban .org/research/publication/reaching-and-enrolling -uninsured-early-efforts-implement-affordable-care-act Accessed January 25, 2021.

11. The Henry J. Kaiser Family Foundation. *Summary of the Affordable Care Act.* April 25, 2013. https://www.kff.org/health -reform/fact-sheet/summary-of-the-affordable-careact/ Accessed August 16, 2021.

12. Courtot B, Coughlin TA, Upadhayay DK. *The Launch of the Affordable Care Act in Selected States: Building ACA-Compliant Eligibility and Enrollment Systems. ACA*

Implementation–Monitoring and Tracking. The Urban Institute. March 2014. https://www.urban.org/sites/default/files/publication/22336/413038-The-Launch-of-the-Affordable-Care-Act-in-Selected-States-Building-ACA-Compliant-Eligibility-and-Enrollment-Systems.PDF Accessed August 16, 2021.

13. Institute of Medicine. *The Impacts of the Affordable Care Act on Preparedness Resources and Programs: Workshop Summary.* Washington, DC: The National Academies Press, 2014. Appendix F: Key Features of the Affordable Care Act by Year. 135–146. https://doi.org/10.17226/18755.

14. Centers for Medicare and Medicaid Services. *Readmissions Reduction Program.* https://www.cms.gov/Medicare/Medicare-Fee-for-Service-Payment/AcuteInpatientPPS/Readmissions-Reduction-Program Accessed August 16, 2021.

15. Centers for Medicare and Medicaid Services. *About the Program.* https://www.cms.gov/Medicare/Medicare-Fee-for-Service-Payment/sharedsavingsprogram/about Accessed January 25, 2021.

16. Chapter 2: How the ACA Will Change the Health Care Delivery System. In: Institute of Medicine. *The Impacts of the Affordable Care Act on Preparedness Resources and Programs: Workshop Summary.* Washington, DC: The National Academies Press, 2014. 15–21. https://doi.org/10.17226/18755

17. Center on Budget and Policy Priorities. *Sabotage Watch: Tracking Efforts to Undermine the ACA.* January 4, 2021. https://www.cbpp.org/sabotage-watch-tracking-efforts-to-undermine-the-aca

18. United States Congress (115th). *Individual Mandate.* H.R.1. https://www.congress.gov/115/bills/hr1/BILLS-115hr1enr.pdf Accessed August 16, 2021.

19. Tolbert J, Diaz M, Hall C, Mengistu S. State Actions to Improve the Affordability of Health Insurance in the Individual Market. Kaiser Family Foundation, July 2019. https://www.kff.org/wp-content/uploads/2019/07/Issue-Brief-State-Actions-to-Improve-the-Affordability-of-Health-Insurance-in-the-Individual-Market.pdf Accessed September 5, 2020.

20. Short-Term, Limited-Duration Insurance; Final Rule. 83 *Federal Register* 150. August 3, 2018. https://www.govinfo.gov/content/pkg/FR-2018-08-03/pdf/2018-16568.pdf

21. Kaiser Family Foundation. *For Consumers Considering Short-Term Policies.* October 2019 Fact Sheet. http://files.kff.org/attachment/Fact-Sheet-ACA-Open-Enrollment-For-Consumers-Considering-Short-term-Policies

22. Internal Revenue Service. *Individual Shared Responsibility Provision.* https://www.irs.gov/affordable-care-act/individuals-and-families/individual-shared-responsibility-provision Updated October 21, 2020. Accessed January 25, 2021.

23. Supreme Court of the United States of America. *National Federation of Independent Business v. Sebelius.* June 28, 2012. https://www.supremecourt.gov/opinions/11pdf/11-393c3a2.pdf

24. Supreme Court of the United States of American. *King v. Burwell.* March 25, 2015. https://www.supremecourt.gov/opinions/14pdf/14-114_qol1.pdf

25. Supreme Court of the United States of America. *Burwell v. Hobby Lobby Stores, Inc.* June 30, 2014. http://www.supremecourt.gov/opinions/13pdf/13-354_olp1.pdf

26. Supreme Court of the United States. 19–431. *Little Sisters of the Poor v. Pennsylvania.* July 8, 2020. https://www.supremecourt.gov/opinions/19pdf/19-431_5i36.pdf

27. Garfield R, Oregera K, Damico A. *The Uninsured and the ACA: A Primer.* Kaiser Family Foundation. January 2019. http://files.kff.org/attachment/The-Uninsured-and-the-ACA-A-Primer-Key-Facts-about-Health-Insurance-and-the-Uninsured-amidst-Changes-to-the-Affordable-Care-Act. Accessed January 25, 2021.

28. Collins SR, Blumenthal D. Coverage and Financial Security Preserved for Millions of Americans in the Supreme Court Ruling for the Government. *The Commonwealth Fund Blog.* June 25, 2015. https://www.commonwealthfund.org/blog/2015/coverage-and-financial-security-preserved-millions-americans-supreme-court-ruling Accessed August 16, 2021.

29. The Henry J. Kaiser Family Foundation. *How Does Where You Work Affect Your Contraceptive Coverage?* October 20, 2014. http://kff.org/womens-health-policy/fact-sheet/how-does-where-you-work-affect-your-contraceptive-coverage/ Accessed September 14, 2020.

30. Collins SR, Rasmussen PW, Doty MM. *Gaining Ground: America's Health Insurance Coverage and Access to Care after the Affordable Care Act's First Open Enrollment Period.* The Commonwealth Fund, July 2014. https://www.commonwealthfund.org/publications/issue-briefs/2014/jul/gaining-ground-americans-health-insurance-coverage-and-access Accessed January 25, 2021.

31. *Status of State Medicaid Expansion Decisions: Interactive Map.* Kaiser Family Foundation, November 2, 2020. https://www.kff.org/medicaid/issue-brief/status-of-state-medicaid-expansion-decisions-interactive-map/ Accessed January 25, 2021.

32. Garfield R, Orgera K, Damico A. The Coverage Gap: Uninsured Poor Adults in States That Do Not Expand Medicaid. *Issue Brief.* January 2020. Kaiser Family Foundation. https://www.kff.org/medicaid/issue-brief/the-coverage-gap-uninsured-poor-adults-in-states-that-do-not-expand-medicaid/ Accessed January 25, 2021.

33. Stephen S, Artiga S, Paradise J. Health Coverage and Care in the South in 2014 and Beyond. The Henry J. Kaiser Family Foundation. *Issue Brief,* June 2014. https://www.kff.org/wp-content/uploads/2014/04/8577-health-coverage-and-care-in-the-south-in-2014-and-beyond-june-2014-update.pdf Accessed January 25, 2021.

34. American Hospital Association. *Health Care Spending Hits Record Low.* https://www.aha.org/guidesreports/2014-03-11-health-care-spending-growth-hits-record-low Accessed January 25, 2020.

35. Centers for Medicare and Medicaid Services. *National Health Expenditures 2019 Highlights.* https://www.cms.gov/files/document/highlights.pdf Accessed January 25, 2021.

LEARNING PORTFOLIO

36. DeLeire T, Karen K, McDonald R. Impact of Insurance Expansion on Hospital Uncompensated Care Costs in 2014. *ASPE Issue Brief.* September 24, 2014. https://aspe.hhs.gov/system/files/pdf/77061/ib_UncompensatedCare.pdf Accessed January 25, 2021.

37. Medicaid and CHIP Payment and Access Commission (MACPAC). *Report to Congress on Medicaid and CHIP.* March 2020. Washington, DC: MACPAC. https://www.macpac.gov/wp-content/uploads/2020/03/March-2020-Report-to-Congress-on-Medicaid-and-CHIP.pdf Accessed August 16, 2021.

38. Coughlin TA, Holahan J, Caswell K, McGrath M. *Uncompensated Care for the Uninsured in 2013: A Detailed Examination.* The Henry J. Kaiser Family Foundation. May 30, 2014. https://www.kff.org/uninsured/report/uncompensated-care-for-the-uninsured-in-2013-a-detailed-examination/ Accessed January 25, 2021.

39. Bachrach D, Boozang P, Herring A, Reyneri D. States Expanding Medicaid See Significant Budget Savings and Revenue Gains. *Issue Brief.* March 1, 2016. Robert Wood Johnson Foundation. https://www.rwjf.org/en/library/research/2015/04/states-expanding-medicaid-see-significant-budget-savings-and-rev.html Accessed August 16, 2021.

40. Brennan N. *Real-Time Reporting of Medicare Readmissions Data.* Centers for Medicare and Medicaid Services. http://www.academyhealth.org/files/2014/monday/brennan.pdf Accessed January 25, 2021.

41. Rau J. Medicare Fines 2,610 Hospitals in Third Round of Readmission Penalties. *Kaiser Health News.* October 2, 2014. https://www.commonwealthfund.org/evidence-decade-innovation-impact-payment-and-delivery-system-reforms-affordable-care-act Accessed August 16, 2021.

42. Lewis C, Abrams M, Seervai S, Blumenthal D. *Evidence from a Decade of Innovation. The Impact of the Payment and Delivery System Reforms of the Affordable Care Act.* April 1, 2020. https://www.commonwealthfund.org/evidence-decade-innovation-impact-payment-and-delivery-system-reforms-affordable-care-act Accessed August 16, 2021.

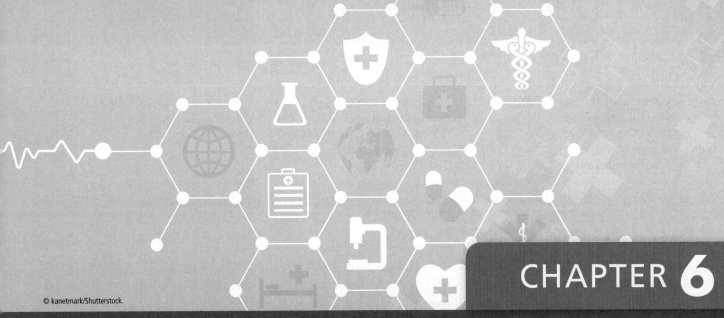

CHAPTER **6**

Medical and Health Information Technology

OBJECTIVES

After studying this chapter, the student should be able to:

- Differentiate between medical and health information technology.
- Name examples of medical terminology innovations.
- List commonly used health information technology solutions.
- Explain the concepts of confidentiality and security in protecting patient health information.

KEY TERMS

3D printing
Apps
Bar coding technology
Billing process
Biomedical engineer
Clinical decision support system
 (CDSS)

Cloud computing
Computerized physician order
 entry system (CPOE)
Confidentiality
Electronic health record (EHR)
Electronic materials
 management

e-prescribing
Functional magnetic resonance
 imaging (fMRI)
Health information technology
 (health IT)
Interoperability
Interventional X-ray machine

Master patient index (MPI)
Medical technology
Mobile technology
Patient portal
Patient registration

Patient registration process
Picture archiving and
    communication system (PACS)
Speech recognition software
Telemedicine

Vendor-neutral archive (VNA)
Vital statistics
Wearable technology

Introduction

The healthcare industry and its many professions have experienced numerous changes over the past century. Among the most striking is the development of medical technology and one of its subsets called health information technology. **Medical technology** refers to the procedures, equipment, and processes by which medical care is delivered. Examples include new medical and surgical procedures (e.g., angioplasty, joint replacements), drugs (e.g., biologic agents), and medical devices (e.g., digestible sensors, pacemakers, computed tomography [CT] scanners, implantable cardioverter-defibrillators). An example of medical technology is seen in FIGURE 6.1.

By contrast, health information technology is focused on the support aspect of delivering patient care. **Health information technology (health IT)** refers to an array of technologies to record, store, retrieve, protect, share, and analyze health information. Examples include support systems such as electronic health records and speech recognition software. Both medical and health information technology are the focus of this chapter.

MEDICAL TECHNOLOGY

Medical technology includes a multitude of products used to diagnose and monitor human conditions and diseases. This technology also is available to treat diseases that were once considered high risk or even fatal and includes instruments used to perform less invasive operations.

The continuing flow of new medical technology results from many factors. Healthcare practitioners are always working to find better ways to treat their patients, and incorporating new technologies is one way to do so. Some healthcare practitioners may feel the need to offer the "latest and greatest" in care because they compete with other providers

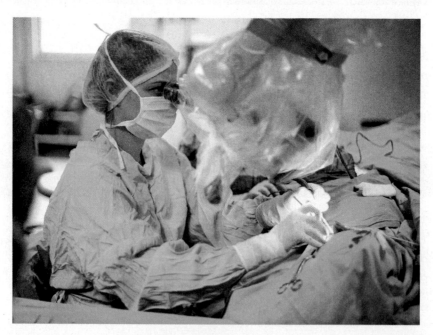

FIGURE 6.1 Doctor operating using a surgical microscope.
© ByeByeTokyo/iStockPhoto.

for patients. Professional goals such as peer recognition, tenure, and prestige may influence healthcare professionals to find ways to improve their practice through use of medical technology.

Consumers also are a prime consideration in the growth of medical technology. Consumer goals to achieve and maintain good health can often be met through advances in medical technology. Consumer demand is also generated by the increased public awareness of advances in medical care achieved through medical technology because of the roles played by the media, the internet, and direct-to-consumer advertising.

Health insurance systems also play a role in advancing medical technology. Medical treatments can be very expensive, and health insurance provides payment for new innovations. Consumers looking for ways to ensure access to the type of medical care they want may increase the demand for health insurance. The promise of better health through improvements in medicine is a strong motivator for consumers.

Much of the work performed in this discipline is done by **biomedical engineers**, professionals who use their knowledge of biology, medicine, technology, and mechanical engineering to research and develop new equipment. These engineers have created miniature robots that are used to perform spinal surgeries considered highly complex and dangerous. They have created miniaturized pacemakers that function without any disturbance to the patient and drugs that can be activated by light to seek out diseased cells. They have created digestible sensors that monitor a patient's body systems and transmit patient information to healthcare providers so they can customize the patient's care.

Technology Innovations

The number and types of medical technology employed in health care could fill an entire textbook. This section addresses some of the innovations that currently play a role in health care and some that show promise to do so in the future.

Many healthcare practitioners are concerned about treating patients whose access to health care may be limited. Telemedicine addresses those concerns. **Telemedicine** is the use of electronic communications and information technologies to provide or support clinical care at a distance.[1] The connection allows the healthcare provider to diagnose, treat, and monitor patients remotely. Examples include transferring diagnostic images to a specialist for a second opinion, virtual visits for patients located thousands of miles away, and collecting medical data from patients outside a clinical setting. Patients can access care via video conferences with physicians to save time and money normally spent on traveling to another geographic location, or they can send health information instantaneously to any specialist or doctor in the world. Remote monitoring devices can track the blood sugar and blood pressure readings of patients, facilitating collaboration between healthcare practitioners and patients on a shared care plan between office visits. An image showing the use of telemedicine equipment is seen in **FIGURE 6.2.**

The use of mobile devices has exploded in the healthcare field, propelled by the use of medical software applications or apps. **Apps** are software programs developed to run on a computer or mobile device to accomplish a specific purpose. Some apps can simulate surgical procedures or can conduct simple medical exams, such as vision and hearing tests. Other apps help the physician develop patient risk

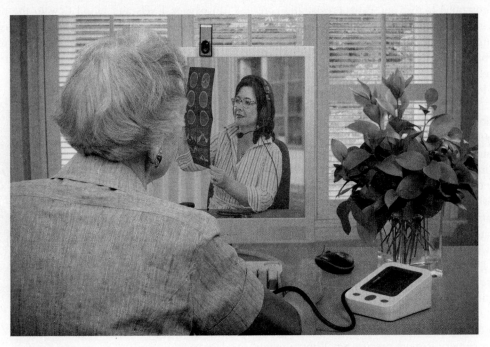

FIGURE 6.2 Doctor using telemedicine.
© verbaska/Shutterstock.

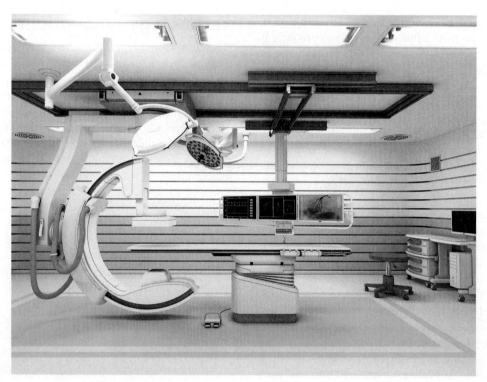

FIGURE 6.3 Interventional X-ray machine.
© 3AlexD/Getty Images.

profiles and provide drug dosage and interaction information. The benefits are numerous, and new apps are created on a daily basis.[2]

Patient registration, not to be confused with the patient registration process (which is discussed later in this chapter), involves creating a set of reference images with medical imaging equipment and recording the images in a digital format for the computer to map out. Patient registration creates a detailed reference about a patient's body and can be used to pinpoint the location of a tumor, for example. This information becomes part of the patient's electronic health record and can be used in the future. For example, a surgeon may use this information in a follow-up appointment to judge whether a tumor has grown or responded to treatment.

Interventional X-ray machines are pieces of high-resolution fixed X-ray equipment that allow physicians to diagnose and perform surgery in a minimally invasive manner. The images are of high clarity and allow the physician to work on the patient based on the images seen on the machine as opposed to looking into the patient's body directly. Patients benefit because both the dose of radiation and the impact on the human body are lower than what might occur with traditional surgery. An example of an interventional X-ray machine is seen in **FIGURE 6.3**.

Robots are another form of technology used in the healthcare setting. Robots can be used to complete daily routine tasks (e.g., restocking, cleaning), dispense medication, and assist during surgeries. The robots used by surgeons can ensure that surgery is more precise. Small instruments attached to a robotic arm are designed to replace traditional

steel tools, allowing these instruments to perform with smoother, feedback-controlled motions than could be achieved by the human hand. An example of surgical tools attached to a robotic arm is seen in **FIGURE 6.4**.

Functional magnetic resonance imaging (fMRI) shows promise to greatly advance knowledge of the brain. fMRIs trace the work of brain cells by tracking changes in oxygen levels and blood flow to the brain. The patient remains awake in the scanner and performs a simple task, like identifying a color or performing a math problem. As the patient performs the task, the fMRI tracks the areas of

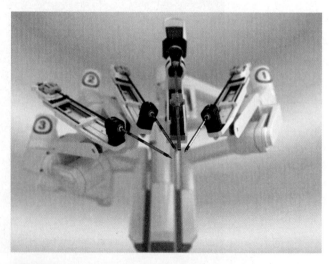

FIGURE 6.4 Surgical robot.
© 3AlexD/iStockPhoto.

the brain that are activated by tracing the speed at which cells metabolize sugar or glucose. These fMRIs are used in the study of depression, brain cancer, autism, and memory disorders, among other areas.

One of the most promising technologies in health care is the use of 3D printing. **3D printing** refers to a manufacturing method whereby three-dimensional objects are quickly made on a machine connected to a computer containing blueprints for the object. Objects made through 3D printing show promise because the blueprints can be customized to the patient's situation through use of patient-specific data to create a physical solution. This method also costs less than comparable objects manufactured in a traditional method, lowers risk to the patient, and can reduce operating time. This new method is currently being used to create prosthetics, orthopedic implants, and lab equipment such as pipettes and minifuge rotors. Research is ongoing for other applications, such as growing human tissue.[3] An example of a human hand generated by a 3D printer is seen in **FIGURE 6.5**.

Not all medical technology advances involve machines. For example, some medications have been created as targeted therapies for cancer and HIV/AIDS. These types of medications typically interfere with the processes that help cells multiply. Other oral medications have their activation delayed by changing the timing or rate of the medicine being released until biological processes break them down as they reach certain organs. This delay can optimize medication therapy or patient compliance.[4] A topical product being researched is an anti-bleeding plant polymer-based gel that works with the body's own blood clotting process to form a web-like structure to halt bleeding instantly.[5] Research on the mix of microbes in the digestive tract has led to development of treatments for obesity.

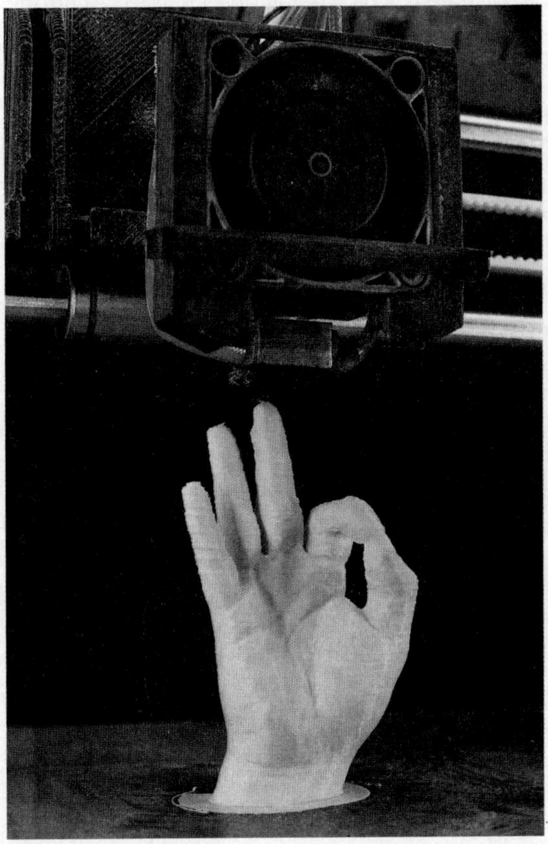

HEALTH INFORMATION TECHNOLOGY

Improving the delivery of patient care and producing optimum outcomes are goals of many healthcare providers and systems. One of the most important ways in which these goals can be accomplished is through use of health IT. Healthcare practitioners need the right information at the right time in order to make the right decisions. Leveraging the many forms of health IT influences the probability of this happening.[6] While the list is not inclusive, examples of commonly used health IT solutions are addressed in this section and listed in **TABLE 6.1**.

The field of health IT bridges several professional disciplines, including medicine, law, informatics, computer science, business, project management, and research. Those who enter this field generally fall into one of two categories: those

FIGURE 6.5 Hand created by 3D printer.
© Suljo/iStockPhoto.

TABLE 6.1 Health IT Applications

Health Information Technology	Examples
Administrative functions	Billing process
	Electronic materials management
	Patient registration process
	Vital statistics reporting
Clinical functions	Clinical decision support systems
	Computerized physician order entry for drugs, labs, and procedures
	Electronic health records
	Electronic prescribing
	Picture archiving and communication systems for filmless imaging
Infrastructure	Bar coding technology for drugs, medical devices, and inventory control
	Cloud computing
	Desktop, laptop, and tablet computers
	Mobile technology
	Speech recognition software
	Wearable technology
	Wireless networks

Professional Profiles

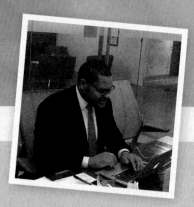

Name: Charles, MHA, RHIA
Job Title: Health Information Technology Consultant
Education: MS in Health Administration; BS in Health Information Management

Q: Tell us about your job and the type of organization you work in.

A: I work for a consulting company in their healthcare division. The clients are health systems such as hospitals, and I meet with the executives. I manage about two projects at a time.

Q: Describe a typical workday.

A: There is no typical workday. I get in at 6:30 AM and start with email. Meetings start at 8 AM, including strategy meetings; there are technical meetings for more servers that the electronic health record system will run on. We discuss the budget. I recently met with the mayor in New York City because the hospital system I am assisting with reports up to state government. I do high-level management and sit with senior-level executives. But I am also in the weeds dealing with a problem—how the product is working for the hospital system—so they can build out the system to meet their needs.

Q: What do you like most about this profession?

A: I love a challenge and doing something different every day. I have worked around the globe with clients—Germany, UK, Amsterdam, Norway, and domestic travel. [It is] 90% travel—home one day a week.

Q: Is there room for advancement in this field, and what kind of academic training is required?

A: Yes, definitely. If you have the drive, dedication, and ambition, you can rise to the top. A master's degree is required.

Q: Name and explain what part of your academic training most prepared you for this profession.

A: Being in student government and being a leader in the organizations that I was part of, as well as leadership positions in college, were essential to prepare me for a career in health IT.

Q: Did you face obstacles in pursuing your goals? If so, describe them and how you overcame them.

A: It is not easy. Long nights and early mornings, good grades, and doing extracurricular activities are required. Time is a big challenge—I needed to prioritize my time.

Q: What do you wish you had known in high school/college about pursuing this career?

A: That it even existed. I did not know about this career. One should look at what is coming, not what is already there.

Q: What advice would you give someone who is considering this career?

A: Be smarter about how you work.

Q: What skills are most essential for being effective in this career?

A: Problem-solving, effective listening, effective communication, and leadership skills are key.

who focus on the information technology in terms of infrastructure (hardware, software, and the systems that surround them) and those who focus on what can be accomplished with the data recorded, reported, and stored by the infrastructure. One talented individual in the field of health IT is the subject of the professional profile in this chapter.

Clinical Applications

The clinical information needed to make informed decisions changes as guidelines and clinical evidence-based medicine evolve. Similarly, the condition of the patient changes over time. The ability of a physician to care for the patient requires not only clinical experience but access to relevant patient data at the appropriate time. Because of the need for clinicians to keep current with medical protocols and patient information and apply them to specific situations, an automated answer arose in the form of a clinical decision support system. A **clinical decision support system (CDSS)** refers to the variety of technologies that provide healthcare practitioners with tools to improve the quality of care through diagnostic and treatment recommendations. Examples include simple alerts, prescription drug interaction warnings, and clinical pathways and protocols. The system applies computable biomedical knowledge to specific patient data and generates information for the clinician to use in treating a specific patient. The information is filtered, organized, and presented in a way that allows the clinician to make an informed decision quickly to act. This system assists the healthcare provider in dealing with what sometimes appears to be an overload of information. It also makes it possible for clinicians to have access to the latest evidence-based knowledge because this knowledge is integrated into the system.[7] Finally, the goal of improving the quality of patient care and enhancing the outcome for the patient is advanced by reducing duplicative testing, ensuring patient safety, and promoting patient engagement.

Most clinical decision support systems are part of a larger health information system that includes an electronic health record system. An **electronic health record (EHR)** refers to an individual patient health record stored in a computer database for easy access by physicians and other healthcare workers regardless of the setting—clinic, hospital, nursing home, or emergency care center. The information contained in the record is real time and offers a snapshot or picture of the patient's condition and treatment. EHRs are easily accessible to those who are treating the patient and serve as a way for clinicians to communicate about the status of a patient.[8]

Implementation of EHRs has grown dramatically and particularly since the inception of the HITECH Act in 2009. This program made physicians and hospitals eligible to receive incentive payments if they proved their use of the EHR systems met criteria set out in the Meaningful Use Program. Among these criteria is a patient portal. A **patient portal** refers to an online application that allows a patient to interact and communicate securely with healthcare providers. With a portal, patients can view, download, and transmit their health information and send messages to their healthcare providers.[9]

A second motivation to employ an EHR is the availability of computerized physician order entry systems. A **computerized physician order entry (CPOE)** system in its most basic form is a medication ordering and fulfillment system. Some more advanced CPOE systems also include the ability to order labs, radiology tests, procedures, discharges, transfers, and referrals. The strength of these systems is that all the orders are entered into the EHR and can be cross-checked in real time for potential errors or problems, such as an allergy. The systems also serve to make prescription orders legible, a difficulty long associated with paper prescription pads or paper forms. When referring solely to writing a prescription and sending it electronically to a pharmacy, CPOE is often called **e-prescribing**.

One significant benefit of EHRs is that information contained within them can be shared with other healthcare providers across different healthcare organizations. To accomplish this, the computer systems of the different healthcare organizations must be able to talk to each other electronically. **Interoperability** refers to the mechanism of electronic communication among organizations so that data can be incorporated from one system into another. Achieving interoperability allows patients' information to follow them to visits with numerous healthcare providers and creates a longitudinal record of a person's health over time.

Currently, interoperability is a significant challenge within the health IT field, as some information systems do not communicate easily with other information systems. The inability for health information to be exchanged electronically between providers impacts patient care and safety. Through the development of standards and rules the federal government is working to address these problems and has made some strides in reducing problems with interoperability.

One challenge with interoperability rests with proper identification of the patient. Medical offices, treatment centers, and hospitals all must maintain a **master patient index (MPI)**, a listing or database of all the patients treated by the healthcare provider, typically arranged according to an identification process. The MPI serves as a permanent record that links information about the patient, both clinical and demographic, across time. The challenge is that some patients share some of the same data characteristics, such as name and birthdate, making it difficult to differentiate between patients. Medical professionals who rely on information that is not properly tied to the right patient can make medical mistakes. Electronic systems containing analytical processes can minimize but not completely address the problem of duplicate entries in the MPI.

Another challenge of interoperability is the need for electronic systems that are developed for different purposes to interact with each other. Pictures and images created from a variety of source machines pose such a problem. A **picture archiving and communication system (PACS)** refers to the technology that captures and integrates diagnostic and radiological images from various devices, stores them, and disseminates them to a health record, a clinical repository, or other points of care. For example, using such a system means the healthcare provider no longer needs to file, retrieve, or transport film jackets of X-rays. To achieve interoperability, many PACS work with a **vendor-neutral archive (VNA)**, a single, consolidated archive platform used to host files from different PACS software. This arrangement allows all types of images stored in separate PACS to be compiled and merged into the same system, increasing the ability to share data internally and externally.

Administrative Applications

While considerable health IT work is focused on clinical functions, other functions are equally important. For example, healthcare providers cannot stay in practice or business unless they have a steady stream of income. This stream of income derives from the billing process. The **billing process** refers to the method of submitting and following up with claims made to government payers, insurance companies, and patients for services rendered to patients.

The Health Insurance Portability and Accountability Act (HIPAA) governs virtually all healthcare billing transactions in the United States. HIPAA establishes security and privacy standards for health information, commonly referred to as the privacy and security rules. These rules establish administrative, technical, and physical safeguards of patient information so that the information may remain confidential, possess integrity, and be electronically formatted for transmission between healthcare providers, insurers, and governmental payers.

HIPAA requires most claims for healthcare services to be submitted via electronic means. Specific codes are assigned to the patient's episode of care. The codes record the patient's diagnosis and any procedures performed during the patient's visit using the most commonly known coding systems such as International Classification of Diseases, Tenth Revision; Clinical Modification (ICD-10 CM); and Current Procedural Terminology (CPT). The codes and other data are transmitted electronically to the government payers and insurance companies. An electronic connection is made from the government payer or insurance company in response to the claims submitted. Those amounts not paid for by the government payers or the insurance companies are then billed to the patient. The IT community has expended considerable effort on following standards and technologies for smooth electronic claims transmission.

Other health record data facilitated for collection and dissemination by health IT involve vital statistics. **Vital statistics** refer to the information that chronicles certain life events of individuals, such as birth and death. An example of a birth certificate is seen in **FIGURE 6.6**. Every state has either a law or set of regulations that requires the reporting of vital statistics; the specifics of what must be reported vary by state. For example, common reporting requirements include

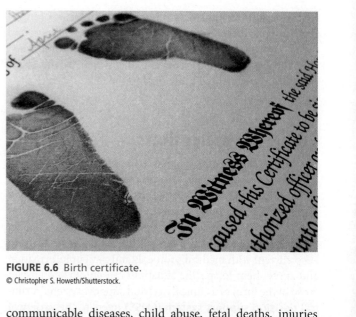

FIGURE 6.6 Birth certificate.
© Christopher S. Howeth/Shutterstock.

communicable diseases, child abuse, fetal deaths, injuries caused by deadly weapons, and cancer. Health IT is used to capture this information and transmit it to the requisite state department of health or similar agency within the specified time period.

Other areas of focus include properly registering patients when they enter the hospital, office, or treatment center. Referred to as the **patient registration process**, this activity involves obtaining pertinent personal, financial, and social information from the patient about their medical history, contact information, and insurance billing data, among other things. This routine activity is generally the first entry in the patient's electronic health record, and the data obtained follows the patient through the entire episode of care and into the billing cycle.

Infrastructure

Efforts have also focused on improving efficiency concerning the many supplies required by healthcare providers when they treat patients. **Electronic materials management** refers to the tracking and managing of inventory of medical supplies, drugs, and other materials. This system allows for paperless ordering of supplies, drugs, and materials; shorter lead times between order and delivery of goods; and a method for automating inventory control.

One way to manage materials involves leveraging bar code labels and technology. **Bar coding technology** refers to the use of an optical scanner to electronically capture information encoded on a product. It is used with medications as a way to match drugs to patients by scanning the bar codes on both the medications and the patient's arm bracelet. This technology is also applied to medical devices, lab, and radiology equipment.

Another significant development in health IT involves **speech recognition software**. This refers to collecting spoken words, analyzing those words, and presenting the results as data. Speech recognition software converts spoken words into text on-screen. This software is very useful for those individuals who cannot use a keyboard or other form of manual input device effectively. It is also useful for dictation and translation of health data.

Most of the equipment used by healthcare providers is either a stationary or mobile object. **Mobile technology** refers to equipment that can be carried or wheeled from place to place. Examples include laptops, tablets, and smartphones. Mobile devices offer many advantages, including the ability to bring them to the patient's bedside and access health information at the place it is needed. Mobile devices facilitate data collection, allowing data to be entered directly without delay. Practitioners have access to any type of information they need within mere seconds, from drug information to research and studies, patient history, records, and more. Disadvantages include the fact that they are particularly prone to being damaged, lost, or stolen because of their smaller size and lighter weight.

As widespread as mobile technology is in health care, the latest trend is the use of wearable technology. **Wearable technology** refers to an electronic device that can be worn on a person. Typically the size of a smartphone or smaller, these devices use wireless technology to perform functions. The use of wearable technology allows for inexpensive, continuous physiological monitoring with little manual intervention by the patient or the healthcare provider. For example, healthcare practitioners can use them to monitor a patient's vital signs and can receive alerts of safety issues and sudden medical emergencies. Some models are set up so that the patient can contact a medical center for advice or push an emergency button that automatically sends an alert to paramedics with the person's status and location.

In addition to the hardware and software present in the delivery of patient care, consideration must also be given to the virtual world. Some healthcare organizations and providers use cloud computing as an administrative aid. **Cloud computing** refers to the virtualization of servers, meaning that servers are not physically present at the healthcare site. Data privacy and security concerns are present with cloud computing, and health IT professionals are working to address those concerns.

Health Information Technology and the Law

As new methods of administering care are developed and technology continues to evolve, the law works in tandem. Numerous HIPAA regulations target concerns about the confidentiality and security of patient information and the steps that must be taken to maintain privacy in the digital world. The regulations establish standards for ensuring confidentiality and security of patient information and protecting patients' health information from unauthorized access and use.

Confidentiality of patient information is protected by both federal and state law. **Confidentiality** refers to the healthcare professional's obligation to maintain patient information in a manner that will not permit dissemination beyond the healthcare provider. HIPAA regulations give patients access to their protected health information (PHI) and protect the privacy of their information by limiting access to it by other parties.

Many of these regulations require that all healthcare providers maintain secure electronic health records. The regulations specify multiple security measures to be employed, including authentication and permission protocols, encryption, and damage prevention techniques. Unfortunately, breaches of protected health information do occur, whether because of identity theft, unauthorized access to data, or theft or loss of laptop computers and mobile devices. The regulations ensure that patients are notified of breaches of protected health information. A healthcare provider that experiences a breach of PHI can be fined by the federal government.

Healthcare practitioners must exercise care when choosing to implement new technologies into their services. They should ensure that all technologies are HIPAA compliant before investing in their implementation.

SUMMARY

Technological innovations in the healthcare industry provide healthcare professionals with new ways to improve the quality of care delivered to their patients and improve the state of health care worldwide. Medical technology can improve access to care for those whose access is limited, improve quality of care through more precise testing and surgical procedures, and offer opportunities to learn more about the human body than ever in history. Health information technology offers better access to patient information at the right time and place, which increases patient safety and improves patient outcomes. Law and technology work together to protect and secure patient information from unauthorized access and use.

Additional Information

For more information about the federal government's efforts with health IT, visit:

- Office of the National Coordinator for Health Information Technology (ONC), https://www.healthit.gov

For more information about private sector initiatives to improve health care through IT, visit:

- The Center for Private Sector Health Initiatives (PSHI), https://pshi.fhi360.org
- The Institute for Healthcare Improvement (IHI), https://www.ihi.org/Pages/default.aspx

For more information about professional associations focused on improving health care through IT, visit:

- American Health Information Management Association (AHIMA), https://www.ahima.org
- Healthcare Information and Management Systems Society (HIMSS), https://www.himss.org

LEARNING PORTFOLIO

Study Points

1. Very little in the field of medicine has not been affected by new technology.

2. Medical technology includes a multitude of products used to diagnose, monitor, and treat human conditions and diseases, including instruments used to perform less invasive operations.

3. The demand for new medical technology springs from consumers, healthcare practitioners, and health insurance systems.

4. Health information technology involves both clinical and administrative applications and infrastructure.

5. An electronic health record documents the patient's condition and treatment.

6. Federal law and regulations serve to protect and secure health information.

CASE STUDY: MEDICAL AND HEALTH INFORMATION TECHNOLOGY

Constance is a recent graduate of the Massachusetts Institute of Technology (MIT) and has been hired by Brigham and Women's Hospital in the position of Assistant Director of Healthcare Technology. She is beginning to map her employee training programs and finds there is some research she first needs to complete.

Based on the information you have read about medical and health information technology, answer the following questions.

1. What is the difference between medical technology and health information technology?

   While designing her training program, Constance decides to develop an activity for participants to help them differentiate between medical technology and health information technology. She lists examples of technology in the hospital and is planning to ask the participants if these examples are forms of medical technology or health information technology.

   Can you answer the following question by filling in the blank with either *medical technology* or *health information technology*?

2. Some examples of common _____ include new surgical procedures and biologic agents. _____ includes the patient registration and billing processes.

   Can you answer the following questions by filling in the blank with the correct terms?

3. One of the goals of training that Constance has set for the medical staff is to ensure they have a logical model to follow when making decisions regarding patient care. The model described in your text is the _____.

4. A(n) _____ refers to an individual patient health record stored in a computer database.

5. The _____ Act introduced the Meaningful Use Program.

6. _____ refers to the virtualization of servers, meaning that servers are not physically present at the healthcare site.

7. Numerous _____ regulations target concerns about the confidentiality and security of patient information and the steps that must be taken to maintain privacy in the digital world.

8. _____ refers to the mechanism of electronic communication among organizations so that data can be incorporated from one system into another.

9. Many healthcare practitioners are concerned about treating patients whose access to health care may be limited. A new technology, _____, addresses those concerns.

10. Software programs developed to run on a computer or mobile device to accomplish a specific purpose are called _____.

Issues for Discussion

1. View the video "Top 10 Medical Technologies of the Future: Ranked!" by visiting the website https://www.youtube.com/watch?v=PXPIu8LazqI. Discuss the types of technological changes you have seen over your lifetime with your instructor and classmates. Speculate on what types of changes may occur in the healthcare field over the remainder of your lifetime.

2. Wearable technologies that have healthcare applications have become common place. Discuss with your instructor and classmates the types of wearable technologies with which you are familiar and whether or how these wearable technologies influence individual behavior.

LEARNING PORTFOLIO

Enrichment Activities

1. Choose one of the technology innovations featured in the text in the "Medical Technology" section. Research more information about this technology and create a presentation (narrative paper, PowerPoint presentation, or infographic) that provides a broader understanding of the technology and its uses.

2. Visit the websites https://www.youtube.com/watch?v=ZnBEVsZSqlk and https://www.youtube.com/watch?v=I9dFMO09wB0 to hear about the field of biomedical engineers and specific career choices.

3. Choose one of the clinical or administrative examples featured in the text in the "Health Information Technology" section. Research more information about this application and create a presentation (narrative paper, PowerPoint presentation, or infographic) that provides a broader understanding of the application and its uses.

References

1. Telecommunications Act of 1996, 47 U.S.C. §§ 254(b) & (h) (2021).

2. Ventola CL. Mobile Devices and Apps for Health Care Professionals: Uses and Benefits, *P T*. 2014 May; 39(5): 356–364. https://www.ncbi.nlm.nih.gov/pmc/articles/PMC4029126/

3. Byers J. 3-D Printing: Healthcare's new edge. Healthcare IT News. http://www.healthcareitnews.com/news/3-d-printing-healthcares-new-edge May 19, 2014; Dunham S. Surgeon's Helper: 3D Printing Is Revolutionizing Health Care (Op-Ed). Live Science. https://www.livescience.com/49913-3d-printing-revolutionizing-health-care.html February 24, 2015; Diana A. 3D Printing Reshapes Healthcare. Information Week. http://www.informationweek.com/healthcare/mobile-and-wireless/3d-printing-reshapes-healthcare/d/d-id/1113893 February 20, 2014.

4. Montero MM, Skalsky B. Advanced Approaches for Delayed-Release Formulations. *ONdrugDelivery*, 2017 July, 77: 4–9. https://www.ondrugdelivery.com/advanced-approaches-delayed-release-formulations/

5. Hickman DA, Pawlowski CL, Sekhon UDS, Marks J, Gupta AS. Biomaterials and Advanced Technologies for Hemostatic Management of Bleeding. *Adv Mater*. 2018;30(4):10.1002/adma.201700859. doi:10.1002/adma.201700859. https://pubmed.ncbi.nlm.nih.gov/29164804/

6. Health Information Technology: A Tool to Help Clinicians Do What They Value Most. Office of the National Coordinator for Health Information Technology. https://www.healthit.gov/sites/default/files/hit_tool_providersfactsheet072013.pdf Published July 2013.

7. What Is Clinical Decision Support (CDS)? Office of the National Coordinator for Health Information Technology. https://www.healthit.gov/topic/safety/clinical-decision-support Updated April 10, 2018.

8. What Is an Electronic Health Record (EHR)? Office of the National Coordinator for Health Information Technology. https://www.healthit.gov/faq/what-electronic-health-record-ehr Updated September 10, 2019.

9. How to Optimize Patient Portals for Patient Engagement and Meet Meaningful Use Requirements. Office of the National Coordinator for Health Information Technology. https://www.healthit.gov/sites/default/files/nlc_how_to_optimizepatientportals_for_patientengagement.pdf May 2013.

PART TWO

Jobs and Careers

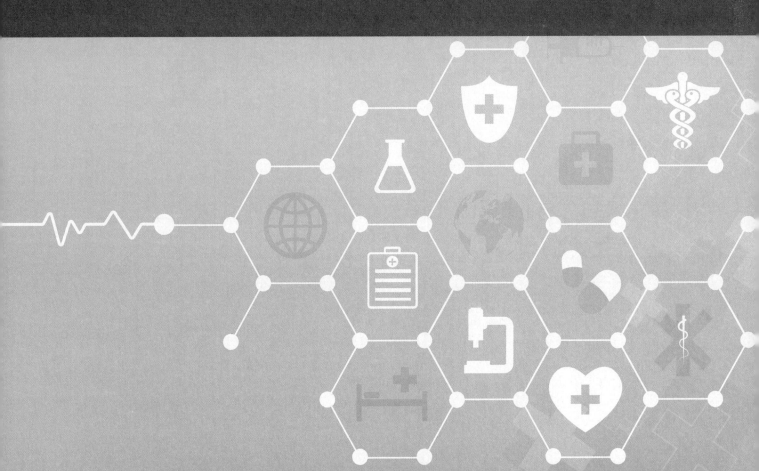

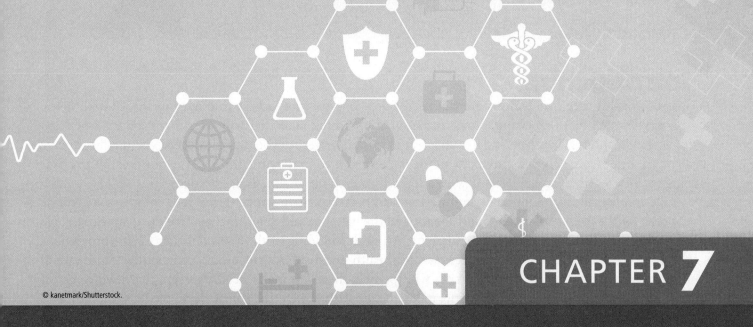
© kanetmark/Shutterstock.

CHAPTER 7

Health Career Planning

OBJECTIVES

After studying this chapter, the student should be able to:

- Obtain all facts pertinent to careers in health services.
- Recognize the specialized knowledge and skills necessary for a given profession.
- Evaluate employment opportunities.
- Find an appropriate health career.
- Select the appropriate school for training.

KEY TERMS

Activities of daily living
Bureau of Labor Statistics (BLS)
Certification
Community and Social Service Occupations
Healthcare Practitioners and Technical Occupations
Health Professional Shortage Areas (HPSAs)

Health Resources and Services Administration (HRSA)
Healthcare Support Occupations
Indian Health Service (IHS)
Licensure
Loan Repayment Program (LRP)
Maldistribution of health personnel
National Health Service Corps (NHSC)

Professional certification
Professional registration
State Loan Repayment Program
Student to Service Loan Repayment Program
U.S. Department of Health and Human Services (DHHS)

Introduction

Because health care occupations are the fastest-growing and the largest employer in the United States, it is appropriate that this chapter assist students in obtaining facts that will steer them toward satisfying careers in health services. The first five chapters in this book were devoted to the development of healthcare services, healthcare delivery, and many of the issues involved in meeting the goals set for health care. This chapter focuses on personnel issues: where and why health professionals are needed.

Desirable traits for individuals considering health careers are a strong desire to help others, a genuine concern for the welfare of patients and clients, and the patience and emotional maturity to deal with people of diverse backgrounds in stressful situations. An understanding of the roles of other health professionals and a collaborative attitude are necessary for health professionals since each contributes to the care of individual patients. If you enjoy working with people, there are many health careers that involve direct contact with clients or patients. Nursing, medicine, dentistry, dietetics, social work, physical therapy, and recreational and occupational therapy are some health career areas that will give you the opportunity to work with and help people of all ages. Workers in other careers have limited direct contact with patients but play a significant role in the health and well-being of patients and clients—for example, laboratory technicians and health information technicians.

If you are considering a career in the healthcare field, there are many opportunities. Some careers require only a high school diploma with on-the-job training while others require graduate degrees plus an internship. This chapter will help the student explore the possibilities and answer these questions: What are the fastest-growing health careers? What are the educational requirements for different health careers? What financial resources are available for students preparing for a health career? How much time are you willing to spend preparing for your career, and how flexible are you about where you live?

WHO ARE THE HEALTHCARE WORKERS?

Employment opportunities for healthcare workers exist along a wide continuum from hospitals and physicians' offices at the medical end through retirement communities and assisted living to adult day care at the social-support end. The continuum of curative and supportive services ranges from diagnosis and treatment such as annual physical exams and surgery to supportive services such as personal care and homemaking services.[1]

The **Bureau of Labor Statistics (BLS)** classifies healthcare occupations into three broad categories based on responsibilities for providing direct clinical care, level of education required, and credentialing (licensure, certification, and registration). The three broad categories are: (1) **Healthcare Practitioners and Technical Occupations**; (2) **Healthcare Support Occupations**; and (3) **Community and Social Service Occupations**.[1]

The first broad category, Healthcare Practitioners and Technical Occupations, is further categorized into those who provide direct clinical care—Diagnosing or Treating Practitioners—and those who support the work of practitioners, Health Technologists and Technicians. Educational and credentialing requirements are higher for practitioners than health technologists and technicians. Typically, the educational requirement for practitioners is a graduate degree and licensure compared to an associate's or bachelor's degree for technologists and technicians. Some examples of practitioners are physicians, registered nurses, dentists, dental hygienists, audiologists, speech-language pathologists, dietitians, chiropractors, physical therapists, and occupational therapists. Examples of health technologists and technicians are clinical laboratory technologists and technicians, diagnostic-related technologists and technicians, medical records specialists, licensed practical and vocational nurses, and dietetic or pharmacy technicians.[1]

The second broad category is Healthcare Support Occupations; this group represents the largest number of healthcare workers. Examples are home health and personal care aides, nursing assistants, medical assistants, dental assistants, massage therapists, phlebotomists, and occupational and physical therapy assistants and aides. Support personnel typically work under the supervision of clinical practitioners such as physicians, registered nurses, physical therapists, and dentists. Educational requirements are lower for this category of healthcare workers and vary from on-the-job training or postsecondary certification to an associate's degree.

The third broad category, Community and Social Service Occupations, includes professionals who often work in healthcare settings. Examples are social workers, substance abuse/behavioral disorders/mental health counselors, and health educators. All work in hospitals and clinics; health educators are also employed in public health settings. All of these require a bachelor's degree to practice at the entry level. Support personnel in this category are community health workers and social service assistants; they support health educators and social workers in various settings. Typically, social service support personnel are required to have a high school diploma and receive on-the-job training.[1]

The healthcare workforce in the United States lacks diversity; that is, the sex, race, and ethnic diversity do not match the diversity of the population and do not match the diversity in the culture or language of the population. Three-quarters of healthcare workers are women.[2] The exceptions are five professions in the Healthcare Practitioners and Technical Occupations where the majority are men: dentists, chiropractors, physicians, optometrists, and emergency medical technicians (EMTs) and paramedics. Male-dominated professions are in the Healthcare Diagnosing or Treating Practitioners category, except for EMTs and paramedics, which are in the Health Technologists and Technicians category. Occupations with the lowest representation of men are dental hygienists and speech-language pathologists.[3]

In terms of racial and ethnic distribution of people in the United States, 76% are White, 13% are Black, 19% are Hispanic, and 6% are Asian.[4] Compare these numbers with the distribution in the healthcare workforce: 64% are White, 12% Black, 16% Hispanic, and 5% Asian. Representation of racial and ethnic minority groups varies by occupational categories; however, Whites represent 50% of workers in almost every healthcare occupation. Minority groups are underrepresented in the Diagnosing or Treating Practitioners category, except for Asians who are dentists, pharmacists, physicians, and optometrists and Blacks who are dietitians and respiratory therapists. In the Community and Social Service category, Asians are underrepresented, while Blacks are employed as counselors and social workers. In the Healthcare Support Occupations category, there is greater diversity; Hispanics are medical assistants, dental assistants, and personal care aides, while Blacks are medical assistants, and nursing, psychiatric, and home health aides. Whites and Asians are underrepresented in this category.[3]

The benefits of having a diverse workforce in healthcare are an improvement in communication between the patient and clinician and greater access to health care for minority (non-White) patients.[3] The **Health Resources and Services Administration (HRSA)** has the responsibility of monitoring the diversity of the healthcare workforce; this information is used by decision makers at the federal, state, and local levels to develop policies to meet the demand for a diverse healthcare workforce. HRSA provides financial support for students in the health professions through grants, loan repayment programs, and scholarships. Some scholarships are designated for disadvantaged students, especially low-income minority students.[5] More detailed information is available under "Additional Information" at the end of this chapter.

PROJECTED DEMAND FOR HEALTHCARE PERSONNEL

As one of the largest and fastest-growing industries in 2018, health care provided 18 million jobs for wage and salary workers and is projected to generate 2.4 million new jobs between 2019 and 2029. The demand for healthcare personnel is expected to increase by 15% between 2019 and 2029 compared to a 4% increase for all occupations. The demand for healthcare workers is expected to continue because of a longer life expectancy and aging of the Baby Boomers (those born between 1946 and 1964). Healthcare practitioners are needed to manage chronic diseases, and home health and personal care aides are needed to provide personal care assistance as seniors age.

According to the U.S. Bureau of Labor Statistics, eight of the 20 fastest-growing occupations are health care–related. Projections are for growth from 25% to 52% between 2019 and 2029 for health-related professions, as shown in **FIGURE 7.1**.[6]

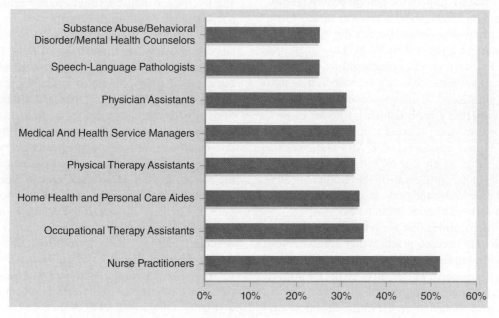

FIGURE 7.1 Projected growth in healthcare employment, 2019–2029.

Data from the Bureau of Labor Statistics, U.S. Department of Labor. *Occupational Outlook Handbook*, 2020. Fastest Growing Occupations. https://www.bls.gov/ooh/fastest-growing.htm

TABLE 7.1 Projections for Numbers of Health-Related Professionals in Highest Demand, 2019–2029

Profession	New Jobs Number	Median Annual Salary May 2020	Educational Requirements
Home health and personal care aides	1,159,500	$ 27,080	Postsecondary non-degree programs
Registered Nurses	221,900	$ 75,330	Bachelor's degree
Nurse practitioners	200,600	$ 111,680	Graduate degree
Medical assistants	139,200	$ 35,850	Postsecondary certificate
Medical and health service managers	133,200	$ 104,280	Graduate degree
Nursing Assistants	116,900	$ 30,830	Postsecondary training
Nursing instructors and teachers, postsecondary	85,700	$ 75,470	Graduate degree
Substance abuse/behavioral disorders/mental health counselors	79,000	$ 47,660	Bachelor's degree
Health specialty teachers, postsecondary	52,100	$ 99,090	Graduate degree

Data from Bureau of Labor Statistics. U.S. Department of Labor. May 2020. National Occupational Employment and Wage Estimate United States. March 31, 2021.http://www.bls.gov/oes/current/oes_nat.htm

Projected growth is anticipated in all three categories of healthcare occupations—for example, substance abuse/behavioral disorders/mental health counselors in the Community and Social Service category; physician assistants, speech-language pathologists, registered nurses, and nurse practitioners in the Healthcare Practitioners and Technical category; and home health and personal care aides and physical and occupational therapy assistants in the Healthcare Support category. Although not considered a category of healthcare workers, postsecondary teachers are needed to train new health professionals, and there is a high demand for both nursing instructors and other health specialty teachers, as shown in **TABLE 7.1**.[7] Both the percent growth (shown in Figure 7.1) and the total number (shown in Table 7.1) are high for home health and personal care aides. Careers are listed in the order of greatest demand between 2019 and 2029 in Figure 7.1, starting with home health and personal care aides with projections for nearly 1.2 million new jobs between 2019 and 2029.

Although projected growth is high for health careers, the total number and the projected number of new positions over the 10 year period between 2019 and 2029 for each profession varies widely. The highest numbers for new positions as well as total numbers are in the Health Care Support category: home health and personal care aides, medical assistants, and nursing assistants (**FIGURE 7.2**).

The largest occupations that are not in the Healthcare Support category are licensed practical and licensed vocational nurses (LPNs) in the Health Technologist and Technician category and registered nurses (RNs) in the Healthcare Practitioners and Technical category (**FIGURE 7.3**).[8]

Generally, occupations in the Healthcare Support category have both low educational requirements and low salaries. Licensed practical nurses and registered nurses have higher educational requirements as well as licensure requirements and are paid higher salaries. (See Table 7.1.) Careers that require graduate degrees—physician assistants, speech-language pathologists, nurse practitioners, and medical and health services managers—also demand higher salaries.

EMPLOYERS OF HEALTH PROFESSIONALS

Healthcare workers are employed in a variety of settings. The five major industries that employ health workers are hospitals, offices of health practitioners, nursing and residential facilities, home health services, and outpatient, laboratory, and other ambulatory services. The majority of healthcare employees work in offices of physicians, dentists, nurse practitioners, physician assistants, and other health practitioners—for example, physical therapists, occupational therapists, chiropractors, audiologists, and speech-language pathologists. These offices tend to be small and also employ healthcare support personnel such as medical assistants and nursing assistants. Both hospitals and nursing homes employ Healthcare Practitioners and Technicians and Healthcare Support personnel; hospitals employ greater numbers of practitioners, while nursing homes employ greater numbers of support personnel. Home health agencies employ Healthcare Practitioners—registered nurses, physical therapists, occupational therapists, dietitians, and social workers—as well as Healthcare Support personnel: nursing assistants and home and personal care assistants. Outpatient services include community health centers and substance use disorder and behavioral health

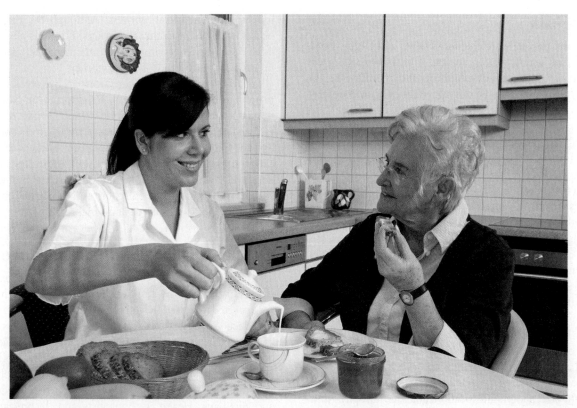

FIGURE 7.2 One of the fastest-growing health professions is home health and personal care aides.
© Lisa S./Shutterstock.

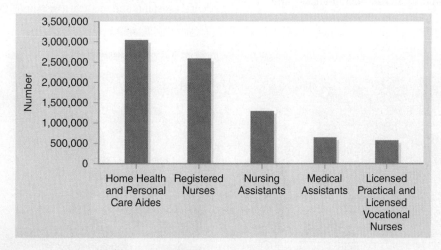

FIGURE 7.3 Largest occupations in health care, May 2020.
Data from U.S. Bureau of Labor Statistics. *Occupational Employment Statistics. Charts of the Largest Occupations in Each Industry.* May 2020. Sector 62: Health Care and Social Assistance. https://www.bls.gov/oes/current/ind_emp_chart/ind_emp_chart.htm

clinics staffed by physicians, dentists, registered nurses, social workers, dietitians, and behavioral and mental health counselors. Healthcare Support personnel include nursing and medical assistants. Laboratory services employ medical technologists and technicians, and other ambulatory services include EMTs.[9]

Growth for healthcare workers is expected to change by industry in the next decade, with fewer jobs available in hospitals in an effort to decrease the cost of healthcare delivery, since care is most expensive in the hospital. Greatest increases will be seen in home health care services as older adults seek ways to remain in their homes. Projections also include an increase in jobs in outpatient, laboratory, and other ambulatory settings; in offices of health practitioners; and in nursing homes and residential facilities (e.g., assisted living and continuing care communities).[3]

Healthcare jobs are found throughout the country, but they are concentrated in metropolitan areas. More details about job opportunities and working conditions for major employers follow.

Hospitals

As a group, hospitals are the best-known and largest single employer of health workers (**FIGURE 7.4**). Hospitals employ workers with all levels of education and training, thereby providing a wider variety of opportunities than is offered by other segments of the healthcare industry. In general, hospitals care for patients with various medical conditions requiring diagnosis and surgical or medical treatment. Hospitalized patients are often acutely ill or are recovering from surgery. Patients in these hospitals generally stay a short time—a few days to a few weeks.[9]

In specialty hospitals, patients are usually limited to those who have a specific illness or condition. Specialty hospitals may treat psychiatric illnesses or chronic diseases such as cancer. Rehabilitation hospitals specialize in the care of patients after a spinal cord injury, traumatic brain injury, or stroke or those with a neurological disorder or chronic pain. Pulmonary care hospitals specialize in care of patients requiring ventilator support. Specialty hospitals are identified as "long-term care facilities" because their patients are usually hospitalized for several weeks to months before they are well enough to return to their homes.[9]

The mix of workers needed by hospitals varies depending on the size, geographic location, goals, philosophy, funding, organization, and management style of the institution. Hospitals employ many practitioners for diagnosing and treatment of patients as well as health technologists and technicians and social workers. Although the majority of hospitals employ healthcare workers, hospitals also employ office support personnel and maintenance, sanitation, housekeeping, and food-service workers.[9]

The majority of healthcare work is shift work since the hospital is open 24 hours a day, 365 days a year. Nurses and nursing assistants typically work 12-hour shifts from 7 AM to 7 PM three days per week and may rotate between day and evening shifts. Clinical laboratory workers also typically work a day, evening, or night shift. Most other hospital employees work a day shift, although some professionals such as radiation technologists or respiratory therapists may be required to work both day and night shifts.[9]

Offices of Health Practitioners

The industry with the second-highest number of healthcare workers is in the offices of health practitioners; the numbers are expected to exceed the numbers working in hospitals in the next decade (**FIGURE 7.5**). Offices of health practitioners employ primarily Diagnosing or Treating Practitioners with high levels of education—for example, physicians, surgeons, podiatrists, dentists, physical therapists, occupational therapists, physician assistants, nurse practitioners, psychologists, registered nurses, and dietitians. Health Technologists and Technicians who work in a group practice include dental hygienists and licensed practical nurses together with Healthcare Support personnel (e.g., dental assistants and medical assistants).[9] Offices of health

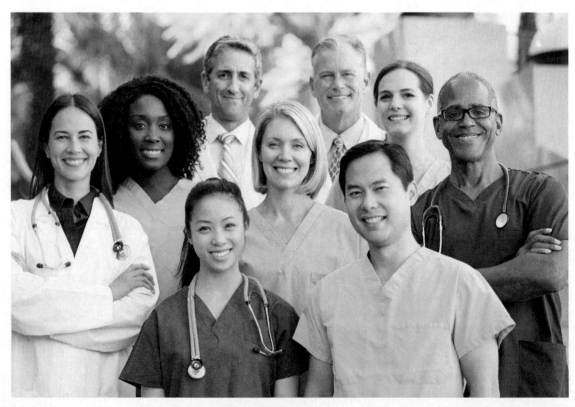

FIGURE 7.4 Hospitals employ the largest number of health professionals.
© Monkey Business Images/Shutterstock.

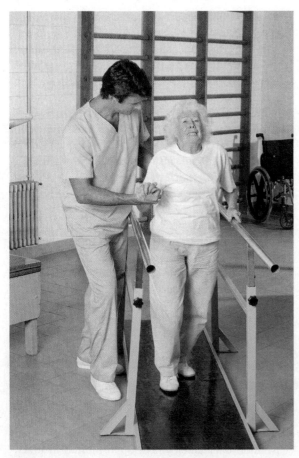

FIGURE 7.5 Offices of health professionals are the second most common employer of health professionals.
© Tyler Olson/Shutterstock.

practitioners also employ practitioners of alternative medicine, such as acupuncturists, massage therapists, homeopaths, hypnotherapists, and naturopaths.

Physicians with a group practice may specialize, for example, in obstetrics and gynecology and diseases of women. Dentists may specialize as orthodontists or oral and maxillofacial surgeons. Other practices may specialize in cardiology and include health practitioners in addition to physicians—for example, exercise physiologists, dietitians, nurses, and psychologists. Physical therapists may work in a practice with a chiropractor and athletic trainer and specialize in treating those with sports injuries.

Nursing and Residential Care Facilities

Nursing homes were almost unknown before the 1930s but have grown rapidly in number since then. By 2019, there were approximately 1.2 million residents in nearly 15,000 nursing homes. An additional 811,500 individuals resided in 28,900 assisted-living facilities.[11] Nursing care facilities provide inpatient nursing, rehabilitation, and health-related personal care to those who need continuous nursing care but do not require medical or surgical treatment. Residential care facilities, also described as assisted-living facilities,

provide around-the-clock social and personal care to older adults and others who have a limited ability to care for themselves, such as those recovering from surgery. The services offered vary from skilled bedside nursing to assistance with **activities of daily living** (bathing, toileting, dressing, eating, and walking). Residents in assisted-living facilities require less nursing and personal care than those residing in nursing care facilities. Most assisted-living facilities provide meals and social and recreational activities. Needs of individual residents vary from assistance with some to all activities of daily living such as bathing, walking, and dressing. However, residents in assisted-living facilities are more independent than those living in nursing care facilities.

In the future, the most growth is expected for healthcare support personnel such as nursing assistants and personal care aides in nursing care facilities.[9] There will continue to be a demand in residential facilities for registered nurses in the Health Diagnosis and Treatment category and for licensed practical nurses, LPNs in the technical category. Other healthcare workers such as physical therapists, social workers, recreation therapists, and dietitians often work as consultants for several facilities and less often as full-time employees for one facility.

Home Health Care Services

Home health care is expected to grow faster than any other healthcare industry in the next decade.[9] The development of in-home medical technologies, substantial cost savings, and patients' preference for care in the home has helped change this once-small segment of the industry into one of the fastest-growing healthcare services. Skilled nursing or medical care is provided in the home primarily to older adults under a physician's supervision. Home healthcare services are provided for patients recovering from surgery or a stroke or for someone receiving treatment for cancer or other conditions requiring ongoing skilled nursing such as treatment of skin wounds.

The majority of healthcare workers in the home care setting are similar to those who work in nursing facilities, registered nurses, licensed practical nurses, home health and personal care aides, and nursing assistants. Depending on the patient's medical condition, other practitioners who may provide services in the home are physical and occupational therapists and assistants, social workers, dietitians, and speech-language therapists. Working schedules for home care workers are usually flexible since workers often make their schedules. Most visits are made during the day between 7 AM and 7 PM and may include weekends.[3] Home care workers are responsible for their transportation to the homes of clients but may be reimbursed for mileage or other travel expenses.

Outpatient, Laboratory, and Other Ambulatory Care Services

In the past, many medical procedures, including certain diagnostic tests and simple surgeries, were done only on an inpatient hospital basis. Now these same procedures are safely and routinely performed on an outpatient basis in an office setting. This greater emphasis on ambulatory care will shift employment opportunities from hospitals to other kinds of health facilities. Examples of these services are clinics where patients go to have blood drawn before surgery by phlebotomists, where a pregnant woman has a sonogram done by a diagnostic medical sonographer, or where a patient with cancer receives radiation therapy from a radiological technician.[9]

Outpatient medical and diagnostic laboratories employ clinical laboratory technologists and technicians, radiological technologists, cardiovascular technologists and technicians, diagnostic medical sonographers, nuclear medical technologists, and magnetic resonance imaging technologists. Healthcare occupations with the most new jobs for this category are registered nurses in the Health Diagnostic and Treatment category, EMTs and paramedics in the technician category, and phlebotomists in healthcare support. Medical and clinical laboratory technicians and medical assistants will also be in demand in this setting.[9] Workers usually have a standard 9 AM to 5 PM shift, which may include Saturdays. The exception would be EMTs and paramedics, who work in shifts to allow coverage 24 hours a day, 365 days a year.

Additional Work Settings for Healthcare Workers

Health workers are employed in vital services that are often overlooked as part of the health industry when career opportunities in the health fields are being evaluated. The following list describes some of these careers:

- Orthotists and prosthetists design medical supportive devices including artificial limbs (arms, hands, legs, and feet), braces, and other medical devices.
- Healthcare workers in blood banks draw, process, store, and distribute human whole blood and its derivatives.
- Dental laboratories provide services to dentists by making and repairing artificial teeth and other dental appliances.
- Family planning services provide physical examinations, laboratory tests, consultations, education, and medications in relation to reproductive health and pregnancy care.
- Health education and promotion departments in large corporations and factories conduct group classes, exercise programs, and health screenings for employees.
- Public health departments at the city, county, and state level work with medical scientists at the Centers for Disease Control and Prevention (CDC) at the federal level to track outbreaks of foodborne illness or influenza.
- Poison control centers provide comprehensive services to the population regarding the effects of toxic substances and the antidotes available.
- Community mental health centers provide comprehensive services to people with mental illness to help them return to satisfying jobs and lifestyles.
- Migrant health programs provide health services to migrant and seasonal farm workers who would not

qualify for health services available to permanent residents.
- Community health centers provide medical, dental, laboratory, radiological, and pharmaceutical and mental health services for people living in a particular geographic area within a city.
- Voluntary health agencies concerned with specific health problems or health services raise funds for medical research, alert the public to specific health problems, and provide health education programs. The American Cancer Society, American Heart Association, American Diabetes Association, and the National Foundation–March of Dimes are examples of voluntary health agencies.
- Several branches of the federal government employ a variety of healthcare workers:
  - Occupational Safety and Health Administration (OSHA) enforces standards related to job health and safety.
  - The U.S. Department of Agriculture (USDA) supervises state-sponsored programs to ensure that agricultural products—including vegetables, fruits, meat, poultry, and eggs—are disease-free and processed under sanitary conditions.
  - The U.S. Food and Drug Administration (FDA) monitors the safety of food, prescription drugs, and medical devices.
  - The U.S. Army, Navy, Air Force, and Veterans Administration offer employment opportunities in practically every health occupation described in this text.

EXPLORING HEALTH CAREERS
Employment Opportunities

Health care continually moves in new and different directions. This movement may alter what health workers will be doing, where they will be working, and how many will be employed in a particular occupation. Opportunities may expand in some areas and diminish in others as the population changes and greater access to health care with healthcare reform is achieved.

No one can predict with absolute certainty the employment outlook for a particular career. The following discussion of current trends gives some clues as to where one might find especially good opportunities today and in the future.

Opportunities in Rural and Inner-City Communities

In some parts of the country, new health workers are finding it difficult to obtain jobs, while in other communities, employers cannot find enough workers to fill existing healthcare jobs. This national problem is often referred to as the **maldistribution of health personnel**. Healthcare workers are not distributed according to the population or health needs in many geographic areas. Low-income and overpopulated inner-city areas and underpopulated rural areas are hardest hit by this maldistribution.

Shortage areas need health professionals of all kinds. This might mean relocation to find the best future opportunities. The federal government has designated areas in each of the 50 states and territories as **Health Professional Shortage Areas (HPSAs)** based on the number of providers of primary care, dental care, and mental health care.[12] To increase the diversity of the health professions workforce and the number of providers working in underserved communities, the HRSA of the **U.S. Department of Health and Human Services (DHHS)** provides funds to accredited U.S. health professions schools. The schools use the money to offer scholarships and low-interest loans to educationally and economically disadvantaged students with financial need. Students who benefit from these programs are often from racial and ethnic minorities underrepresented in the health workforce.[13] The **National Health Service Corps (NHSC) Loan Repayment Program (LRP)** offers primary care medical, dental, and mental and behavioral health care providers the opportunity to have their student loans repaid while earning a competitive salary in exchange for providing health care in urban, rural, or tribal communities with limited access to care.[13]

The National Health Service Corps (NHSC) Loan Repayment Program (LRP) offers primary care medical, dental, and mental and behavioral health care providers the opportunity to have their student loans repaid while earning a competitive salary, in exchange for providing health care in urban, rural, or tribal communities with limited access to care.[13]

Scholarships and loans are administered through the NHSC. Scholarships are available for students planning a career in primary care including nurse practitioners, physician assistants, mental health professionals, and dentists.[14] Loans are offered under three separate programs: (1) **State Loan Repayment Program**, available in 30 states for students in a variety of healthcare training programs; (2) the NHSC LRP for those already practicing in primary care, dentistry, and behavioral health in urban, rural, or tribal communities with limited access to care and making a two-year commitment;[15] and (3) the **Student to Service Loan Repayment Program** for students in the last year of school training as a physician, dentist, nurse practitioner, or certified nurse-midwife. Loan repayment is in exchange for serving three years in a HPSA. Applicants are required or strongly encouraged to have work experience after completion of training before being assigned to a location.[16]

Career Exploration—the Process

Career exploration can be a learning experience as you make new discoveries about the world of work and yourself. The reality of the work world is always different from what you learn in school or from research in books. One good way to gain firsthand information is to visit several facilities. Make appointments and visit several departments within the facilities. Compare different types of facilities and what people with the same job titles are doing in each. Some helpful strategies include:

- If you have a particular interest, set up interviews with a health worker in that discipline. This is usually very rewarding for you both. Most health professionals enjoy talking to students and answering questions about their particular fields.
- Visit laboratories, both private and hospital based. Visit practitioners in private practice and those in salaried positions. Learn all you can about community-based programs and special services offered by clinics and hospitals.
- Ask about the philosophy of each facility you visit. Does it provide in-service education for its employees and offer continuing education programs? Does it subscribe to patient education concepts? What are the general amenities offered to workers in different kinds of facilities?

Before you go exploring, do your homework. View video clips of health professionals available on the websites listed at the end of this chapter as well as the websites of professional organizations. Do some more reading in the library. Be prepared to ask pertinent questions that will help you make decisions.

Also, visit schools that offer majors in the health careers. You can find out much about the professions by talking to students and instructors and by spending some time on campus and possibly in classes (most schools permit such visits). Another way to learn more about health careers is to join student health professions organizations in high school or community college.

Some professions stipulate that students have some experience in the field before they are considered for admission to an academic program. Experience can be obtained by summer work, part-time jobs, or volunteer work in a facility. The firsthand experience you gain from such an endeavor will not only help you make decisions about your career but may also help you get into the school of your choice. For example, if you are considering a career as a registered nurse, consider working as a nursing assistant, or work in a hospital lab if you are considering a career as a lab technician. Investigate many careers, not just those with which you are familiar. The more information you have, the easier it will be for you to make career decisions.

Selecting a School

Next to choosing a career, selecting the right school for training is the most important career decision you will need to make. As you read the job requirements for the many careers detailed in Parts three to five of this text, you will discover that health career training is available in many kinds of schools, including two- and four-year colleges and universities. Training programs are also available in vocational or trade schools and the military.

The secret to selecting the right school lies in answering two important questions: (1) Will the school you are interested in prepare you for the career you want? and (2) What will be the cost of your education, and what are the sources of financial support? The "Additional Information section at the end of this chapter lists resources to locate accredited programs for the health professions. Before you seek the answer to these questions, you should understand three basic terms related to employment in the health field: "licensure," "certification," and "registration."

Licensure, Certification, and Registration

Obtaining and maintaining **licensure** or in some professions, **certification**, is necessary to practice legally in individual states. Obtaining continuing education hours within a specified time period—for example, every two years—is required to maintain licensure or certification.

Licensure

Before you can work in many health professions, a state license is legally required. The qualifications for licensure vary. In general, a student must graduate from a school that has a program approved by the state licensing agency and then prove that he or she is qualified to give health services by passing a special licensing examination. Licensure is the state's way of protecting the public from unqualified health practitioners. Health professions that are licensed vary within each state, and individual state licensing requirements for each profession also vary by state. Some professions, such as registered nurse, practical nurse, physician, dentist, optometrist, podiatrist, pharmacist, social worker, and veterinarian, are licensed in all states. The Education Department, Department of Higher Education, and Department of Health are usually the agencies responsible for testing and issuing licenses. A state agency and a specialty board, such as the Board of Nursing or the Board of Dentistry, may also grant licenses jointly.

Certification

Professional certification is voluntary for individual health professionals and ensures the employer and the public that a health professional meets an established level of competence in their field. Certification is granted by national professional organizations and is recognized in all states. In health professions for which there is no state licensure, professional certification may be required for employment. However, even when certification is not required, it is a strong asset. Most employers prefer to hire certified professionals, and in a tight job market, certification may be the key to getting a job. In general, to qualify for certification, a student must first complete a program of training that is recognized by the profession. Usually this means graduating from an accredited (approved by the professional organization) program. After graduation, the student must pass a special certification examination.

Registration

Technically, **professional registration** means the listing of certified health professionals on an official roster kept by a state agency or health professional organization. In practical terms, some health professional organizations use the term "registration" interchangeably with "certification."

HEALTH CAREERS: SOMETHING FOR EVERYONE

The health field, perhaps more than any other career area, offers wide-ranging opportunities to match almost any interest. For example:

- Do you like to work with your hands? Dental technicians, ophthalmic technicians, biomedical equipment technicians, orthotists and prosthetists, and many other health professionals work with their hands.
- Are you interested in working with machines? Respiratory therapists and radiologic technologists are examples of professionals who work with patients and medical machines.
- Are you an artist, musician, or professional dancer? Does sharing your art with individuals or small groups of people appeal to you? Combining a career in the arts and psychotherapy may be the career for you.
- Do you enjoy working with people? Nursing, medicine, dentistry, dietetics, optometry, social work, rehabilitation, and mental health are some health career areas that will give you the opportunity to work with and help people of all ages.

These careers only begin to enumerate the possibilities. Health careers do offer something for everyone, but too often students say "no" to health careers simply because they do not have the facts. Some common assumptions students make when talking about health careers include such statements as the following:

I couldn't work around sick people in a hospital. That's depressing. Besides, I can't stand the sight of blood.

A health career does not automatically mean a hospital job or care of the sick. You can work in health care in research, health planning and administration, health education, disease prevention, environmental protection, and other important areas. But don't judge hospital work until you try it, either as a hospital volunteer or as a part-time employee. You may discover by working there and observing trained health professionals that you can learn to accept the less pleasant parts of helping people get well. You will also find that even in hospitals many jobs are "behind the scenes," with little or no direct contact with patients.

You need science and math for health careers. That's not for me.

Science and mathematics are required for some healthcare jobs, but many others do not emphasize these subjects. Health education and mental health are just a few areas where psychology and the social sciences are stressed. However, even when science and math are needed, different levels of skills are required. Some occupations such as optometrist and medical scientist require in-depth knowledge, while many other careers require just good basic skills and working knowledge of science and math.

Training takes too long.

Some careers do take eight or more years of preparation. Professional occupations, such as physicians and surgeons, dentists, occupational therapists, social workers, and physical therapists, require a graduate degree. However, many health occupations require two or fewer years of preparation to practice. For example, physical and occupational therapy assistants and laboratory technicians may enter through an associate's degree,

Training costs too much.

The cost of training must be balanced against what one can earn. Figures show that lifetime earnings generally increase with years of education. Most students today need and can find financial aid for training. Scholarships, loans, and loan repayment programs are available to students who are willing to make a commitment to working in underserved areas. The HRSA, National Health Service Corps, and the **Indian Health Service (IHS)** provide financial assistance in the form of scholarships, loans, and loan repayment for students who agree to serve in designated HPSAs or with the Indian Health Service for a specified period, usually two to three years depending on the amount of the loan. More details about financial assistance are listed under "Additional Information" at the end of this chapter.

Training is too hard.

Don't sell yourself short. Many students who felt the same way are now working as doctors, nurses, therapists, technologists, or other health professionals. If you fear that training may be too hard for you, then think twice. A change of attitude, a special remedial program, or additional study may be all you need to succeed. Most community colleges and educational centers offer the special studies needed to prepare you for education in a health career. Each year, many interested, qualified students give up on a health career simply because they did not explore alternatives when their first career choice was not possible. A prime example is the aspiring physician who is not admitted to a medical or osteopathic school and drops out of the health field entirely. The health field is vast; in it you will find many related careers where you can contribute and find personal satisfaction. Your talents are definitely needed in the health field.

USING THIS TEXT TO SELECT AND PLAN A HEALTH CAREER

Parts three to five of this text describe in detail the requirements, including registration, licensure, and certification, of the well-known health professions. In addition to information about requirements, each of the chapters on health careers describes the work and the work environment, employment opportunities and trends, and earnings for a specific category of patient care career. The chapters also discuss related occupations and additional sources of information about the particular career. Taken together, the career descriptions present a practical, detailed "road map"

of the vast healthcare field. Appendix A lists annual salaries for many health professions, and Appendix B has an extensive list of places to begin collecting information on careers and job opportunities. Appendix C will help you with job hunting, writing résumés, and successful interviewing.

Additional Information

The U.S. government and professional organizations involved in education and training programs in the health professions are excellent resources for students exploring health careers. General information on health careers is available from:

- Health Resources and Services Administration. 5600 Fishers Ln., Rockville, MD 2085 https://www.hrsa.gov/about/contact/index.html

Video clips describing a variety of health careers are available from government and nonprofit websites:

- U.S. Department of Labor. CareerOneStop. *Career Videos.* https://www.careeronestop.org/Videos/CareerVideos/career-videos.aspx

Students interested in pursuing a medical career should contact:

- Association of American Medical Colleges, 655 K Street, NW, Suite 100, Washington, DC, 20001-2399. https://students-residents.aamc.org/

For a list of accredited programs for dentists, dental hygienists, and dental assistants, contact:

- Commission on Dental Accreditation, American Dental Association, 211 East Chicago Avenue, Chicago, IL 60611. http://www.ada.org/en/coda/find-a-program/

For a list of accredited programs in allied health fields, contact:

- Commission on Accreditation of Allied Health Education Programs, 25400 US Highway 19 North, Suite 158, Clearwater, FL 33763. https://www.caahep.org/Students/Find-a-Program.aspx

Financial aid in the form of scholarships, loans, and loan repayment programs for healthcare workers in underserved areas is available from:

- Indian Health Service (IHS). *Loan Repayment.* http://www.ihs.gov/careeropps/loanrepayment/
- National Health Services Corps (NHSC). Health Resources and Service Administration (HRSA). *Program Areas and Resources.* https://nhsc.hrsa.gov/

Scholarships and loan repayments for disadvantaged students can be found at:

- Bureau of Health Workforce. Health Resources and Service Administration (HRSA). *For Schools: Apply for a Loan Program.* https://bhw.hrsa.gov/funding/schools-apply-loan-program#lds

LEARNING PORTFOLIO

Study Points

1. Desirable traits for healthcare workers are patience and empathy and the ability to work with people from diverse backgrounds in stressful situations.

2. The healthcare industry provides a variety of careers requiring different levels of education, from a high school diploma with on-the-job training or postsecondary training to a two-year associate's degree, four-year bachelor's degree, or six to eight years of graduate school.

3. In general, salaries are higher for healthcare practitioners and technical occupations that also require more education.

4. The expected growth for healthcare and personal assistance careers in the next decade is close to 15% compared to 4% for all other occupations.

5. The high demand for healthcare workers is related to longevity and the aging of the population who require management of chronic diseases and personal assistance with activities of daily living.

6. The group of healthcare workers projected to have the highest numbers in the next decade is home health and personal care aides.

7. The U.S. Bureau of Labor Statistics classifies healthcare workers into three broad categories: (1) Healthcare Practitioners and Technical, (2) Healthcare Support, and (3) Community and Social Service.

8. The healthcare workforce in the United States lacks diversity by gender, race, and ethnicity. The majority of workers are White women. More White males and Asians are employed in the Healthcare Practitioners and Technical category, occupations that require graduate degrees. In comparison, Blacks and Hispanics are employed in Healthcare Support occupations—those that require on-the-job training or one to two years of training—as medical and nursing assistants and home and personal care aides.

9. The benefits of a diverse healthcare workforce are improvements in communication between the healthcare worker and the patient and greater access to healthcare for minority (non-White) patients. The Health Resources and Services Administration provides financial support for minority students in the health professions.

10. The majority of healthcare workers are employed in hospitals, offices of health professionals (for example, a group practice of physicians or physical therapists), and nursing and residential facilities, including assisted-living facilities. In the next decade, more healthcare workers are expected to work in offices of health professionals, outpatient laboratory and ambulatory centers, and home care instead of hospitals.

11. There is a maldistribution of healthcare workers and a shortage of primary care providers (physicians, physician assistants, and nurse practitioners), dentists, registered nurses, and mental health clinicians in rural areas and inner cities, designated as Health Professional Shortage Areas. The National Health Service Corps and the Indian Health Service provide scholarships, loans, and loan repayment opportunities for students in exchange for working in these areas for at least two years.

12. Two important questions for students to answer when exploring a health career are: Will the degree program prepare me for the career that I want? What financial resources are available for obtaining the training or degree?

13. Most health careers require either state licensure or certification to legally practice within a state. Requirements to become licensed are completion of a training or educational program and successfully passing a licensing exam. Certification is granted by professional organizations and requires completion of an accredited education program and successfully completing a qualifying exam. Certified employees are more competitive in a tight job market.

Issues for Discussion

1. Review the requirements for becoming a dentist, dental hygienist, and dental assistant. Review dental careers in Chapter 12, the Commission on Dental Accreditation (https://www.ada.org/en/coda/find-a-program), and other resources to find out the educational requirements for each career. Compare the requirements for preparing for these three careers in terms of length of training, cost of training, job opportunities, and lifetime income. Which of these dental careers best matches your career goals?

2. Select two health careers that you are interested in pursuing—for example, massage therapist and physical therapist. Search for an educational program for each to determine the entrance requirements. What advice would you give a high school student to prepare for each career to improve their chances of being admitted to the program?

LEARNING PORTFOLIO

3. Go to the National Health Service Corps Job Center website to review jobs available to students who make a commitment to work in a Health Professional Shortage Areas (HPSA) in exchange for school loans. Are there jobs in your state? Are there locations that you are interested in pursuing? https://nhsc.hrsa.gov/

Enrichment Activities

1. Review videos of members who have served in the National Health Service Corps. Listen to members describe their experiences. Choose a specific type of loan or scholarship program, location, and discipline by using the filters on the web page.

2. Go to the website ExploreHealthCareers.org, review the section "Why Diversity Matters in Health Care," and link to workforce diversity to learn more about why the workforce needs to reflect the races and ethnicities of the population of the United States. https://explorehealthcareers.org/career-explorer/diversity-matters-health-care/#Workforce

CASE STUDY: HEALTH CAREER PLANNING

Felix is a junior in high school and is interested in pursuing a career in physical therapy. However, he is concerned about the cost and the amount of time that he will be required to be in college to become a physical therapist. Felix will be the first in his family to pursue a college degree. His parents immigrated to the United States from Mexico and were married for five years before he was born.

Based on the information you have read about career planning, answer the following questions.

1. True or false? Felix will need to obtain a doctor of physical therapy to be able to work in the field of physical therapy.

2. True or false? Felix would qualify for a college scholarship as a disadvantaged student through a school-based scholarship.

3. High school courses that would provide a good foundation for coursework for the physical therapy field are:
   A. Physics, physiology
   B. Speech, debate
   C. English composition, literature
   D. Art drawing, sculpture

4. Median yearly salaries for a physical therapy assistant (PTA) and physical therapist (DPT) in the United States are:
   A. PTA: $55,000   DPT: $ 75,000
   B. PTA: $57,000   DPT: $ 70,000
   C. PTA: $59,000   DPT: $ 90,000
   D. PTA: $70,000   DPT: $100,000

5. Healthcare workers are employed in a variety of settings. What are the major industries that employ healthcare workers?
   A. Hospitals
   B. Home health services
   C. Offices of health practitioners
   D. Nursing and residential facilities
   E. All of these are correct.

References

1. Bovbjerg R., McDonald E. Literature Review: Healthcare Occupational Training and Support Programs under the ACA—Background and Implications for Evaluating HPOG, OPRE Report #2014-29, Washington, DC: Office of Planning, Research and Evaluation, Administration for Children and Families, U.S. Department of Health and Human Services; 2014. https://www.acf.hhs.gov/sites/default/files/documents/opre/hpog_litreviewessay_policybackground_final.pdf Accessed August 24, 2021.

2. Cheeseman Day J, Christnacht C. *Women Hold 76% of All Health Care Jobs, Gaining in Higher-Paying Occupations.* August 14, 2019. U.S. Census Bureau. https://www.census.gov/library/stories/2019/08/your-health-care-in-womens-hands.html

3. U.S. Department of Health and Human Services Administration. Health Resources and Services Administration, National Center for Workforce Analysis. 2017. *Sex, Race, and Ethnic Diversity of the U.S. Health Occupations (2011–2015),* Rockville, MD. https://bhw.hrsa.gov/sites/default/files/bhw/nchwa/diversityushealthoccupations.pdf

4. United States Census Bureau. *Quick Facts.* Population Estimates. July 1, 2019. https://www.census.gov/quickfacts/fact/table/US/PST045219

5. Health Resources and Services Administration. *About Us.* https://bhw.hrsa.gov/about-us Reviewed December 2020. Accessed August 23, 2021.

6. Bureau of Labor Statistics, U.S. Department of Labor, *Occupational Outlook Handbook, 2020.* Fastest Growing Occupations. https://www.bls.gov/ooh/fastest-growing.htm

7. Bureau of Labor Statistics, U.S. Department of Labor. May 2019. *National Occupational Employment and Wage Estimate United States*. March 31, 2020. http://www.bls.gov/oes/current/oes_nat.htm

8. U.S. Bureau of Labor Statistics. Occupational Employment Statistics. *Charts of the Largest Occupations in Each Industry, May 2020. Sector 62: Health Care and Social Assistance.* https://www.bls.gov/oes/current/ind_emp_chart/ind_emp_chart.htm Accessed August 23, 2021.

9. Torpey E. Healthcare: Millions of Jobs Now and in the Future. *Occup Outlook Q*. March 2014. http://www.bls.gov/careeroutlook/2014/spring/art03.pdf

10. Kaiser Family Foundation. *State Health Facts. Providers and Service Use.* https://www.kff.org/state-category/providers-service-use/nursing-facilities/ Accessed October 20, 2020.

11. National Center for Assisted Living. *Assisted Living: A Growing Aspect of Long-Term Care.* https://www.ahcancal.org/Advocacy/IssueBriefs/NCAL_Factsheet_2019.pdf Accessed August 24, 2021.

12. Health Workforce. Health Resources and Services Administration. *What is Shortage Designation?* https://bhw.hrsa.gov/shortage-designation Shortage Designation. Reviewed February 2021. Accessed August 23, 2021.

13. Health Workforce. Health Resources and Services Administration. *Loans for Disadvantaged Students (LDS).* https://bhw.hrsa.gov/funding/schools-manage-loan-programs#LDS Reviewed January 2021. Accessed August 23, 2021.

14. National Health Services Corp. Health Resources and Services Administration. *How to Meet Eligibility Requirements for the NHSC Scholarship Program.* https://nhsc.hrsa.gov/scholarships/eligibility-requirements.html Reviewed May 2021. Accessed August 23, 2021.

15. Health Resources and Services Administration. National Health Services Corps. National Health Services Corps. Health Resources and Services Administration. *National Health Service Corps Loan Repayment Program.* Reviewed May 2021. Accessed August 23, 2021.

16. National Health Service Corps. *Students to Service Loan Repayment Program FY 2021 Application and Program Guidance.* September 2020. https://nhsc.hrsa.gov/sites/default/files/NHSC/loan-repayment/nhsc-students2service-LRP-application-program-guidance.pdf Accessed August 24, 2021.

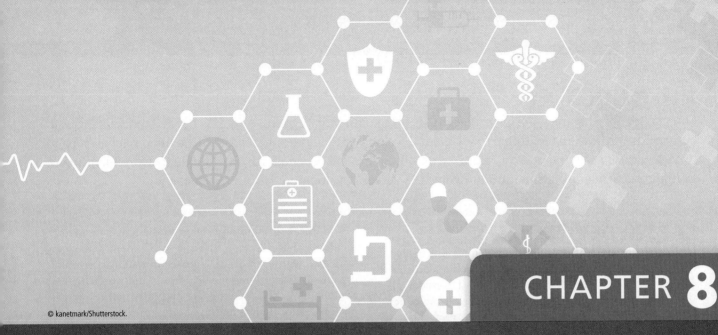

© kanetmark/Shutterstock.

CHAPTER 8

Career Development

Introduction

Often students who are choosing careers focus on the immediate future—what is needed today in order to become the professional of tomorrow. Career development includes that initial focus but stretches beyond it. **Career development** refers to an organized planning method used to form an individual's work identity. An example of the many considerations involved in career development is seen in **FIGURE 8.1**.

CAREER DEVELOPMENT

In developing one's career, an individual must understand what must be studied and understood to become successful initially and over time. The individual must consider all aspects of professionalism, including those involving ethics and confidentiality. Because some healthcare professionals have derailed their careers by acting in a negligent manner with patients, healthcare practitioners must understand legal issues affecting themselves and the patients with whom they interact. Healthcare practitioners must understand not only the need but also the mechanisms for continuing their education so that they may learn the most recent information in their field. How these concerns have played out for one healthcare practitioner is the subject of the professional profile in this chapter.

COMMON CORE KNOWLEDGE

Health care is a dynamic and complex field that requires training in not only the sciences but also the intricacies of interpersonal skills. In completing their training and in performing their careers, healthcare professionals share a common core of knowledge. Because entire courses are devoted to the following subjects, they are described briefly as a way of introduction to the common core of knowledge.[1]

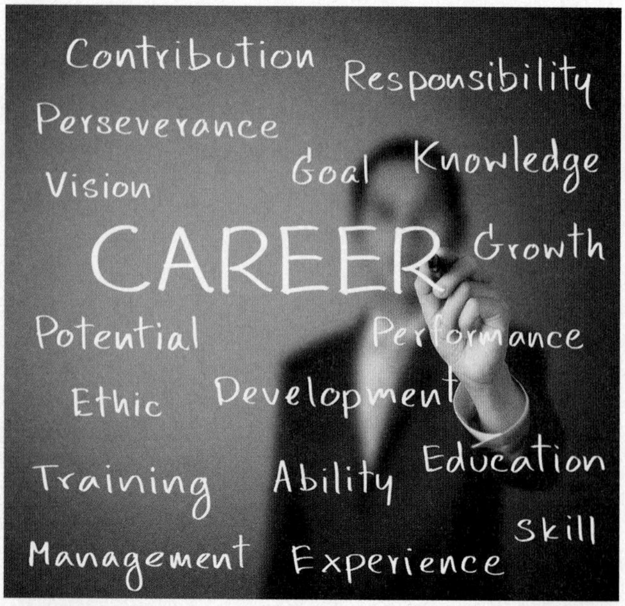

FIGURE 8.1 There are many factors that can impact career development in a positive way.
© Dusit/Shutterstock.

Medical terminology refers to the language used in medicine that allows healthcare professionals to communicate with each other. Courses in medical terminology involve identifying medical terms and words by their component parts, defining the body's structures and its systems, and understanding body orientation, health, wellness, disease terms, and appropriate medical abbreviations and symbols. Upon mastering the subject, healthcare professionals can communicate with precision and accuracy about the medical issues associated with their patients.

Anatomy and physiology (A&P) are courses common in the healthcare professional curriculum. **Anatomy** refers to the structure of organisms and their parts. **Physiology** focuses on how organisms and their parts carry out the normal physical functions that allow them to exist. Often taken in combination or sequentially, A&P courses provide a comprehensive understanding of how the human body works and allow professionals to describe diseases and disorders of each body system.

Technical skills are part of every curriculum in healthcare specialties that involve direct patient contact. Students typically learn procedures for measuring and recording vital signs. They commonly learn first aid, cardiopulmonary resuscitation (CPR), how to use an automated external defibrillator (AED), and how to clear a foreign body airway obstruction (FBAO). They learn additional technical skills depending on their career specialty.

Safety is of paramount importance in health care, including to patients, visitors, and healthcare providers themselves. **Infection control** deals with preventing the spread of healthcare-associated infections. The focus rests on preventing or halting the spread of infection within the healthcare setting, whether that spread is among patients, among patients and healthcare providers, or among healthcare providers. Once an infection is present, focus rests on monitoring its spread in the healthcare setting and managing the outbreak.

Safety also refers to applying procedures and protocols to reduce the potential for bodily injury. Healthcare students learn about body mechanics and the proper ways in which to move patients so as to avoid injury to patients and themselves. Most learn about the proper use and disposal of body fluids, pharmaceutical products, dressings, syringes, needle sticks, lancets, and hazardous materials. Proper methods of sterilization, such as using liquid or solid cleaning solutions, are learned and employed in the school and work settings. Also offered are training on

Professional Profiles

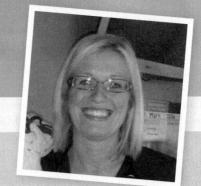

Name: Amanda, RN
Job Title: Charge Nurse
Education: ADN; enrolled for BSN

Q: Tell us about your career progression.

A: After graduating from nursing school, I hired on at a local hospital with 113 beds and soon after found myself a charge nurse on a 31-bed high acuity telemetry unit. Diagnoses of our patients varied from congestive heart failure, myocardial infarction, cardiomyopathy, and many chest pain rule-outs that resulted in other various outcomes.

I recently took a position on a 40-bed medical floor as a free charge nurse. My job now allows me to focus on the hospital's quality indicators and outcomes. I get to round on patients in the morning to determine the needs of my colleagues and the floor. I love the role I am currently in because I can advocate for patients by discussing the care they are receiving and learning ways to improve our delivery.

Q: What challenges you about your profession?

A: Nursing has been a very challenging yet fulfilling career for me. It has allowed me to develop a professional skill set, build relationships with patients, and learn on a daily basis from my peers. I have recently become engaged in community events while sitting on the Young Professional Advisory Board in my county. I have had many great opportunities while working as a registered nurse and look forward to many to come.

Q: How have you demonstrated professionalism in your career?

A: Over the years, my career has presented me with many opportunities to grow as a professional. The hospital has a clinical development program that allows nurses to put together a portfolio representing their work over time. There are many requirements including service in the community, continuing education, awards or recognition from patients, and participation in committees or improvement events that take place in the hospital. Developing this portfolio and committing to the work that it entails encourages me to view my job as a nurse as something much more. Nursing is a profession and has been elevated to that over time. As a nurse, I feel it's my obligation to continue to engage myself into my community and help represent what the profession of nursing is.

Q: Without disclosing protected health information, describe an ethical challenge you've faced and how you addressed it.

A: As a nurse I often am witness to ethical dilemmas within the acute care setting. When taking care of an elderly patient who had decided to go on hospice, I witnessed many family members who came in to visit who were not in agreement with the patient's decision. Over the course of a few days, the patient had become very weak and unable to communicate. Many family members began to demand that the decision to start hospice care be reversed and that [hospital staff] resume treatment for the patient's cancer. When involved in caring for large families and patients with terminal illness, it is important to advocate for the patient. At times, it can be emotionally taxing, and your own beliefs may not agree with those of the patient; however, it's important to keep your own beliefs out of it. Ultimately, in this particular situation, my patient had paperwork that reflected his wants and needs for end-of-life care. He had made a decision to die peacefully, and my job was to allow him just that. We called a chaplain in to comfort the family and help them understand that the patient was clear about his wishes. In this case, the family just needed support to accept his wishes. Death is hard for all parties involved, but as a nurse, my first priority was advocacy for my patient.

Q: Describe the continuing education requirements for your profession.

A: Continuing education is mandated each year and can be different from unit to unit. My floor must participate in a skills lab that ensures that we are proficient in a number of clinical skills. We must also obtain eight hours of continuing education hours that we can do online or take classes within the hospital. Throughout the hospital, there are multiple types of equipment to safely transfer patients who need assistance with ambulation, so every year we have to demonstrate proficiency in safe patient handling. It is also mandatory to maintain a current BLS (basic life support) card to keep up to date a BLS (basic life support) card and in some areas a ACLS (advanced cardiac life support) card.

emergency procedures and protocols in the event of a fire or other disaster and compliance with safety techniques in the work environment.

Math courses are common across the healthcare professions. Frequently referred to as **medical math**, these courses teach students how to apply mathematical computations related to healthcare procedures. Students learn to record time using the 24-hour clock and to analyze charts, diagrams, graphs, and tables to interpret healthcare results. Examples of math used by some healthcare professionals are given in **TABLE 8.1**.

Students sometimes express worry about medical math, concerned that it may be too hard to master. The reality is that medical math builds on basic mathematical concepts such as addition, subtraction, multiplication, and division. Students learn to express math results as whole numbers, fractions, degrees, angles, decimals, ratios, and percentages. Students learn to convert between systems of measurement, such as metric, household, and apothecary, and between Fahrenheit and Celsius. The understanding of basic math skills and the ways to express and convert numbers makes it possible for healthcare professionals to perform their duties.

Knowledge of healthy behaviors is central to a healthcare provider's success with patients. A **healthy behavior** refers to an action taken to attain, maintain, or regain good health and to prevent illness. Common healthy behaviors include weight control, exercise, and good sleep habits. Students learn strategies that promote health and wellness and integrate them into their activities with patients. These activities may be seen in outreach programs to the community, screenings for diseases and disorders, and stress management offerings.

Communication refers to the sharing of information between two or more people as a way to convey meaning. Healthcare professionals must communicate with and relate to a wide variety of individuals, including patients, family members and visitors, other members of the healthcare team, administrators, and, on occasion, vendors. Honing active listening skills, which focus on what the speaker is saying, is a requirement of a successful healthcare professional.

Verbal communication is essential to the delivery of high-quality patient care. Patients must be able to address their health complaints and concerns with healthcare professionals who can process that information in a manner that will work to respond to the patient's complaints and concerns. Additionally, healthcare professionals use verbal communication skills to convey instructions to patients on measures to take to treat their current illness, prevent future illness, and maintain a healthy lifestyle. They also employ these skills to report to other healthcare providers the condition and progress of the patients for whom they care.

Communication includes more than verbal skills but also the ability to write and effectively present information. Writing in health care frequently refers to documenting in the patient's health record. A **health record** is an ordered set of documents or a collection of data that contains a complete and accurate description of a patient's history, condition, diagnostic and therapeutic treatment, and results of treatment. Health records are considered the primary source to document patient care and to communicate between the healthcare team. The process of entering this description is referred to as **documentation**. The documentation process may consist of traditional paper, an electronic health record, or a hybrid of both.

Written communication might also take the form of health literacy presentations, whether through graphs, narratives, infographics, or other means. Healthcare professionals may need to "tell a story" to an audience, whether that story is the progression of care provided to patients for a given disease or disorder or to convey how a patient may typically interact with providers in a healthcare environment, among numerous topics. Working to improve one's communication skills can educate current and future patients so that they can take a strong role in addressing their own healthcare needs.

The manner in which health care is delivered to patients is commonly taught to healthcare students. Many different healthcare delivery systems exist, including governmental, nonprofit, for-profit, public, and private. Each of these systems influences how care is delivered by healthcare providers and paid for by insurers, the government, and patients. Students study healthcare economics and common methods of payment, the structure and relationships of healthcare systems, and the responsibilities of consumers in the healthcare system.

TABLE 8.1 Examples of Medical Math Used by Healthcare Professionals

Healthcare Professional	Activities
Administrators	Prepare bills; create budgets.
Diagnostic medical sonographers	Determine angles needed to create a three-dimensional image.
Health information managers	Develop and report descriptive and vital statistics; analyze case mix.
Nurses and aides	Record vital signs; administer medications.
Pharmacists	Calculate medication dosages.
Psychologists	Analyze diagnostic surveys and studies.
Technicians and therapists (laboratory, occupational, physical, radiation, and respiratory)	Perform tests; record results.

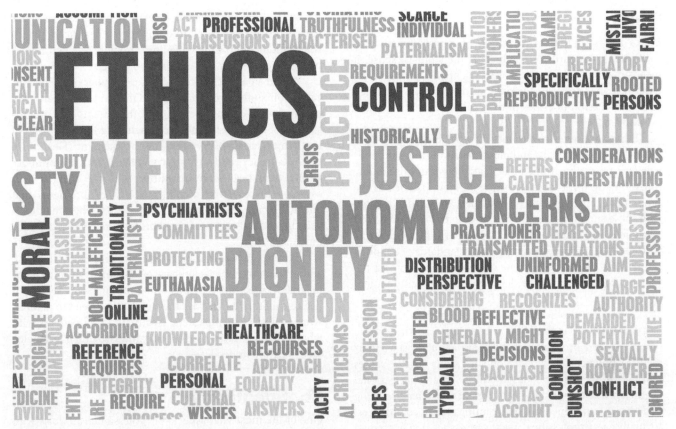

FIGURE 8.2 Having a strong code of ethics helps promote the welfare of patients and the delivery of high-quality patient care.
© kentoh/Shutterstock.

Students also study the impact of emerging technologies in health care. They learn about new technologies that affect their ability to care for patients. They learn basic computer concepts, terminology, and skills and what is considered appropriate use of social media and email in the healthcare workplace. They learn about electronic health records, the data that is entered into them, and the fundamentals of securing that data from unlawful access.

PROFESSIONALISM

To sustain their careers over time, healthcare practitioners must be prepared to act in a professional manner at all stages. A **professional** is a person with specialized learning who is engaged in a specified activity as an occupation. Those professionals who specialize in the healthcare realm are referred to as healthcare professionals. **Professionalism** refers to the conduct, character, skill, and judgment of a trained person. Healthcare professionals who act in an accountable and ethical manner in the workplace and maintain a steady composure in the face of adversity demonstrate professionalism.

The manner in which healthcare professionals conduct themselves on the job influences the confidence patients have in the care they receive. Placing the patient's welfare first and treating everyone with common courtesy are signs of a professional attitude. Similarly, dressing and looking like a professional is often seen by patients as a sign of respect.

A critical feature of professionalism is the achievement of a high level of skill in the discipline in which the healthcare provider is trained. Maintaining a healthy balance between caring for patients without becoming emotionally attached is essential to a professional approach to delivering health care.

The professional manner in which healthcare providers conduct themselves on the job also influences their opportunities for advancement. Those individuals who merely "do their job" without any further commitment limit their opportunities for promotion. By contrast, those individuals who contribute positively to the workplace through interaction with their patients and coworkers and address work-related problems as opportunities to demonstrate problem-solving skills present themselves as good candidates for advancement. Performing at the highest professional standards positions an individual for further progress in his or her career.

The need to handle conflict in the workplace in an appropriate manner is a sign of professionalism. **Conflicts** are serious disagreements or arguments. Conflicts can arise for numerous reasons, whether because of personality clashes; differences in culture, values, or work style; competition between people; or a host of other reasons. Utilizing communication skills is essential to resolving conflicts. Addressing conflicts in a calm manner, actively listening to a coworker's concerns, defining the essence or cause of the conflict, and finding areas of agreement can go a long way to resolving a conflict and demonstrating professionalism.

Ethics

Ethics refers to the formal study of moral choices that conform to standards of conduct. In the simplest sense, it means making judgments between right and wrong or listening to one's conscience. Many of the concepts included in any discussion of ethics in the healthcare field are listed in **FIGURE 8.2**.

Ethics are interwoven into the professional lives of healthcare professionals, and many situations these individuals face pose ethical dilemmas. Situations can arise at any time, ranging from the time before an infant is born to the time a patient dies. Healthcare providers are aided in dealing with these situations not only by their internal compass but by professional codes of ethics. A **code of ethics** refers to a written list of a profession's values and standards of conduct. In the healthcare context, these codes of ethics promote the welfare of patients and the delivery of high-quality patient care.

Codes of ethics have existed for thousands of years. The best-known code is the Hippocratic Oath, an ethical code typically taken by physicians who are about to start their medical practice. This oath contains many of the values that form the basis for codes of ethics of many professional healthcare associations: acting to benefit the patient, refusing to do harm to patients, and maintaining patient confidences. Virtually every professional healthcare association has issued a code of ethics, and members of those associations are bound by the terms of those codes.

Many codes of professional conduct address the issue of disparagement, a form of professional misconduct. **Disparagement** refers to belittling or criticizing the skills, knowledge, or qualifications of another professional. It is often seen in the form of personal attacks upon a fellow professional instead of a focus on the merits of the issue under consideration. Healthcare practitioners who exercise care to avoid disparagement increase the possibility of persuading others of the merits of an issue and avoid accusations of professional misconduct.

Similarly, many codes of ethics address the issue of conflict of interest. A **conflict of interest** means a clash between an individual's selfish interests and his or her obligations to an organization, group, or person. Conflicts of interest arise when the healthcare practitioner places his or her interests ahead of the patient's interests. For example, sexual relations between a healthcare practitioner and a patient are seen as a conflict of interest because the healthcare practitioner has advantage over the patient in terms of knowledge, power, and status. Such advantage results in a power imbalance, making true consent impossible to measure and raising questions of ethically inappropriate conduct.

Ethical issues may impact the safety and welfare of patients, and when they do, healthcare professionals are obligated to address those issues. For example, healthcare practitioners who experience substance abuse problems place their patients' safety at risk. Healthcare practitioners who

recognize a fellow colleague impaired by substance abuse have an obligation to act. In doing so, the healthcare practitioner should follow the guidelines and policies of both their professional association and their employer.

When a patient, visitor, or other member of the healthcare team suffers from an adverse incident, the healthcare provider may create a report that documents the circumstances of the adverse incident, including the condition of the subject and observations of the incident. Healthcare providers may address ethical issues with committees within their healthcare institution who are charged with assisting in resolving complicated ethical problems that affect the care and treatment of patients. They may consult the code of ethics of their professional association for guidance.

Ethical practice also includes addressing cultural, social, and ethnic diversity. Healthcare professionals need to demonstrate respect for religious and cultural values related to health care that differ from their own. They need to demonstrate civility and empathetic treatment to all patients with whom they come in contact, regardless of their ethnicity, race, religion, or gender.

Confidentiality

One of the most vital aspects of professionalism deals with confidentiality of patient information. **Confidentiality** refers to the healthcare professional's obligation to maintain patient information in a manner that will not permit dissemination beyond the healthcare provider. A major fear of patients is that they will become the subject of gossip or social conversations among healthcare providers overheard by others. Healthcare professionals are taught to only discuss

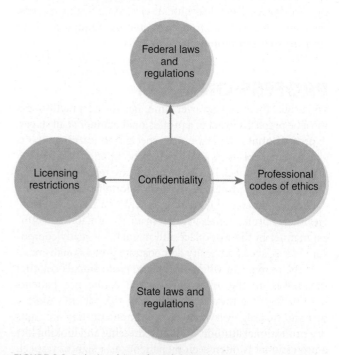

FIGURE 8.3 Relationships of confidentiality with law and ethics.

confidential patient information with those medical personnel who are involved in treating the patient. Professionals know not to make comments in public areas about patient information.

Healthcare professionals who breach confidentiality not only damage their relationship with the patient, but they may also violate the law and professional requirements. Each state has laws addressing patient confidentiality and allows for lawsuits against those who breach those laws. At the federal level, regulations issued pursuant to the Health Insurance Portability and Accountability Act (HIPAA) establish many confidentiality restrictions, identify what constitutes improper disclosure of protected health information, and specify fines and other penalties that may be imposed if confidentiality is violated. Additionally, most regulatory and licensing bodies that govern the health professions have similar requirements, and healthcare professionals who violate those requirements may face discipline, including removal of their license to practice in the healthcare field. Finally, professional associations to which healthcare providers belong publicize codes of ethics that contain confidentiality restrictions, and healthcare providers risk discipline, including expulsion, from those associations for violating patient confidentiality. The relationship between and among confidentiality, law, licensing, and professional codes of ethics is seen in **FIGURE 8.3**.

Healthcare Teams

The concept of **health teams** in all types of health services has brought about changes in healthcare delivery. The health team consists of a variety of health personnel, each with a specialized function. The membership of the health team varies in accordance with the needs of the client and his or her family. Team members are usually doctors, nurses, dietitians, therapists, and other direct-care providers. The diverse knowledge, skills, and talents of these team members and the collaborative manner in which they work can result in the delivery of improved patient care and a better patient experience.

There are two general types of health teams: functional and patient-centered. Both depend on the kind of problem to be solved, and teams may dissolve at any given point and regroup to meet special problems. Functional teams are formed to take care of specific problems. Examples include a mental health team or a coronary care team. Patient-centered teams include patients and their families who are involved in making healthcare decisions together with their doctor and other healthcare professionals. Medical technologists, radiologic technologists, and pathologists may form a backup medical care team for the patient. They are not in close contact with the patient but deal with parts of the patient's service, such as his or her X-rays, blood samples, and cultures.

At the outside edge of the interrelated teams are the people who concentrate on the delivery, costs, quality, and availability of services. This healthcare team is composed of public health agents, hospital administrators, health information managers, health educators, sanitarians, and others.

People working in the health professions understand the changing nature of the teams and recognize that the combined skills of many professionals contribute to modern health care.

LEGAL ISSUES IN HEALTH CARE

In terms of career development, the focus rests on two main legal issues: obtaining the legal right to practice in a particular health profession and staying out of trouble that might result in a lawsuit.

Right to Practice

Once an individual completes his or her course of study, he or she generally feels competent to set off into the workforce. Like some other professions, those involved in health care are highly regulated, meaning that in order to practice a given health profession, an individual must determine if they need a license or certification.

Licensing refers to a right conferred by a governmental body to practice an occupation or provide a service. Each state decides what professions to license; occupations commonly subject to licensure include medicine; podiatry; pharmacy; nursing; occupational, physical, and respiratory therapy; and osteopathy, among others. Licensing serves as a way to control the number of individuals who practice a particular calling. To be licensed, one generally must present proof of specialized education and pass an examination administered by the appropriate state board. If one practices a given profession without a license, the individual does so at his or her own risk because that practice is considered illegal under state law.

The licensing process extends beyond individuals to healthcare facilities. State regulatory bodies have developed basic minimum standards for healthcare facilities to meet in order to obtain and maintain a license to operate. In addition, healthcare facilities often seek accreditation status. **Accreditation** refers to the process by which an external entity reviews an organization or program of study to determine if the organization or program meets certain predetermined standards. Healthcare facilities are motivated to achieve accreditation status because this status is linked with the ability to receive financial reimbursement for services and recognition of the delivery of high-quality services.

Certification refers to the action or process of providing an individual with an official document attesting to his or her status or level of achievement. In contrast to licensure, certification is conferred by private organizations and not state governmental bodies. To become certified, an individual must pass an examination administered by an accredited body that monitors and upholds prescribed standards for the industry involved. Occupations commonly subject to certification include addiction or behavior specialists, health information administrators and technicians, mental health aides, and home health aides, among others. Individuals without certification who attempt to practice in professions that commonly require certification may experience trouble getting a job; however, practicing without certification generally does not violate state law.

Avoiding Lawsuits

Lawsuits are a hallmark of American life because they attempt to resolve disputes that were not resolved by other means. Healthcare professionals are subjects of lawsuits for a number of reasons.

The most common accusation leveled in a lawsuit against a healthcare practitioner is malpractice. **Malpractice** refers to professional misconduct. Numerous forms of malpractice exist, but the most common type is negligence. **Negligence** refers to someone failing to do something that a reasonably prudent person would do in the same or a similar situation or, alternatively, doing something that a reasonably prudent person would not do in the same or a similar

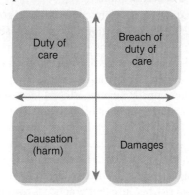

FIGURE 8.4 Elements of a negligence claim.

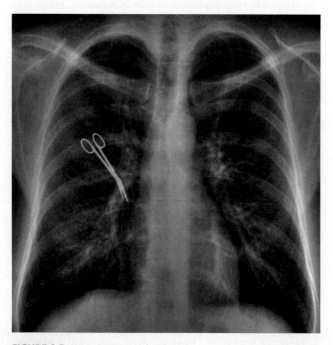

FIGURE 8.5 X-ray image with scissors.
© luk/Shutterstock.

situation. Negligence is characterized by carelessness, inattentiveness, or neglectfulness as opposed to intentionally trying to cause harm. Four elements constitute a negligence claim, and the individual bringing the lawsuit must prove all elements to succeed, absent a successful defense. These elements are listed in **FIGURE 8.4**.

Numerous forms of negligence exist. Perhaps a sponge was left inside the patient following surgery. In the regular course of surgery, a foreign object would not be left in the patient. In that instance, the patient could sue under the legal theory of *res ipsa loquitor*, meaning the thing speaks for itself. An example of a foreign body left in a patient is seen in **FIGURE 8.5**. Alternatively, a healthcare provider may not observe confidentiality restrictions and improperly disclose protected patient information to someone not treating the patient. In that instance, the patient could sue for breach of confidentiality. Then again, a psychologist may fail to take steps to protect an innocent third party from a dangerous patient.[2] In that instance, the injured third party could sue for failure to warn. In each of these examples, the healthcare provider possessed a duty of care that wasn't properly exercised (the breach) and caused harm to another person, resulting in damages.

Not all forms of malpractice are nonintentional; some are arguably committed by healthcare professionals with the intent to cause harm. For example, a physician may act in a manner beyond that to which the patient originally agreed or consented, such as performing a mastectomy when the patient only agreed to exploratory surgery.[3] In that instance, the patient could sue for technical battery. Alternatively, a physician may unilaterally end a relationship with a patient without giving notice when the patient continues to need care.[4] In that instance, the patient could sue for medical abandonment.

Another possibility for a malpractice lawsuit involves the use of social media. Healthcare professionals must exercise care in using blogs, online forums, wikis, chat rooms, and similar forms of social media. For example, a healthcare professional may dispense inadequate medical advice based on material received through social media that is not as thorough as what may have been gathered in a face-to-face encounter, thereby reducing the healthcare provider's understanding of the patient's condition. In that instance, the patient could sue for negligence. Alternatively, a healthcare provider may respond to a patient's social media inquiry with patient-specific, protected health information but not do so in a secure fashion, such as using encryption technology. In this instance, the patient could sue for breach of confidentiality. Finally, a healthcare professional may treat patients through social media who do not reside in the same state in which the professional is licensed. Most states issues licenses that are limited to practice within a state's boundaries. In that instance, the patient could sue for the unauthorized practice of the healthcare practitioner's profession.

While many lawsuits involving health care focus on treatment of the patient, some lawsuits focus on

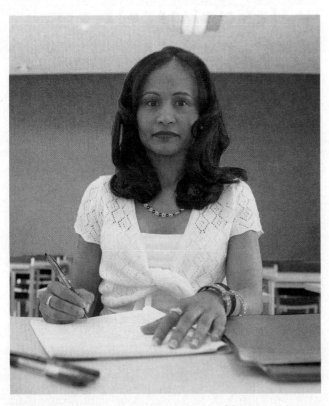

FIGURE 8.6 Continuing education is a part of career development.
© Blend Images/Shutterstock.

administrative matters. Fraud and abuse are the most frequently alleged legal issues related to administrative matters in health care. **Fraud** refers to the intentional deception of another person to that person's detriment. **Abuse** refers to a pattern of practices or customs that are unsound or inconsistent with ethical business, fiscal, or healthcare practices or customs. Actions involving fraud and abuse cover a wide range, including misrepresentation in the marketing of pharmaceuticals and failure to submit medical device reports to the Food and Drug Administration. These actions may also include filing false cost reports to Medicare, conspiracy to fraudulently bill Medicare or Medicaid, or payment of bribes. Lawsuits alleging fraud and abuse are often brought by a governmental entity or an insurance company against the healthcare practitioner.

Each of these examples illustrate how healthcare professionals have experienced legal trouble and been sued for some form of malpractice or allegations of fraud and abuse. While not every lawsuit can be avoided, healthcare practitioners can reduce the chance they will be sued by exercising care in treating patients, complying with acceptable standards of care, and taking only those actions they are authorized to take by state law.

CONTINUING EDUCATION REQUIREMENTS

Because the healthcare field evolves so rapidly and frequently, healthcare professionals are called upon to learn the most recent information in their professional field. Additionally, state licensing boards and professional associations may require the healthcare professional to continually learn. The process by which a professional seeks recurrent learning activities and training beyond that required for the initial license or certificate is referred to as **continuing education**. Continuing education is seen as an integral part of career development and an example is shown in **FIGURE 8.6**.

Continuing education can take many forms. Individuals may take a degree credit course, pursue nondegree career training, engage in sponsored workforce training or experiential learning, or participate in self-directed learning. In each instance, the individuals may be trying to better their understanding, improve their technique, or learn a new skill or technology. This form of growth can in turn be applied to the delivery of patient care.

Additionally, individuals may seek to meet the requirements of their state licensing board or professional association. In those situations, the licensing board or professional association possesses authority to decide how much continuing education is required over a specific period of time in order to maintain or renew a license or credential, which forms of continuing education it will recognize as acceptable, and how the individual must report or show evidence of meeting the continuing education requirement. Failure of healthcare professionals to meet the established requirements may result in jeopardizing their licenses and certifications to practice their profession.

SUMMARY

Career development is a continuum. It extends beyond the common core of knowledge needed initially to enter into a healthcare profession and lasts through all stages of the profession. During the span of a given career, healthcare professionals may encounter difficult situations that require taking action in keeping with ethical norms. They may be faced with concerns over patient confidentiality or the possibility of being sued in court. Additionally, they need to continually learn about their discipline, as health care is a rapidly changing field.

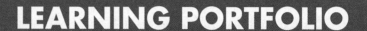

LEARNING PORTFOLIO

Study Points

1. Career development stretches beyond what is needed initially to enter into a healthcare profession.

2. Training for healthcare students includes similarities across disciplines, referred to as a common core of knowledge.

3. Healthcare professionals who act in an accountable and ethical manner in the workplace and maintain a steady composure in the face of adversity demonstrate professionalism.

4. Codes of ethics are common across virtually every healthcare discipline.

5. Healthcare professionals who breach confidentiality not only damage their relationship with the patient, but they may also violate the law and professional requirements.

6. Many healthcare practitioners contribute to the successful treatment of patients through health teams.

7. Malpractice is professional misconduct.

8. Continuing education is an integral part of career development.

Issues for Discussion

1. At one time or another, most everyone has encountered someone who has acted in a less-than-professional manner. Discuss with your instructor and classmates examples you have experienced of this phenomenon. Describe what actions you think should have been taken in these examples that could have turned the nonprofessional situation into a professional situation.

2. Math anxiety has played a role in discouraging students from pursuing entry into the health professions. Brainstorm with your classmates and instructor the reasons math anxiety exists, considering whether timed tests and the risk of public embarrassment play a role. Discuss what actions can be taken to lessen or eliminate math anxiety.

Enrichment Activities

1. Safety of healthcare professionals is an important function of the job. Research the Internet for the rates of injury to registered nurses, physicians, nurse's aides, dietitians, physical therapists, respiratory therapists, and housekeeping staff. Create a chart comparing the types and rates of injury among these healthcare professionals.

2. Codes of ethics exist in virtually every healthcare profession. Research the websites of any of the professional associations listed in subsequent chapters to see what they include in their code of ethics. Create a chart identifying the similarities and differences between the codes of ethics of various professional associations.

3. Continuing education is usually a central tenet of a professional association. Research the websites of some professional associations listed in subsequent chapters to see what types and how much continuing education activity are required over a specified period of time. Create a chart comparing this information for each profession chosen.

4. Educating patients about various healthcare topics is increasingly important to the quality of health care. Thinking of yourself as a future healthcare professional, brainstorm ideas of what topics you might use to educate patients so that they can play a larger role in their own health care. Discuss these ideas with your classmates and instructor.

CASE STUDY: PROFESSIONALISM

Montez is a medical assistant at a physician's office whose role is to greet patients, collect information from them, make patients comfortable, and answer questions about their appointment at the physician's office. Montez is particularly fond of a video game that he plays on his phone when there is downtime in the office. One afternoon, Montez was so engrossed in the video game he was playing that he ignored a patient when the patient approached Montez's desk and only acknowledged the patient after the patient got loud and demanded Montez's attention. When he did speak with the patient, Montez acted preoccupied, as though he was still thinking of his video game instead of the patient before him. Montez failed to collect any information from the patient beyond the patient's name and asked the patient to sit in the waiting room until being called.

1. Did Montez act as a professional in this situation? Why or why not?

2. Did Montez use effective communication skills in this situation? Why or why not?

3. Did Montez act in an ethical manner? Why or why not?

4. Was any conflict of interest present? Why or why not?

LEARNING PORTFOLIO

References

1. Material related to the common core of knowledge arises from two sources: the National Health Science Standards, National Consortium for Health Science Education (2019) available at https://www.healthscienceconsortium.org/wp-content/uploads/2019/05/NATIONAL_HEALTH_SCIENCE_STANDARDS.pdf and Health Science Alignment—Common Core Mathematics, Department of Elementary and Secondary Education, State of Missouri (2011) available at https://dese.mo.gov/sites/default/files/HealthSciMath.pdf

2. *Tarasoff v. Regents of University of California*, 529 P.2d 553 (Cal. 1974), *reargued*, 551 P.2d 334 (Cal. 1976).

3. *Corn v. French*, 289 P.2d 173 (Nev. 1955).

4. *Katsetos v. Nolan*, 368 A.3d 172 (Conn. 1976).

PART THREE

Health Practitioners and Technicians

This section includes the most popular health careers and newer careers as a result of technology, research, changes in reimbursement policies, or greater access to health care. Greater demands are expected for community health workers, substance abuse and behavior disorder counselors, genetic counselors, and advanced practice registered nurses. New specialty areas for physicians are hospitalists and palliative and hospice care.

OBJECTIVES

The following objectives are for all chapters in Part Three. After studying the chapters in this part, the student should be able to:

- Describe the responsibilities and work of each profession.
- Classify the types of specialties in each profession.
- Discuss the environment in which the work takes place.
- Identify any healthcare personnel who assist the professionals with their work.
- Compare and contrast the following factors among the professions: educational requirements, employment trends, opportunities for advancement, salary potential, and career ladders.
- Describe the differences in licensing, certification, and registration for careers of interest.
- Identify the professionals who do similar tasks or have similar responsibilities.
- Explain the concept and process of interprofessional education (IPE) and interprofessional practice (IPP) in healthcare.

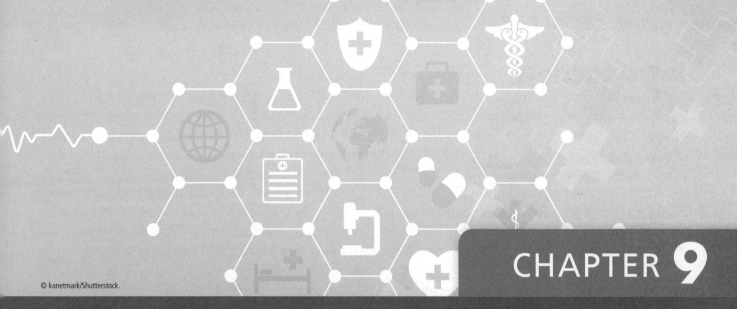

© kanetmark/Shutterstock.

CHAPTER 9

Physicians, Surgeons, and Podiatrists*

KEY TERMS

Advanced Practice Registered Nurse (APRN)

Allopathic physician

American Board of Medical Specialties (ABMS)

American Board of Podiatric Medicine (ABPM)

American Board of Podiatric Surgery (ABFAS)

American Osteopathic Association (AOA)

American Podiatric Medical Licensing Exam (APMLE)

Comprehensive Osteopathic Medical Licensing Examination (COMLEX-USA)

Council on Podiatric Medical Education (CPME)

Doctor of Osteopathy (DO)

Doctor of Podiatric Medicine (DPM)

Group practice

Hospice and palliative medicine (HPM)

Hospitalist

Liaison Committee on Medical Education (LCME)

Medical College Admissions Test (MCAT)

Medical Doctor (MD)

Medical home

Osteopathic Manipulative Medicine (OMM)

Osteopathic physician

Palliative care

Physician Assistant (PA)

Primary care provider (practitioner) (PCP)

Solo practitioner

U.S. Medical Licensing Examination (USMLE)

* All information in this chapter, unless otherwise indicated, was obtained from Bureau of Labor Statistics. *Occupational Outlook Handbook 2020–2021 Edition.* Washington, DC: U.S. Department of Labor; 2021.

Introduction

Although only one of many career paths available to those with an interest in and aptitude for a career involving patient care, the profession of physician is one that most readily comes to mind when one thinks of a career in health care. The title "Doctor" traditionally inspires respect—and perhaps envy. Media portrayal through the years has contributed to a popular perception of doctors as public servants of rare intelligence, compassion, and skill.

Although public perceptions of physicians will undoubtedly persist, individuals approaching a career choice should be guided by realities rather than perceptions. The cost of training is a serious consideration for would-be physicians, and like other healthcare professionals, physicians must adjust to changes in the healthcare system, some of which are potentially constraining to autonomy and earning power.

PHYSICIANS AND SURGEONS: THE PERCEPTIONS
Significant Points

- Many physicians and surgeons work long, irregular hours.
- Acceptance to medical school is highly competitive.
- Formal education and training requirements are among the most demanding of any occupation, but earnings are among the highest. Training is typically four years of undergraduate school, four years of medical school, one year of internship, and two to seven years of residency and fellowship.
- Job opportunities should be very good, particularly in rural and low-income areas.

DOCTORS AND SURGEONS: THE REALITIES
Projected Shortage of Primary Care Practitioners

The demand for physicians is projected to exceed supply by 2032 because of the aging population and because seniors have more chronic diseases requiring more health care.[1] **Primary care providers or practitioners (PCPs)** include physicians, **Advanced Practice Registered Nurses (APRNs)**, and **Physician Assistants (PAs)** practicing in family medicine, general pediatrics, internal medicine, and geriatrics. There is also a shortage of PCPs because many physicians train to be specialists who do not see patients for common health problems. The number of APRNs and PAs is projected to grow faster than physicians through 2029; both APRNs and PAs can extend primary care services.[2] Having sufficient numbers of PCPs is important because they coordinate care for individual patients and the U.S. healthcare system requires that referrals to physician specialists be made through PCPs (**FIGURE 9.1**).

The primary care model includes a **medical home** to provide ongoing preventive care such as health screening and immunizations, treatment of common health problems such as upper respiratory infections and minor injuries as needed, and making referrals to physician specialists for diagnosis and treatment of complex health problems. For example, a PCP might refer a patient with angina— symptoms of coronary artery disease—to a cardiologist to conduct balloon angioplasty or stent placement.[3]

Work Description

Physicians and surgeons diagnose illnesses and prescribe and administer treatment for people suffering from injury or disease. Physicians examine patients, obtain medical histories, and order, perform, and interpret diagnostic tests. They also counsel patients on preventive health care.

There are two types of physicians: **Medical Doctor (MD)** and **Doctor of Osteopathy (DO)**. MDs also are known as **allopathic physicians**, and DOs are known as **osteopathic physicians**. Although both MDs and DOs may use all accepted methods of treatment, including drugs and surgery, DOs place special emphasis on the body's musculoskeletal system, preventive medicine, and holistic patient care. DOs are more likely to work in primary care, although they can be found in all specialties. About half of DOs practice general or family medicine, general internal medicine, or general pediatrics. Medical school training that is unique to DOs is **Osteopathic Manipulative Medicine (OMM)**, a hands-on approach used to treat discomfort, pain, or limited range of motion from injury or disease. Examples of conditions treated by OMM are headaches; lower back, neck, or shoulder pain; and stress or athletic injuries. Some DOs choose an internship or residency program that incorporates OMM, usually a DO residency. Other DOs apply to an MD residency (**FIGURE 9.2**).[4]

Physicians work in one or more of several specialties, including (but not limited to) anesthesiology, family and general medicine, general internal medicine, general pediatrics, obstetrics and gynecology, psychiatry, and surgery. These areas of practice are required rotations for all medical students. Two relatively new specialties—hospitalist and hospice and palliative medicine—will also be reviewed.

Anesthesiologists focus on the care of surgical patients and pain relief. Like other physicians, they evaluate and treat patients and direct staff members. Through continual monitoring and

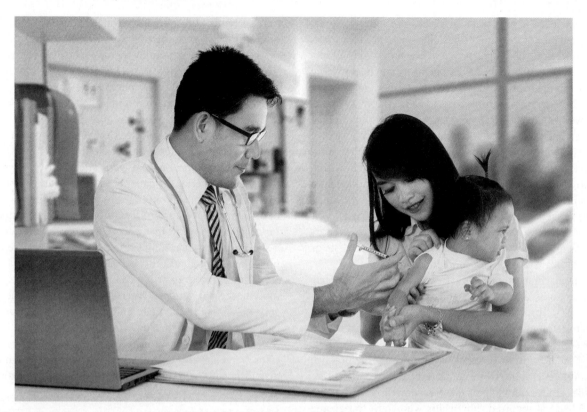

FIGURE 9.1 Pediatricians are primary care providers for children and adolescents.
© Creativa Images/Shutterstock.

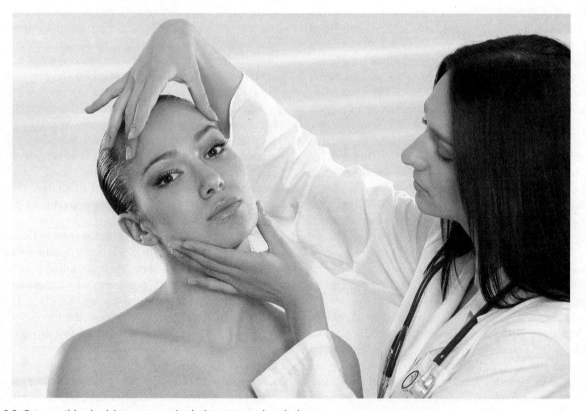

FIGURE 9.2 Osteopathic physicians use manipulation to treat headaches.
© lenetstan/Shutterstock.

assessment, these critical care specialists are responsible for the maintenance of the patient's vital life functions—heart rate, body temperature, blood pressure, and breathing—during surgery. They also work outside the operating room, providing pain relief in the intensive care unit, during labor and delivery, and for those who suffer from chronic pain. Anesthesiologists confer with other physicians and surgeons about appropriate treatments and procedures before, during, and after operations.

Family medicine physicians often provide the first point of contact for people of all ages seeking health care by acting as the traditional family physician. They assess and treat a wide range of conditions, from sinus and respiratory infections to broken bones. Family and general physicians typically have a base of regular, long-term patients. These doctors refer patients with more serious conditions to specialists or other healthcare facilities for more intensive care.

General internists usually treat adult patients. They make diagnoses and provide nonsurgical treatment for a wide range of problems that affect internal organ systems, such as the stomach, kidneys, liver, and digestive tract. Internists use a variety of diagnostic techniques to treat patients through medication or hospitalization. Like family practice physicians, general internists commonly act as primary care specialists. They refer patients to other specialists when more complex care is required. Physicians who train to become specialists usually complete training in general medicine first before applying for a fellowship—for example, in endocrinology, neurology, or rheumatology.

General pediatricians care for the health of infants, children, and adolescents. They specialize in the diagnosis and treatment of a variety of ailments specific to children and teens and track growth to adulthood. Like most physicians, pediatricians work with different healthcare workers, such as nurses and other physicians, to assess and treat children with various ailments. Most of the work of pediatricians involves treating day-to-day illnesses—minor injuries, infectious diseases, and immunizations—that are common to children, much as a general internist treats adults. Some pediatricians specialize in pediatric surgery or serious medical conditions, such as asthma or diabetes.

Obstetricians and gynecologists (OB/GYNs) specialize in women's health. They are responsible for women's general medical care, and they also provide care related to pregnancy and the reproductive system. Like general practitioners, they diagnose and treat general health problems, but they focus on ailments specific to the female anatomy, such as cancers of the breast or cervix, urinary tract and pelvic disorders, and hormonal disorders. OB/GYNs also specialize in childbirth, which includes treating and counseling women throughout their pregnancy, from giving prenatal care to assisting with delivery and providing postpartum care.

Psychiatrists are the primary mental health providers; they assess and treat mental illnesses through a combination of psychotherapy, psychoanalysis, hospitalization, and medication. Individual psychotherapy involves regular counseling sessions with patients about their problems; the psychiatrist helps patients find solutions through changes in their behavioral patterns, explores their past experiences, and makes referrals to group and family therapy sessions. Psychoanalysis involves long-term psychotherapy and counseling. In many cases, the psychiatrist prescribes medications to correct chemical imbalances that cause emotional and behavioral problems.

Surgeons specialize in the treatment of injury, disease, and deformity through surgery. Using a variety of instruments and with patients under anesthesia, a surgeon corrects physical deformities, repairs bone and tissue after injuries, or performs preventive surgeries on patients with debilitating diseases or disorders. The most common preventive surgery is removal of benign or cancerous tumors. Although a large number perform general surgery, many surgeons choose to specialize in a specific area. After completing a general surgery residency, physicians may choose to specialize and complete a fellowship—for example, in orthopedic surgery, the treatment of the musculoskeletal system. Other specialties include neurosurgery (treatment of the brain and nervous system), cardiovascular surgery, otolaryngology (treatment of the ear, nose, and throat), and plastic or reconstructive surgery. Like other physicians, surgeons also examine patients, perform and interpret diagnostic tests, and counsel patients on preventive health care.

Hospitalists

A relatively new specialty for physicians is that of a **hospitalist**. The professional society for hospitalists, the Society of Hospital Medicine, was established as recently as 1997. The majority of hospitalists specialize in general internal medicine or family practice, with a smaller percentage focusing on pediatrics.[5] Some hospitalists only work the night shift, others work only weekends, and others serve as a hospitalist for a skilled nursing facility (**FIGURE 9.3**).[6]

Before hospitalists developed into a specialty, physicians admitted patients to the hospital only to make referrals to surgeons or other specialists for treatment. Hospitalists do not have an office practice. Instead, they serve as the single point of contact for a patient moving through the hospital, from the time of admission until discharge. Hospitalists perform medical procedures, design treatment plans, and communicate and coordinate with patients and hospital staff. For patients, having a hospitalist reduces the confusion of a hospital stay and provides access to a staff member who can answer questions about their condition and treatment options. The hospitalist coordinates with the primary physician to ensure that treatment fits with the patient's medical history and health needs and keeps the physician updated on the patient's condition. Hospitalists also may recommend a discharge treatment plan, such as temporary home care, or prescribe medications or physical therapy to ensure a safe transition home. The hospitalist connects patients with resources in their communities that help with recovery or ongoing treatment by referring patients to the hospital's discharge specialists, usually social workers or nurses, who link patients with rehab centers.[5] Some hospitalists are also

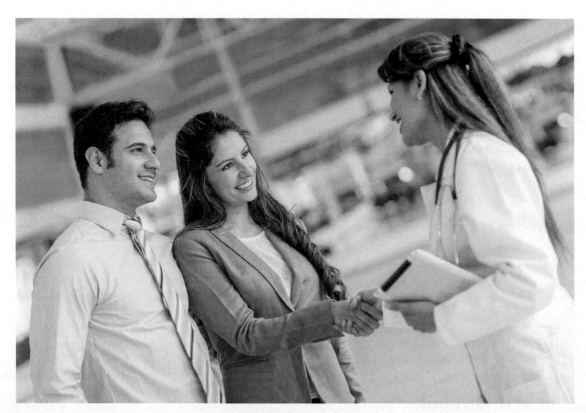

FIGURE 9.3 Hospitalists are a single point of contact from admission to discharge from the hospital.
© Andresr/Shutterstock.

responsible for establishing and monitoring patient safety and quality assurance programs in an effort to reduce the length of hospital stays and readmissions.[6]

Hospice and Palliative Medicine (HPM)

Another emerging specialty for physicians is **Hospice and Palliative Medicine (HPM)**. There is a need for physicians trained to counsel patients near the end of life, since 20% of the population is projected to be 65 years of age and older by 2030.[7] This medical specialty focuses on patients with life-limiting or serious health conditions with a goal of managing pain and other symptoms to the greatest extent possible. Hospice has existed in the United States since 1974 and has focused on treating symptoms such as pain, fear, and anxiety associated with a life-limiting illness.[8] **Palliative care** is a relatively new field for physicians and is part of hospice care but also an important part of care to treat symptoms associated with a serious chronic illness. Examples are neurological diseases, such as Parkinson's disease or amyotrophic lateral sclerosis (ALS), that limit the ability to move, talk, or swallow and eventually result in death and Guillain-Barré syndrome (GBS), a disease that causes whole-body paralysis and requires a long recovery time.

Referrals are made to palliative care physicians when patients have a severe illness or are near the end of life. Both hospice and palliative care address the spiritual, emotional, and social concerns of patients as well as those of the patient's family and significant others. A multidisciplinary team of health professionals provide hospice and palliative services in a nursing facility or hospital. Additional sites for hospice services are in-patient hospice centers and in patients' homes.

The **American Board of Medical Specialties (ABMS)** and the **American Osteopathic Association (AOA)** began certifying physicians in this specialty in 2008. There are now HPM residency training programs, and as of June 6, 2018, there were 8,198 physicians certified in HPM.[9]

WORK ENVIRONMENT

Many physicians—primarily family practice physicians, general internists, pediatricians, OB/GYNs, and psychiatrists—work in small, private offices or clinics, often assisted by a small staff of nurses and other administrative personnel. Increasingly, physicians are practicing in groups or healthcare organizations that provide backup coverage and allow for more time off. Physicians in a **group practice** or healthcare organization often work as part of a team that coordinates care for a number of patients; they are less independent than the **solo practitioners** of the past. A growing number of physicians are partners or wage-and-salary employees of group practices. Organized as clinics or as associations of physicians, medical groups can more easily afford expensive medical equipment, share support staff, and benefit from other business advantages. Hospitalists usually work for a salary and share shifts with other hospitalists at the same hospital.

Surgeons and anesthesiologists usually work in well-lit, sterile environments while performing surgery and often stand for long periods. Most work in hospitals or in surgical outpatient centers.

Many physicians and surgeons work long, irregular hours. Physicians and surgeons travel between an office and a hospital to care for their patients. While on call, a physician will deal with many patients' concerns over the phone and make emergency visits to hospitals or nursing homes.

Employment Opportunities

Physicians and surgeons held about 752,400 jobs in 2019; according to Bureau of Labor Statistics in 2019, 29% of physicians in patient care were in primary care: family medicine, pediatrics, internal medicine, and obstetrics and gynecology; 5% were general surgeons, and the remaining 65% practiced in other specialties such as oncology, dermatology, psychiatry, anesthesiology, and cardiology (**TABLE 9.1**).

Educational and Legal Requirements

The common path to practicing as a physician is eight years of education beyond high school and three to eight additional years of internship and residency. All states, the District of Columbia, and U.S. territories license physicians.

Education and Training

The minimum educational requirement for entry into medical school is three years of college; most applicants, however, have at least a bachelor's degree, and many have advanced degrees. Although no specific major is required, all students must complete undergraduate work in biology, chemistry,

TABLE 9.1 Distribution of U.S. Physicians by Specialty, 2019

Medical Fields	Percent
Family medicine/general practice	16%
General pediatrics	4%
General internal medicine	6%
Obstetrics and gynecology	3%
Anesthesiology	4%
Psychiatry	4%
General surgery	5%
Other specialties	57%

Data from Bureau of Labor Statistics. *Occupational Outlook Handbook.* U.S. Department of Labor; 2020.

physics, mathematics, and English. Students also take courses in the humanities and social sciences. Some students volunteer at local hospitals or clinics to gain experience in a healthcare setting.

In 2020, there were 138 medical schools in the United States and Puerto Rico and 17 in Canada accredited by the **Liaison Committee on Medical Education (LCME)**. The LCME is the accrediting body for MD medical education programs in the United States and Canada. The American Osteopathic Association accredits schools that award a DO degree; there were 37 accredited osteopathic medical schools in 2021. There has been a dramatic increase in the number of osteopathic medical students from 6,614 in 1988–1989[10] to 33,800 in 2020—2021 or 25% of all medical students.[11]

Medical schools are highly competitive. Most applicants must submit transcripts, scores from the **Medical College Admission Test (MCAT)**, and letters of recommendation. Schools also consider an applicant's personality, leadership qualities, and participation in extracurricular activities. Most schools require applicants to interview with members of the admissions committee.

Students spend most of the first two years of medical school in laboratories and classrooms, taking courses such as anatomy, biochemistry, pharmacology, psychology, medical ethics, and the laws governing medicine. They also gain practical skills, learning to take medical histories, examine patients, and diagnose illnesses.

During their last two years, medical students work with patients under the supervision of experienced physicians in hospitals and clinics. Through rotations in internal medicine, family practice, obstetrics and gynecology, pediatrics, psychiatry, and surgery, they gain experience in diagnosing and treating illnesses in a variety of areas.

Formal education and training requirements for physicians are among the most demanding of any occupation—four years of undergraduate school, four years of medical school, and three to eight years of internship and residency, depending on the specialty selected. A few medical schools offer combined undergraduate and medical school programs that last six or seven years rather than the customary eight years. Following medical school, almost all MDs enter a residency—graduate medical education in a specialty that takes the form of paid on-the-job training, usually in a hospital. Most DOs serve a 12-month rotating internship after graduation before entering a residency, which may last two to six years.

Licensure

All states require physicians and surgeons to be licensed; requirements vary by state. To qualify for a license, candidates must graduate from an accredited medical school, complete residency training in their specialty, and pass written and practical exams. All physicians and surgeons must pass a standardized national licensure examination. MDs take the **U.S. Medical Licensing**

Examination **(USMLE)**. DOs take the **Comprehensive Osteopathic Medical Licensing Examination (COMLEX-USA)**. Although physicians licensed in one state usually can get a license to practice in another without further examination, some states limit reciprocity. Graduates of foreign medical schools generally can qualify for licensure after passing an examination and completing a U.S. residency. For specific information on licensing in a given state, contact that state's medical board.

Certification and Other Qualifications

Certification is not required for physicians and surgeons; however, it may increase their employment opportunities. MDs and DOs seeking board certification in a specialty may spend up to seven years in residency training; the length of time varies with the specialty. An examination after residency is required for certification by the American Board of Medical Specialties (ABMS) or the American Osteopathic Association (AOA). A final examination immediately after residency or after one or two years of practice is also necessary for certification by a member board of the ABMS or the AOA. The ABMS represents 24 boards related to medical specialties ranging from allergy and immunology to urology. The AOA has approved 18 specialty boards, ranging from anesthesiology to surgery. For certification in a subspecialty, physicians usually need another one to two years of residency training in the specialty area. For information about different options for specialties and subspecialties to become board-certified, review information from the ABMS listed under "Additional Information" at the end of this chapter.

Desirable characteristics for people who wish to become physicians are a desire to serve patients, self-motivation, emotional stability, and the ability to survive the pressures and long hours of medical education and practice. Physicians also must demonstrate compassion and patience when caring for the sick or injured, who may be in extreme pain or distress. Excellent communication skills are necessary in order to communicate effectively with patients and other health professionals. Other important qualities are attention to detail to ensure appropriate treatment, leadership skills to direct the work of staff members, and problem-solving skills to evaluate the patient's symptoms and administer appropriate treatment in emergencies. Prospective physicians must be willing to study throughout their career.

Advancement

Some physicians and surgeons advance by gaining expertise in specialties and subspecialties and by developing a reputation for excellence among their peers and patients. Physicians and surgeons may also start their own practice or join a group practice. Others teach residents and other new doctors, and some advance to supervisory and managerial roles in hospitals, clinics, and other settings.

Employment Trends

Employment is expected to grow faster than the average for all occupations. Job opportunities should be very good, particularly in rural and low-income areas.

Employment Change

Employment of physicians and surgeons is projected to grow 4 percent from 2019 to 2029, about as fast as average for all occupations. Job growth will occur because of the continued expansion of healthcare-related industries. The growing and aging population will drive overall growth in the demand for physician services, as consumers continue to demand high levels of care using the latest technologies, diagnostic tests, and therapies. Many medical schools are increasing their enrollments based on a perceived new demand for physicians.

Despite growing demand for physicians and surgeons, some factors will temper growth. For example, new technologies allow physicians to be more productive. This means physicians can diagnose and treat more patients in the same amount of time. The rising cost of health care can dramatically affect the demand for physicians' services. PAs and APRNs can perform many of the routine duties of physicians at a fraction of the cost and may be increasingly used. Furthermore, the demand for physicians' services is highly sensitive to changes in healthcare reimbursement policies. If changes to health coverage result in higher out-of-pocket costs for consumers, this could result in fewer visits to the doctor and lower demand for physicians' services.

Job Prospects

Opportunities for individuals interested in becoming physicians and surgeons are expected to be very good because almost all graduates of domestic medical schools are matched to residencies (their first jobs as physicians) immediately after graduating. In addition to job openings from employment growth, openings will result from the need to replace the relatively high number of physicians and surgeons expected to retire in the next decade.

Job prospects should be particularly good for physicians willing to practice in rural and low-income areas because these medically underserved areas typically have difficulty attracting these workers. Job prospects will also be especially good for physicians in specialties that afflict the rapidly growing elderly population. Examples of such specialties are cardiology and radiology because the risks for heart disease and cancer increase as people age. Neurologists and geriatricians will also be in demand because of the elderly population with diseases of aging requiring diagnosis and management. Most experts expect that the number of physicians and surgeons will increase by 27,300 from 752,400 in 2019 to 779,700 in 2029.

TABLE 9.2 Practice Area and Median Salaries of Physicians, 2020	
Specialty	**Median Salary**
Hospitalist	$285,569
Anesthesiologists	$271,440
Surgeons	$251,650
Obstetricians/gynecologists	$239,120
Psychiatrists	$217,100
Family and general practitioner	$214,370
Hospice and palliative medicine	$207,500
Internist, General	$210,960
Pediatrician, General	$184,570

Data from Number of hospitalists: Wachter RM, Goldman L. Zero to 50,000 — The 20th Anniversary of the Hospitalist. *NEJM* 2016;375:1109–1011. DOI: 10.1056/NEJMp1607958.[12] Data Source on hospitalist salary: Gesensway D. Is the bull market for compensation over? Today's Hospitalist, November 2019.[13] Data Source on number of hospice and palliative physicians: American Academy of Hospice and Palliative Medicine. Workforce Data and Reports. http://aahpm.org/career/workforce-study#HPMphysicians.[14] Data Source on salary for hospice and palliative physicians: American Academy of Hospice and Palliative Medicine. A Profile of New Hospice and Palliative Medicine Physicians, January 2019. https://aahpm.org/uploads/Profile_of_New_HPM_Physicians_2018_June_2019.pdf

Earnings

Earnings of physicians and surgeons are among the highest of any occupation. Self-employed physicians—those who own or are part owners of their medical practice—generally have higher median incomes than salaried physicians. Earnings vary according to number of years in practice, geographic region, hours worked, skill, personality, and professional reputation. Physicians who are board certified in a specialty or subspecialty usually earn higher salaries, and those with additional responsibilities, such as the administrator of a medical group, also earn higher salaries. Self-employed physicians and surgeons must provide for their own health insurance and retirement.

Median salaries by specialty are listed in **TABLE 9.2**. The Bureau of Labor Statistics does not collect information for all subspecialties; data for hospitalists and hospice and palliative medicine were obtained from other sources.

Related Occupations

Physicians work to prevent, diagnose, and treat diseases, disorders, and injuries. Other healthcare practitioners who need similar skills who exercise critical judgment include chiropractors, dentists, optometrists, physician assistants, podiatrists, advanced practice registered nurses, and veterinarians.

PODIATRISTS
Significant Points

- Formal training for podiatrists is similar to that of physicians and surgeons with four years of undergraduate school, four years of podiatry school, and one year of residency. Specialization requires an additional year or more.
- Podiatrists are needed to treat wounds associated with diabetes and peripheral arterial disease of the lower limbs and to treat bone deformities of the foot and ankle.
- Job opportunities should be excellent for podiatrists, especially for those with certification in wound care and preservation and reconstruction of the ankle and foot.

Work Description

Podiatrists have training similar to MDs and DOs but specialize in the medical and surgical care of foot, ankle, and lower leg problems. They diagnose illnesses, treat injuries, and perform surgery involving the lower extremities. Podiatrists review the patient's medical history and perform a physical exam and X-rays, laboratory tests, and other diagnostic methods to make a diagnosis and develop a treatment plan (**FIGURE 9.4**).

Podiatrists treat a variety of foot and ankle ailments, including calluses, ingrown toenails, heel spurs, and arch problems. They also treat foot and leg problems associated with diabetes and other diseases. Some podiatrists spend most of their time performing advanced surgeries, such as foot and ankle reconstruction. Others may choose a specialty such as sports medicine or pediatrics.

Treatment may include prescribing shoe inserts (orthotics) to improve mobility or performing foot or ankle surgery to remove bone spurs or to correct foot and ankle deformities such as hammer toes or bunions. Another significant area of

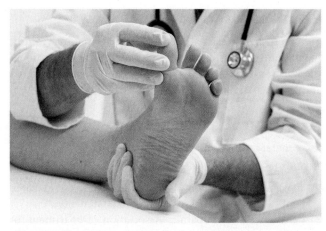

FIGURE 9.4 Podiatrists specialize in medical and surgical treatment of the ankle and feet.
© gajdamak/Shutterstock.

practice is treatment of wounds of the foot, ankle, or lower leg, often associated with diabetes or peripheral arterial disease of the lower legs. Wounds often take several weeks or months to completely heal and require surgical debridement. Podiatrists coordinate medical treatment with other physicians—for example, endocrinologists when working with a patient with diabetes or a cardiologist for patients with peripheral arterial disease.

Podiatrists also give advice and instruction on foot and ankle care and on general wellness techniques, including choosing appropriate footwear to prevent callouses and bunions. They may provide routine foot care for the elderly who are no longer able to properly care for their feet and are at greater risk for falls.

Work Environment

Most podiatrists work in offices of other health professionals or in group practices with physicians. Others work in private and public hospitals and outpatient care centers and routinely care for residents in nursing and assisted-living facilities.

Self-employed podiatrists either solely own or are partners in a medical practice. Most podiatrists work full time. Podiatrists' offices may be open in the evenings or on weekends to accommodate patients. In hospitals, podiatrists may have to work occasional nights or weekends or may be on call. Podiatrists who own their practice may spend time on business-related activities, such as hiring employees and managing inventory.

Employment Opportunities

There were 10,500 podiatrists in the United States in 2019. Podiatry provides excellent opportunities as a health career because of the need for lower limb and feet care in those with diabetes and peripheral vascular disease and general podiatric care for the aging population.

Education and Legal Requirements

Podiatrists must earn a **Doctor of Podiatric Medicine (DPM)** degree and complete a three-year residency program. Podiatrists must be licensed.

Education and Training

Podiatrists must have a Doctor of Podiatric Medicine (DPM) degree from an accredited college of podiatric medicine. A DPM degree program takes four years to complete. In 2020, there were nine colleges of podiatric medicine accredited by the **Council on Podiatric Medical Education (CPME)**. Admission to podiatric medicine programs requires at least three years of undergraduate education, including specific courses in laboratory sciences such as biology, chemistry, and physics, as well as general coursework in subjects such as English. In practice, nearly all prospective podiatrists earn a bachelor's degree before attending a college of podiatric medicine. Admission to DPM programs usually requires taking the Medical College Admission Test (MCAT), the same exam required for medical students.

Courses for a Doctor of Podiatric Medicine degree are similar to those for other medical degrees. They include anatomy, physiology, pharmacology, and pathology, among other subjects. During their last two years, podiatric medical students gain supervised experience by completing clinical rotations.

After earning a DPM, podiatrists must apply to and complete a podiatric medical and surgical residency (PMSR) program, which lasts three years. Residency programs take place in hospitals and provide both medical and surgical experience. For a list of residencies available in the United States, go to the CPME website. Podiatrists may do additional training in specific fellowship areas. Some of the specialties are sports medicine, wound care, diabetic foot, complex lower limb extremity surgery, diabetic limb salvage and preservation, and reconstruction of the foot and ankle. For more information about specific fellowships, visit the CPME website listed at the end of this chapter.

Licensure

Podiatrists in every state must be licensed. Usually, podiatrists must pay a fee and pass the **American Podiatric Medical Licensing Exam (APMLE)**. Some states also require podiatrists to take a state-specific exam. Licenses must typically be renewed periodically, and podiatrists must take continuing medical education to maintain licensure.

Certification and Other Qualifications

Many podiatrists choose to become board certified. The **American Board of Foot and Ankle Surgery (ABFAS)** is the certifying agency in podiatric surgery, and the **American Board of Podiatric Medicine** is the certifying agency in orthopedics and primary care podiatry. Certification requires a combination of work experience and passing scores on exams.

Desirable qualities for podiatrists include compassion, since many patients that seek the services of a podiatrist are in pain. Since podiatrists spend most of their time interacting with patients excellent interpersonal skills—the ability to listen and put patients who are in pain or undergoing surgery at ease—are necessary. They also need to have critical thinking skills to correctly diagnose the patient's medical problems and to develop an appropriate treatment plan. Attention to detail is also important to make an accurate diagnosis and to monitor patients during and after treatment.

Advancement

Podiatrists who obtain additional training through a fellowship and become certified in a subspecialty can expect higher salaries.

Employment Trends

As the U.S. population both ages and increases, the number of people expected to have mobility and foot-related problems will rise. Growing rates of chronic conditions such as diabetes and obesity also may limit mobility of those with these conditions and lead to problems such as poor circulation in the feet and lower extremities. More podiatrists will be needed to provide care for these patients.

In addition, podiatrists are increasingly working in group practices along with other healthcare professionals. Continued growth in the use of outpatient surgery also will create new opportunities for podiatrists.

Employment Change

Employment of podiatrists is projected to remain unchanged from 2019 to 2029, slower than the average for all occupations. However, because it is a small occupation, growth will result in only about 500 new jobs over the 10-year period.

Job Prospects

Job prospects for trained podiatrists should be good given that there are a limited number of colleges of podiatry. In addition, the retirement of currently practicing podiatrists in the coming years is expected to increase the number of job openings for podiatrists.

Earnings

The median annual wage for podiatrists was $134,300 in May 2020. Podiatrists who worked for the federal government earned the highest salary; the median salary was $163,000. Self-employed podiatrists may earn more than salaried doctors, but they are also responsible for the costs of running a business, such as providing benefits for themselves and employees.

Related Occupations

Other health professionals that have similar training requirements and responsibilities are chiropractors, occupational therapists, physicians and surgeons, optometrists, orthotists and prosthetists, and physical therapists.

Additional Information

For general information on physicians, contact:

- American Medical Association, AMA Plaza, 330 N. Wabash Ave., Suite 39300, Chicago, IL 60611-5885. https://www.ama-assn.org/residents-students
- American Osteopathic Association, Department of Communications, 142 East Ontario St., Chicago, IL 60611. http://www.osteopathic.org

For a list of allopathic medical schools and residency programs as well as general information on premedical education, financial aid, and medicine as a career, contact:

- Association of American Medical Colleges (AAMC), 655 K St., NW, Suite 100, Washington, DC, 20001-2399. https://students-residents.aamc.org/

For information about osteopathic medical schools, contact:

- American Association of Colleges of Osteopathic Medicine, 7700 Old Georgetown Rd., Suite 250, Bethesda, MD 20814. https://www.aacom.org/

For a list of both MD and DO residencies and fellowships listed with the Electronic Residency Application Service (ERAS) of the American Association of Medical Colleges, visit:

- ERAS 2016 Participating Specialties & Programs. https://services.aamc.org/eras/erasstats/par/

For information on licensing, contact:

- Federation of State Medical Boards, 400 Fuller Wiser Rd., Euless, TX 76039. http://www.fsmb.org

For information about specialties and subspecialties in medicine and requirements for obtaining board certification, contact:

- American Board of Medical Specialties (ABMS), 353 North Clark St., Suite 1400, Chicago, IL 60654. http://www.abms.org/member-boards/specialty-subspecialty-certificates/

Information on federal scholarships and loans is available from the directors of student financial aid at schools of medicine. Information on licensing is available from state boards of examiners.

For more information about podiatrists, visit:

- American Podiatric Medical Association, 9312 Old Georgetown Rd., Bethesda, MD, 20814. https://www.apma.org/

For information on colleges of podiatric medicine and their entrance requirements, curricula, and student financial aid, visit:

- American Association of Colleges of Podiatric Medicine, 15850 Crabbs Branch Way, Suite 320, Rockville, MD, 20855. http://www.aacpm.org/

For a list of accredited podiatric programs and residency programs, visit:

- Council on Podiatric Medical Education, 9312 Old Georgetown Rd., Bethesda, MD 20814. https://www.cpme.org/

For more information about the podiatric licensing exam, visit:

- The National Board of Podiatric Medical Examiners, Prometric/NBPME, 7941 Corporate Dr., Nottingham, MD 21236. http://apmle.com/talk-us

For more information about board certification for podiatrists, visit:

- American Board of Foot and Ankle Surgery, 445 Fillmore St., San Francisco, CA 94117. https://www.abfas.org/become-board-qualified/certification-process
- American Board of Podiatric Medicine, 1060 Aviation Blvd. #100, Hermosa Beach, CA 90254. https://www.abpmed.org/pages/exam-info/board-certification

LEARNING PORTFOLIO

Issues for Discussion

1. What are some of the reasons for a possible doctor shortage within the next decade? How can physician assistants and advanced practice registered nurses be used to extend the care of physicians?

2. Review the four main categories of core competencies (interpersonal, intrapersonal, thinking and reasoning, and science) used to evaluate applicants to medical school. Choose two core competencies within two different main categories and describe how you would demonstrate those competencies through coursework, paid work, or volunteer experience as a high school or undergraduate college student. Core Competencies for Entering Medical Students. Association of American Medical Colleges. https://students -residents.aamc.org/applying-medical-school /what-medical-schools-are-looking-understanding- 15-core-competencies

3. Read the article "A 'hospitalist plus': Grace C. Huang, MD" from the March 2, 2021, issue of The Hospitalist. What are the areas of job responsibility for this hospitalist? What does the hospitalist like and dislike about her job? https://www.the-hospitalist.org/hospitalist /article/236622/leadership-training/hospitalist-plus -grace-c-huang-md

4. Go to the American Board of Medical Specialties website and choose one specialty you might be interested in pursuing. What are the requirements for certification in one specialty of your choosing? Choose a specialty (e.g., internal medicine) and identify subspecialties within the specialty. https://www.abms.org/member-boards/specialty -subspecialty-certificates/

Enrichment Activities

1. Go to the website and read stories written about the path of medical students to medical school. Select two stories you find inspiring and explain why the stories are inspiring. Association of American Medical Colleges. *Inspiring Stories*. https://students-residents.aamc .org/choosing-medical-career/inspiring-stories

2. View videos of medical students as they describe how they made the choice to apply for medical school or their experiences as a medical student. View and report on at least one of the students during class. Association of American Medical Colleges. *Ask a Med Student Video Series*. https://students-residents.aamc.org /choosing-medical-career/ask-med-student-video-series

3. Go to the Council on Podiatric Medical Education website to review the list of approved fellowships offered for licensed podiatrists. Identify the specialty area for each fellowship (e.g., sports medicine or wound care). https://www.cpme.org/fellowships/content.cfm?Item Number=2441&navItemNumber=2246

CASE STUDY: SPECIALTY PHYSICIANS AND PODIATRISTS

Bill is a junior in biology at the state university who is completing the requirements for pre-med. He plans to take the MCAT this summer as well as visit several medical schools before completing his application. Bill always thought that he wanted to be a family doctor but wants to consider all options before applying for medical school. Bill has a friend who is enrolled in osteopathic medicine, and one of his classmates has decided to apply to a school of podiatry.

   The following questions are based on the information about Bill and the decision-making process about choosing a medical school.

1. What are other career options for Bill—in addition to medical school—if he has a desire to be the primary care provider for individuals and families?

2. In which areas of medicine do physicians act as a primary care provider?

3. Explain to Bill why a college of osteopathy would be a good choice for medical school.

LEARNING PORTFOLIO

References

1. Association of American Medical Colleges. *Physician Supply and Demand A 15-Year Outlook: Key Findings, April, 2019.* https://www.aamc.org/system/files/2020-07/aamc-2020-workforce-projections-15-year-outlook-key-findings-f2.pdf Accessed July 2, 2020.

2. U.S. Department of Health and Human Services, Health Resources and Services Administration, National Center for Health Workforce Analysis. *Projecting the Supply and Demand for Primary Care Practitioners through 2020.* Rockville, Maryland: U.S. Department of Health and Human Services, 2013. https://bhw.hrsa.gov/sites/default/files/bureau-health-work force/data-research/projecting-primary-care.pdf Accessed August 3, 2021.

3. Patient-Centered Primary Care Collaborative. *Defining the Medical Home. A Patient-Centered Philosophy That Drives Primary Care Excellence.* https://www.pcpcc.org/about/medical-home Accessed July 2, 2020.

4. American Osteopathic Association. *What Is Osteopathic Medicine?* https://osteopathic.org/what-is-osteopathic-medicine Accessed July 2, 2020.

5. Royster S. You're a what? Hospitalist. *Career Outlook.* July 2015. http://www.bls.gov/careeroutlook/2015/youre-a-what/hospitalist.htm Accessed August 27, 2021.

6. Hall AM, Sanyal-Dey P, Chang D, Kwan B, Seymour P. The branching tree of hospital medicine. Diversity of training backgrounds. *The Hospitalist.* December 13, 2019.

7. Ortman JM, Velkhoff VA. An Aging Nation: The Older Population in the United States. *Current Population Reports.* P25-1140. May 2014. U.S. Census Bureau.

8. National Hospice and Palliative Care Organization. History of Hospice. https://www.nhpco.org/hospice-care-overview/history-of-hospice Accessed August 3, 2021.

9. American Academy of Hospice and Palliative Medicine. *Workforce Data and Reports.* http://aahpm.org/career/workforce-study#HPMphysicians Accessed July 2, 2020.

10. American Osteopathic Association. *OMP Osteopathic Medical Profession Report 2018.* https://osteopathic.org/wp-content/uploads/2018-OMP-Report.pdf Accessed July 2, 2020.

11. American Osteopathic Association. *Osteopathic Medical Profession Report, 2020-21.* https://osteopathic.org/wp-content/uploads/OMP-Report-2020-21.pdf Accessed July 30, 2021.

12. Gesensway D. Is the bull market for compensation over? *Today's Hospitalist,* November 2019.

13. American Academy of Hospice and Palliative Medicine. *A Profile of New Hospice and Palliative Medicine Physicians,* January 2019. https://aahpm.org/uploads/Profile_of_New_HPM_Physicians_2018_June_2019.pdf Accessed July 2, 2020.

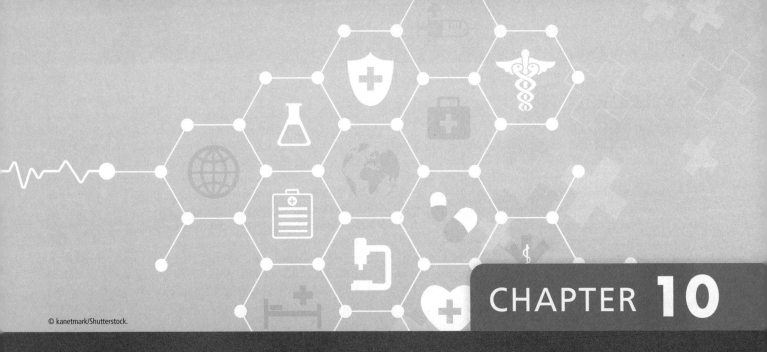

CHAPTER **10**

Physician Assistant*

KEY TERMS

Emergency medicine
Family practice
Geriatrics
Gynecology
Internal medicine
Middle-level health workers

National Commission on
  Certification of Physician
  Assistants (NCCPA)
Pediatrics
Physician Assistant National
  Certifying Examination (PANCE)

Primary care
Psychiatry
Surgery
Telemedicine

* All information in this chapter, unless otherwise indicated, was obtained from Bureau of Labor Statistics. *Occupational Outlook Handbook 2020–2021 Edition*. Washington, DC: U.S. Department of Labor; 2021.

A RELATIVELY NEW PROFESSION

The occupation of physician assistant (PA) came into being during the mid-1960s in response to a shortage of primary care physicians. The purpose of the PA in **primary care** is to help physicians provide personal health services to patients under their care. PAs are skilled health practitioners, qualified through academic and clinical training to serve patients with and under the supervision of a doctor of medicine (MD) or osteopathy (DO), who is responsible for the performance of that particular assistant. PAs are also responsible for their own actions and are considered **middle-level health workers**.

PHYSICIAN ASSISTANT

Significant Points

- Requirements for admission to training programs vary; most applicants have a college degree and some health-related work experience.
- Physician assistants must complete an accredited education program and pass a national exam to obtain a license.
- Employment is projected to grow much faster than average.
- Job opportunities should be good, particularly in rural and inner-city healthcare facilities.

Work Description

Physician assistants are formally trained to provide routine diagnostic, therapeutic, and preventive healthcare services under the direction and supervision of a physician. They take medical histories, examine patients, order and interpret laboratory tests and X-rays, and make preliminary diagnoses.

They also treat minor injuries by suturing, splinting, and casting (**FIGURE 10.1**). PAs record progress notes, instruct and

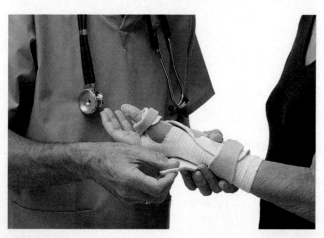

FIGURE 10.1 Splinting a patient's wrist.
© AnnBaldwin/iStockPhoto.

counsel patients, and order or carry out therapy. In all 50 states and the District of Columbia, physician assistants may prescribe medications. PAs may have managerial duties, too. Some order medical and laboratory supplies and equipment; others supervise technicians and assistants.

Physician assistants always work under the supervision of a physician. The extent of supervision, however, depends on the work setting. For example, PAs working in rural or inner-city clinics, where a physician may be available just one or two days each week, may provide most of the health care for patients and consult with the supervising physician and other medical professionals as needed or required by law. Other PAs may make house calls or go to hospitals and nursing homes to check on patients and report to the physician.

Physician assistants assist physicians in a variety of practice settings and specialty areas. Settings that see the most physician assistants employed are hospitals, clinics, and physicians' offices. Leading medical specialties using PAs are **family practice**, **internal medicine**, general **surgery**, **emergency medicine**, **pediatrics**, orthopedic surgery, thoracic surgery, and **geriatrics**.

The duties of physician assistants are determined by the supervising physician and by state law. Aspiring PAs should investigate the laws and regulations in the states where they wish to practice.

Work Environment

Although PAs generally work in a comfortable, well-lit environment, they often must stand for long periods and do considerable walking. The workweek and schedule vary according to practice setting. Some emergency room PAs work 24-hour shifts twice weekly, and others work three 12-hour shifts each week. The workweek of PAs who work in physicians' offices may include weekends, night hours, or early-morning hospital rounds to visit patients. PAs in clinics usually work a 5-day, 40-hour week. A collage of activities in which PAs engage is shown in **FIGURE 10.2**.

Employment Opportunities

Physician assistants held about 125,500 jobs in 2019. The number of jobs is greater than the number of practicing PAs because some hold two or more jobs. For example, some PAs work with a supervising physician but also work in another practice, clinic, or hospital. According to the American Academy of Physician Assistants, PAs can expect to earn higher salary if employed as independent contractors or in roles at private healthcare industries excluding clinics and hospitals.[1]

Around 54% of jobs for PAs were in the offices of physicians. About 26% were in public or private hospitals. The rest were mostly in outpatient care centers, including health maintenance organizations, the federal government, and public or private colleges, universities, and professional schools. Very few PAs were self-employed.

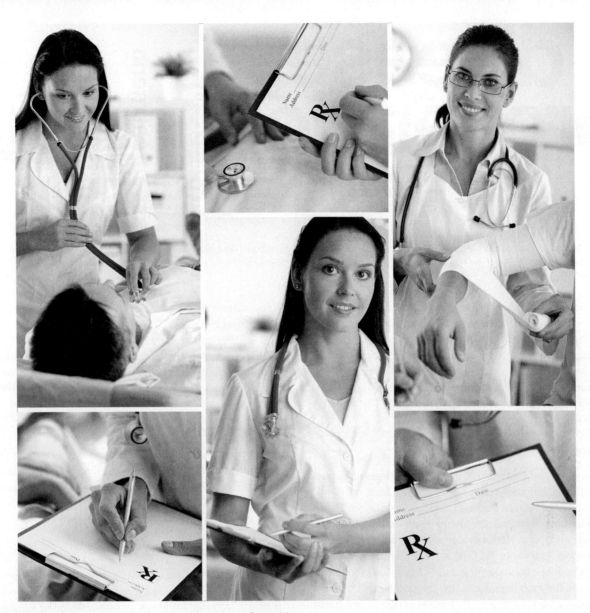

FIGURE 10.2 Physician assistants perform a wide variety of activities.
© Pressmaster/Shutterstock.

Educational and Legal Requirements

Physician assistant programs usually last at least two years in a postgraduate setting. Admission requirements vary by program, but many require at least two years of college and some healthcare experience. All states require that PAs complete an accredited, formal education program and pass a national exam to obtain a license.

Education and Training

Physician assistant education programs usually last at least two years and are full time. Most programs are in schools of allied health, academic health centers, medical schools, or four-year colleges; a few are in community colleges, the military, or hospitals. Many accredited PA programs have clinical teaching affiliations with medical schools.

In 2021, 277 education programs for physician assistants were accredited or provisionally accredited by the Accreditation Review Commission on Education for the Physician Assistant, Inc.[2] Depending on the program, one might earn a master's, bachelor's, or associate's degree or a certificate upon completion of the study requirements.

Admission requirements vary, but many programs require two to four years of college and some work experience in the healthcare field. Students should take courses in biology, English, chemistry, mathematics, psychology, and the social sciences. Many PAs have prior experience as registered nurses, and others come from varied backgrounds, including military corpsmen or medics and allied health occupations, such as respiratory therapists, physical therapists, and emergency medical technicians and paramedics.

PA education includes classroom instruction in biochemistry, pathology, human anatomy, physiology, microbiology, clinical pharmacology, clinical medicine, geriatric and

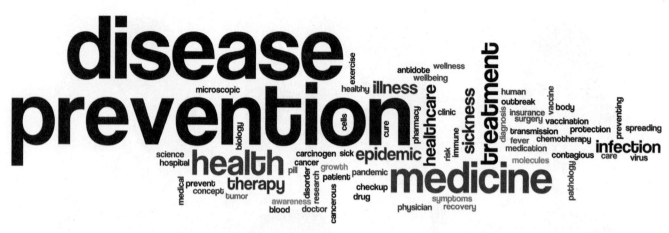

FIGURE 10.3 As a part of their educational experience, physician assistant students obtain supervised clinical training in several areas as well as classroom instruction around many critical topics including disease prevention.
© ibreakstock/Shutterstock.

home health care, disease prevention, and medical ethics. Students obtain supervised clinical training in several areas, including family medicine, internal medicine, surgery, pre-natal care and **gynecology**, geriatrics, emergency medicine, **psychiatry**, and pediatrics (**FIGURE 10.3**). Sometimes, PA students serve one or more of these rotations under the supervision of a physician who is seeking to hire a PA. The rotations often lead to permanent employment.

Licensure

All states and the District of Columbia have legislation governing the qualifications or practice of physician assistants. All jurisdictions require physician assistants to pass the **Physician Assistant National Certifying Examination (PANCE)**, administered by the **National Commission on Certification of Physician Assistants (NCCPA)** and open only to graduates of accredited PA education programs.[3] Only those successfully completing the examination may use the credential "Physician Assistant–Certified" (PA-C). To remain certified, PAs must complete 100 hours of continuing medical education every two years. Physician assistants must pass a recertification examination or complete an alternative program combining learning experiences and a take-home examination every 10 years.

Other Qualifications

Physician assistants must have a desire to serve patients and be self-motivated. PAs also must have a good bedside manner, emotional stability, and the ability to make decisions in emergencies. Physician assistants must be willing to study throughout their career to keep up with medical advances.

Certification and Advancement

Some PAs pursue additional education in a specialty such as surgery, neonatology, or emergency medicine. PA postgraduate educational programs are available in areas such as internal medicine, rural primary care, emergency medicine, surgery, pediatrics, neonatology, and occupational medicine.

Candidates must be graduates of an accredited program and be certified by the NCCPA.

As they attain greater clinical knowledge and experience, PAs can advance to added responsibilities and higher earnings. However, by the very nature of the profession, clinically practicing PAs always are supervised by physicians.

Employment Trends

Employment is expected to grow much faster than average as healthcare establishments increasingly use physician assistants to contain costs. Job opportunities for PAs should be good, particularly in rural and inner-city clinics, as these settings typically have difficulty attracting physicians.

Employment Change

Employment of physician assistants is expected to grow 31% from 2019 to 2029, much faster than the average for all occupations. Projected rapid job growth reflects the expansion of healthcare industries and an emphasis on cost containment, which results in the increasing use of PAs by healthcare establishments.

Physicians and institutions are expected to employ more PAs to provide primary care and to assist with medical and surgical procedures because PAs are cost-effective and productive members of the healthcare team. Physician assistants can relieve physicians of routine duties and procedures. **Telemedicine**—using technology to facilitate interactive consultations between physicians and physician assistants—also will expand the use of physician assistants.

Besides working in traditional office-based settings, PAs should find a growing number of jobs in institutional settings such as hospitals, academic medical centers, public clinics, and prisons. PAs also may be needed to augment medical staffing in inpatient teaching hospital settings as the number of hours physician residents are permitted to work is reduced, encouraging hospitals to use PAs to supply some physician resident services.

TABLE 10.1 Projection Data for Physician Assistants, 2019–2029				
			Change, 2019–2029	
Occupational Title	Employment, 2019	Projected Employment, 2029	Number	Percentage
Physician assistants	125,500	164,800	39,300	31%

Data from Bureau of Labor Statistics, U.S. Department of Labor. *Occupational Outlook Handbook*. U.S. Department of Labor; 2020.

Job Prospects

Job opportunities for PAs should be good, particularly in rural and inner-city clinics because those settings have difficulty attracting physicians. In addition to job openings from employment growth, openings will result from the need to replace physician assistants who retire or leave the occupation permanently. Opportunities will be best in states that allow PAs a wider scope of practice. **TABLE 10.1** shows some projection data provided by the U.S. Department of Labor.

Earnings

Median annual earnings of wage-and-salary physician assistants were $115,390 in 2020. The lowest 10% earned less than $76,700, and the highest 10% earned more than $162,4270. Median annual wages in the industries employing the largest numbers of physician assistants in May 2020 are shown in **TABLE 10.2**.

According to the American Academy of Physician Assistants' 2020 Census Report, median income for physician assistants in full-time clinical practice was $111,000 in 2019; approximately half of physician assistants earned a bonus, at a median pay of $5,500. Income varies by specialty, practice setting, geographic location, and years of experience. Employers often pay for their employees' liability insurance, registration fees with the Drug Enforcement Administration, state licensing fees, and credentialing fees.

Related Occupations

Other healthcare workers who provide direct patient care that requires a similar level of skill and training include audiologists, occupational therapists, physical therapists,

TABLE 10.2 Median Annual Earnings in the Industries Employing the Largest Numbers of Physician Assistants, May 2019	
Hospitals: state, local, and private	$118,600
Outpatient care centers	$124,610
Offices of physicians	$113,460
Employment services	$115,780

Data from Bureau of Labor Statistics, U.S. Department of Labor. *Occupational Outlook Handbook*. U.S. Department of Labor; 2020.

registered nurses, nurse-midwives, nurse anesthetists, nurse practitioners, and speech-language pathologists.

Additional Information

For information on a career as a physician assistant, including a list of accredited programs, contact:

- American Academy of Physician Assistants Information Center, 2318 Mill Rd., Suite 1300, Alexandria, VA 22314. https://www.aapa.org

For a list of accredited physician assistant, programs, contact:

- Accreditation Review Commission on Education for the Physician Assistants, 12000 Findley Rd., Suite 275, Johns Creek, GA 30097. https://www.arc-pa.org

For eligibility requirements and a description of the Physician Assistant National Certifying Examination, contact:

- National Commission on Certification of Physician Assistants, Inc., 12000 Findley Rd., Suite 100, Johns Creek, GA 30097. https://www.nccpa.net

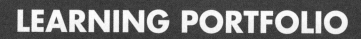

LEARNING PORTFOLIO

Issues for Discussion

1. Every state's licensing board requires physician assistants to work under the supervision of a physician. Brainstorm why state licensing boards believe a physician's supervision might be needed.

2. The physician assistant field is relatively new to health care, beginning in the 1960s and becoming more prevalent in the twenty-first century. Not all patients want to be seen by a physician assistant, with some preferring to be seen by a physician instead. Brainstorm the reasons why patients might resist receiving care from a physician assistant.

Enrichment Activities

1. Use the Internet to research national organizations associated with nurses, physician assistants, medical doctors, and doctors of osteopathy. Compare and contrast the responsibilities of a physician assistant with a nurse, a medical doctor, or a doctor of osteopathy. Create an infographic to show this information.

Alternatively, create a Venn diagram to show how the responsibilities in these professions overlap and what responsibilities are distinct to a profession.

2. Using the Internet, research the history and development of the physician assistant profession. Identify the reason(s) why the profession was created and when and how the federal government and insurance companies decided to reimburse care provided by physician assistants. Prepare a written narrative or infographic of this information for your instructor.

3. View the infographic titled "What Is a PA?" found at https://www.aapa.org/download/80021/ and the steps to becoming a PA at https://www.aapa.org/career-central/become-a-pa/ Discuss your impressions with your instructor and classmates.

4. Create a one-page infographic or flyer for students who are thinking of a career as a physician assistant. The pamphlet should inform students what a PA is, what a PA does, and of both the benefits and drawbacks of this occupation.

CASE STUDY: FAMILY PRACTICE APPOINTMENT

You are currently employed by a group of family practice physicians. This practice includes physician assistants who routinely provide care to patients. Your duties include signing patients in as they arrive for their appointments and gathering their demographic and insurance information. When Mrs. Smith sits down in your office to provide her information, she states that she has a question about the doctor's "assistants." You respond that you will be more than happy to answer her questions or direct her to someone who can. Mrs. Smith asks the following questions.

Based on the information you have read about physician assistants, answer the following questions:

1. Are the physician assistants qualified to take care of me?
   A. Some are better than others.
   B. PAs are qualified through both academic and clinical training.
   C. Physicians review the work of PAs on a monthly basis.
   D. PAs are responsible for their own practice.

2. Who decides what job duties the physician assistant will be able to perform?
   A. The government does this
   B. The school where the PA received their diploma

   C. The PAs job duties are determined by the supervising physician and the laws in the state in which they practice.
   D. The PA may do whatever they feel comfortable doing.

3. Are physician assistants licensed?
   A. No, but they are certified.
   B. No, but they must complete on-the-job training.
   C. Yes, they must pass a national certification exam to be licensed.
   D. No, only physicians are required to be licensed.

4. How are physician assistants different from registered nurses?
   A. Nurses are certified, and physician assistants are licensed.
   B. A PA must complete the same type of program as a registered nurse.
   C. Many PAs have prior experience as registered nurses, and others come from varied backgrounds, including military corpsmen or medics and allied health occupations.
   D. Both can perform the same job duties, but a physician must directly supervise a PA, and a nurse can work independently.

LEARNING PORTFOLIO

References

1. 2020 AAPA Physician Assistant Census Report, available at https://www.aapa.org/shop/salary-report/ Accessed August 1, 2021.

2. Accreditation Review Commission on Education for the Physician Assistant, Inc. Accredited PA Programs. http://www.arc-pa.org/accreditation/accredited-programs/ Accessed August 1, 2021.

3. Physician Assistant National Certifying Examination. PANCE Eligibility Requirements. https://www.nccpa.net/become-certified/#pance-resources Accessed August 1, 2021.

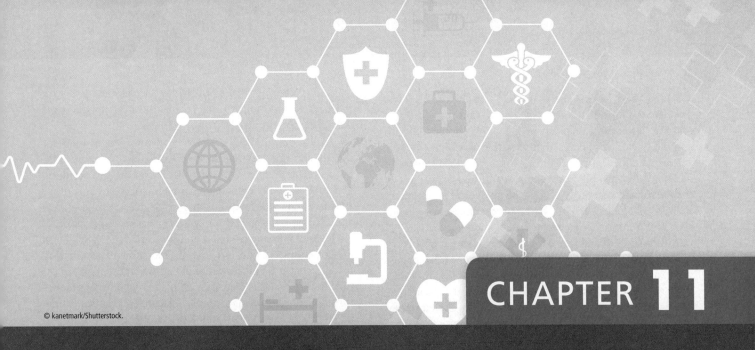

© kanetmark/Shutterstock.

CHAPTER 11

Nursing*

KEY TERMS

Accreditation Commission for
    Midwifery Education (ACME)
ADN-to-BSN
ADN-to-MSN
Advanced Practice Registered
    Nurse (APRN)
American Academy of Nurse
    Practitioners Certification
    Board (AANPCB)
American Midwifery
    Certification Board (AMCB)
American Nursing Credentialing
    Center (ANCC)
Associate's Degree in Nursing
    (ADN)
Bachelor of Science in Nursing
    (BSN)
Certified Midwives (CM)
Certified Nurse-Midwives (CNM)

Certified Registered Nurse
    Anesthetists (CRNAs)
Clinical Nurse Specialist (CNS)
Consensus Model for APRN
    Regulation
Council on Accreditation of
    Nurse Anesthesia Educational
    Programs (COA)
Interprofessional education (IPE)
Licensed Practical Nurses (LPNs)
Licensed Vocational Nurses
    (LVNs)
LPN-to-BSN
Master of Science in Nursing
    (MSN)
National Board of Certification
    and Recertification for Nurse
    Anesthetists (NBCRNA)

National Council Licensure
    Examination (NCLEX-PN)
National Council Licensure
    Examination (NCLEX-RN)
National Council of State Boards
    of Nursing (NCSBN)
National Federation of Licensed
    Practical Nurses (NFLPN)
National League for Nursing
    (NLN)
Nurse anesthetists
Nurse-midwives
Nurse Practitioners (NPs)
Pediatric Nursing Certification
    Board (NPCB)
Pediatric oncology
Registered Nurses (RNs)
RN-to-BSN
RN-to-MSN

* All information in this chapter, unless otherwise indicated, was obtained from Bureau of Labor Statistics. *Occupational Outlook Handbook 2020–2021 Edition*. Washington, DC: U.S. Department of Labor; 2021.

THE FUTURE OF NURSING

The demand for skilled nurses is at an all-time high for three reasons. First, the expansion of the aging population with complex health problems increases the number of people requiring skilled nursing care. Second, greater numbers of newly insured people are seeking health care as a result of the Affordable Care Act (ACA).[1] Third, Medicare reimbursement rates to hospitals are based on readmission rates for six conditions or procedures: heart failure, heart attack, pneumonia, hip and knee replacement surgery, chronic obstructive pulmonary disease, and coronary artery bypass graft surgery,[2] and there is evidence that employing nurses with higher education is linked to improved patient outcomes. There is also a greater need for highly skilled nurses to assume new and expanded roles in community settings—primary care, public health, and long-term care. Nurses in these settings are needed to serve as care coordinators, case managers, chronic care specialists, and patient educators.[1,3] In addition, because of a shortage of primary care physicians, **Nurse Practitioners (NPs)** are assuming the role of primary care providers in outpatient settings. However, a barrier that limits the practice of nurses is state regulations that prohibit an independent practice of **Advanced Practice Registered Nurses (APRNs)**; in these states, APRNs are required to work under the supervision of a licensed physician.

Projected employment for **Registered Nurses (RNs)** in 2029 is 3.3 million, more than any other healthcare practitioner, and yet educational requirements for RNs are lower than any other practitioner with similar job responsibilities. Nurses can become registered after completing a two- to three-year associate's degree. The educational requirement for many entry-level healthcare practitioners is a master's degree—for example, medical social workers, occupational therapists, and speech therapists—and the entry-level requirement for audiologists and physical therapists is a doctorate. Also, in the past, nurses' training has focused on acute hospital care, while current needs are preventing and managing chronic disease in community settings.

The 2010 Institute of Medicine (IOM) report "The Future of Nursing: Leading Change, Advancing Health" identified a need to make changes in nursing education: a need not only to increase the number of nurses but also to increase the skills of RNs—necessary to deliver safe, high-quality care across all settings from primary care to community and public health. Three recommendations to ensure that nurses receive high-quality education were to (1) increase the number of RNs with a bachelor's degree from 50% to 80% by 2020, (2) double the number with doctorate degrees by 2020, and (3) require a nurse residency program after completing pre-licensure or an advanced practice degree program.[4] In addition, the IOM report recommended **interprofessional education (IPE)** through collaboration among the schools of nursing and other health professional schools in designing and implementing joint classroom and clinical training opportunities. The goal of IPE is to train students from various health professions to work together as a team. Students learn the contributions of individual professions and how to integrate and modify input from all team members while delivering patient care.[4]

Since one of the barriers to advanced education for nurses was the cost and lack of work flexibility, the IOM report recommended that employers cover the cost of tuition and provide benefits for part-time employees to encourage RNs to obtain a bachelor's or higher degree.[4] Several professional organizations including the American Association of Colleges of Nursing (AACN) and the American Association of Community Colleges (AACC) recommend structuring bridge programs and educational pathways that are seamless to allow graduates to transition into a higher level of practice through education. For example, a **Licensed Practical Nurse (LPN)** or **Licensed Vocational Nurse (LVN)** can transition to a **Bachelor of Science in nursing (BSN)** program (**LPN-to-BSN**), and an associate's degree nursing graduate can transition into a bachelor's program (**ADN-to-BSN**) or **Master of Science in Nursing (MSN)** program (**ADN-to-MSN**). Many RNs who graduate from ADN programs do not complete a bachelor's program.[3] Another pathway to becoming an RN is by first working as a certified nursing assistant (CNA); many nursing programs require applicants to have work experience in the field before being accepted into an ADN or RN educational program.[5] There is also a need for nurses to obtain master's and doctorate degrees, both a doctorate in nursing practice (DNP) to provide care in advanced practice roles and a doctor of philosophy (PhD) to assume leadership positions and serve as faculty in nursing schools for teaching as well as conducting research.[3]

Since the IOM report in 2010, enrollment in graduate nursing programs has increased by 161% for DNP programs and 15% for PhD programs.[6] As of 2018, the majority of nurses held a bachelor's degree (45%) followed by an associate's degree (30%), but only 19% of nurses held graduate degrees and only 2% held doctorate degrees.[7] The number of years of education required to become employed in the nursing field is shown in **FIGURE 11.1**.

LPNs provide a variety of direct care services—administering medication, taking medical histories, recording symptoms and vital signs, and other tasks as delegated by RNs, physicians, and other healthcare providers. LPNs typically receive training for a year beyond high school. The route to becoming an RN is to complete a two-year associate's degree, a diploma from an approved nursing program, or a bachelor's degree in nursing. The scope of RN responsibilities is more complex and analytical than that of LPNs. RNs provide a wide array of direct-care services, such as administering treatments, care coordination, disease prevention, patient education, and health promotion for individuals, families, and communities. RNs may choose to obtain advanced clinical education and training to become APRNs; who usually have a master's degree, although some complete doctoral-level training, and often focus on a clinical specialty area.[8]

For both LPNs and RNs, the majority of jobs are expected to be in skilled nursing, rehabilitation, and residential facilities,

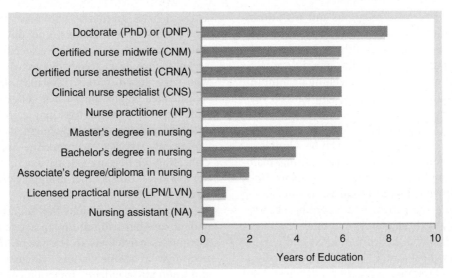

FIGURE 11.1 Educational pathways for nursing professionals.

Data from Institute of Medicine. *The Future of Nursing: Leading Change, Advancing Health.* The National Academies Press; 2011.

home health care, and ambulatory care because of shorter hospital stays. Job growth is expected in long-term care facilities that provide care for patients after a stroke or head injury and for those with Alzheimer's disease. Since surgical procedures and chemotherapy for oncology patients routinely take place in ambulatory settings, more jobs for nurses will be available in these settings. Nurses also may provide basic health care to patients outside healthcare settings in such venues as correctional facilities, schools, summer camps, manufacturing plants, and the military. Both LPNs and RNs work as private duty nurses for those living at home who need 24-hour-a-day care because of physical or mental disabilities. Some RNs travel around the United States and throughout the world providing care to patients in areas with shortages of healthcare workers or during an emergency such as weather-related disasters—a hurricane or tornado.

For students interested in a nursing career, there are many choices available for training—one year for an entry-level career as an LPN or two to four years to become an RN. Nurses work with all ages from premature infants in a neonatal intensive care unit to elderly women living at home on hospice care. Opportunities for advancement are through additional experience and education. Specializing in a clinical area and working more independently requires a master's degree. APRNs work as nurse anesthetists, midwives, or nurse practitioners specializing in pediatrics, psychiatry, or gerontology. There are many possibilities for a nursing career depending on the preferred work environment and educational goals. In the future, nurses will be expected to have completed a minimum of a bachelor's degree, and a graduate degree will be required to specialize or to assume supervisory responsibilities, teaching, or research.

The focus of this chapter is the RN, the APRN—nurse anesthetist, nurse-midwife, clinical nurse specialist, and nurse practitioner—and the LPN/LVN. For information on educational requirements and responsibilities of nursing assistants, review Chapter 33.

REGISTERED NURSES (RNs)
Significant Points

- Registered Nurses (RNs) constitute the largest healthcare occupation, with 3.4 million jobs.
- About 60% of RN jobs are in hospitals.
- The three typical educational paths to becoming an RN are a diploma from an approved nursing program, an associate's degree from a community college, or a bachelor's degree from a four-year college.
- Clinical nurse specialists provide direct patient care to a certain population of people and/or within a specific medical or surgical specialty and usually are required to have a master's degree.
- Overall job opportunities are expected to be excellent, especially for RNs with a bachelor's degree, but may vary by employment and geographic setting; some employers report difficulty in attracting and retaining an adequate number of RNs, usually in underserved urban or rural areas.

Work Description

Registered Nurses (RNs), regardless of specialty or work setting, treat and educate patients and the public about various medical conditions. RNs also give advice and emotional support to the patient as well as family members. RNs record medical histories and symptoms, help perform diagnostic tests and analyze results, operate medical equipment, administer treatment and medications, consult and collaborate with other health professionals, and help with patient follow-up and rehabilitation.

RNs teach patients and their families how to manage injuries or illness by explaining post-treatment home care such as diet and exercise programs and self-administration of medication and physical therapy. Some RNs may work to promote general health by educating the public on warning signs and symptoms of a disease. RNs also might conduct general health screening or immunization clinics, blood drives, and public seminars on various conditions.

When caring for patients, RNs establish a care plan that may include numerous activities, such as administering medication; carefully checking dosages; starting, maintaining, and discontinuing intravenous (IV) lines for fluid, medication, blood, and blood products; administering treatments; observing the patient and recording observations; and consulting with physicians and other healthcare clinicians. Some RNs direct the work of LPNs and nursing assistants regarding patient care. RNs with advanced educational preparation and training may perform diagnostic and therapeutic procedures.

Specific work responsibilities will vary; duties and titles are often determined by the work setting or patient population served. RNs can specialize in one or more areas of patient care. RNs may work in a specific workplace such as a trauma nurse who works in a hospital emergency room or a school nurse who works in an elementary, middle, or high school. RNs may specialize in specific health conditions,

as do diabetes specialists who assist patients in managing blood glucose, medications, and physical activity. Other RNs specialize in working with a specific part of the body or organ, such as dermatology nurses, who work with patients who have skin disorders. RNs may also specialize with a well-defined population, such as geriatric nurses, who work with the elderly. Some RNs may combine specialties. For example, **pediatric oncology** nurses deal with children and adolescents who have cancer. The opportunities for specialization for RNs are extensive with 104 nursing specialties.[9] **TABLE 11.1** lists other examples of specialty areas and responsibilities.

Some nurses have jobs that require little or no direct patient care but still require an active RN license. Forensics nurses participate in the scientific investigation and treatment of abuse victims, violence, criminal activity, and traumatic accidents. Infection control nurses identify, track, and control infectious outbreaks in healthcare facilities and develop programs for outbreak prevention and response to biological terrorism. Nurse educators plan, develop, implement, and evaluate educational programs and curricula for the professional development of student nurses and RNs.

Nurses also may work as healthcare consultants, public policy advisors, pharmaceutical and medical supply

TABLE 11.1 Specialty Areas and Responsibilities for Registered Nurses

Specialty Area	Responsibilities
Cardiac care nurse	Cares for patients with heart disease from coronary artery disease to heart failure and recovery from heart surgery
Critical care nurse	Cares for patients with critical conditions or recovery from serious illness or injury in a hospital intensive care unit
Hospice nurse	Cares for terminally ill patients to manage pain and other symptoms that accompany the dying process
Military nurse	Members of the armed services who care for the military all over the world and veterans in the United States
Neonatal intensive care nurse	Cares for premature and critically ill newborns in a neonatal intensive care unit in the hospital
Obstetrics nurse	Cares for women during pregnancy, labor, childbirth, or other reproductive issues
Psychiatric nurse	Cares for patients with psychiatric disorders such as mental illness or substance use disorders
Rehabilitation nurse	Cares for patients who have chronic illnesses or long-term disabilities
School nurse	Cares for students from pre-K to college who become sick or injured while in school
Substance abuse nurse	Cares for patients who are addicted to drugs, alcohol, or other substances
Transplant nurse	Cares for patients who are donating or receiving an organ or tissue through the transplant procedure

Data from Johnson & Johnson. *Nursing. Nursing Specialties.* Accessed July 20, 2021. https://nursing.jnj.com/specialty

researchers and salespersons, and medical writers and editors. Nursing informatics integrates nursing science with information management and analytical science to manage and communicate nursing data to improve decision-making by consumers, patients, nurses, and other healthcare providers. The majority of nurses, however, work in hospitals, ambulatory care, home health care, and long-term care, and some of the roles of nurses in each of these settings are described in this section.

Ambulatory care nurses provide preventive care and treat patients with a variety of illnesses and injuries in physicians' offices or clinics including public health clinics. Holistic nurses provide care—such as acupuncture, massage and aromatherapy, and biofeedback—meant to treat mental and spiritual health in addition to physical health. Diabetes management nurses help those with diabetes manage their disease by teaching them proper nutrition and showing them how to test blood sugar levels and administer insulin injections. Oncology nurses care for patients with various types of cancer and may assist in the administration of radiation and chemotherapies and follow-up monitoring. Occupational health nurses work in large manufacturing plants, such as automobile factories, where there is a high risk for employee injury; they recognize and prevent health effects from hazardous exposure to chemicals, prevent job-related injuries and illnesses, provide monitoring and emergency care services, and help employers implement health and safety standards. Some ambulatory care nurses are involved in telehealth, providing care and advice through electronic communications such as video conferencing, email, or telephone.

Hospital nurses provide care to patients with serious, complex, and acute illnesses or injuries that require very close monitoring and extensive medication protocols and therapies. Emergency or trauma nurses work in the emergency room of a hospital or stand-alone emergency departments, providing initial assessment and care for patients with life-threatening conditions—for example, after a heart attack, car accident, or gunshot wound. Some emergency nurses may become qualified to serve as transport nurses, who provide medical care to patients transported by helicopter or airplane to the nearest medical facility, especially in rural areas. Medical-surgical nurses provide health promotion and basic medical care to patients before and after surgery. Perioperative nurses assist surgeons by selecting and handling instruments, controlling bleeding, and suturing incisions. Wound, ostomy, and continence nurses treat patients with wounds caused by traumatic injury, ulcers, or arterial disease; provide postoperative care for patients with openings that allow for alternative methods of bodily waste elimination; and treat patients with urinary and fecal incontinence.

Home healthcare nurses provide at-home nursing care for patients, often as follow-up care after discharge from a hospital or a rehabilitation, long-term care, or skilled nursing facility. Infusion nurses administer medications, fluids, and blood to patients through the patients' veins. Nurses provide wound care for patients with pressure ulcers; they also monitor medication compliance for patients with serious medical problems, such as asthma or heart failure. Other nurses who make home visits are psychiatric nurses, who monitor medication compliance and provide counseling for those with mental illness, and public health nurses, who provide education and support for new mothers.

Long-term care nurses provide healthcare services for patients with chronic physical or mental disorders, often in nursing or assisted-living facilities, adult day care, intermediate care facilities for those with intellectual disabilities, or inpatient psychiatric services for those under age 21. Rehabilitation centers and skilled nursing facilities provide in-patient, short-term services for those recovering from surgery—for example, a hip replacement—or from complications of a lung disease requiring respiratory support.

Work Environment

Most RNs work in well-lit, comfortable healthcare facilities. Other nurses travel to patients' homes, schools, community centers, and other sites. RNs may spend considerable time walking, bending, stretching, and standing. Patients in hospitals and nursing care facilities require 24-hour care; consequently, nurses in these institutions may work nights, weekends, and holidays. RNs also may be on call, available to work on short notice.

Nurses who work in offices, schools, and other settings that do not provide 24-hour care are more likely to work regular business hours. Nurses who work in hospitals, rehabilitation centers, and skilled nursing facilities work in shifts. The most common shift for hospitals is three 12-hour shifts per week. Those in skilled nursing facilities are more likely to work five 8-hour shifts. The newest employee usually works the night shift or a rotating shift, which may interfere with regular sleep patterns. Nurses in ambulatory settings usually work a day shift; however, the hours can be from 7 AM to 7 PM. Nurses in home care usually have the flexibility of scheduling appointments.

RNs may be in close contact with individuals who have infectious diseases and with toxic, harmful, or potentially hazardous compounds, solutions, and medications. RNs must observe rigid, standardized guidelines to guard against disease and other dangers, such as those posed by radiation, accidental needle sticks, chemicals used to sterilize instruments, and anesthetics. In addition, they are vulnerable to back injury when moving or lifting patients.

Most nurses work as part of a team of other health professionals such as physicians, respiratory therapists, dietitians, occupational and physical therapists, and others. Some teams have regular team meetings with the patient to discuss treatment plans. Some registered nurses oversee licensed practical nurses, nursing assistants, and home health aides.

Employment Opportunities

As the largest healthcare occupation, RNs held about 3.1 million jobs in 2019, and hospitals employed the majority of RNs, with 60% of such jobs. About 18% of jobs were in ambulatory health care and 7% in nursing and residential care facilities.

Educational and Legal Requirements

Educational paths to becoming an RN are a bachelor's degree, an associate's degree, or a diploma from an approved nursing program. Individuals then must complete a national licensing examination to obtain a nursing license. Specializing in a clinical specialty often requires a master's degree.

Education and Training

There are three typical educational paths to becoming an RN—a **Bachelor of Science in Nursing (BSN)**, which takes four years to complete; an **Associate's Degree in Nursing (ADN)**; or a diploma. BSN programs are offered by colleges and universities and take four years to complete. ADN programs are offered by community colleges and take about two to three years to complete. Diploma programs, administered by hospitals, last about three years. Generally, licensed graduates of any of the three types of educational programs qualify for entry-level positions as staff nurses. There are hundreds of registered nursing programs that result in an ADN or BSN; however, there are relatively few diploma programs, and in 2018, only 6% of RNs received their nursing education through a diploma program.[7]

For high school students interested in becoming a nurse, recommended courses are biology, chemistry, physics, computer science, algebra, and geometry. Two years of a foreign language are also recommended, since English is not the first language for many patients. In all nursing education programs, students take courses in anatomy, physiology, microbiology, chemistry, nutrition, psychology, and other social and behavioral sciences as well as in liberal arts.

All programs also include supervised clinical experience provided in hospital departments such as pediatrics, psychiatry, maternity, and surgery. Some programs include clinical experience in nursing care facilities, public health departments, home health agencies, and ambulatory clinics.

Many registered nurses with an ADN or diploma choose to go back to school to earn a bachelor's degree through an **RN-to-BSN** degree program, an **RN-to-MSN** degree program, or a program for those who wish to enter the nursing profession but hold a bachelor's degree in another field. Accelerated BSN programs last 12 to 18 months and provide the fastest route to a BSN for individuals who already hold a degree.

Individuals considering a career in nursing should carefully weigh the advantages and disadvantages of enrolling in each type of education program. Advancement opportunities may be more limited for ADN and diploma holders compared to RNs who obtain a BSN or higher. Individuals who complete a BSN receive more training in areas such as communication, leadership, and critical thinking, all of which are becoming more important as nursing practice becomes more complex. Additionally, a BSN offers more clinical experience in nonhospital settings. A BSN is often necessary for administrative positions, research, consulting, and teaching.

Licensure

In all states, the District of Columbia, and U.S. territories, students must graduate from an approved nursing program and pass a national licensing examination, known as the **National Council Licensure Examination (NCLEX-RN)**, to obtain an RN nursing license. Other requirements for licensing vary by state. Each state's board of nursing can give details. For more on the NCLEX-RN examination and a list of state boards of nursing, visit the **National Council of State Boards of Nursing (NCSBN)** website.

Certification and Other Qualifications

Certification is optional for RNs; however, nurses with certification will be recognized as having additional qualifications, which will be an advantage when applying for jobs. The **American Nursing Credentialing Center (ANCC)** offers certification for specialty areas for nurses—for example, nursing informatics, ambulatory care nursing, and cardiac rehabilitation nursing. The **Pediatric Nursing Certification Board (PNCB)** certifies nurses who work in pediatrics, and the **National League for Nursing (NLN)** certifies nurse educators. For specific specialty areas and eligibility requirements, go to the credentialing resources listed at the end of the chapter under "Additional Information."

Desirable personal qualities for RNs are to be caring, sympathetic, responsible, and detail-oriented. Critical thinking skills are necessary to correctly assess patients' conditions and determine when to take corrective action and when to make referrals to other health professionals. RNs need emotional stability to cope with human suffering, emergencies, and other stressors. Because most nurses work with multiple patients with different health needs, organizational skills are critical to ensure that each patient receives the correct treatment at the right time. Speaking skills are necessary as nurses must be able to talk with patients to assess their health conditions and to instruct patients to take medications correctly as well as perform other self-care activities. Nurses also need to communicate patient needs and update the status of patients with other health team members. RNs must be able to direct or supervise others.

Advancement

Most RNs begin as staff nurses in hospitals and, with experience and good performance, often move to other settings or are promoted to positions with more responsibility. Another path to advancement is specialty certification, which is usually voluntary but demonstrates adherence to a higher standard; some employers may require it.[9] In management, nurses can advance from assistant unit manager or head nurse to more senior-level administrative roles of assistant director, director, vice president, or chief of nursing. Increasingly, management-level nursing positions require a graduate or an advanced degree in nursing or health services administration. Administrative positions require leadership, communication and negotiation skills, and good judgment. Some nurses move into the business side of health care. Their nursing expertise and experience on a healthcare team equip them to manage ambulatory, acute, home-based, and chronic care businesses. Employers—including hospitals, insurance companies, pharmaceutical manufacturers, and managed care organizations—need registered nurses for jobs in health planning and development, marketing, consulting, policy development, and quality assurance (**FIGURE 11.2**).

Employment Trends

Job opportunities may vary by employment and geographic setting. Employment of RNs is expected to grow faster than average, and because the occupation is very large, 221,900 new jobs are projected by 2029, among the largest number of new jobs for any occupation. Additionally, hundreds of thousands of job openings will result from the need to replace experienced nurses who leave the occupation.

Employment Change

Employment of RNs is expected to grow by 7% from 2019 to 2029, faster than the average for all occupations. Demand for healthcare services will increase because of the aging population, since older people typically have more medical problems than younger people. Nurses also will be needed to educate and care for geriatric patients with various chronic conditions, such as arthritis, dementia, diabetes, and obesity.

Employment of RNs will not grow at the same rate in every industry; growth is expected to be slower in hospitals—health care's largest industry—than in most other healthcare industries. Growth will be driven by technological advances in patient care, which permit a greater number of health problems to be treated, and by an increasing emphasis on preventive care. Although the intensity of nursing care is likely to increase, requiring more nurses per patient, the number of inpatients (those who remain in the hospital for more than 24 hours) is not likely to grow by much. The financial pressure on hospitals to discharge patients as soon as possible may result in more people receiving care in outpatient care centers, such as those providing same-day surgery, rehabilitation, and chemotherapy; because many older people prefer to

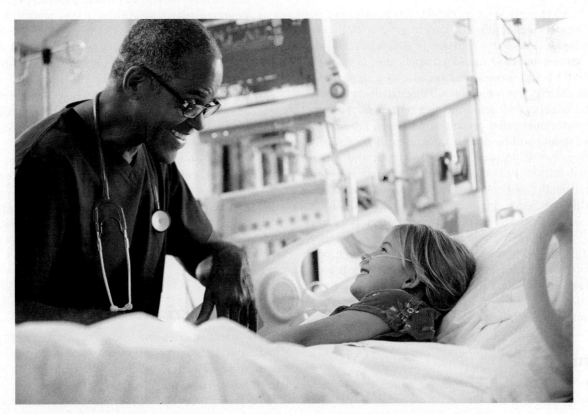

FIGURE 11.2 A registered nurse can become certified as a pediatric nurse.
© Monkey Business Images/Shutterstock.

TABLE 11.2 Projections Data for Registered Nurses, 2019–2029

Occupational Title	Employment, 2019	Projected Employment, 2029	Change, 2019–2029	
			Number	Percentage
Registered nurses	3,096,700	3,318,700	221,900	7%

Data from Bureau of Labor Statistics. *Occupational Outlook Handbook*. U.S. Department of Labor; 2020.

TABLE 11.3 Median Annual Wages in the Industries Employing the Largest Numbers of Registered Nurses, May 2020

Government	$84,490
Hospitals	$76,840
Ambulatory healthcare services	$72,340
Nursing and residential care facilities	$68,450
Educational services	$64,630

Data from Bureau of Labor Statistics. *Occupational Outlook Handbook*. U.S. Department of Labor; 2020.

be treated at home or in residential care facilities, registered nurses will be in demand in those settings.

Job Prospects

Overall, job opportunities are expected to be excellent for RNs. Competition for jobs may vary by geographic area— for example, Texas has a shortage of RNs while Florida has a surplus of RNs.[8] Qualified applicants to nursing schools are being turned away because of a shortage of nursing faculty. The need for nursing faculty will only increase as many instructors are near retirement. Despite the slower employment growth in hospitals, job opportunities should still be excellent because of the relatively high turnover of hospital nurses. To attract and retain qualified nurses, hospitals may offer signing bonuses, family-friendly work schedules, or subsidized training. Although faster employment growth is projected in physicians' offices and outpatient care centers, RNs may face greater competition for these positions because they generally offer regular working hours and more comfortable working environments. Generally, RNs with at least a BSN will have better job prospects. **TABLE 11.2** shows the projections data through 2029 from the national employment matrix.

Earnings

The median annual wages of registered nurses were $75,330 in May 2020. Median annual wages in the industries employing the largest numbers of registered nurses in May 2020 are shown in **TABLE 11.3**.

Related Occupations

Because of the number of specialties for RNs and the variety of responsibilities and duties, many other healthcare occupations are similar in some aspects of their job. Some healthcare occupations with similar levels of responsibility that work under the direction of physicians or dentists are dental hygienists, diagnostic medical sonographers, emergency medical technicians and paramedics, LPNs, and physician assistants.

ADVANCED PRACTICE REGISTERED NURSES (APRNs)
Significant Points

- Advanced Practice Registered Nurses (APRNs)— clinical nurse specialists, nurse anesthetists, nurse-midwives, and nurse practitioners—require a master's degree; most are also certified in a specialty area.
- Projected growth for APRNs is 45%, much faster than other occupations, as a result of greater numbers of people having health insurance, an increased emphasis on preventive care, and greater health needs of the aging population.
- Changes in state laws governing APRN practice authority have allowed APRNs to perform more services without the direct supervision of a physician to meet primary care needs.
- Overall job opportunities are expected to be excellent, particularly in medically underserved rural and urban areas where there is a shortage of primary care physicians. In addition, APRNs can expect to be in demand as clinical specialists and consultants in hospitals and other healthcare systems because of advanced clinical training.

Work Description

Nurse anesthetists, nurse-midwives, nurse practitioners, and clinical nurse specialists, also referred to as APRNs, coordinate patient care and provide primary and specialty health care. The scope of practice varies from state to state. APRNs work independently or in collaboration with physicians. In most states, they can prescribe medications, order medical tests, and diagnose health problems.

APRNs provide primary and preventive care and may specialize in care for certain groups of people, such as children, pregnant women, or patients with mental health disorders. APRNs who work with patients typically perform many of the same duties as RNs, gathering information about a patient's condition and taking action to treat or manage the patient's health. However, in most states, they perform many additional functions that are beyond the scope of the RN, including prescribing medications, ordering tests and evaluating test results, referring patients to specialists, and diagnosing and treating injuries and illnesses. APRNs focus on patient-centered care, which means understanding a patient's concerns and lifestyle before choosing a course of action.

APRNs may also conduct research or teach the nursing staff about new policies or procedures. Others may provide consultation services based on a specific field of knowledge, such as oncology. Following are examples of the four main types of APRNs.

Certified Registered Nurse Anesthetists (CRNAs)

Certified Registered Nurse Anesthetists (CRNAs) provide anesthesia and related care before, during, and after surgical, therapeutic, diagnostic, and obstetrical procedures. They also provide pain management and some emergency services. Before a procedure begins, **nurse anesthetists** discuss with a patient any medications the patient is taking as well as any allergies or illnesses the patient may have so that anesthesia can be safely administered. CRNAs then give a patient general anesthesia to put the patient to sleep or regional or local anesthesia to numb an area of the body. They remain with the patient throughout a procedure to monitor vital signs and adjust the anesthesia as necessary.

Nurse anesthetists have practiced in the United States since providing care for wounded soldiers during the Civil War. Currently they work in all settings where anesthesia is delivered, either in collaboration with anesthesiologists or independently. These settings include hospital surgical suites and obstetrical delivery rooms; ambulatory surgical centers; offices of dentists, podiatrists, ophthalmologists, plastic surgeons, and pain management specialists; and healthcare facilities in the military, Public Health Services, and Veteran's Administration hospitals and clinics.[10] CRNAs are the sole providers of anesthesia in two-thirds of rural hospitals and are sole providers in 100% of rural hospitals in some states. CRNAs who practice in rural areas make it possible for these hospitals to offer surgical, obstetrical, and trauma care. As APRNs, they are given a high degree of autonomy and professional respect[10,11] (**FIGURE 11.3**).

Certified Nurse-Midwives (CNMs)

Certified Nurse-Midwives (CNMs) and **Certified Midwives (CMs)** provide care to women, including gynecological exams, family planning services, prenatal care, attendance in labor and delivery, and postpartum care. They deliver

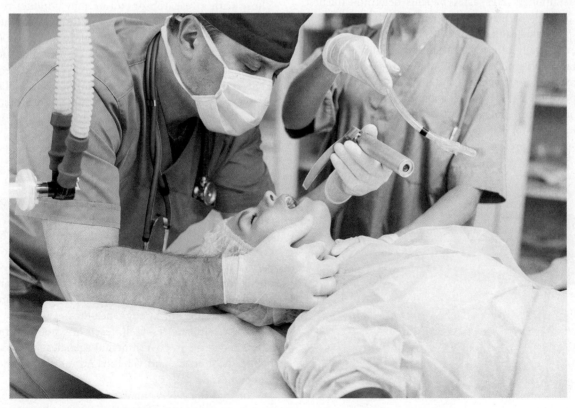

FIGURE 11.3 Nurse anesthetists are the sole provider of anesthesia in some rural areas.
© ProStockStudio/Shutterstock.

babies, manage emergencies during labor, and repair lacerations and may provide surgical assistance to physicians during cesarean births. They may act as primary care providers for women and newborns. Many **nurse-midwives** provide wellness care, educating their patients on how to lead healthy lives by discussing topics such as nutrition and disease prevention. Nurse-midwives also provide care to their patients' partners for sexual or reproductive health issues.

Today, CNMs and their colleagues, CMs, provide family-centered primary health care to women throughout their reproductive lives. Skilled midwifery can reduce the need for high-tech interventions for most women in labor, but midwives also are trained in the latest scientific procedures to assist in normal deliveries and work in collaboration with physicians.

In 2019, CNMs/CMs attended 14% of all births; for all births, 89% were in hospitals, 9% in free-standing birthing centers, and 8% at home. The majority consider their practice to be exclusively reproductive care (76%) while 49% consider their practice to be primary care.[12]

Midwifery began in the United States in the 1920s when British-educated women provided health care in the remote mountains of Kentucky; the Manhattan Midwifery School was established in New York City in 1925. Challenges to the practice of midwifery include restrictive legislation related to requirements for physician supervision, hospital delivery, and third-party reimbursement.[13]

Nurse Practitioners (NPs)

Nurse Practitioners (NPs) assess patients, determine the best way to improve or manage a patient's health, and discuss ways to integrate health promotion strategies into a patient's life. They typically care for a certain population of people. For instance, NPs may work in adult and geriatric health, pediatric health, or psychiatry and mental health. Although the scope of their duties varies some by state, many nurse practitioners work independently, prescribe medications, and order laboratory tests. All NPs consult with physicians and other health professionals when needed (**FIGURE 11.4**).

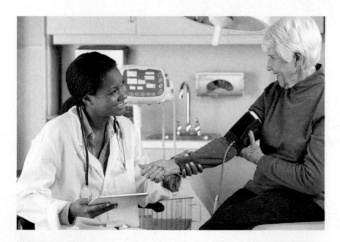

FIGURE 11.4 Nurse practitioners can specialize in gerontology.
© Monkey Business Images/Shutterstock.

NPs complete comprehensive physical examinations; diagnose and treat common acute illnesses and injuries such as colds and sprained ankles; provide immunizations; manage chronic diseases; order and interpret diagnostic tests including X-rays, ECGs, and laboratory tests; prescribe medications and therapies; and perform procedures and educate patients on a healthy lifestyle and management of chronic diseases.[14] The majority of NPs are certified in an area of primary care; some have additional certification in a specialty area such as pediatric primary care, gerontology primary care, or mental health.[15]

Clinical Nurse Specialists (CNSs)

Clinical Nurse Specialists (CNSs) are a type of APRN. They provide direct patient care in one of many nursing specialties, such as psychiatric-mental health or pediatrics. CNSs provide direct patient care to a certain population of people, such as pediatric patients, within one of many nursing specialties, such as orthopedic nursing or oncology nursing—thus, a CNS might specialize, for example, in pediatric oncology. CNSs also provide indirect care by working with other nurses, healthcare teams, and various other staff to improve the quality of care that patients receive. They also work at the system or organizational level in hospitals or ambulatory centers to improve the quality of nursing care throughout a facility or system related to their specialty. The requirement for a CNS credential is a master's degree. Those with a research doctorate may conduct research. Examples of clinical specialties in nursing are certification in Pediatric Nursing, Medical-Surgical Nursing, or Nursing Case Management. CNS credentialing for RNs is available from the American Nursing Credentialing Center for clinical certification and the National League for Nursing for certification of nurse educators. These organizations are listed at the end of the chapter under "Additional Information."

Work Environment

APRNs work in a variety of settings, including physicians' offices, hospitals, nursing care and assisted-living facilities, schools, and clinics. Nurse-midwives also work in birthing centers, and nurse anesthetists work in ambulatory surgery centers and offices of dentists and podiatrists. APRNs often work in underserved urban or rural areas and may also travel long distances to help care for patients in places where there are not enough healthcare workers. APRNs perform healthcare research, teach in schools and universities, and serve in governmental agencies: health departments, the military, and Veterans Administration hospitals and clinics.

In addition, NPs may work in worksite employee health centers and for healthcare technology companies (e.g., pharmaceutical manufacturers). Approximately 15%

of all NPs have private practice, and others manage outpatient health centers.[14] APRNs' work can be both physically and emotionally demanding. Some APRNs spend much of their day on their feet. They are vulnerable to back injuries because they must lift and move patients. APRNs' work can also be stressful, as they may make critical decisions about care.

Because of the environments in which they work, APRNs may come in close contact with infectious diseases and potentially harmful drugs. Therefore, they must follow strict, standardized guidelines to guard against diseases and other dangers, such as accidental needle sticks.

APRNs working in physicians' offices or schools typically work during normal business hours. Those working in hospitals and various other healthcare facilities may work in shifts to provide round-the-clock patient care. They may work nights, weekends, and holidays. Nurse anesthetists and nurse-midwives may also be on call.

Employment Opportunities

Employment of APRNs is expected to grow 45% from 2019 to 2029, much faster than the average for all occupations. The demand is expected to be greater for NPs than for other APRNs. Growth will occur because of an increase in the demand for healthcare services. Several factors, including healthcare legislation and the resulting increase in newly insured persons, an increased emphasis on preventive care, and the large, aging Baby Boom population, will contribute to this demand.

APRNs can perform many of the same services as physicians and may be needed to provide primary care services. As states change their laws governing APRN practice authority, APRNs are being allowed to perform more services. They are also becoming more widely recognized by the public as a source for primary health care.

APRNs will also be needed to care for the aging Baby Boom generation. As Baby Boomers age, they will experience ailments and complex conditions that require medical care. APRNs will be needed to keep these patients healthy and to treat the growing number of patients with chronic conditions. The percentage of APRNs in different work settings in 2019 is shown in **TABLE 11.4**.

TABLE 11.4 Work Settings with the Largest Number of Advanced Practice Registered Nurses, 2019

Offices of physicians	47%
Hospitals	27%
Outpatient care centers	8%
Offices of other health practitioners	3%

Data from Bureau of Labor Statistics. *Occupational Outlook Handbook*. U.S. Department of Labor; 2020.

Education and Legal Requirements

APRNs must earn a master's degree from an accredited program. These programs include both classroom education and clinical experience. APRNs must also be licensed RNs in their state and pass a national certification exam.

Education and Training

Nurse-midwives, clinical nurse specialists, and nurse practitioners must earn a master's degree from an accredited program. These programs include both classroom education and clinical experience. Courses in anatomy, physiology, and pharmacology are common as well as coursework specific to the chosen APRN role.

Programs for nurse anesthetists require one year of work experience as a registered nurse in a critical care setting; also, beginning January 1, 2022, all students matriculating into an accredited nurse anesthetist program must be enrolled in a doctoral program.[16] A master's degree is the most common form of entry-level education, although many APRNs have a Doctor of Nursing Practice (DNP) or a PhD and education programs for clinical nurse specialists and nurse practitioners are moving to the DNP degree.[17]

Most APRN programs prefer candidates who have a bachelor's degree in nursing. However, some schools offer bridge programs for registered nurses with an associate's degree or diploma in nursing. Graduate-level programs are also available for individuals who did not obtain a bachelor's degree in nursing but in a related health science field. These programs prepare the student for the RN licensure exam in addition to the APRN curriculum.

As of September 2020, there were 124 accredited nurse anesthesia programs in the United States and Puerto Rico approved by the **Council on Accreditation of Nurse Anesthesia Educational Programs (COA)**. Of these, 102 programs award doctoral degrees for entry-level practice.[16] Nurse anesthesia programs range from 24 to 51 months in length. All programs include clinical training in university-based or large community hospitals.[16]

There are 38 programs for midwifery accredited by the **Accreditation Commission for Midwifery Education (ACME)**. There are two educational pathways for those interested in midwifery as a career. Programs that require students to be RNs lead to the CNM credential while programs not requiring students to be an RN lead to the CM credential. A bachelor's degree is required for application. Training programs for midwives are concentrated in the Northeast and on the East and West coasts, and the shortage of nursing faculty makes it difficult to increase the number of graduates. However, 21% of the programs are offered through a distance-learning format and 45% are hybrid programs using a combination of classroom and distance learning.[18]

There were over 400 nurse practitioner programs in the United States as of 2020 that offered degrees at the master's or doctorate level. The American Association of Nurse Practitioners website lists all nurse practitioner programs and tips for applying to programs. For more information about NP programs, go to the American Association of Nurse Practitioners website listed at the end of the chapter under "Additional Information." CNSs must earn a master's degree in nursing, which usually requires two years. CNSs who conduct research typically need a doctoral degree.

Licensure

Most states recognize all of the APRN roles. In states that recognize some or all of the roles, APRNs must be licensed as an RN, complete an approved graduate-level program, and pass a national certification exam. Each state's board of nursing can provide details.

The **Consensus Model for APRN Regulation**, a document developed by a wide variety of professional nursing organizations, including the National Council of State Boards of Nursing, aims to standardize APRN requirements. The model recommends all APRNs complete a graduate degree from an accredited program, be a licensed RN, pass a national certification exam, and earn a second license specific to one of the APRN roles specific to a certain group of patients—for example, gerontology. CNMs have prescriptive authority in all 50 states and are defined as primary care providers under federal law; however, the CMs are not recognized as independent health providers in all states.[12]

Certification and Other Requirements

Certification is required in the vast majority of states to use an APRN title. Certification is used to show proficiency in an APRN role and is often a requirement for state licensure. The **National Board of Certification and Recertification for Nurse Anesthetists (NBCRNA)** offers the National Certification Examination (NCE). CRNAs must recertify every two years, which includes 40 hours of continuing education. The **American Midwifery Certification Board (AMCB)** offers the Certified Nurse-Midwife (CNM) and Certified Midwife (CM) designations. Individuals with these designations must recertify every five years.

There are a number of certification exams for NPs and CNSs because of the large number of populations with which they may work and the number of specialty areas in which they may practice. Certifications are available from a number of professional organizations, including the **American Nursing Credentialing Center (ANCC)**. NPs can also obtain certification through the **American Academy of Nurse Practitioners Certification Program (AANPCB)**.

Personal qualities that are important for all APRNs include the ability to communicate with patients and other health professionals to ensure that the appropriate course of action is followed. Critical thinking skills are necessary to assess the patient's status quickly, to determine appropriate treatment, and to identify when consultation with other health professionals is needed. APRNs need to have excellent interpersonal skills and demonstrate compassion to successfully work with patients, families, and other health professionals and to be able to work as part of a team. Other important qualities are to be detail-oriented and able to notice changes in a patient's status; also needed is resourcefulness—being able to find answers—to diagnose and treat health problems. Many APRNs lead teams of healthcare workers and need to be able to successfully lead the team.

Advancement

Because the APRN designation is in itself an advancement of one's career, many APRNs choose to remain in this role for the duration of their career. Some APRNs may take on managerial or administrative roles, while others go into academia. Further advancement for APRNs may be achieved by earning a doctoral degree and conducting independent research or working as part of an interprofessional research team.

Employment Trends

Greater numbers of individuals with access to health insurance because of federal health insurance reform legislation will increase the demand for APRNs in outpatient settings. APRNs can perform many of the same services as physicians and may be needed to meet primary care needs. The shortage of obstetrics and gynecology specialty physicians is expected to increase the demand for midwives.

As states change their laws governing APRN practice authority, APRNs are being allowed to perform more services and able to receive reimbursement from Medicare, Medicaid, and private insurance. They are also becoming more widely recognized by the public as a source for primary health care.

APRNs will also be needed to care for the aging Baby Boom generation. APRNs will be needed to keep these patients healthy and to treat the growing number of patients with chronic conditions.

Employment Change

Employment of nurse anesthetists, nurse-midwives, and nurse practitioners is expected to grow 45% from 2019 to 2029, much faster than the average for all occupations. Growth will occur because of an increase in the demand for healthcare services. Several factors, including healthcare legislation and the resulting newly insured, an increased emphasis on preventive care, and the large, aging Baby Boom population, will contribute to this demand.

Job Prospects

Overall, job opportunities for APRNs are expected to be excellent. APRNs will be in high demand, particularly in medically underserved areas such as inner cities and rural areas. The demand will be greatest for NPs and CNMs/CMs who work in primary care settings because of a shortage of primary care and maternity care physicians. In addition,

TABLE 11.5 Projections Data for Advanced Practice Registered Nurses, 2019–2029

Occupational Title	Employment, 2019	Projected Employment, 2029	Change, 2019–2029	
			Number	Percentage
Nurse anesthetists, nurse-midwives, and nurse practitioners	263,400	381,100	117,700	45%
Nurse anesthetists	44,900	51,000	6,200	14%
Nurse-midwives	7,200	8,100	800	12%
Nurse practitioners	211,300	322,000	110,700	52%

Data from Bureau of Labor Statistics. *Occupational Outlook Handbook*. U.S. Department of Labor; 2020.

CRNAs are in demand in rural areas, and NPs and CNSs are in demand to provide consultation and support as clinical specialists in hospitals and long-term care facilities. Job opportunities may also exist from attrition. **TABLE 11.5** provides projected needs for APRNs through 2029.

Earnings

The median annual wage for nurse anesthetists is higher than for nurse-midwives or nurse practitioners; however, all APRNs command higher salaries than RNs because of advanced education and increased responsibilities. Median salaries for 2029 are listed in **TABLE 11.6**.

Related Occupations

Other healthcare occupations with similar educational requirements and job responsibilities are physicians and surgeons, physician assistants, audiologists, speech therapists, occupational therapists, physical therapists, and RNs.

LICENSED PRACTICAL AND LICENSED VOCATIONAL NURSES
Significant Points

- Most training programs last about one year and are offered by vocational or technical schools or community or junior colleges.
- Overall job prospects are expected to be very good, but job outlook varies by industry.
- Replacement needs will be a major source of job openings, as many workers leave the occupation permanently.

Work Description

Licensed Practical Nurses (LPNs) and Licensed Vocational Nurses (LVNs) care for people who are sick, injured,

TABLE 11.6 Median Annual Salary for Advanced Practice Registered Nurses, May 2020

Nurse anesthetists	$183,580
Nurse practitioner	$111,680
Nurse-midwives	$111,130

Data from Bureau of Labor Statistics, U.S. Department of Labor. *Occupational Employment and Wages*; May 2019. http://www.bls.gov/oes/#data/

convalescent, or disabled under the direction of physicians and registered nurses. The nature of the direction and supervision required varies by state and job setting.

LPNs care for patients in many ways. Often, they provide basic bedside care. Many LPNs measure and record patients' vital signs such as height, weight, temperature, blood pressure, pulse, and respiration. They also prepare and give injections and enemas, monitor catheters, dress wounds, and give alcohol rubs and massages. To help keep patients comfortable, they assist with bathing, dressing, personal hygiene, moving in bed, standing, and walking. They might also feed patients who need help eating. Experienced LPNs may supervise nursing assistants and aides (**FIGURE 11.5**).

As part of their work, LPNs collect samples for testing, perform routine laboratory tests, and record food and fluid intake and output. They clean and monitor medical equipment. Sometimes, they help physicians and registered nurses perform tests and procedures. Some LPNs help deliver, care for, and feed infants.

LPNs also monitor their patients and report adverse reactions to medications or treatments. They gather information from patients, including their health history and how they are currently feeling. They may use this information to complete insurance forms, pre-authorizations, and referrals, and they share information with RNs and doctors to help determine the best course of care for a patient. LPNs

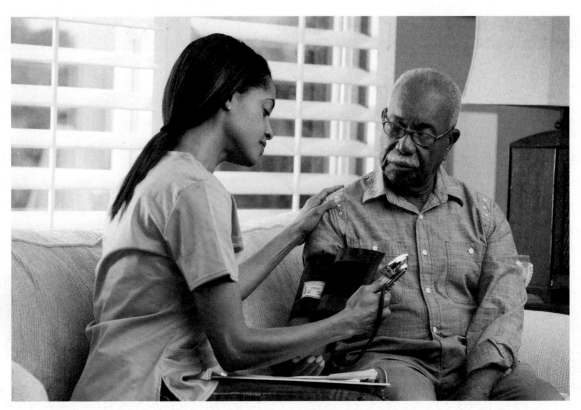

FIGURE 11.5 LPNs take vital signs, including blood pressure.
© Monkey Business Images/Shutterstock.

often teach family members how to care for a relative or teach patients about good health habits.

Most are generalists and will work in any area of health care. However, some work in a specialized setting, such as a nursing or assisted-living facility, in a doctor's office, or in home health care. LPNs in nursing care facilities help evaluate residents' needs, develop care plans, and supervise the care provided by nursing aides. In doctors' offices and clinics, they may be responsible for making appointments, keeping records, and performing other clerical duties. LPNs who work in home health care may prepare meals and teach family members simple nursing tasks. In some states, LPNs are permitted to administer prescribed medicines, start intravenous fluids, and provide care to ventilator-dependent patients.

Work Environment

Employment projections are that LPNs will work primarily in homecare and ambulatory settings as well as nursing care and assisted-living facilities. LPNs/LVNs often wear scrubs, a type of medical clothing that usually consists of a shirt and drawstring pants.

Nurses must often be on their feet for much of the day and may have to lift patients who have trouble moving in bed, standing, or walking. These duties can be stressful, as can dealing with ill and injured people. Many work nights, weekends, and holidays because medical care takes place at all hours. They may be required to work shifts of longer than eight hours.

LPNs/LVNs may face hazards from caustic chemicals, radiation, and infectious diseases and are subject to back injuries when moving patients. They often must deal with the stress of heavy workloads. In addition, the patients for whom they care may be confused, agitated, or uncooperative.

Employment Opportunities

LPNs/LVNs held about 721,700 jobs in 2019. About 38% worked in nursing and assisted-living facilities, 15% worked in hospitals, 13% in physicians' offices, and 13% in home health care.

Educational and Legal Requirements

Most practical nursing training programs last about one year and are offered by vocational and technical schools or community or junior colleges. LPNs must be licensed to practice.

Education and Training

LPNs must complete a state-approved nondegree training program in practical nursing to be eligible for licensure.

Contact your state's board of nursing for a list of approved programs. Most training programs are available from technical and vocational schools or community colleges. Other programs are available through high schools, hospitals, and colleges and universities. A high school diploma or its equivalent usually is required for entry, although some programs accept candidates without a diploma and some programs are part of a high school curriculum.

Most yearlong LPN programs include both classroom study and supervised clinical practice (patient care). Classroom study covers basic nursing concepts and subjects related to patient care, including anatomy, physiology, medical-surgical nursing, pediatrics, obstetrics nursing, pharmacology, nutrition, and first aid. Clinical practice usually is in a hospital but sometimes includes other settings.

Licensure

The **National Council Licensure Examination (NCLEX-PN)** is required to obtain licensure as an LPN. The exam is developed and administered by the National Council of State Boards of Nursing. The NCLEX-PN is a computer-based exam and varies in length. The exam covers four major client-needs categories: safe and effective care environment, health promotion and maintenance, psychosocial integrity, and physiological integrity. Eligibility for licensure may vary by state; for details, contact your state's board of nursing.

Other Qualifications

LPNs should have a caring, sympathetic nature. They should be emotionally stable because working with the sick and injured can be stressful. They also need to be observant and have good decision-making and communication skills. As part of a healthcare team, they must be able to follow orders and work under close supervision.

LPNs should enjoy learning because some states and/or employers require continuing education credits at regular intervals. Career-long learning is a distinct reality for LPNs.

Advancement

In some employment settings, such as nursing homes, LPNs can advance to become charge nurses who oversee the work of other LPNs and nursing aides. LPNs may become credentialed in specialties like IV therapy and gerontology through the **National Federation of Licensed Practical Nurses (NFLPN)**. Some LPNs also choose to become RNs through LPN-to-RN training programs.

Employment Trends

Employment of LPNs is projected to grow much faster than average. Overall job prospects are expected to be very good, but job outlook varies by industry.

Employment Change

Employment of LPNs is expected to grow by 9% between 2019 and 2029, much faster than the average for all occupations, in response to the long-term care needs of an increasing elderly population and the general increase in demand for healthcare services.

Demand for LPNs will be driven by the increase in the share of the older population. Older persons have an increased incidence of injury and illness, which will increase their demand for healthcare services. In addition, with better medical technology, people are living longer, increasing the demand for long-term health care. Job growth will occur in all healthcare settings, but especially those that service the geriatric population like nursing care facilities, community care facilities, and home healthcare services.

In order to contain healthcare costs, many procedures once performed only in hospitals are being performed in physicians' offices and in outpatient care centers, largely because of advances in technology. As a result, the number of LPNs should increase faster in these facilities than in hospitals. Nevertheless, hospitals will continue to demand the services of LPNs.

Job Prospects

In addition to projected job growth, job openings will result from replacement needs, as many workers retire. Very good job opportunities are expected. Rapid employment growth is projected in most healthcare industries, with the best job opportunities occurring in nursing care facilities and in home healthcare services. There is a perceived inadequacy of available health care in many rural areas, so LPNs willing to locate in rural areas should have good job prospects. Projections data from the National Employment Matrix are shown in **TABLE 11.7**.

TABLE 11.7 Projections Data for Licensed Practical and Licensed Vocational Nurses, 2019–2029

Occupational Title	Employment, 2019	Projected Employment, 2029	Change, 2019–2029	
			Number	Percentage
Licensed practical and licensed vocational nurses	721,700	787,400	65,700	9%

Data from Bureau of Labor Statistics. *Occupational Outlook Handbook.* U.S. Department of Labor; 2020.

Professional Profiles

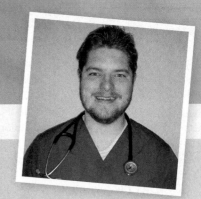

Name: Andrew, RN
Job Title: Registered Nurse
Education: BS in Nursing

Q: Describe your job and organization.

A: I work in a suburban community hospital that is part of a larger hospital system in a metropolitan area. The hospital has 380 beds with an average occupancy of 250. I work on a floor that averages 20 to 36 patients and has a high turnover of patients as well as staff. After I was hired, I spent three months of orientation and training to prepare me for patient care.

Q: Describe a typical workday.

A: A typical workday is quite rigorous and begins with checking patient equipment, passing out medications, completing assessments, reviewing new orders, and attending patient conferences with case managers and physicians. I communicate with other hospital departments for patients having diagnostic or treatment procedures, such as the cath lab, GI lab, radiology, and even the emergency room or doctor's office for newly admitted patients. By afternoon I might be arranging for kidney dialysis or receiving, transferring, or discharging a patient. Throughout the day peripheral IV lines may need to be replaced or feeding tubes may need to be adjusted. I may need to call the cafeteria to order a meal tray for a newly admitted patient or a patient returning to the floor from a procedure. Before ending my shift, I give a report on patients to the oncoming nurse.

Q: Why did you choose this profession?

A: I chose nursing because I wanted to help people create a better life, live longer, or have a better quality of life. Also, I have always been intrigued by the human body.

Q: What challenges you most about this profession?

A: I struggle with patients who are noncompliant with medications, diet, or other restrictions. I understand that it is difficult to make lifestyle changes; however, when patients are noncompliant, they are often readmitted to the hospital, and their health condition worsens.

Q: Is there room for advancement in this field?

A: There are many job opportunities for me since I have a BSN. Opportunities expand exponentially for registered nurses who obtain a master's degree or a nursing doctorate.

Q: Name and explain what part of your academic training most prepared you for this profession.

A: The courses that provided the foundation for a nursing career were nursing assessment, medical-surgical nursing, and pathophysiology. These courses teach critical thinking as it relates to different disease processes.

Q: Did you face obstacles in pursuing your goals? If so, describe them and how you overcame them.

A: It took me five years to complete a BSN because I changed colleges and majors, so not all courses were accepted by the BSN program. Although changing majors and colleges was difficult, it helped me appreciate the nursing profession even more. Initially it was difficult to find a job after completing the BSN because I lacked experience. However, once I found a hospital that was hiring new graduates, they hired me the same day that I interviewed. It took two months to find a hospital that was hiring in the area that I wanted to live; with perseverance and multiple applications, I was successful.

Q: What advice would you give someone who is considering this career?

A: Be able to deal with people at their worst. Most people are nice, but some are mean or rude. However, the work itself is rewarding when you see a smile on a patient's face when they are able to go home after extensive surgery or when a patient cries tears of joy when they realize they will be okay. Be prepared for the worst, such as when a patient receives news of a terminal illness, and provide emotional support in the difficult times. Skills that are important are listening to patients and trusting your instincts. If you notice a change in the patient, inform the physician. I discovered an active heart attack even though the patient had no chest pain; my quick action prevented serious heart damage.

TABLE 11.8 Median Annual Wages in the Industries Employing the Largest Numbers of Licensed Practical and Licensed Vocational Nurses, May 2020

Government	$51,700
Nursing and residential care facilities	$50,100
Home healthcare services	$49,430
Hospitals	$46,560
Offices of physicians	$44,830

Data from Bureau of Labor Statistics. *Occupational Outlook Handbook*. U.S. Department of Labor; 2020.

Earnings

Median annual wages of LPNs/LVNs were $48,820 in May 2020. Median annual wages in the industries employing the largest numbers of LPNs/LVNs in May 2020 are shown in **TABLE 11.8.**

Related Occupations

LPNs work closely with people while helping them. Other healthcare occupations that work closely with patients and have similar educational and experience requirements include surgical technicians, physical therapy assistants and aides, occupational therapy assistants and aides, nursing assistants and aides, psychiatric technicians and aides, and RNs.

Additional Information

For information on baccalaureate and graduate nursing education, nursing career options, and financial aid, contact:

- American Association of Colleges of Nursing, 655 K St., NW, Suite 750, Washington, DC 20036. https://www.aacnnursing.org/

For additional information on registered nurses, including credentialing, contact:

- American Nurses Association, 8515 Georgia Ave., Suite 400, Silver Spring, MD 20910. http://nursingworld.org/

For information on a career in nursing education, certification for nursing education, and nursing education scholarships, contact:

- National League for Nursing, The Watergate, 2600 Virginia Ave., NW, Eighth Floor, Washington, DC 20037. http://www.nln.org

For information on scholarships and loan repayment for nurses and nursing faculty, contact:

- Health Resources & Services Administration, Health Workforce, 5600 Fishers Ln., Rockville, MD 20857.

https://bhw.hrsa.gov/funding/apply-loan-repayment/faculty-lrp

For information on becoming certified in pediatric nursing, a pediatric nurse practitioner, or a pediatric mental health specialist, contact:

- Pediatric Nursing Certification Board, 9605 Medical Center Dr., Suite 250, Rockville, MD 20850. https://pncb.org/certified-pediatric-nurse

For information on accredited educational programs to become a certified registered nurse anesthetist (CRNA), contact:

- Council on Accreditation of Nurse Anesthesia Educational Programs (COA), 222 S. Prospect Ave., Park Ridge, IL 60068. https://www.coacrna.org/

For information on the National Council Licensure Examination for registered nurses (NCLEX-RN) and licensed practical nurses (NCLEX-PN) and a list of individual state boards of nursing, contact:

- National Council of State Boards of Nursing, 111 E. Wacker Dr., Suite 2900, Chicago, IL 60601. https://www.ncsbn.org/index.htm

For a list of accredited clinical nurse specialist programs, contact:

- American Nurses Credentialing Center, 8515 Georgia Ave., Suite 400, Silver Spring, MD 20910. https://www.nursingworld.org/our-certifications/
- National Association of Clinical Nurse Specialists, 11130 Sunrise Valley Dr., Suite 350, Reston, VA 20191. http://www.nacns.org/

For additional information on registered nurses in all fields and specialties and to search for jobs in nursing, contact:

- American Society of Registered Nurses, 1001 Bridgeway, Suite 233, Sausalito, CA 94965. https://www.asrn.org/

For information on nurse anesthetists, including a list of accredited programs, contact:

- American Association of Nurse Anesthetists, 222 S. Prospect Ave., Park Ridge, IL 60068. http://www.aana.com/

For information on becoming certified as a certified registered nurse anesthetist, contact:

- National Board of Certification and Recertification for Nurse Anesthetists, 8725 W. Higgins Rd., Suite 525, Chicago, IL 60631. https://www.nbcrna.com/

For information on a list of accredited programs in midwifery, contact:

- American College of Nurse-Midwives. 8403 Colesville Rd., Suite 1550, Silver Spring, MD 20910.

https://portal.midwife.org/education/education
-pathway

For information on becoming certified as a nurse-mid-wife, contact:

- American Midwifery Certification Board, 849 International Dr., Suite 120, Linthicum, MD 21090. http://www.amcbmidwife.org/

For information on nurse practitioners, including a list of accredited programs and certification, contact:

- American Academy of Nurse Practitioners, P.O. Box 12846, Austin, TX 78711. http://www.aanp.org/
- American Academy of Nurse Practitioners Certification Board, Capital Station, LBJ Building, P.O. Box 12926, Austin, TX 78711-2926.

For information about practical nursing and specialty credentialing, contact

- National Association for Practical Nurse Education and Service, Inc., 2071 N Bechtle Ave., PMB 307, Springfield, OH 45504. http://www.napnes.org

LEARNING PORTFOLIO

Issues for Discussion

1. Review the video "Be a Nurse" from the Washington Center for Nursing. List the roles and responsibilities of four different nurses described in the video: public health nurse, school nurse, nurse educator, and military nurse. What were the recommendations for reducing health disparities? https://www.youtube.com/watch?v=gJlxRGFGlbQ

2. Review the two-minute video "Nurse Practitioner." Based on the information from the video, list three typical areas of practice or populations served. Describe the educational requirements of a Nurse Practitioner. https://youtu.be/smiXChYIRUU

3. Review the three-minute video "The Nurse Practitioner Will See You Now" from ConsumerReports.org. What are some of the barriers for nurse practitioners to practice independently? http://www.consumerreports.org/cro/magazine/2013/08/the-nurse-practitioner-will-see-you-now/index.htm

4. What are the advantages and disadvantages of each of the nursing professions discussed in this chapter: LPN/LVN, RN, APRN?

5. Choose one nursing profession and select a training program in your state. What are the entrance requirements? What is the length of the training program? What is the cost of the program? Are there scholarships or loans available for students?

Enrichment Activities

1. View the YouTube video "CRNAs: The Future of Anesthesia Care Today," which describes the work of a certified registered nurse anesthetist (CRNA). Explain why the patient in this video required anesthesia. https://www.youtube.com/watch?v=BF0mnxAeIr4

2. View the four-minute video "Midwives & the Care They Provide" from the American College of Nurse-Midwives. What are some of the benefits for women who use a certified nurse-midwife? https://www.youtube.com/watch?v=MLVwdmlZU_8_

3. View the following videos that discuss different career paths of three nurses. The women explain what led to their decision to become a nurse, how their roles changed over time, and how they became leaders in the nursing field. How did each begin their career in nursing, either through volunteer experience or their first job as a nurse?

- https://campaignforaction.org/nursing-journeys-started-candy-striper/
- https://campaignforaction.org/nursing-journeys-a-former-army-nurse-on-how-she-became-a-nurse-leader/
- https://campaignforaction.org/nursing-journeys-voice-profession/

CASE STUDY: NURSING

Jeff has been a licensed practical nurse for almost five years. He went to the local trade school to receive his training. Although Jeff really enjoys his job and the people he works with, he feels he is ready to further his career in nursing. He is researching the possibilities and has many questions.

The following questions relate to nursing careers. Please help Jeff answer them based on what you have learned from this chapter.

1. What are the educational requirements for a registered nurse?
   A. One can become a registered nurse by attending a diploma, associate's degree, or bachelor's degree program.
   B. One must complete a master's degree in order to become a registered nurse.
   C. All careers in nursing require a minimum of an associate's degree.
   D. All careers in nursing require a minimum of a bachelor's degree.

2. Jeff is concerned about repayment of school loans should he decide to continue his education to become a registered nurse. Can you choose the most accurate statement regarding job opportunities for registered nurses?
   A. Only advanced practice registered nurses can expect to have many job opportunities.
   B. Overall job opportunities for RNs are expected to be excellent.
   C. Job opportunities in the hospital setting are usually filled by LPNs and LVNs.
   D. Registered nurses are being phased out in most healthcare settings.

LEARNING PORTFOLIO

References

1. Spetz J. How will health reform affect demand for RNs? *Nursing Econ.* 2014; *323*:42–44.2.

2. Centers for Medicare and Medicaid Services. *Hospital Readmissions Reduction Program (HRRP).* https://www.cms.gov /Medicare/Medicare-Fee-for-Service-Payment/AcuteInpa tientPPS/Readmissions-Reduction-Program Accessed July 2, 2020.

3. Gorski MS, Gerardi T, Giddens J, Meyer D, Peters-Lewis A. Nursing education transformation. Building infrastructure for the future. *Am J Nursing.* 2015; *115*:53–57.

4. Institute of Medicine. *The Future of Nursing: Leading Change, Advancing Health*, 2011. Washington, DC: The National Academies Press. doi.org/10.17226/12956.

5. Nursing Licensure.org. *Nursing Bridge: CNA to RN.* https:// www.nursinglicensure.org/articles/cna-rn.html Accessed July 2, 2020.

6. National Academies of Sciences, Engineering, and Medicine. *Assessing Progress on the Institute of Medicine Report The Future of Nursing*, 2016. Washington, DC: The National Academies Press. doi.org/10.17226/21838.

7. National Center for Health Workforce Analysis. *Brief Summary Results from the 2018 National Sample Survey of Registered Nurses.* U.S. Department of Health and Human Services, Health Resources and Services Administration. Rockville, MD; 2019.

8. National Center for Health Workforce Analysis. *National and Regional Supply and Demand Projections of the Nursing Workforce: 2014–2030.* U.S. Department of Health and Human Services, Health Resources and Services Administration, National Center for Health Workforce Analysis. Rockville, MD; 2017.

9. Johnson & Johnson. *Nursing. Nursing Specialties.* https:// nursing.jnj.com/specialty Accessed July 20, 2021.

10. ExploreHealthCareers.org. *Nurse Anesthetists.* https:// explore healthcareers.org/career/nursing/nurse-anesthetist/ Accessed July 2, 2020.

11. American Association of Nurse Anesthetists. *Certified Registered Nurse Anesthetists Fact Sheet.* https://www .aana.com/membership/become-a-crna/crna-fact-sheet Accessed July 2, 2020.

12. American College of Nurse-Midwives. *Essential Facts about Midwives.* https://www.midwife.org/acnm/files/cclibraryfiles /filename/000000008273/EssentialFactsAboutMidwives _Final_June_2021_new.pdf Updated June 2021. Accessed July 28, 2021.

13. Walker D, Lannen B, Rossie D. Midwifery practice and education: Current challenges and opportunities. *OJIN: The Online Journal of Issues in Nursing.* 2014; *19*(2): Manuscript 4. **DOI:** 10.3912/OJIN.Vol19No02Man04

14. Explore Health Careers.org. *Nurse Practitioner.* https://explore healthcareers.org/career/nursing/nurse-practitioner/ Accessed July 2, 2020.

15. American Association of Nurse Practitioners. *NP Fact Sheet.* February 2020. https://www.aanp.org/about/all-about-nps /np-fact-sheet Accessed July 2, 2020.

16. American Association of Nurse Anesthetists. *Certified Registered Nurse Anesthetists Fact Sheet.* https://www .aana.com/membership/become-a-crna/crna-fact-sheet Accessed July 28, 2021.

17. American Association of Colleges of Nursing. *Fact Sheet: The Doctor of Nursing Practice (DNP).* https://www.aacnnursing .org/Portals/42/News/Factsheets/DNP-Factsheet.pdf Accessed July 28, 2021.

18. Accreditation Commission for Midwifery Education. *Midwifery Education Trends Report, 2019.* https://www.mid wife.org/acnm/files/cclibraryfiles/filename/000000007637 /Midwifery_Education_Trends_Report_2019_Final.pdf Accessed September 1, 2021.

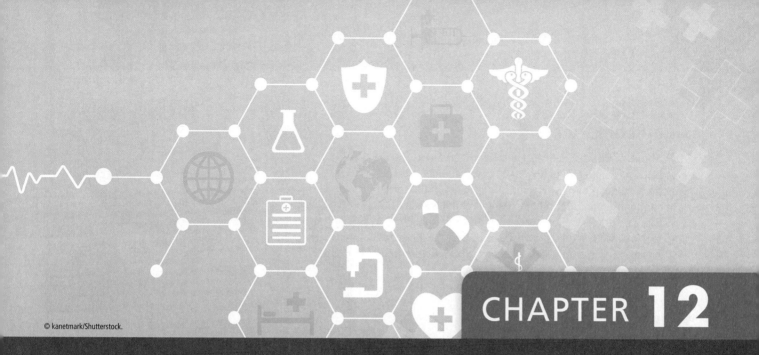

© kanetmark/Shutterstock.

CHAPTER 12

Dentistry*

KEY TERMS

American Dental Association (ADA)
Dental assistant
Dental ceramist
Dental hygienist
Dental laboratory technician

Dental public health specialist
Dentist
Endodontist
Oral and maxillofacial surgeon
Oral pathologist
Orthodontist

Pediatric dentist
Periodontist
Pit and fissure sealants
Prosthodontist

* All information in this chapter, unless otherwise indicated, was obtained from Bureau of Labor Statistics. *Occupational Outlook Handbook 2020–2021 Edition*. Washington, DC: U.S. Department of Labor; 2021.

DENTISTS
Significant Points

- About one-half of dentists are solo practitioners.
- Dentists must graduate from an accredited dental school and pass written and practical examinations; competition for admission to dental school is keen.
- Fast as average employment growth is projected.
- Job prospects should be good, reflecting the need to replace the large number of dentists expected to retire.

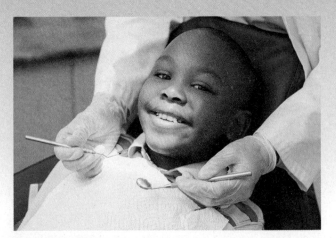

FIGURE 12.1 Dental examination of a child.
© wavebreakmedia/Shutterstock.

Work Description

Dentists diagnose and treat problems with teeth and tissues in the mouth, along with giving advice and administering care to help prevent future problems. They provide instruction on diet, brushing, flossing, the use of fluorides, and other aspects of dental care. They remove tooth decay, fill cavities, examine X-rays, place protective plastic sealants on children's teeth, straighten teeth, and repair fractured teeth. They also perform corrective surgery on gums and supporting bones to treat gum diseases. Dentists extract teeth and make models and measurements for dentures to replace missing teeth. They also administer anesthetics and write prescriptions for antibiotics and other medications.

Dentists use a variety of equipment, including X-ray machines, drills, mouth mirrors, probes, forceps, brushes, and scalpels. Lasers, digital scanners, and other computer technologies also may be used. Dentists wear masks, gloves, and safety glasses to protect themselves and their patients from infectious diseases.

Dentists in private practice oversee a variety of administrative tasks, including bookkeeping and the buying of equipment and supplies. They may employ and supervise dental hygienists, dental assistants, dental laboratory technicians, and receptionists.

Many dentists are general practitioners, handling a variety of dental needs. Other dentists practice in any of nine specialty areas. **Orthodontists**, the largest group of specialists, straighten teeth by applying pressure to the teeth with braces or other appliances. The next-largest group, **oral and maxillofacial surgeons**, operates on the mouth, jaws, teeth, gums, neck, and head. The remainder may specialize as **pediatric dentists** (focusing on dentistry for children and special-needs patients); **periodontists** (treating gums and bone supporting the teeth); **prosthodontists** (replacing missing teeth with permanent fixtures, such as crowns and bridges, or with removable fixtures such as dentures); **endodontists** (performing root-canal therapy); **oral pathologists** (diagnosing oral diseases); oral and maxillofacial radiologists (diagnosing diseases in the head and neck through the use of imaging technologies); or **dental public health specialists** (promoting good dental health and preventing dental diseases within the community). An example of a pediatric dentist working on a patient is shown in **FIGURE 12.1**.

Work Environment

Many dentists are solo practitioners, meaning that they own their own businesses and work alone or with a small staff. Some dentists have partners, and some work for other dentists as associate dentists.

Most dentists work four or five days a week. Some work evenings and weekends to meet their patients' needs. The number of hours worked varies greatly among dentists. Most full-time dentists work between 35 and 40 hours a week. Others, especially those who are trying to establish a new practice, work more hours. Also, experienced dentists often work fewer hours. It is common for dentists to continue in part-time practice well beyond the usual retirement age.

Dentists usually work in the safety of an office environment. Nonetheless, work-related injuries can occur, such as those resulting from the use of handheld tools when performing dental work on patients.

Employment Opportunities

Dentists held about 151,600 jobs in 2019. Employment was distributed among general practitioners and specialists, as shown in **TABLE 12.1**. Approximately 15% of all dentists were specialists. Very few salaried dentists worked in hospitals

TABLE 12.1 Employment Distribution among General Practitioners and Specialists

Specialties	Distribution
Dentists, general	132,100
Orthodontists	7,200
Oral and maxillofacial surgeons	5,600
Prosthodontists	600
Dentists, all other specialists	6,200

Data from Bureau of Labor Statistics. *Occupational Outlook Handbook. U.S.* Department of Labor; 2020.

and offices of physicians. Almost three-quarters of dentists work in private practice. According to the **American Dental Association (ADA)**, about three out of four dentists in private practice own their own practices, and the remaining belong to a partnership.[1] Solo practices were the norm at one time in dentistry, but that has changed over the past two decades. Now approximately half of dentists are solo practitioners.[2]

Educational and Legal Requirements

All 50 states and the District of Columbia require dentists to be licensed. To qualify for a license in most states, candidates must graduate from an accredited dental school and pass written and practical examinations.

Education and Training

In 2021, there were 67 dental schools in the United States accredited by the ADA's Commission on Dental Accreditation.[3] Dental schools require a minimum of two years of college-level, pre-dental education prior to admittance. Most dental students have at least a bachelor's degree before entering dental school, although a few applicants are accepted to dental school after two or three years of college and complete their bachelor's degree while attending dental school.

High school and college students who want to become dentists should take courses in biology, chemistry, physics, health, and mathematics. College undergraduates planning on applying to dental school are required to take many science courses. Because of this, some choose a major in a science, such as biology or chemistry, whereas others take the required science coursework while pursuing a major in another subject.

All dental schools require applicants to take the Dental Admissions Test (DAT).[4] When selecting students, schools consider scores earned on the DAT, applicants' grade point averages, and information gathered through recommendations and interviews. Competition for admission to dental school is keen.

Dental school usually lasts four academic years. Studies begin with classroom instruction and laboratory work in science, including anatomy, microbiology, biochemistry, and physiology. Beginning courses in clinical sciences, including laboratory techniques, are also completed. During the last two years, students treat patients, usually in dental clinics, under the supervision of licensed dentists. Most dental schools award the degree of Doctor of Dental Surgery (DDS). Others award an equivalent degree, Doctor of Dental Medicine (DMD).

Licensure

Licensing is required to practice as a dentist. In most states, licensure requires passing written and practical examinations in addition to having a degree from an accredited dental school. Candidates may fulfill the written part of the state licensing requirements by passing the National Board Dental Examinations. Individual states or regional testing agencies administer the written or practical examinations.

Individuals can be licensed to practice any of the nine recognized specialties in all 50 states and the District of Columbia. Requirements include two to four years of postgraduate education and, in some cases, the completion of a special state examination. A postgraduate residency term also may be required, usually lasting up to two years. Most state licenses permit dentists to engage in both general and specialized practice.

Other Qualifications

Dentistry requires diagnostic ability and manual skills. Dentists should have good visual memory; excellent judgment regarding space, shape, and color; a high degree of manual dexterity; and scientific ability. Good business sense, self-discipline, and good communication skills are helpful for success in private practice.

Advancement

Dentists and aspiring dentists who want to teach or conduct research full time usually spend an additional two to five years in advanced dental training in programs operated by dental schools or hospitals. Many private practitioners also teach part time, including supervising students in dental school clinics.

Some dental school graduates work for established dentists as associates for one to two years to gain experience and save money to equip an office of their own. Some dental school graduates, however, purchase an established practice or open a new one immediately after graduation.

Employment Opportunities

Employment is projected to grow as fast as the average for all occupations. Job prospects should be good, reflecting the need to replace the large number of dentists expected to retire.

Employment Change

The employment of dentists is projected to grow by 3% through 2029, which is as fast as the average for all occupations. The demand for dental services is expected to continue to increase. The overall U.S. population is growing, and the elderly segment of the population is growing even faster; these phenomena will increase the demand for dental care. Many members of the Baby Boom generation will need complicated dental work. In addition, older adults are more likely to retain their teeth than were their predecessors, so they will require much more care than in the past. The younger generation will continue to need preventive checkups despite an overall increase in the dental health of

TABLE 12.2 Some Projection Data for Dentists, 2019–2029

Occupational Title	Employment, 2019	Projected Employment, 2029	Change, 2019–2029	
			Number	Percentage
Dentists	151,600	155,500	4000	3
Dentists, general	132,100	135,700	3,700	3
Oral and maxillofacial surgeons	5,600	5,700	100	2
Orthodontists	7,200	7,300	100	2
Prosthodontists	600	600	0	2
Dentists, all other specialists	6,200	6,200	0	0

Data from Bureau of Labor Statistics. *Occupational Outlook Handbook*. U.S. Department of Labor; 2020.

the public over the past few decades. Recently, some private insurance providers have increased their dental coverage. If this trend continues, people with new or expanded dental insurance will be more likely to visit a dentist than in the past. Also, although they are currently a small proportion of dental expenditures, cosmetic dental services, such as providing teeth-whitening treatments, will become increasingly popular. This trend is expected to continue as new technologies allow these procedures to take less time and be much less invasive.

Nonetheless, the employment of dentists is not expected to keep pace with the increased demand for dental services. Productivity increases from new technology, as well as the tendency to assign more tasks to dental hygienists and assistants, will allow dentists to perform more work than they have in the past. As their practices expand, dentists are likely to hire more hygienists and dental assistants to handle routine services.

Demand for dentists with minority backgrounds is seen by the ADA as critical. The ADA reports in 2020 that the dental student body has diversified over time, making up 46% of the dental student population. Data from the ADA shows that minority dentists treat the highest number of minority patients. As underrepresented groups constitute a larger percentage of the population over time, the ADA hopes that dentists from a minority background will work to eliminate barriers to oral care.[5]

Dentists will increasingly provide care and instruction aimed at preventing the loss of teeth rather than simply providing treatments such as fillings. Improvements in dental technology also will allow dentists to offer more effective and less painful treatment to their patients. Studies establishing the link between oral health and overall health will increase demands for dental care.

Job Prospects

As an increasing number of dentists from the Baby Boom generation reach retirement age, many of them will retire or work fewer hours and stop taking on new patients. Furthermore, the number of applicants to apply to and graduate from dental schools has increased in recent years. Job prospects should be good because younger dentists will be able to take over the work of older dentists who retire or cut back on hours as well as provide dental services to accommodate the growing demand.

Demand for dental services tends to follow the business cycle, primarily because these services usually are paid for either by the patient or by private insurance companies. As a result, during slow times in the economy, demand for dental services can decrease; consequently, dentists may have difficulty finding employment, or if they are already in an established practice, they may work fewer hours because of reduced demand. **TABLE 12.2** shows some projection data provided by the U.S. Department of Labor.

Earnings

Median annual wages of salaried general dentists were $164,010 in May 2020. Earnings vary according to number of years in practice, location, hours worked, and specialty. Self-employed dentists in private practice tend to earn more than salaried dentists.

Dentists who are salaried often receive benefits paid by their employer, with health insurance and malpractice insurance being among the most common. Like other business owners, self-employed dentists must provide their own health insurance, life insurance, retirement plans, and other benefits.

Related Occupations

Dentists examine, diagnose, prevent, and treat diseases and abnormalities. Other workers who perform similar tasks include chiropractors, optometrists, physicians and surgeons, podiatrists, and veterinarians.

Additional Information

For information on dentistry as a career, a list of accredited dental schools, and a list of state boards of dental examiners, contact:

- American Dental Association, Commission on Dental Accreditation, 211 E. Chicago Ave., Chicago, IL 60611. https://www.ada.org

For information on admission to dental schools, contact:

- American Dental Education Association, 655 K St. NW, Suite 1100, Washington, DC 20005. https://www.adea.org

For more information on general dentistry or on a specific dental specialty, contact:

- Academy of General Dentistry, 560 W. Lake St., Sixth Floor, Chicago, IL 60661. https://www.agd.org
- American Association of Orthodontists, 401 North Lindbergh Blvd., St. Louis, MO 63141. https://www.aaoinfo.org/
- American Association of Oral and Maxillofacial Surgeons, 9700 West Bryn Mawr Ave., Rosemont, IL 60018. https://www.aaoms.org
- American Academy of Pediatric Dentistry, 211 East Chicago Ave., Suite 1600, Chicago, IL 60611. https://www.aapd.org
- American Academy of Periodontology, 737 North Michigan Ave., Suite 800, Chicago, IL 60611. https://www.perio.org
- American Academy of Prosthodontists, 211 East Chicago Ave., Suite 1000, Chicago, IL 60611. https://www.prosthodontics.org
- American Association of Endodontists, 180 N. Stetson Ave., Suite 1500, Chicago, IL 60611. https://www.aae.org
- American Academy of Oral and Maxillofacial Radiology, P.O. Box 359, Winfield, IL 60190. https://www.aaomr.org/
- American Association of Public Health Dentistry, P.O. Box 7317, Springfield, IL 62791. https://www.aaphd.org

People interested in practicing dentistry should obtain the requirements for licensure from the board of dental examiners of the state in which they plan to work.

To obtain information on scholarships, grants, and loans, including federal financial aid, prospective dental students should contact the office of student financial aid at the schools to which they would like to apply.

DENTAL HYGIENISTS
Significant Points

- A degree from an accredited dental hygiene school and a state license are required for this job.
- Dental hygienist growth is expected to grow faster than average for all occupations.
- Job prospects are expected to be favorable in most areas, but strong competition for jobs is likely in some areas.
- Many dental hygienists work part time, and flexible scheduling is a distinctive feature of this job.

Work Description

Dental hygienists clean teeth and provide other preventive dental care; they also teach patients how to practice good oral hygiene. Hygienists examine patients' teeth and gums, recording the presence of diseases or abnormalities. They remove tartar, stains, and plaque from teeth; take and develop dental X-rays; and apply cavity-preventive agents such as fluorides and **pit and fissure sealants**. In some states, hygienists administer local anesthetics and anesthetic gas; place and carve filling materials, temporary fillings, and periodontal dressings; remove sutures; and smooth and polish metal restorations.

Dental hygienists also help patients develop and maintain good oral health. For example, they may explain the relationship between diet and oral health, inform patients how to select toothbrushes, and show patients how to brush and floss their teeth. Dental hygienists use hand and rotary instruments, lasers, and ultrasonics to clean teeth; X-ray machines to take dental pictures; syringes with needles to administer local anesthetics; and models of teeth to explain oral hygiene. Dental hygienists often wear safety glasses, surgical masks, and gloves to protect themselves and their patients from disease, as shown in **FIGURE 12.2**.

The nature of the work may vary by practice setting. In school-based settings, for example, hygienists may assist the dentist in examining children's teeth to determine the dental treatment required. Hygienists who have advanced training may teach or conduct research.

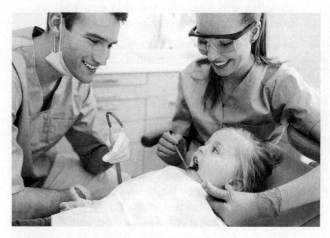

FIGURE 12.2 Dental hygienist assisting in care.
© Edyta Pawlowska/Shutterstock.

Professional Profiles

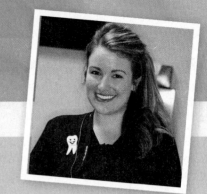

Name: Chelsea, RDH
Job Title: Dental Hygienist
Education: AAS in Dental Hygiene

Q: Tell us about your job and the organization in which you work.

A: I'm a dental hygienist. I work with a general dentist in a suburban area (population 47,000 people). The office I work at is busy, producing $1–2 million each year. It is state of the art; we try to stay up to date on the newest technology. There are six treatment rooms. I am a full-time hygienist, and we have three part-time hygienists.

I have worked for this dental practice for two years, but I have worked at this office for one year. My dental practice was able to transfer me when I moved from one state to another because it had offices in both states.

Q: Describe a typical workday.

A: I work Monday through Friday with varying hours. Some days I see patients as early as 7 AM; some days I see patients until 7 PM. I usually work 38 hours per week. I see a wide variety of patients ranging from 3 years old to 101 years old, from different cultures and walks of life. I perform a mixture of different services to my patients: child prophylaxis cleanings, adult prophylaxis cleanings, scaling and root planning, laser bacterial reduction for periodontal treatment, antibiotic placement for periodontal treatment, sealant placement on adults and children, fluoride treatments, and desensitizer treatments.

Q: Why did you choose this profession, and what do you like most?

A: I chose this profession because I was amazed by the results I got from orthodontic treatment. Correcting my crowded and crooked teeth improved my self-esteem—after that, the dental world fascinated me. I went to college to pursue hospitality management, this right in the midst of the recession. I remember during my first semester an instructor was brutally honest when explaining that the industry was struggling, I realized I should pursue a career that was always going to be needed—health care. Since I was already fascinated by teeth, it was a no-brainer that I should consider a career in dentistry. After researching different dental careers, I chose dental hygiene because it would allow me to work with a variety of different people while allowing me to make a difference in someone's life and health.

What I like most about this profession is seeing an improvement in the periodontal health and overall health of my patients. There is nothing more satisfying than when a patient is able to save their teeth because of the oral hygiene instructions I taught them and treatment I performed (SRP, laser, Arestin). The relationships and trust that I form with my patients are the best part of my job.

Q: What part of your training prepared you for your position?

A: The part that most prepared me was the dental hygiene clinic at my college. The dental hygiene clinic is the only dental hygiene clinic in the area that is completely free. We would see a variety of patients for prophylaxis cleanings and periodontal treatment. The periodontal cases I saw there were some of the most advanced periodontal cases I've seen. It was helpful to treat those advanced cases with the hands-on support and instruction from the instructors that had been practicing dental hygiene for many years.

Q: What obstacles have you faced?

A: I did face obstacles during the final stages of getting licensed to practice dental hygiene. I took three exams to become licensed in my state: Jurisprudence, Clinical Exam, Written Exam. I passed the Jurisprudence and Clinical Exams with 100% and 98%. However, I failed the written test by 1%. Failing that test was a huge letdown; it caused me to question the path I was on and whether or not I should be a hygienist. I scheduled to take the test again, studied nonstop, studied with other hygienists that I went to school with—and I passed. I feel I value my dental hygiene license more because of the obstacles I faced.

Q: What advice would you give to someone considering this career?

A: Follow other hygienists to ensure that this is a career you would enjoy. Volunteer as much as possible with groups like Give Kids A Smile. Start networking immediately; this will help out tremendously when looking for a job.

Work Environment

Dental hygienists usually work in clean, well-lit offices. Important health safeguards for those in this occupation include regular medical checkups; strict adherence to proper radiologic procedures; compliance with required infection control procedures, including the latest safety precautions; and the use of appropriate protective devices when administering nitrous oxide/oxygen analgesia. The occupation is one of several covered by the Consumer-Patient Radiation Health and Safety Board, which sets uniform standards for the training and certification of individuals who perform medical and dental radiologic procedures.

Most hygienists work 30 to 35 hours per week in jobs that may include Saturday or evening hours. Flexible scheduling is a distinctive feature of this job.

Employment Opportunities

Dental hygienists held about 226,400 jobs in 2019. Because holding multiple jobs is common in this field, the number of jobs exceeds the number of hygienists. Almost all jobs for dental hygienists—about 93%—were in offices of dentists. A very small number worked for employment services, in physicians' offices, or in other industries.

Educational and Legal Requirements

Prospective dental hygienists must become licensed in the state in which they wish to practice. A degree from an accredited dental hygiene school is required along with licensure examinations.

Education and Training

A high school diploma and college entrance test scores are usually required for admission to a dental hygiene program. High school students interested in becoming a dental hygienist should take courses in biology, chemistry, and mathematics. Also, some dental hygiene programs require applicants to have completed at least one year of college. Specific entrance requirements vary from one school to another.

In 2021, there were 325 dental hygiene programs accredited by the Commission on Dental Accreditation.[6] Most dental hygiene programs grant an associate's degree, although some also offer a certificate, a bachelor's degree, or a master's degree. A minimum of an associate's degree or a certificate in dental hygiene is generally required for practice in a private dental office. A bachelor's or master's degree usually is required for research, teaching, or clinical practice in public or school health programs.

Schools offer laboratory, clinical, and classroom instruction in subjects such as anatomy, physiology, chemistry, microbiology, pharmacology, nutrition, radiography, histology (the study of tissue structure), periodontology (the study of gum diseases), pathology, dental materials, clinical dental hygiene, and social and behavioral sciences.

Licensure

Dental hygienists must be licensed by the state in which they practice. Nearly all states require candidates to graduate from an accredited dental hygiene school and pass both a written and clinical examination. The American Dental Association's Joint Commission on National Dental Examinations administers the written examination, which is accepted by all states and the District of Columbia. State or regional testing agencies administer the clinical examination. In addition, most states require an examination on the legal aspects of dental hygiene practice. Alabama is the only state that allows licensure candidates to take its examinations if they have been trained through a state-regulated, on-the-job program in a dentist's office.

Other Qualifications

Dental hygienists should work well with others because they work closely with dentists and dental assistants as well as deal directly with patients. Hygienists also need good manual dexterity because they use dental instruments within a patient's mouth with little room for error. Assessing and evaluating patients requires strong critical thinking skills and conveying patient information to dentists and educating patients about oral health requires strong communication skills.

Advancement

Advancement opportunities usually come from working outside a typical dentist's office and usually require a bachelor's or master's degree in dental hygiene. Some dental hygienists may choose to pursue a career teaching in a dental hygiene program, working in public health, or working in a corporate setting.

Employment Trends

Dental hygienist ranks as a fast-growing occupation, and job prospects are expected to be favorable in most areas; competition for jobs is likely in some areas.

Employment Change

Employment of dental hygienists is expected to grow 6% through 2029, which is much faster than the average for all occupations. This projected growth ranks dental hygienist among the fastest-growing occupations, in response to increasing demand for dental care and the greater use of hygienists.

The demand for dental services will grow because of population growth, older people increasingly retaining

TABLE 12.3 Projections Data for Dental Hygienists, 2019–2029

Occupational Title	Employment, 2019	Projected Employment, 2029	Change, 2019–2029	
			Number	Percentage
Dental hygienists	226,400	239,700	13,300	6%

Data from Bureau of Labor Statistics. *Occupational Outlook Handbook.* U.S. Department of Labor; 2020.

more teeth, and a growing focus on preventive dental care. To meet this demand, facilities that provide dental care, particularly dentists' offices, will increasingly employ dental hygienists, and more hygienists per office, to perform services that have been performed by dentists in the past. Ongoing research indicating a link between oral health and general health also will spur the demand for preventive dental services, which are typically provided by dental hygienists.

Job Prospects

Job prospects are expected to be favorable in most areas but will vary by geographical location. Because graduates are permitted to practice only in the state in which they are licensed, hygienists wishing to practice in areas that have an abundance of dental hygiene programs may experience strong competition for jobs. Older dentists, who have been less likely to employ dental hygienists, are leaving the occupation and will be replaced by recent graduates, who are more likely to employ one or more hygienists. In addition, as dentists' workloads increase, they are expected to hire more hygienists to perform preventive dental care, such as cleaning, so that they may devote their own time to more complex procedures. **TABLE 12.3** shows some projection data provided by the U.S. Department of Labor.

Earnings

Median annual wages of dental hygienists were $77,090 in May 2020. The lowest 10% earned less than $54,200, and the highest 10% earned more than $104,420.

Earnings vary by geographic location, employment setting, and years of experience. Dental hygienists may be paid on an hourly, daily, salary, or commission basis. Benefits vary substantially by practice setting and may be contingent upon full-time employment. A dental hygienist's benefits package may include health insurance coverage, membership dues for professional associations, paid vacation, sick leave, and tuition aid for continuing dental education.

Related Occupations

Other workers supporting health practitioners in an office setting include dental assistants, medical assistants, occupational therapist assistants and aides, physical therapist assistants and aides, physician assistants, and registered nurses. Dental hygienists sometimes work with radiation technology, as do radiation therapists.

Additional Information

For information on a career in dental hygiene, including educational requirements, contact:

- American Dental Hygienists Association (ADHA), 444 N. Michigan Ave., Suite 400, Chicago, IL 60611. https://www.adha.org

For information about accredited programs and educational requirements, contact:

- Commission on Dental Accreditation, American Dental Association, 211 E. Chicago Ave., Chicago, IL 60611. https://www.ada.org/en/coda

The State Board of Dental Examiners in each state can supply information on licensing requirements.

DENTAL ASSISTANTS
Significant Points

- Job prospects should be excellent.
- Dentists are expected to hire more assistants to perform routine tasks so dentists may devote their time to more complex procedures.
- Many assistants learn their skills on the job, although an increasing number are trained in dental-assisting programs; most programs take one year or less to complete.
- Most dental assistants work full time, with some work on evenings and weekends.

Work Description

Dental assistants perform a variety of patient care, office, and laboratory duties. They work alongside the dentists as they examine and treat patients. They make patients as comfortable as possible in the dental chair, prepare them for treatment, and obtain dental records. Assistants hand instruments and materials to dentists and keep patients' mouths dry and clear by using suction or other devices. They also sterilize and disinfect instruments and equipment, prepare tray setups for dental procedures, and instruct patients on

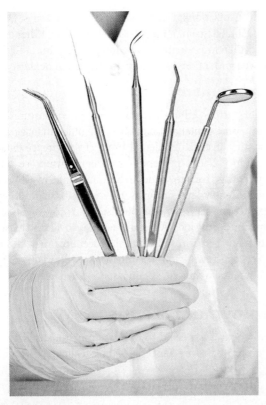

FIGURE 12.3 Dental tools.
© Africa Studio/Shutterstock.

postoperative and general oral health care. Examples of the types of tools used to assist dentists are shown in **FIGURE 12.3**.

Some dental assistants prepare materials for making impressions and restorations, expose radiographs, and process dental X-ray film as directed by the dentist. State law determines which clinical tasks a dental assistant may perform, but in most states they may remove sutures, apply anesthetic and caries-preventive agents to the teeth and oral tissue, remove excess cement used in the filling process, and place rubber dams on the teeth to isolate them for individual treatment. Some states are expanding dental assistants' duties to include tasks such as coronal polishing and restorative dentistry functions for those assistants who meet specific training and experience requirements.

Those with laboratory duties make casts of the teeth and mouth from impressions taken by dentists, clean and polish removable appliances, and make temporary crowns. Dental assistants with office duties arrange and confirm appointments, receive patients, keep treatment records, send bills, receive payments, and order dental supplies and materials. Dental assistants should not be confused with dental hygienists, who are licensed to perform a wider variety of clinical tasks.

Work Environment

Dental assistants work in a well-lit, clean environment. Their work area is usually near the dental chair so they can arrange instruments, materials, and medication and hand them to the dentist when needed. Dental assistants wear gloves and

masks to protect themselves from infectious diseases. Following safety procedures minimizes the risks of handling radiographic equipment.

Most dental assistants work full time. Many dental assistants have variable schedules. Depending on the hours of the dental office where they work, assistants may have to work on Saturdays or evenings. Some dental assistants hold multiple jobs by working at dental offices that are open on different days or by scheduling their work at a second office around the hours they work at their primary office.

Employment Opportunities

Dental assistants held about 354,600 jobs in 2019. About 90% of all jobs for dental assistants were in dentists' offices. A small number of jobs were in the federal, state, and local governments or in offices of physicians. Some dental assistants worked part time, sometimes in more than one dental office.

Educational and Legal Requirements

Many assistants learn their skills on the job, although an increasing number are trained in dental-assisting programs offered by community and junior colleges, trade schools, technical institutes, or the armed forces. Most programs take one year to complete. For assistants to perform more advanced functions or to have the ability to complete radiological procedures, many states require assistants to obtain a license or certification.

Education and Training

Some states have no formal education or training requirements to become an entry-level dental assistant. High school students interested in a career as a dental assistant should take courses in biology, chemistry, health, and office practices. For those wishing to pursue further education, the Commission on Dental Accreditation (CODA) approved 240 dental-assisting training programs in 2021.[7] Programs include classroom, laboratory, and preclinical instruction in dental-assisting skills and related theory. In addition, students gain practical experience in dental schools, clinics, or dental offices. Most programs take one year or less to complete and lead to a certificate or diploma. Two-year programs offered in community and junior colleges lead to an associate's degree. All programs require a high school diploma or its equivalent, and some require science or computer-related courses for admission. A number of private vocational schools offer four- to six-month courses in dental assisting, but the Commission on Dental Accreditation does not accredit these programs.

Many dental assistants learn through on-the-job training. In these situations, the employing dentist or other dental assistants in the dental office teach the new assistant dental terminology, the names of the instruments, how to perform daily duties, how to interact with patients, and other things necessary to help keep the dental office running smoothly. Although some things can be picked up easily, it may be a few months before new dental assistants are completely knowledgeable about their duties and comfortable doing all of their tasks without assistance.

A period of on-the-job training is often required even for those who have completed a dental-assisting program or have some previous experience. Different dentists may have their own styles of doing things that need to be learned before an assistant can be comfortable working with them. Office-specific information, such as where files are kept, will need to be learned at each new job. Also, as dental technology changes, dental assistants need to stay familiar with the tools and procedures that they will be using or helping dentists use. On-the-job training is often sufficient to keep assistants up to date on these matters.

Licensure

Most states regulate the duties that dental assistants are allowed to perform. Some states require licensure or registration to perform expanded functions or to perform radiological procedures within a dentist's office. Licensure may include attending an accredited dental-assisting program and passing a written or practical examination. There are a variety of schools offering courses—approximately 10 to 12 months in length—that meet their state's requirements. Other states require dental assistants to complete state-approved continuing education courses of 4 to 12 hours in length. Some states offer the registration of other dental-assisting credentials with little or no education required. Some states require continuing education to maintain licensure or registration. A few states allow dental assistants to perform any function delegated to them by the dentist. Individual states have adopted different standards for dental assistants who perform certain advanced duties; in some states, for example, dental assistants who perform radiological procedures must complete additional training. Completion of the Radiation Health and Safety examination offered by Dental Assisting National Board (DANB) meets the standards in more than 30 states. Some states require the completion of a state-approved course in radiology as well. Twelve states have no formal requirements to perform radiological procedures.

Certification and Other Qualifications

Certification is available through the DANB and is recognized or required in the majority of states. Certification is an acknowledgment of an assistant's qualifications and professional competence and may be an asset when one is seeking employment. Candidates may qualify to take the DANB certification examination by graduating from an ADA-accredited dental-assisting education program or by having two years of full-time or four years of part-time experience as a dental assistant. In addition, applicants must have current certification in cardiopulmonary resuscitation. For annual recertification, individuals must earn continuing education credits.

Other organizations offer registration, most often at the state level. Dental assistants must be a second pair of hands for a dentist; therefore, dentists look for people who are reliable, work well with others, and have good manual dexterity.

Advancement

Without further education, advancement opportunities are limited. Some dental assistants become office managers, dental-assisting instructors, dental product sales representatives, or insurance claims processors for dental insurance companies. Others go back to school to become dental hygienists. For many, this entry-level occupation provides basic training and experience and serves as a stepping-stone to more highly skilled and higher-paying jobs. Assistants wishing to take on expanded functions or perform radiological procedures may choose to complete coursework in those functions as allowed under state regulation or, if required, obtain a state-issued license.

Employment Trends

Employment is expected to increase much faster than average; job prospects are expected to be excellent.

Employment Change

Employment is expected to grow 7% from 2019 to 2029, which is faster than the average for all occupations.

Population growth, greater retention of natural teeth by middle-aged and older people, and an increased focus on preventive dental care for younger generations will fuel demand for dental services. Federal health legislation has expanded the number of individuals with access to health insurance, and those with new or expanded dental insurance coverage are expected to visit a dentist more often than they have in the past. Older dentists, who have been less likely to employ assistants or have employed fewer assistants, are leaving the occupation and will be replaced by recent graduates, who are more likely to use one or more assistants. In addition, as dentists' workloads increase, they are expected to hire more assistants to perform routine tasks so that they may devote their time to more complex procedures.

Job Prospects

Job prospects for dental assistants should be excellent, as dentists continue to need the aid of qualified dental assistants. There will be many opportunities for entry-level positions, which may offer on-the-job training, but some dentists prefer to hire experienced assistants, those who have completed a dental-assisting program, or those who have met state requirements to take on expanded functions within the office. In addition to job openings due to employment growth, numerous job openings will arise out of the need to replace assistants who transfer to other occupations, retire, or leave for other reasons. TABLE 12.4 shows some projection data provided by the U.S. Department of Labor.

TABLE 12.4 Projections Data for Dental Assistants, 2019–2029

Occupational Title	Employment, 2019	Projected Employment, 2029	Change, 2019–2029	
			Number	Percentage
Dental assistants	354,600	378.000	23,400	7%

Data from Bureau of Labor Statistics. *Occupational Outlook Handbook.* U.S. Department of Labor; 2020.

Earnings

Median annual wages of dental assistants were $41,180 in May 2020. The lowest 10% earned less than $28,940, and the highest 10% earned more than $58,390.

Benefits vary substantially by practice setting and may be contingent upon full-time employment. According to a 2018–19 survey by the Dental Assisting National Board, the top work benefits dental assistants received from their employers were paid vacation, paid holidays, a retirement plan, health insurance, and paid sick leave.[8]

Related Occupations

Other workers supporting health practitioners include dental hygienists, medical assistants, surgical technologists, pharmacy aides, pharmacy technicians, occupational therapist assistants and aides, and physical therapist assistants and aides.

Additional Information

Information about career opportunities and accredited dental-assisting programs is available from:

- Commission on Dental Accreditation, American Dental Association, 211 East Chicago Ave., Suite 1900, Chicago, IL 60611. https://www.ada.org/en/education-careers

For information on becoming a certified dental assistant and a list of state boards of dentistry, contact:

- Dental Assisting National Board, Inc., 444 N. Michigan Ave., Suite 900, Chicago, IL 60611. https://www.danb.org

For more information on a career as a dental assistant and general information about continuing education, contact:

- American Dental Assistants Association, 35 East Wacker Dr., Suite 1730, Chicago, IL 60601. http://www.dentalassistant.org

DENTAL LABORATORY TECHNICIANS
Significant Points

- Most technicians learn their craft on the job, but many employers prefer to hire those with formal training.
- Faster-than-average employment growth is expected for dental laboratory technicians.
- Job opportunities should be favorable because few people seek these positions.

Work Description

Dental laboratory technicians fill prescriptions from dentists for crowns, bridges, dentures, and other dental prosthetics. First, dentists send a specification of the item to be manufactured, along with an impression or mold of the patient's mouth or teeth. With new technology, a technician may receive a digital impression rather than a physical mold. Then dental laboratory technicians, also called dental technicians, create a model of the patient's mouth by pouring plaster into the impression and allowing it to set. They place the model on an apparatus that mimics the bite and movement of the patient's jaw. The model serves as the basis of the prosthetic device. Technicians examine the model, noting the size and shape of the adjacent teeth as well as gaps within the gum line. Based on these observations and the dentist's specifications, technicians build and shape a wax model of the tooth or teeth, using small hand instruments called wax spatulas and wax carvers. The wax model is used to cast the metal framework for the prosthetic device.

After the wax tooth has been formed, dental technicians pour the cast, form the metal, and, using small handheld tools, prepare the surface to allow the metal and porcelain to bond. They then apply porcelain in layers to arrive at the precise shape and color of a tooth. Technicians place the tooth in a porcelain furnace to bake the porcelain onto the metal framework and then adjust the shape and color, with subsequent grinding and addition of porcelain to achieve a sealed finish. The final product is a nearly exact replica of the lost tooth or teeth.

In some dental laboratories, technicians perform all stages of the work, whereas in other labs, each technician works on only a few. Dental laboratory technicians can specialize in one of five areas: orthodontic appliances, crowns and bridges, complete dentures, partial dentures, or ceramics. Job titles can reflect specialization in these areas. For example, technicians who make porcelain and acrylic restorations are called **dental ceramists**.

In small laboratories, technicians usually handle every phase of the operation. In large ones, in which virtually every phase of the operation is automated, technicians may be responsible for operating computerized equipment. Technicians also inspect the final product for quality and accuracy. An example of a dental laboratory technician working with an articulator device is seen in **FIGURE 12.4.**

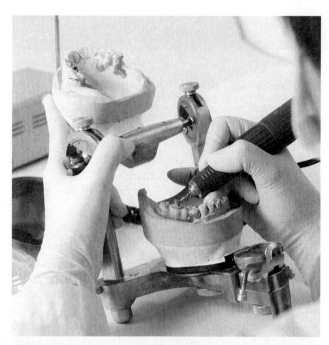

FIGURE 12.4 Dental lab technician working with an articulator device.
©pixs4u/Shutterstock.

Work Environment

Dental laboratory technicians generally work in clean, well-lit, and well-ventilated laboratories. They have limited contact with the public. Salaried laboratory technicians usually work 40 hours a week, but some work part time. At times, technicians wear goggles to protect their eyes, gloves to handle hot objects, or masks to avoid inhaling dust. They may spend a great deal of time standing. Dental technicians should be particularly careful when working with tools because there is a risk of injury.

Dental technicians usually have their own workbenches, which can be equipped with Bunsen burners, grinding and polishing equipment, and hand instruments, such as wax spatulas and wax carvers. Some dental technicians have computer-aided milling equipment to assist them with creating artificial teeth.

Employment Opportunities

Dental laboratory technicians held about 36,200 jobs in 2019. Many of the salaried jobs were in medical equipment and supply manufacturing laboratories, which usually are small, privately owned businesses with fewer than five employees. Some laboratories are large; a few employ more than 1,000 workers. In addition to manufacturing laboratories, many dental laboratory technicians worked in offices of dentists. Some dental laboratory technicians open their own offices.

Educational and Legal Requirements

Most dental laboratory technicians learn their craft on the job; many employers, however, prefer to hire those with formal training or at least a high school diploma.

Education and Training

High school students interested in becoming dental laboratory technicians should take mathematics, metal and wood shop, and drafting. Dental laboratory technicians usually begin as helpers and gradually learn new skills as they gain experience.

Dental laboratory technicians begin by learning simple tasks, such as pouring plaster into an impression, and progress to more complex procedures, such as making porcelain crowns and bridges. Becoming a fully trained technician requires an average of three to four years, depending on the individual's aptitude and ambition, but it may take a few years more to become an accomplished technician. High school students interested in becoming dental laboratory technicians should take courses in art, metal and wood shop, drafting, and sciences. Courses in management and business may help those wishing to operate their own laboratories.

Training in dental laboratory technology also is available through universities, community and junior colleges, vocational-technical institutes, and the armed forces. Formal training programs vary greatly both in length and in the level of skill they impart. In 2021, the Commission on Dental Accreditation, in conjunction with the American Dental Association, accredited 14 programs in dental laboratory technology.[9] These programs provide classroom instruction in materials science, oral anatomy, fabrication procedures, ethics, and related subjects. In addition, each student is given supervised practical experience in a school or an associated dental laboratory. Accredited programs normally take two years to complete and lead to an associate's degree. A few programs take about four years to complete and offer a bachelor's degree in dental technology. Graduates of two-year training programs need additional hands-on experience to become fully qualified.

Each dental laboratory owner operates in a different way, and classroom instruction does not necessarily expose students to techniques and procedures favored by individual laboratory owners. Students who have taken enough courses to learn the basics of the craft usually are considered good candidates for training, regardless of whether they have completed a formal program. However, many employers will train someone without any classroom experience.

General information on grants and scholarships is available from individual schools. State employment service offices can provide information about job openings for dental laboratory technicians.

Other Qualifications

Dental technicians need a high degree of manual dexterity, good vision, and the ability to recognize very fine color shadings and variations in shape. An artistic aptitude for detailed and precise work also is important.

Certification and Advancement

In large dental laboratories, dental technicians may become supervisors or managers. Experienced technicians may teach

TABLE 12.5 Projections Data for Dental Laboratory Technicians 2019–2029

Occupational Title	Employment, 2019	Project Employment, 2029	Change, 2019–2029	
			Number	Percentage
Dental laboratory technicians	36,200	39,600	3,400	9%

Data from Bureau of Labor Statistics. *Occupational Outlook Handbook.* U.S. Department of Labor; 2020.

or take jobs with dental suppliers in such areas as product development, marketing, and sales. Opening one's own laboratory is another, and more common, way to advance and earn more.

The National Board for Certification in Dental Laboratory Technology, an independent board established by the National Association of Dental Laboratories, offers certification in dental laboratory technology. Certification, which is voluntary except in three states, can be obtained in six specialty areas: crowns and bridges, ceramics, partial dentures, complete dentures, implants, and orthodontic appliances.[10] Certification may increase chances of advancement.

Employment Trends

Overall, faster-than-average growth is expected for employment of dental laboratory technicians, but projections vary by detailed occupation. Job opportunities should be favorable because few people seek these positions.

Employment Change

Employment of dental laboratory technicians is expected to grow 9%, which is faster than the average for all occupations. During the past few years, demand has arisen from an aging public that is growing increasingly interested in cosmetic prostheses. For example, many dental laboratories are filling orders for composite fillings that are the same shade of white as natural teeth to replace older, less attractive fillings. It is possible the job growth for dental laboratory technicians will be limited. The overall dental health of the population has improved because of the fluoridation of drinking water and greater emphasis on preventive dental care, which has reduced the incidence of dental cavities. As a result, full dentures will be less common, as most people will need only a bridge or crown. An increase in the need for dental appliances is anticipated due to the increased risk of oral cancer due to age.

Job Prospects

Job opportunities for dental laboratory technicians should be favorable. Those with formal training in a dental laboratory technology program will have the best job prospects. In addition to openings from job growth, many job openings also will

arise from the need to replace technicians who transfer to other occupations or who leave the labor force. **TABLE 12.5** shows some projection data provided by the U.S. Department of Labor.

Earnings

Median annual earnings of wage and salary dental laboratory technicians were $42,110 in May 2020. The lowest 10% earned less than $25,770, and the highest 10% earned more than $63,910. In the two industries that employed the most dental laboratory technicians—medical equipment and supplies manufacturing and offices of dentists—median annual earnings were $39,300 and $43,670, respectively.

Related Occupations

Dental laboratory technicians manufacture and work with the same devices that are used by dispensing opticians, orthotists, prosthetists, and medical and ophthalmic laboratory technicians. Other occupations that work with or manufacture goods using similar tools and skills are precision instrument and equipment repair and textile, apparel, and furnishings occupations.

Additional Information

For a list of accredited programs in dental laboratory technology, contact:

- Commission on Dental Accreditation, American Dental Association, 211 E. Chicago Ave., Chicago, IL 60611. https://www.ada.org

For information on requirements for the certification of dental laboratory technicians, contact:

- National Board for Certification in Dental Technology, 325 John Knox Rd., L103, Tallahassee, FL 32303. https://nbccert.org/homepage.cfm

For information on career opportunities in commercial dental laboratories, contact:

- National Association of Dental Laboratories, 325 John Knox Rd., L103, Tallahassee, FL 32303. https://www.nadl.org

LEARNING PORTFOLIO

Issues for Discussion

1. Which of the jobs discussed in this chapter would you be most likely to recommend to a friend or acquaintance interested in working in the healthcare field? Explain your selection and rationale.

2. Choose one of the professions discussed in this chapter. Discuss the most important personal attribute this profession should have. Why do you feel this is so important?

Enrichment Activities

1. Many in the dental community believe a connection exists between a person's diet and tooth decay and other mouth disorders. Search the Internet for information about this connection and create a presentation about your findings.

2. Visit https://www.webmd.com/oral-health/healthy-teeth-14/brushing-teeth-mistakes to learn about toothbrush mistakes and how to fix them. Name any of the identified mistakes that surprised you.

3. Develop a chart to compare and contrast the following factors among the professions discussed in this chapter: educational requirements, employment trends, opportunities for advancement, salary potential, and possible career ladders.

4. Use the Internet to research your state's requirements for any of the professions discussed in this chapter. List these requirements, if they exist. Compare and contrast licensing, certification, and registration for this career with any other career you have examined in this course.

5. View the following videos: "Dentists, General Career Video About (Dentist)" at https://www.careeronestop.org/videos/careeronestop-videos.aspx?videocode=29102100 and "Dental Hygienists Career Video" at https://www.careeronestop.org/videos/careeronestop-videos.aspx?videocode=29129200 Discuss the roles of a dentist and a dental hygienist with your instructor and classmates.

CASE STUDY: DENTAL PRACTITIONERS

Diego is studying to be a dentist. He will complete his educational program in May of next year. His goal is to work in a small private practice. Today, Diego is shadowing in a small dental practice where he will see exactly how the dentists and dental hygienists perform their job duties.

Based on the information you have read about dentists and dental hygienists, answer the following questions:

1. Identify the service Diego would see the dentist perform during his shadowing.
   A. Cleaning teeth
   B. Taking X-rays
   C. Setting up the patient room for a service
   D. Applying sealants to a child

2. Determine the appropriate reason for Diego to wear personal protective equipment while observing patient care.
   A. To look professional
   B. To protect against infections
   C. To protect his clothes
   D. To follow the practice's dress code

3. While shadowing, Diego may be introduced to other employees. Identify any employees Diego may encounter.
   A. Dental assistant
   B. Dental hygienist
   C. Laboratory technician
   D. All of these are correct.

4. A new employee has been recently hired to clean teeth and provide other preventive dental care. This employee is a ____.
   A. laboratory technician
   B. dental hygienist
   C. receptionist
   D. dentist

5. One patient appointment was to take an initial impression of the upper and lower jaw for dentures. Identify the occupation that is responsible for creating the wax mold from the impression.
   A. Dentist
   B. Dental assistant
   C. Dental hygienist
   D. Laboratory technician

At the end of the shadowing experience, Diego interviews the dentist. During the interview, the dentist shares her education, steps to become licensed, and thoughts on working in a small practice.

Based on the information you have read about dentists, answer the following questions:

6. Skills in dentistry include ____.
   A. All of these are correct.
   B. communication skills
   C. diagnostic ability
   D. manual skills

LEARNING PORTFOLIO

7. The dentist recommended that the Dental Admissions Test (DAT) be completed ___ before applying to an accredited dental school.
   A. twelve months
   B. six months
   C. nine months
   D. three months

8. To obtain her license, the dentist had to have a degree from an accredited dental school and pass ____.
   A. None of the answers are correct.
   B. an oral exam and written exam
   C. a written exam and practical exam
   D. a practical exam and oral exam

9. The dentist stated in her interview that to meet the needs of the patient she had office hours ___.
   A. during weekdays
   B. in the evenings
   C. on the weekend
   D. All of these are correct.

10. The demand for dental services is expected to increase with a focus on ____.
    A. filling cavities
    B. making crowns
    C. preventive care
    D. emergency care

References

1. American Dental Association. *Dental Practice Ownership is Declining.* https://www.ada.org/~/media/ADA/Science%20and%20Research/HPI/Files/HPIgraphic_0121_2.pdf?la=en Accessed August 11, 2021.

2. American Dental Association. *How Many Dentists are in Solo Practice?* https://www.ada.org/~/media/ADA/Science%20and%20Research/HPI/Files/HPIGraphic_0121_1.pdf?la=en Accessed August 11, 2021.

3. American Dental Association, Commission on Dental Accreditation. *Search for Dental Programs.* https://www.ada.org/en/coda Accessed August 1, 2021.

4. American Dental Association. *Dental Admission Test (DAT).* https://www.ada.org/en/education-careers/dental-admission-test Accessed August 1, 2021.

5. American Dental Association. *Racial and Ethnic Mix of Dental Students in the U.S.* https://www.ada.org/~/media/ADA/Science%20and%20Research/HPI/Files/HPIgraphic_0421_2.pdf?la=en Accessed August 1, 2021.

6. Commission on Dental Accreditation. *Dental Hygiene Programs.* https://www.ada.org/en/coda Accessed August 1, 2021.

7. Commission on Dental Accreditation. *Dental Assistant Programs.* http://www.ada.org/en/coda/find-a-program/search-dental-programs#t=us&sort=relevancy&f:ProgramName=[Dental%20Assisting] Accessed August 1, 2021.

8. Dental Assisting National Board. *2018–2019 Dental Assistants Salary & Satisfaction Survey.* https://www.danbcertified.org/wp-content/uploads/2019/06/2018-Salary-Survey-visual-report-1.pdf Accessed August 1, 2021.

9. Commission on Dental Education. *Dental Laboratory Technician Programs.* https://www.ada.org/en/coda Accessed August 1, 2021.

10. National Board for Certification in Dental Laboratory Technology. https://nbccert.org/homepage.cfm Accessed August 1, 2021.

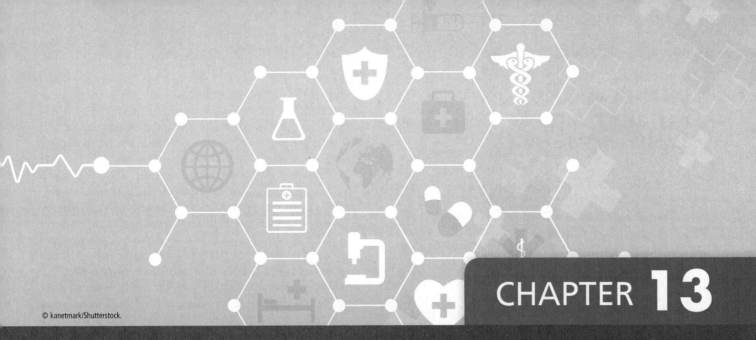

© kanetmark/Shutterstock.

CHAPTER 13

Dietetics*

KEY TERMS

Academy of Nutrition and Dietetics (AND)

Accreditation Council for Education in Nutrition and Dietetics (ACEND)

Association of Nutrition and Foodservice Professionals (ANFP)

Business dietitian nutritionists

Centers for Medicare and Medicaid Services (CMS)

Certified Diabetes Care and Education Specialist (CDCES)

Certified Dietary Manager (CDM)

Certified Nutrition Specialist (CNS)

Certified Nutrition Support Clinician (CNSC)

Clinical dietitian nutritionists

Commission on Dietetic Registration (CDR)

Community dietitian nutritionists

Consultant dietitian nutritionists

Coordinated Program in Dietetics (CP)

Didactic Program in Dietetics (DPD)

Dietetic educator

Dietetic Internship (DI)

Individualized Supervised Practice Pathways (ISPPs)

The Joint Commission

Management dietitian nutritionists

Medical nutrition therapy

National Board of Nutrition Support Certification (NBNSC)

Nutrition and Dietetic Technician, Registered (NDTR)

Registered Dietitian (RD)

Registered Dietitian Nutritionist (RDN)

Research dietitian nutritionists

School Nutrition Specialist (SNS)

Specialty board certification

* All information in this chapter, unless otherwise indicated, was obtained from Bureau of Labor Statistics. *Occupational Outlook Handbook 2020–2021 Edition*. Washington, DC: U.S. Department of Labor; 2021.

DIETITIANS AND NUTRITIONISTS
Significant Points

- Most dietitians and nutritionists work in hospitals and outpatient and ambulatory care centers, including offices of physicians and other healthcare professionals, and in long-term care, including nursing care and assisted-living facilities.
- Dietitians and nutritionists need at least a bachelor's degree; licensure, certification, or registration requirements vary by state. However, new graduates will need a master's degree to be eligible for registration beginning January 1, 2024. One-half of dietitians and nutritionists hold a master's degree.
- Most dietitians who become certified through the Academy of Nutrition and Dietetics use the title Registered Dietitian Nutritionist (RDN).
- Applicants with specialized training, an advanced degree, or certifications beyond the particular state's minimum requirement should enjoy the best job opportunities.

Work Description

Registered Dietitian Nutritionists (RDNs) are experts in food and nutrition. They advise people on what foods to eat in order to lead a healthy lifestyle or achieve a specific health-related goal. They counsel individuals and groups; supervise foodservice systems for institutions such as schools, hospitals, and prisons; promote sound eating habits through education; and conduct research. Some RDNs are self-employed, working as consultants to facilities such as hospitals and nursing care facilities and food- and nutrition-related businesses, or have a private practice providing medical nutrition therapy for individuals. Federal government jobs are with the U.S. Department of Veteran Affairs (VA) hospitals and the U.S. Department of Defense in different branches of the armed services. RDNs also work in the U.S. Department of Agriculture and the National Cancer Institute, in either research or program planning and evaluation. Some work as consultants to facilities such as hospitals and nursing care facilities. Some RDNs are employed in special food services, an industry made up of firms providing food services on contract to facilities such as school lunch programs, colleges and universities, airlines, correctional facilities, and company cafeterias.

Although many RDNs do similar tasks, there are several specialties in the occupation. Major areas of specialization include clinical, management, community, business and industry, and consultant dietetics. RDNs also work in academia as educators and researchers. **Clinical dietitian nutritionists** provide nutrition services for patients in hospitals, long-term care facilities, outpatient clinics, or the offices of physicians and other healthcare practitioners. They assess the patient's nutritional needs based on their medical condition, develop and implement nutrition care plans, and evaluate and document the results. Clinical dietitians confer with doctors and nurses to coordinate the nutritional and medical needs of patients.

Expanding knowledge in medical science has led to practice specialties in dietetics. Increasingly, clinical dietitians specialize in such areas as geriatrics, pediatrics, oncology, care of the critically ill, renal care, and diabetes care. Those who care for critically ill patients select or recommend formulas for patients who require tube or intravenous feedings. RDNs who specialize in renal dietetics evaluate and counsel patients with kidney disease who are on chronic dialysis; those who specialize in diabetes assist patients in managing diet, physical activity, and insulin or other medications to keep blood sugar at optimum levels (**FIGURE 13.1**).

Pediatric RDNs specialize in the nutritional care of infants, children, and adolescents during hospitalization and in outpatient clinics for follow-up, especially for children with developmental disabilities or chronic diseases such as cystic fibrosis, diabetes, or celiac disease. Oncology dietitians are challenged with helping patients find foods concentrated in protein and calories that they find palatable with the changes in appetite and altered taste that sometimes accompany chemotherapy. Gerontology specialists work in long-term care facilities and other programs for the elderly at the local, state, or national level. Aside from assessing nutritional needs and developing a plan of treatment for individual patients, clinical dietitians may also perform administrative and managerial duties. In a nursing home or small hospital, the RDN may also manage the foodservice department.

Consultant dietitian nutritionists work under contract with healthcare facilities or in their own private practices. Consulting has become a significant specialty in dietetics. It has appeal for RDNs who need flexible work schedules and have a desire to be autonomous. Some work for

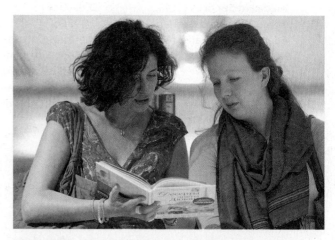

FIGURE 13.1 A clinical dietitian helps a client with diabetes select recipes for meal planning to manage blood glucose.
© Lilyana Vynogradova/Shutterstock.

wellness programs, sports teams, supermarkets, and other nutrition-related businesses. They may consult with food-service managers to provide expertise in food sanitation and safety, menu development, and budgeting. They advise food and pharmaceutical industries; speak at professional seminars; author food and nutrition books; counsel patients for a group practice of physicians; plan food service systems; and tailor nutrition regimens within fitness programs for athletes, dancers, and others.

Community dietitian nutritionists counsel individuals and groups on sound nutrition practices to prevent disease and to promote good health. Community RDNs may be employed by a city or county health department or federal health clinics. Many RDNs work for Women, Infants, and Children (WIC), a government-funded supplemental nutrition program; eligibility is based on income and nutritional risk. WIC dietitians and nutritionists do nutrition screening and counseling of women during pregnancy and mothers of infants and young children at nutritional risk (**FIGURE 13.2**).

They also conduct nutrition education classes, including breastfeeding support. Their job is to evaluate individual nutritional needs, establish care plans, and communicate the principles of good nutrition in a way that individuals and their families can understand.

RDNs are employed by home health and hospice agencies and by human service agencies that provide group and home-delivered meals through government-supported elderly nutrition programs at senior centers. Many community RDNs work for local or regional food banks to monitor food sanitation and safety and to provide nutrition education for clients. They coordinate nutrition awareness and disease prevention programs in settings such as farmers' markets, public health agencies, child day care centers, and health clubs. They may also collaborate with nurses and health educators in conducting information sessions on such subjects as alcoholism, smoking, or hypertension. Community RDNs counsel clients on food selection in relation to culture and lifestyle. Potential clients might be, for example, a truck

driver who has diabetes and limited access to healthy food or an elderly woman with heart failure who is on a low-sodium diet but who eats mostly high-sodium canned and frozen foods because she doesn't have the energy to cook. In addition to evaluating clients, RDNs working in a home health setting may provide informal instruction on nutrition, menu planning, grocery shopping, food safety and sanitation, or preparation of special infant formulas. In ambulatory settings, dietitians provide **medical nutrition therapy** for clients with a variety of medical conditions, including obesity, diabetes, and cardiovascular disease, and for parents of infants or children with special dietary needs because of metabolic disorders or other chronic disease.

Practice opportunities for clinical and community RDNs are becoming more diverse because of increased interest in nutrition and fitness on the part of the public and the medical profession alike. This new awareness has resulted in opportunities for private practitioners in areas such as food manufacturing, advertising, and marketing. Those who work for food manufacturers or grocery store chains may analyze the nutritional content of foods for labeling or marketing. Those working for grocery stores often conduct tours for groups with special dietary needs—for example, those with celiac disease who must avoid gluten—to assist in label reading and choosing gluten-free foods. They may also prepare literature for distribution to customers, students, or other interested parties. Those employed by magazines may determine the nutrient content of new recipes, analyze and report on the effectiveness of new diets, or report on important topics in nutrition, such as the importance of dietary fiber or the value of vitamin supplements.

Business dietitian nutritionists work as a professional resource for corporations in product development, food styling, menu design, and nutrient analysis. As businesses become more aware of the public's desire for accurate nutrition information, they are eager to hire RDN experts. Other roles for the business RDN are the sales professional or purchasing agent representing food, equipment, or nutrition product accounts or as a food, nutrition, or marketing expert in public relations and the media.

Management dietitian nutritionists are responsible for large-scale food services in a variety of settings: hospitals, long-term care, company cafeterias, prisons, elementary and secondary schools, and colleges and universities. They supervise the planning, preparation, and service of meals; select, train, and direct foodservice supervisors and workers; budget for and purchase food, equipment, and supplies; enforce sanitary and safety regulations; and prepare records and reports. Increasingly, RDNs use computer programs to plan meals that satisfy nutrition requirements and are economical at the same time. Directors also decide on departmental policy, coordinate dietetic services with the activities of other departments, and are responsible for the dietetics department budget, which in large organizations may amount to millions of dollars annually. Directors are responsible for all employees and functions in the department, including hiring

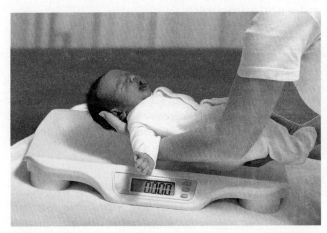

FIGURE 13.2 Community RDNs monitor weight as part of nutrition screening in the WIC program.
© Beneda Miroslav/Shutterstock.

and evaluating employees and quality control, and, depending on the size of the department, may delegate some of these responsibilities to assistant directors or supervisors.

Military dietitians work for a branch of the U.S. Armed Services—the air force, army, or navy—and have many of the same responsibilities as civilian dietitians. They provide medical nutrition therapy for both active and retired military personnel on military bases and hospitals. In addition, the dietitian teaches active duty personnel how to achieve optimum physical fitness with appropriate food choices to meet nutrient and fluid needs.

Research dietitian nutritionists usually are employed in academic medical centers or universities and federal nutrition programs, although some work in community health programs. Using established research methods and analytical techniques, they conduct studies in areas that range from basic science to practical applications. Research RDNs may examine changes in the way the body uses food and nutrients over the course of a lifetime, for example, or the interaction of medications and diet. They may investigate the nutritional needs of persons with particular diseases, behavior modification for those on a weight loss program, or applied topics such as foodservice systems and equipment. Often research RDNs collaborate with life scientists, physicians, nurses, biomedical engineers, and researchers from other disciplines.

As a **dietetic educator**, the RDN teaches the science of nutrition and foodservice systems management in colleges, universities, and hospitals. RDNs have always recognized the need to teach, whether in clinical practice, in community settings, or for corporations, and some are specifically interested in pursuing careers as educators. In academia, the RDN conducts nutrition and foodservice systems research and writes articles and books on nutrition and foodservice systems. Many educators in the field are directors of dietetic internships. RDNs in education usually hold advanced degrees and have considerable experience.

Work Environment

Most RDNs work 40 hours per week. About 20% worked part time in 2019.[1] Those employed in hospitals sometimes work on weekends, while those in commercial food services tend to have irregular hours. Clinical RDNs working in ambulatory settings and in private practice may work evenings and weekends to accommodate working hours of their clients and for community programs such as health fairs. Those involved in consulting spend a significant amount of time traveling. Consulting RDNs and those in private practice may need to spend time on marketing and other business-related tasks, such as scheduling appointments and preparing informational materials for clients.

Employment Opportunities

RDNs held about 74,200 jobs in 2019. According to a 2019 survey by the **Academy of Nutrition and Dietetics (AND)**,

TABLE 13.1 Practice Areas of Dietitians and Nutritionists, 2019	
Clinical nutrition, hospital inpatient	40%
Clinical nutrition, ambulatory care/outpatient	14%
Clinical nutrition, long-term care facilities	6%
Community	9%
Food and nutrition management	9%
Consultation and business	9%
Education and research	6%

Data from Griswold K, Rogers D. Compensation and benefits survey 2019. *J Acad Nutr Diet.* 2020;120(3):448–464. doi:10.1016/j.jand.2019.12.015

latory care, and long-term care facilities including assisted care facilities. Others worked in community programs such as public health or WIC, food and nutrition management positions, and private practice. The majority worked in for-profit (39%) and nonprofit (37%) settings; about 15% worked for the government, and 8% were self-employed (**TABLE 13.1**).[1]

Experienced RDNs may advance to assistant, associate, or director of a clinical nutrition department or food and nutrition services in a hospital or in long-term care. Some RDNs specialize in areas such as renal, diabetes, or pediatric dietetics. Others become sales representatives for equipment, pharmaceutical, or food manufacturers. Advancement to higher-level positions in teaching and research requires graduate education; public health nutritionists usually earn a graduate degree. Graduate study in institutional or business administration is valuable to those interested in management dietetics. Clinical specialization offers another path to career advancement. Specialty areas for clinical RDNs include kidney disease, diabetes, oncology, pediatrics, gerontology, and obesity and weight management.

Educational and Legal Requirements

RDNs need at least a bachelor's degree. However, new graduates will need a master's degree to be eligible for registration beginning January 1, 2024. Licensure, certification, and registration requirements vary by state.

Education and Training

Becoming an RDN requires at least a bachelor's degree in dietetics, foods and nutrition, foodservice systems management, or a related area plus supervised clinical experience. College students in these majors take courses in foods, nutrition, institution management, chemistry, biochemistry, biology,

Professional Profiles

Name: Eecole, MS, RDN, LD
Job Title: Dietitian Nutritionist—
Sustainable Food Programs Coordinator
Education: MS in Nutrition, BS Biology

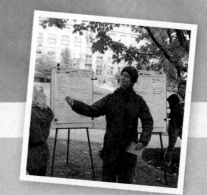

Q: Describe your job and organization.

A: I am the sustainable food programs coordinator at a large academic hospital in an urban setting. My work is seasonal. During the spring and summer, I manage a farmers' market for the hospital—our consumers are from the hospital and the wider community.

Q: Describe a typical workday.

A: Managing the farmers' market in the spring and summer involves marketing, finding and enrolling vendors, cost accounting, and overall task management. In the hospital, I am responsible for the food prescriptions pharmacy and recommend foods based on health components. In the food and nutrition department that prepares healthy meals, I work with the executive chef and the food buyer to ensure that all categories of food—meat, dairy products, fruits, and vegetables—are grown sustainably. The department uses a closed-loop system by composting all food waste to generate energy for the hospital.

Q: Why did you choose this profession?

A: I am passionate and believe in the philosophy that food is medicine and that healthy food is produced without antibiotics for animals and without pesticides for fruits, vegetables, and grains. I work with both food and people, and I'm able to change systems. I conduct sustainability training for staff and teach how sustainability relates to their job.

Q: What challenges you most about this profession?

A: There is much hidden information behind the scenes in food production, both misinformation and contradictory information. My job is to shed light on misguided and hidden information. People are resistant to change—and the current industrial food system provides relatively inexpensive processed food because of heavy government subsidies for corn and soy products. Unsubsidized fresh fruits and vegetables are more expensive, so it's a hard sell to get the public to buy the more expensive foods.

Q: Name and explain what part of your academic training most prepared you for this profession.

A: A master's degree in nutrition—especially environmental policy and nutrition education. Of course, basic nutrition is important. I had a lot of life experience around waste management and environmentalism. My current position requires a master's degree. Other paths to the field of sustainability are certification programs or a degree in engineering or sustainability.

Q: What do you wish you had known in high school or college about pursuing this career?

A: That this career existed! My first degree was in biology.

Q: What advice would you give someone who is considering this career?

A: You can't be afraid to get your hands dirty or face a lot of resistance. It helps to be passionate and know that you will often need to lead the way, since this is a very new territory for most. Sustainability is a new field—about 10 years young!

Q: What personal characteristics are needed for this work?

A: Personal characteristics needed for my position are courage, persistence, curiosity, open-mindedness, and passion. Excellent communication skills are also necessary.

Q: What websites do you recommend as resources?

A: The Hunger and Environmental Nutrition Practice Group within the Academy of Nutrition and Dietetics (http://www.hendpg.org/), Health Care Without Harm (https://noharm.org/), and Practice Green Health (https://practicegreenhealth.org/). Two films that provide background on the industrial food system are *Food, Inc.* and *Forks over Knifes*.

microbiology, and physiology. Other suggested courses include business, statistics, computer science, psychology, sociology, and economics. High school students interested in becoming an RDN should take courses in biology, chemistry, mathematics, health, and communications. Most RDNs have a love for food—growing food, developing recipes, and preparing food—and communicate this passion to clients as part of promoting a healthy lifestyle or managing chronic health conditions.

The **Accreditation Council for Education in Nutrition and Dietetics (ACEND)** of the AND is the body that accredits programs in dietetics education, including the **Didactic Program in Dietetics (DPD)**, **Coordinated Program in Dietetics (CPD)**, and **Dietetic Internship (DI)**.[2]

To complete requirements for the **Commission on Dietetic Registration (CDR)** registration examination required for licensure or certification, graduates must have completed supervised clinical training. Clinical training is incorporated into CPD or is obtained through a DI.[2]

As of 2019, there were 63 accredited CPDs. Some are bachelor's programs, and others are master's programs; the area of emphasis varies from clinical to food systems management. The number of positions available varies with each program and requires application at least one year before starting the program.[2] Students accepted into a CPD are not required to apply for a DI since the CPD incorporates supervised clinical training.

Students graduating from a DPD typically apply for a DI during their last year of the DPD. The DI includes clinical supervision and upon completion interns are eligible to take the registration exam administered by CDR. In 2019, there were 213 DPDs in the United States. Competition is keen for internships, and graduation from a DPD program does not guarantee obtaining an internship. There are 261 accredited DIs. These internships may be full-time programs lasting 6 to 12 months or part-time programs lasting two years. DIs are offered by a variety of colleges and universities, hospitals, WIC programs, and other agencies. The emphasis of each internship varies. Some examples are community nutrition, school nutrition, medical nutrition therapy, health promotion and disease prevention, mental health, communication, research, sports nutrition, and food systems management and child nutrition programs. Some programs offer a graduate degree and require admission to graduate school as well as admission to the internship program. Application for DIs is completed online and can be submitted for matching in either April or November. Students interested in exploring internship options can view available internships online.[2] Applicants to DIs are computer matched to one internship program.[3] For more information on internships, go to "Additional Information" at the end of this chapter.

Because of the competition for DIs by graduates of DPD programs, in 2011 the AND developed **Individualized Supervised Practice Pathways (ISPPs)**—referred to as "iss-pees"—to allow ACEND-accredited dietetics programs to add supervised practice into the degree program to meet the 1,200 hours of supervised clinical experience required to be able to sit for the registration exam. ISSPs allow students

unable to match for a DI after obtaining a bachelor's degree through a DPD program to be able to obtain the needed clinical experience.[4]

Beginning in 2012, ACEND conducted meetings to obtain recommendations for the future educational needs of dietetic practitioners. Individuals representing employers, practitioners, educators, administrators, professionals working with nutrition and dietetic professionals, and students met with ACEND staff members to provide input. Based on this input and the expected roles of future dietetics professionals, ACEND made these recommendations for educational requirements: (1) master's degree preparation for entry-level generalist dietitian nutritionists, (2) bachelor's degree preparation for entry-level nutrition and dietetics technicians, and (3) an associate's degree for nutrition health workers—a new category. ACEND will develop new standards for each of the three degree programs. Dietetic education programs will be given the opportunity to voluntarily adopt these new degree-based standards.[5]

Those interested in a career in nutrition and dietetics need to be knowledgeable about the requirement for a master's degree to be eligible for registration and to use the title, Registered Dietitian (RD) or Registered Dietitian Nutritionist (RDN) as of January 1, 2024.[6] Also, because of ACEND recommendations, many dietetic programs are in the process of changing the curriculum and the requirements for students applying for programs. A change in the educational requirements for dietitians and nutritionists is in line with other allied health professions, which require a master's degree at the entry level—for example, occupational therapy, clinical social work, and speech-language pathology—and doctoral-level training—physical therapy and audiology.

Licensure

Of the 52 states and jurisdictions with laws governing dietetics, all except four require certification or licensure to practice. Requirements vary by state.[7] As a result, interested candidates should determine the requirements of the state in which they want to work before sitting for any exam. In states that require licensure, only people who are licensed can work as RDNs. States that require statutory certification limit the use of occupational titles to people who meet certain requirements; individuals without certification can still practice as a dietitian or nutritionist, but without using certain titles. Registration is the least restrictive form of state regulation of dietitians and nutritionists. In some states, those who are not registered are allowed to practice as RDNs.

Certification and Other Qualifications

Although not required, the CDR of AND awards the Registered Dietitian (RD) or Registered Dietitian Nutritionist (RDN) credential to those who pass an exam after completing academic coursework and a supervised internship. This certification is different from the statutory certification regulated by some states discussed in the previous section. To maintain RDN status, at least 75 credit hours of CDR-approved continuing education must be obtained every five years.

Another route to certification (other than the AND) is through the Board for Certification of Nutrition Specialists (BCNS) as a **Certified Nutrition Specialist (CNS)**. Eligibility requirements for the CNS are a graduate degree, supervised clinical experience, and successfully completing a certification examination.[8]

Advancement

Experienced RDNs may advance to management positions, such as assistant director, associate director, or director of a dietetic department, or may become self-employed. Some become sales representatives for equipment, pharmaceutical, or food manufacturers. A master's degree can help some workers advance their careers, particularly in career paths related to research, advanced clinical positions, or public health. For those interested in management positions, a master's in business administration may be desirable. Clinical RDNs who become board certified in one of the seven specialties demand higher salaries.[1] The CDR offers **specialty board certification** in the following specialty areas:

- Gerontological Nutrition (GSG)
- Oncology Nutrition (CSO)
- Pediatric Nutrition (CSP)
- Pediatric Critical Care Nutrition (CSPCC)
- Renal Nutrition (CSR)
- Sports Dietetics (CSSD)
- Obesity and Weight Management (CSOWM)[9] (**FIGURE 13.3**)

Eligibility requirements to become board certified include a specified number of practice hours in the specialty area and successfully completing a certifying exam.[9] RDNs can also become either a **Certified Diabetes Care and Education Specialist (CDCES)**, conferred by the National Certification Board for Diabetes Educators (NCBDE),[10] or a **Certified Nutrition Support Clinician (CNSC)**, conferred by the **National Board of Nutrition Support Certification (NBNSC)**, an independent board established by the American Society for Parenteral and Enteral Nutrition (ASPEN).[11]

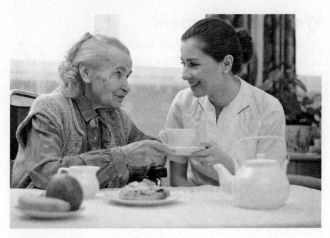

FIGURE 13.3 RDNs can obtain specialty board certification in gerontological nutrition (CSG).
© Alexander Raths/Shutterstock.

Employment Trends

Above-average employment growth is projected. Good job opportunities are expected, especially for RDNs with specialized training, an advanced degree, or certifications beyond the particular state's minimum requirement.

Employment Change

Employment of RDNs is expected to increase 8% during the 2019–2029 projection decade, much faster than average. Job growth will result from an increasing emphasis on disease prevention because of the high incidence of obesity and diseases that accompany obesity: diabetes and cardiovascular disease. As the Baby Boom generation grows older and seek ways to stay healthy, there will be greater demand for dietetic services. The aging population will increase the need for RDNs in long-term care facilities and home health care. In recent years, interest in the role of food and nutrition in promoting health and wellness has increased, particularly as a part of preventative health care in medical settings.

Employment growth, however, may be constrained if some employers substitute other workers, such as health educators, foodservice managers, and dietetic technicians, to do work related to nutrition. Also, demand for medical nutritional therapy services is related to the ability of patients to pay, either out of pocket or through health insurance, and although more insurance plans now cover medical nutrition therapy services, the extent of such coverage varies among plans. Growth may be curbed by limitations on insurance reimbursement for dietetic services.

Hospitals will continue to employ a large number of RDNs to provide medical nutrition therapy and to manage the foodservice department. Hospitals also will continue, however, to contract with outside agencies for food service and move medical nutritional therapy to outpatient care facilities, slowing job growth related to food service in hospitals and outpatient facilities and with other employers.

The number of positions in nursing care facilities is expected to decline, as these establishments continue to contract with outside agencies for food services. Another reason for the decline is the desire for elderly to receive care in their home. However, employment is expected to grow rapidly in contract providers of food services, in outpatient care centers, in offices of physicians and other health practitioners, and in home health.

Job Prospects

Overall, job opportunities for RDNs are expected to be favorable. RDNs who have earned advanced degrees or certification in a specialty area may enjoy better job prospects. In addition to employment growth, job openings will result from the need to replace experienced workers who retire or leave the occupation for other reasons. RDNs with specialized training, an advanced degree, or certifications beyond the particular state's minimum requirement will experience the best job opportunities. Those specializing in renal and diabetes or gerontological nutrition will benefit from the increased incidence of diabetes and the aging of the population. **TABLE 13.2** shows some projection data provided by the U.S. Department of Labor.

TABLE 13.2 Projections Data for Dietitians and Nutritionists, 2019–2029

Occupational Title	Employment, 2019	Projected Employment, 2029	Change, 2019–2029	
			Number	Percentage
Dietitians and nutritionists	74,200	80,100	5,900	8%

Data from Bureau of Labor Statistics. *Occupational Outlook Handbook.* U.S. Department of Labor; 2020.

Earnings

According to AND, the median annual wage for RDNs was $68,600 in 2019. The median annualized wages varied by practice area (**TABLE 13.3**). Those working in consultation and business earned the highest salary ($85,000), and clinical dietitians working in the community earned the lowest salaries ($60,000). Clinical dietitians working in outpatient settings and in long-term care earned around $67,500. Those in education and research—many with doctoral degrees—earned the highest salaries, $86,000.[1] Salaries also vary by years in practice, educational level, and geographic region.

Related Occupations

Workers in other occupations who have similar educational and job requirements are foodservice managers, health educators, dietetic technicians, rehabilitation counselors, and registered nurses.

DIETETIC TECHNICIANS
Significant Points

- Most jobs are in hospitals and long-term care including nursing care and assisted-living facilities and in foodservice management in these settings.

TABLE 13.3 Median Annual Wages in the Industries Employing the Largest Numbers of Dietitians and Nutritionists, 2019

Education and research	$86,000
Consultation and business	$85,000
Food and nutrition management	$81,200
Outpatient/ambulatory care	$67,000
Long-term care (nursing and assisted-living facilities)	$67,900
Inpatient (hospital)	$64.500
Community	$60,000

Data from Griswold K, Rogers D. Compensation and benefits survey 2019. *J Acad Nutr Diet.* 2020;120(3):448–464. doi:10.1016/j.jand.2019.12.015

- The Nutrition and Dietetic Technician, Registered (NDTR) needs at least an associate's degree; only the state of Maine requires licensure.
- Applicants with experience in foodservice management will enjoy the best job opportunities.

Work Description

A **Nutrition and Dietetic Technician, Registered (NDTR)** works as a member of the foodservice management and healthcare team, independently or in consultation with a registered dietitian. The NDTR works under the supervision of an RDN when conducting medical nutrition therapy as a part of nutrition care planning. In other settings, the NDTR does not necessarily work under the supervision of an RDN.[12] The NDTR supervises support staff, monitors cost-control procedures, interprets and implements quality assurance procedures, and screens patients/clients for nutritional risk. An NDTR helps supervise food production and service; plans menus; tests new products for use in the facility; and selects, schedules, and conducts orientation programs for personnel. The technician may also be involved in selecting personnel and providing on-the-job training. The NDTR obtains, evaluates, and uses diet histories to plan nutritional care for patients. Using this information, the technician guides families and individuals in selecting and preparing food and planning menus based on nutritional needs. In a clinical setting, the dietetic technician often monitors and documents calorie and protein intakes of patients or residents.

Work Environment

Most NDTRs work 40 hours per week. They may work weekends as well as early or late shifts depending on the facility in which they are employed. They spend some of their time in clean, well-lit, ventilated areas and some time in hot, steamy kitchens and serving areas. They may be on their feet for most of their working day and may be required to do some lifting.

Employment Opportunities

Job opportunities for NDTRs vary depending on the geographic area and the number of hospitals within that area. Job opportunities are available in hospitals, day care centers,

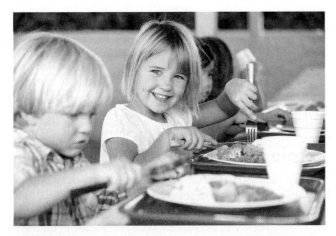

FIGURE 13.4 DTRs work in child care and school lunch programs.
© Monkey Business Images/Shutterstock.

restaurants, health clubs, WIC programs, Meals on Wheels programs, community health programs, and long-term care facilities. NDTRs also work in university foodservice operations, some commercial food establishments, correctional facilities, public schools, health clubs, weight management clinics, food companies, and contract food management companies (**FIGURE 13.4**).

Based on a 2019 survey conducted by the AND, 42% of dietetic technicians worked in hospitals, 20% worked in food and nutrition management, and 18% worked in community settings such as a WIC (women infants and children) nutritionist.[1] Depending on the size of the facility, NDTRs often are responsible for both clinical and foodservice management in long-term care facilities (**TABLE 13.4**).

Educational and Legal Requirements

The requirement for the NDTR is completion of at least an associate's degree, which includes clinical training and successful completion of the qualifying exam.

TABLE 13.4 Most Common Positions of Nutrition Dietetic Technicians, Registered, 2019

Dietetic technician, clinical	41%
Nutritionist, women, infants, and children	12%
Dietetic technician, foodservice management	10%
Dietetic technician, long-term care	8%
Director of food and nutrition services	5%

Modified from Griswold K, Rogers D. Compensation and benefits survey 2019. *J Acad Nutr Diet.* 2020;120 (3):448–464. doi:10.1016/j.jand.2019.12.015

Education and Training

Individuals interested in becoming an NDTR should expect to study a wide variety of topics focusing on foods, nutrition, food sanitation and safety, and management. These areas of study are supported by communication, and by the sciences: biological, physiological, behavioral, and social. Becoming a dietetic technician involves a combination of academic preparation and 450 hours of supervised practice culminating in, at minimum, an associate's degree in an institution sponsoring a program accredited by ACEND of AND. Clinical practice in both food service operations and clinical nutrition are required. Graduates from one of the 31 ACEND-accredited programs are eligible to take the CDR registration examination for dietetic technicians. In addition, graduates of a DPD program (usually with a bachelor's degree) who have completed 450 hours of supervised practice are eligible to take the registration exam to become an NDTR.[12]

Licensure

In 2020, Maine was the only state that recognized the NDTR as a licensed practitioner. In California, the law exempts NDTRs from licensure but specifies that the NDTR must work under the supervision of the RDN when providing medical nutrition therapy.[12]

Certification and Other Qualifications

NDTRs are certified by CDR and are required to complete 75 hours of continuing education every five years to maintain registration status. Another option for NDTRs who work in school lunch and child care programs is to become certified as a **School Nutrition Specialist (SNS)** through the School Nutrition Association. Requirements are an associate's degree, one year of work experience in the area of school or child care nutrition programs, and successfully completing the qualifying exam. Continuing education hours are required to maintain certification.[13]

Employment Trends

There were 30,200 NDTRs in 2019, with a projected growth rate of 6% between 2019 and 2029.[14] Growth rate for NDTRs is expected to be about as fast as average for all occupations through the year 2029 because of increased emphasis on disease prevention, a growing and aging population, and public interest in nutrition. NDTRs can expect to be employed in food service management in hospitals, school lunch programs, and long-term care facilities.

Earnings

According to AND, the median annual wage for NDTRs was $46,700 in 2019. The salary levels vary with region, employment setting, geographical location, scope of responsibility, and so on (**FIGURE 13.5**).[1]

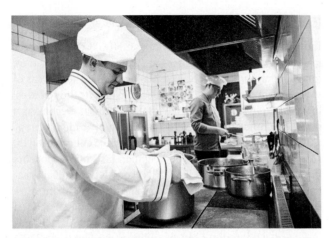

FIGURE 13.5 Salaries for NDTRs working in foodservice management can expect higher salaries than in other positions.
© Dmitry Kalinovsky/Shutterstock.

Related Occupations

Workers with duties similar to those of NDTR include associate's degree nurses, licensed practical nurses, and certified dietary managers.

DIETARY MANAGER
Significant Points

- Certified Dietary Managers (CDM) work primarily in long-term care facilities and hospitals and are responsible for foodservice operations.
- Certified Dietary Managers work in consultation with an RDN in tasks related to clinical dietetics, food preparation and service.

Work Description

The **Certified Dietary Manager (CDM)** is the third level among personnel involved in the provision of nutritional care. The CDM works in a variety of foodservice operations including hospitals, nursing homes and assisted-living facilities, schools, correctional facilities, and the military. In hospitals and long-term care facilities, the CDM works in cooperation with residents/patients, the RDN, physicians and other facility staff, and vendors. The CDM develops appropriate dietary plans in consultation with the RDN and in compliance with physicians' orders. In other settings, the CDM ensures that menus are planned to meet the nutrient needs of the population served and that proper sanitation and safety practices are followed in food preparation, service, and storage. The CDM manages all aspects of the foodservice operation—personnel management, budgeting, and cost control—while meeting the standards of local, state, and federal regulations.

Work Environment

According to a 2018 survey conducted by the **Association of Nutrition and Foodservice Professionals (ANFP)**, about 47% of dietary managers worked in skilled nursing facilities/nursing home care and 22% worked in hospitals.[15] The majority of CDMs work full time and often work weekends. Working as a foodservice manager requires physical stamina because much of the day is spent standing and moving from station to station in a hot kitchen as well as lifting heavy items.

Employment Opportunities

Dietary managers who are certified will have many opportunities as a food service supervisor in large facilities or as a foodservice director in smaller facilities or community feeding programs. The demand for CDMs is expected to increase as a result of the September 28, 2019, final ruling by the **Centers for Medicare and Medicaid Services (CMS)** regarding management of food and nutrition services in long-term care facilities. The ruling states that the facility must employ a qualified director of food and nutrition services—a person with CDM certification or an associate's degree graduate from a foodservice management program—when an RDN is employed either part time or as a consultant by the facility.[16]

Educational and Legal Requirements

The CDM works in noncommercial foodservice operations that require third-party oversight—**The Joint Commission** for hospitals and the CMS for nursing homes—as well as city and state health departments. These foodservice operations are in hospitals, nursing homes, schools, correctional facilities, and the military.[17]

Education and Training

There are several different pathways for becoming eligible to sit for the certification exam to become a Certified Dietary Manager. The ANFP lists over 100 approved educational programs in the United States in a variety of delivery formats from online to classroom based. Students with no college credits can expect to spend two semesters taking courses in foodservice management, human resource management, nutrition and medical nutrition therapy, and food safety/sanitation together with 150 hours of field experience in dietary management.[18] Educational programs may offer a fast track to certification for graduates with an associate's or bachelor's degree in foodservice management, nutrition, culinary arts, or hotel-restaurant management. Current and former members of the U.S. military who have graduated from an approved military dietary manager training program may also be eligible for certification.[17]

Licensure

CDMs are not required to be licensed; however, some state health departments regulate staffing requirements for long-term care and hospitals and require that the foodservice supervisor in these facilities be a CDM. For further clarification, contact the state health department.[19]

Certification and Other Qualifications

Requirements for maintaining certification are completion of 45 hours of continuing education every three years, including nine hours of sanitation and safety and one hour of professional ethics.[20]

Advancement

CDMs with education beyond certification requirements, either an associate's or bachelor's degree in food and nutrition or a graduate degree in business management, can expect to advance to higher levels of responsibility including director of food service.

Employment Change

The majority of CDMs belong to their professional organization—Association of Nutrition and Food Service Professionals (ANFP)—with a membership of 15,000. This number is expected to increase with the recent ruling by the CMS requiring foodservice directors in long-term care facilities and hospitals be certified. Nutrition and Dietetic Technicians, Registered (NDTRs) have similar training and job responsibilities in foodservice operations and may compete for the same positions as CDMs. RDNs may compete for positions in larger hospitals or continuing care communities.

Job Prospects

Those with the nationally recognized CDM credential are in demand due to regulatory requirements by both the federal and state governments. CDMs have the training and experience to supervise foodservice operations in long-term care facilities and hospitals.

Earnings

Foodservice managers earned an average salary of $53,116 according to a 2018 survey conducted by the ANFPA. Salaries increased with greater responsibility for other employees and larger budgets. Managers with CDM credentials earned more than those without the credential; those with a bachelor's or master's degree earned the highest salaries. Those employed by hospitals and continuing care communities also earned higher salaries.[15]

Related Occupations

Similar occupations are Nutrition and Dietetic Technicians, Registered (NDTRs), chefs, and hotel and restaurant managers.

Additional Information

For information about a career in dietetics, contact:

- Academy of Nutrition and Dietetics (AND), 120 South Riverside Plaza, Suite 2000, Chicago, IL 60606-6995. https://www.eatrightpro.org/about-us/become

For a list of academic programs to become either a registered dietitian or a dietetic technician, registered, contact:

- Accreditation Council for Education in Nutrition and Dietetics (ACEND), Academy of Nutrition and Dietetics, 120 South Riverside Plaza, Suite 2000, Chicago, IL 60606-6995. https://www.eatrightpro.org/acend/accredited-programs/about-accredited-programs

For information on taking the qualifying exam to become certified as a registered dietitian nutritionist or nutrition and dietetic technician, registered, contact:

- Commission on Dietetic Registration (CDR), Academy of Nutrition and Dietetics. 120 South Riverside Plaza, Suite 2000, Chicago, IL 60606-6995. https://www.cdrnet.org/

For information about becoming a board-certified specialist in dietetics, contact:

- Commission on Dietetic Registration (CDR), Academy of Nutrition and Dietetics. 120 South Riverside Plaza, Suite 2000, Chicago, IL 60606-6995. https://www.cdrnet.org/certifications/board-certified-specialist

For information on becoming a certified nutrition specialist (CNS), contact:

- American Nutrition Association, 211 West Chicago Ave., Suite 217, Hinsdale, IL 60521. https://theana.org/certify

For information about certification as a school nutrition specialist (SNS), contact:

- School Nutrition Association, 2900 S. Quincy St., Suite 700, Arlington, VA 22206. https://schoolnutrition.org/certificate-and-credentialing/credentialing-program/

For information on educational programs for dietary managers, contact:

- The Association of Nutrition and Foodservice Professionals, 406 surrey Woods Dr., St. Charles, IL 60174. https://www.anfponline.org

For information about certification as a dietary manager, contact:

- Certifying Board for Dietary Managers, 406 Surrey Woods Dr., St. Charles, IL 60174. https://www.cbdmonline.org/

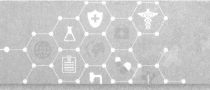

LEARNING PORTFOLIO

Issues for Discussion

1. Go to the website for the Academy of Nutrition and Dietetics to link to the fact sheets "Becoming an RDN" and "Becoming an NDTR" under the section for students. Compare the educational and professional requirements for each. Which career path would you prefer, and why? https://www.eatrightpro.org/acend/students-and-advancing-education/information-for-students

2. View the five-minute video "Exploring a Career in Dietetics" and the six-minute video "RDNs: The Passion to Create Positive Change" to learn about different careers in dietetics. Which of the careers described in the videos appeals to you? https://www.eatrightpro.org/about-us/become-an-rdn-or-dtr/high-school-students/exploring-a-career-in-dietetics; https://www.youtube.com/watch?v=oXVmXm2-WC8

3. Review NDTR videos to learn more about the career of the NDTR. Summarize the videos for your classmates. https://www.cdrnet.org/dtr-videos

4. Go to the Accreditation Council for Education in Nutrition and Dietetics (ACEND) website to review different internship programs. Which of the internships appeals to you? Are there internships where you now live? https://www.eatrightpro.org/acend/accredited-programs/accredited-programs-directory

5. Discuss different options for a graduate of a DPD program who didn't match for a dietetic internship to obtain the necessary supervised practice to be eligible to sit for the registration exam.

6. Compare the educational and certification requirements for the RDN, NDTR, and CDM by going to the Academy of Nutrition and Dietetics (AND) website (https://www.eatrightpro.org) and the Association of Nutrition & Food Service Professionals website (https://www.anfponline.org). List the professionals in order of the amount of education and training required from the least to the most.

Enrichment Activities

1. View bios of school foodservice directors to learn about their jobs. School Nutrition Association. *What It Means to Be a School Nutrition Professional* (not all are RDNs or NDTRs). http://schoolnutrition.org/school-meals/careers/what-it-means-to-be-a-school-nutrition-professional/

2. Review the two-minute video that explains different pathways to becoming a certified Dietary Manager/Certified Food Protection Professional. Describe at least four pathways to becoming a Certified Dietary Manager shown in the video. https://www.anfponline.org/become-a-cdm/cdm-cfpp-credential

3. Review the following YouTube videos to learn how to obtain certification as a dietary manager as well as different positions held by a Certified Dietary Manager.

- "Discover the Power of the CDM, CFPP Credential." https://www.youtube.com/watch?v=J32oq2ls6gU&t=4s
- "What It Means to Be a CDM, CFPP." https://www.youtube.com/watch?v=F-Ilny_DPpc

CASE STUDY: DIETETICS

Jill is a junior in high school and is interested in pursuing a career in food and nutrition. She has been active in the community organic garden at her high school and has taught cooking classes for middle school children. Jill would like to combine her interests in food and nutrition and teaching children about gardening and healthy eating as a career and is considering working in a school lunch program or hospital. She is researching the possibilities and has many questions.

The following questions relate to careers in food and nutrition. Please help Jill answer them based on what you have learned from this chapter.

1. What are the educational requirements for a registered dietitian nutritionist?
   A. One-year certification program
   B. Associate's degree
   C. Bachelor's degree
   D. Master's degree

2. Jill is interested in learning more about specializing in school food service. Which of the following professional organization offers certification as a school nutrition specialist (SNS)?
   A. Academy of Nutrition and Dietetics
   B. Association of Nutrition & Food Service Professionals
   C. School Nutrition Association
   D. American Nutrition Association

3. The median annual salary range for the registered dietitian nutritionist (RDN) is:
   A. $30,000 to $39,000
   B. $40,000 to $49,000
   C. $50,000 to $59,000
   D. $60,000 to $69,000

4. Two other career paths for Jill if she decides that she would prefer a shorter training program are _____ and _____
   _____.

LEARNING PORTFOLIO

References

1. Griswold K, Rogers D. Compensation and benefits survey 2019. *J Acad Nutr Diet.* 2020;*120*(1):448–464.

2. Accreditation Council for Education in Nutrition and Dietetics. *About Accredited Programs.* https://www.eatrightpro.org/acend/accredited-programs/about-accredited-programs Accessed July 2, 2020.

3. Accreditation Council for Education in Nutrition and Dietetics. *Dietetic Internship Match Students.* https://www.eatrightpro.org/acend/students-and-advancing-education/dietetic-internship-match-students Accessed July 2, 2020.

4. Commission on Dietetic Registration. Academy of Nutrition and Dietetics. *Individualized Supervised Pathways.* https://www.eatrightpro.org/acend/students-and-advancing-education/ispp-for-students Accessed July 2, 2020.

5. Accreditation Council for Education in Nutrition and Dietetics, *Rationale for Future Education Preparation of Nutrition and Dietetics Practitioners.* November 2017. http://www.eatrightpro.org/~/media/eatrightpro%20files/acend/futureeducationmodel/finalrationale.ashx Accessed July 2, 2020.

6. Commission on Dietetic Registration. 2024 *Graduate Degree Requirement-Registration Eligibility.* http://www.cdrnet.org/graduatedegree Accessed July 2, 2020.

7. Commission on Dietetic Registration. Academy of Nutrition and Dietetics. *Licensure and Professional Regulation.* https://www.eatrightpro.org/advocacy/licensure/professional-regulation-of-dietitians#state Accessed July 2, 2020.

8. American Nutrition Association. *What Is the CNS Credential?* https://theana.org/certify/CNScandidate Accessed July 2, 2020.

9. Commission on Dietetic Registration. Academy of Nutrition and Dietetics. *Board Certified Specialist Home.* https://www.cdrnet.org/certifications/board-certified-specialist Accessed July 2, 2020.

10. Certification Board for Diabetes Care and Education (CBDCE). *Eligibility.* https://www.cbdce.org/eligibility Accessed July 31, 2021.

11. The National Board of Nutrition Support Certification (NBNSC). *Why Certify?* http://www.nutritioncare.org/NBNSC/Certification/Certification_Main_Page/ Accessed July 2, 2020.

12. Commission on Dietetic Registration. Academy of Nutrition and Dietetics. *Becoming a Nutrition and Dietetics Technician, Registered.* https://www.eatrightpro.org/about-us/what-is-an-rdn-and-dtr/what-is-a-nutrition-and-dietetics-technician-registered/becoming-a-nutrition-dietetics-technician-registered Accessed July 2, 2020.

13. School Nutrition Association. *SNS Credentialing.* https://schoolnutrition.org/certificate-and-credentialing/credentialing-program/ Accessed July 31, 2021.

14. Bureau of Labor Statistics, U.S. Department of Labor, *Occupational Outlook Handbook, Data for Occupations Not Covered in Detail.* https://www.bls.gov/ooh/about/data-for-occupations-not-covered-in-detail.htm#Healthcare%20practitioners%20and%20technical%20occupations Accessed August 11, 2021.

15. Certifying Board for Dietary Managers. *Discover the Power of the Credential.* January 2020. https://www.cbdmonline.org/docs/default-source/legacy-docs/docs/careerguide.pdf?sfvrsn Accessed June 21, 2021.

16. Association of Nutrition & Foodservice Professionals. *CDM, CFPP Credential Meets New CMS LTC Requirement.* https://www.anfponline.org/docs/default-source/cbdm/cms-regulations-revised.pdf Accessed July 31, 2021.

17. Certifying Board for Dietary Managers. *Eligibility.* https://www.cbdmonline.org/get-certified/eligibility Accessed July 2, 2020.

18. Association of Nutrition and Foodservice Professionals. *ANFP Approved Training Programs.* https://www.anfponline.org/become-a-cdm/anfp-approved-programs Accessed July 31, 2021.

19. Association of Nutrition and Food Service Professionals. *State Regulations.* https://www.anfponline.org/news-resources/regulations/regulations Accessed July 31, 2021.

20. Certifying Board for Dietary Managers. *Maintaining Your Credentials.* https://www.cbdmonline.org/maintain-your-credentials/maintaining-your-credentials Accessed July 2, 2020.

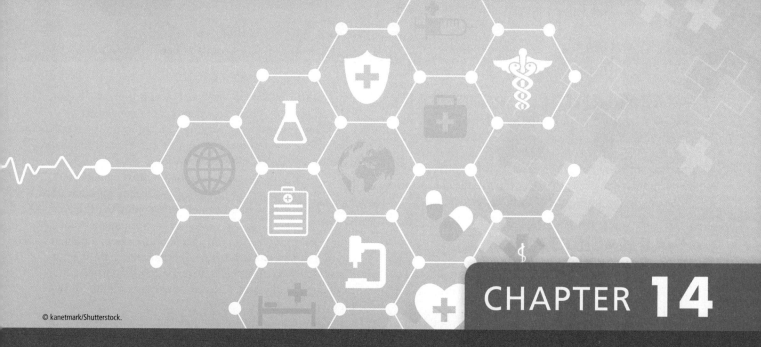

© kanetmark/Shutterstock.

CHAPTER **14**

Pharmacy*

* All information in this chapter, unless otherwise indicated, was obtained from Bureau of Labor Statistics. *Occupational Outlook Handbook 2020–2021 Edition*. Washington, DC: U.S. Department of Labor; 2021.

PHARMACEUTICAL PARTNERS

One of the main tools of physicians treating patients is medication. Medicines are prescribed to prevent, treat, and cure illnesses and diseases. Although doctors prescribe **pharmaceuticals**, the professionals who dispense the medication are pharmacists. The details of the pharmacist's profession follow in the rest of this chapter.

PHARMACISTS
Significant Points

- Pharmacists counsel patients and plan drug therapy programs.
- Pharmacists have direct patient contact in both clinical and retail settings.
- Earnings are relatively high, but some pharmacists are required to work nights, weekends, and holidays.
- Pharmacists must graduate from an accredited college of pharmacy and pass a series of examinations to be licensed.

WORK DESCRIPTION

Pharmacists advise health professionals and the public on the proper selection and use of medicines. The special knowledge of the pharmacist is needed because of the complexity and potential **side effects** of the large and growing number of pharmaceutical products on the market.

In addition to providing information, pharmacists dispense drugs and medicines prescribed by physicians, dentists, and other health professionals. Pharmacists must understand the use, composition, and effects of drugs and how they are tested for purity and strength. Because of the introduction of new medications and the complexity of these medications, pharmacists must engage in continuing education activities. **Compounding**—the actual mixing of ingredients to form powders, tablets, capsules, ointments, and solutions—is now only a small part of a pharmacist's practice, as most medicines are produced by pharmaceutical companies in the dosage and form used by the patient.

Pharmacists practicing in community or retail pharmacies have many duties. They counsel patients and answer questions about prescription drugs, such as those regarding possible adverse reactions or interactions. An example of a pharmacist explaining medication to a patient is shown in **FIGURE 14.1**. They provide information about over-the-counter drugs and make recommendations after asking a series of health questions, such as whether the customer is taking any other medications. Such pharmacists also give advice about durable medical equipment and home healthcare supplies. Pharmacists must work in coordination with insurance companies on behalf of the patient, completing and submitting necessary paperwork to ensure eligible medication costs are covered under the patient's insurance policy. Those pharmacists who own or manage community pharmacies may sell non-health-related merchandise, hire and supervise personnel, and oversee the general operation of the pharmacy.

Many pharmacists working in a community or retail setting are called upon by patients to provide patient care activities, such as immunizations and simple diagnostic tests, along with some forms of therapy management.[1] Pharmacy departments often make space for a private area way from the flow of customer traffic, allowing the pharmacist to meet with the customer to complete a medication review, provide a yearly flu shot, or assess a patient's blood pressure to determine the patient's health status. These specialized services help patients manage conditions such as diabetes, asthma, smoking cessation, or high blood pressure.

The widespread use of computers in community and retail settings allows pharmacists to create **medication profiles** for their customers. A medication profile is a computerized record of the customer's drug therapy. Pharmacists use these profiles to ensure that harmful drug interactions do not occur and to monitor a patient's compliance with the doctor's instructions by comparing how long it takes the patient to finish the drug against the recommended daily dosage.

Pharmacists in hospitals and clinics dispense medications and advise the medical staff on the selection and side effects of drugs. They may make sterile solutions, buy medical supplies, teach students majoring in health-related disciplines, and perform administrative duties. They also may be involved in patient education, monitoring of drug regimens, and drug use evaluation. In addition, pharmacists work as consultants to the medical team on drug therapy and patient care. In some hospitals, they make hospital rounds with physicians, talking to patients and monitoring pharmaceutical use. Their role is crucial to safe, efficient, and proper therapeutic care.

Not all clinical pharmacists work in a traditional hospital or clinic setting. Pharmacists who work in home health care monitor drug therapy and prepare infusions—solutions that are injected into patients—and other medications for use in the home.

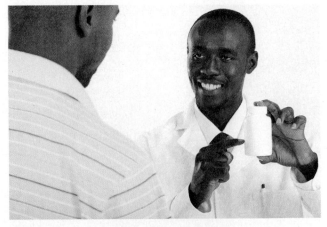

FIGURE 14.1 Pharmacist explaining medication to a patient.
© michaeljung/Shutterstock.

Pharmacotherapists specialize in drug therapy and work closely with physicians. They may make hospital rounds with physicians, talking to patients and monitoring pharmaceutical use.

Nutrition support pharmacists help determine and prepare the drugs needed for nutrition. Some pharmacists work in oncology (cancer) and psychiatric drug treatment.

Some pharmacists prepare and dispense radioactive pharmaceuticals. Called **radiopharmacists** or **nuclear pharmacists**, they apply the principles and practices of pharmacy and radiochemistry to produce radioactive drugs that are used for diagnosis and therapy.

Pharmaceutical industry pharmacists work in the sales, research and development, or marketing divisions of pharmaceutical companies. Because pharmacists understand patients and how patients use their medications, their insight is valuable to pharmaceutical companies. These pharmacists may work to develop new drugs, designing and running clinical trials to determine the safety and effectiveness of these new drugs. They may work to establish safety regulations and ensure quality control of the drugs manufactured by the pharmaceutical companies.

Pharmacists use their basic educational backgrounds in a host of federal and state positions. At the federal level, pharmacists hold staff and supervisory posts in the U.S. Public Health Service, the Veterans Administration, and the Food and Drug Administration and in all branches of the armed services. Certain of these posts provide commissioned officer status; others come under the heading of civil service.

State and federal boards are boards charged with regulating the practice of pharmacy to preserve and protect public health. These legal boards governing pharmacy practice usually employ pharmacists as full-time executive officers. One or more inspectors, frequently also pharmacists, serve each state. As state health agencies consolidate their purchases, pharmacists are often engaged as purchasers of medical and pharmaceutical supplies on a mass scale.

Nearly every state has an active pharmaceutical association that employs a full-time executive officer. This officer is usually a graduate of a college of pharmacy. Several national professional associations are also guided by pharmacists with an interest and special talent in organizational work.

Other pharmacists are engaged in highly specialized tasks. There are pharmacists in advertising, packaging, technical writing, magazine editing, and science reporting. Pharmacists with legal training serve as patent lawyers or as experts in pharmaceutical law. Pharmacists are found in U.S. space laboratories, aboard ships such as the *S.S. Hope*, and directing giant manufacturing firms.

Work Environment

Pharmacists usually work in clean, well-lit, and well-ventilated areas that resemble small laboratories. Shelves are lined with hundreds of different drug products. An example

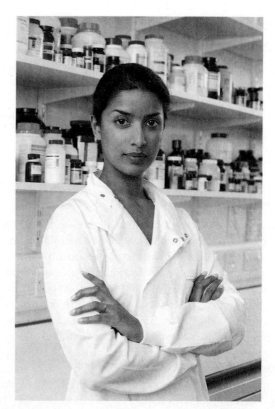

FIGURE 14.2 Pharmacist in pharmacy setting.
© bikeriderlondon/Shutterstock.

of a pharmacist in a pharmacy setting is shown in **FIGURE 14.2**. In addition, some items are refrigerated, and many substances (narcotics, depressants, and stimulants) are kept under lock and key. Pharmacists spend much time on their feet. When working with dangerous pharmaceutical products, pharmacists must take the proper safety precautions, such as wearing gloves and masks and working with special protective equipment.

Many community and hospital pharmacies are open around the clock, so pharmacists may be required to work nights, weekends, and holidays. **Consultant pharmacists** may travel to nursing homes or other facilities to monitor patients' drug therapy. Although most pharmacists work full time, some pharmacists work part time.

Employment Opportunities

Pharmacists held about 321,700 jobs in 2019. About 42% worked in retail settings, which include community pharmacies that were either independently owned or part of a drugstore chain, grocery store, department store, or mass merchandiser. Most of these community pharmacists were salaried employees, but some were self-employed owners. About 26% of pharmacists worked in hospitals. A small proportion worked in mail order and Internet pharmacies, pharmaceutical wholesalers, offices of physicians, and the federal government.

Educational and Legal Requirements

A license is required in all states, the District of Columbia, and all U.S. territories. In order to obtain a license, pharmacists must earn a Doctor of Pharmacy (PharmD) degree from a college of pharmacy and pass several examinations. There are 141 Doctor of Pharmacy programs fully accredited by the Accreditation Council for Pharmacy Education (ACPE) as of 2020.[2]

Education and Training

Pharmacists must earn a PharmD degree from an accredited college or school of pharmacy. The PharmD degree has replaced the Bachelor of Pharmacy degree, which is no longer being awarded. To be admitted to a PharmD program, an applicant must have completed at least two years of specific professional study. This requirement generally includes courses in mathematics and natural sciences, such as chemistry, biology, and physics, as well as courses in the humanities and social sciences. In addition, most applicants have completed three or more years at a college or university before moving on to a PharmD program, although this is not specifically required. Most PharmD programs require applicants to take the Pharmacy College Admissions Test (PCAT).[3] Many pharmacy schools also interview prospective students to determine their fit and enthusiasm for the pharmacy program. PharmD programs generally take four years to complete.

Courses offered at colleges of pharmacy are designed to teach students about all aspects of drug therapy. In addition, students learn how to communicate with patients and other healthcare providers about drug information and patient care. Students also learn professional ethics, concepts of public health, and medication distribution systems management. In addition to receiving classroom instruction, students in PharmD programs spend about one-fourth of their time in a variety of pharmacy practice settings under the supervision of licensed pharmacists.

Some colleges of pharmacy also award a Master of Science degree or PhD degree. Both degrees are awarded after the completion of a PharmD and are designed for those who want additional clinical, laboratory, and research experience. Areas of graduate study include **pharmaceutics** and **pharmaceutical chemistry** (physical and chemical properties of drugs and dosage forms), **pharmacology** (effects of drugs on the body), and **pharmacy administration**. Many master's and PhD degree holders go on to do research for a drug company or teach at a university.

Other options for pharmacy graduates who are interested in further training include one- or two-year residency programs or fellowships. Pharmacy residencies are postgraduate training programs in pharmacy practice and usually require the completion of a research project. These programs are often mandatory for pharmacists who wish to work in hospitals. Pharmacy fellowships are highly individualized programs designed to prepare participants to work in a specialized area of pharmacy, such as clinical practice or research laboratories. Some pharmacists who own their own pharmacy obtain a master's degree in business administration (MBA). Others may obtain a degree in public administration or public health.

Licensure

A license to practice pharmacy is required in all states, the District of Columbia, and all U.S. territories. To obtain a license, a prospective pharmacist must graduate from a college of pharmacy that is accredited by the ACPE and pass a series of examinations. All states, U.S. territories, and the District of Columbia require the North American Pharmacist Licensure Exam (NAPLEX), which tests pharmacy skills and knowledge.[4] The vast majority of states and the District of Columbia also require the Multistate Pharmacy Jurisprudence Exam (MPJE), which tests pharmacy law. Both exams are administered by the National Association of Boards of Pharmacy (NABP). Of the states and territories that do not require the MPJE, each has its own pharmacy law exam. In addition to the NAPLEX and MPJE, some states and territories require additional exams that are unique to their jurisdiction.

A pharmacist who wishes to specialize in an area of medical care may become certified from a national association as one who possesses an advanced level of knowledge in the respective area. For example, the Certification Board for Diabetes Educators may certify those pharmacists with advanced knowledge of diabetes.[5] Similarly, the Board of Pharmacy Specialties offers certification in specialty areas such as nutrition, oncology, critical care, and pediatrics.[6] These certification boards require varying degrees of work experience in addition to passing an exam and paying a fee.

All jurisdictions except California currently grant license transfers to qualified pharmacists who already are licensed by another jurisdiction. Many pharmacists are licensed to practice in more than one jurisdiction. Most jurisdictions require continuing education for license renewal. Those interested in a career as a pharmacist should check with individual jurisdiction boards of pharmacy for details on license renewal requirements and license transfer procedures.

Graduates of foreign pharmacy schools may also qualify for licensure in some U.S. states and territories. These individuals must apply for certification from the Foreign Pharmacy Graduate Examination Committee (FPGEC).[7] Once certified, they must pass the Foreign Pharmacy Graduate Equivalency Examination (FPGEE), Test of English as a Foreign Language (TOEFL) exam, and Test of Spoken English (TSE) exam. They then must pass all of the exams required by the licensing jurisdiction, such as the NAPLEX and MPJE.

Other Qualifications

Prospective pharmacists should possess scientific aptitude, good interpersonal skills, and a desire to help others. They also must be conscientious and pay close attention to detail, because the decisions they make affect human lives.

Advancement

In community pharmacies, pharmacists usually begin at the staff level. Pharmacists in chain drugstores may be promoted to pharmacy supervisor or manager at the store level, then to manager at the district or regional level, and later to an executive position within the chain's headquarters. Hospital pharmacists may advance to supervisory or administrative positions. After they gain experience and secure the necessary capital, some pharmacists become owners or part owners of independent pharmacies. Pharmacists in the pharmaceutical industry may advance into marketing, sales, research, quality control, production, or other areas.

Employment Trends

Employment is expected to decrease overall through 2029. As a result of job growth, the replacement of workers leaving the occupation, and the limited capacity of training programs, job prospects are mixed.

Employment Change

Employment of pharmacists is expected to decline by 3% between 2019 and 2029. Where a pharmacist works drives in part whether there is an increasing or decreasing need for a pharmacist. The advent of fulfilling prescriptions via mail order or online has decreased the demand for pharmacists working in retail settings. Some tasks previously performed by pharmacists in a retail setting, such as collecting patient information and preparing select medications, have been delegated to pharmacy technicians, allowing pharmacists to focus on patient care but lessening the need for as many pharmacists as before. Conversely, hospitals and clinics have seen a need to increase the number of pharmacists on their staffs and have asked pharmacists to assume some patient care tasks such as testing blood sugar or cholesterol.

The increasing numbers of middle-aged and older people—who use more prescription drugs than younger people—will continue to spur demand for pharmacists throughout the projection period. As the population ages, assisted-living facilities and homecare organizations should see particularly rapid growth. Other factors likely to impact the demand for pharmacists include scientific advances that will make more pharmaceutical products available, higher rates of chronic diseases, and increasing coverage of prescription drugs by health insurance plans and Medicare. Demand will also be impacted as cost-conscious insurers, in an attempt to improve preventive care, use pharmacists in areas such as patient education and the administration of vaccines.

Demand may increase in managed care organizations where pharmacists analyze trends and patterns in medication use and in **pharmacoeconomics**—the cost and benefit analysis of different drug therapies. New jobs also are being created in disease management—the development of new methods for curing and controlling diseases—and in sales and marketing. Rapid growth is also expected in *pharmacy informatics*—the use of information technology to improve patient care through medication use.

Job Prospects

The number of pharmacy schools has grown in recent years, producing a greater number of pharmacy school graduates. With larger graduating classes, there is more competition for pharmaceutical jobs. Students who choose to complete residency programs or certification from the Board of Pharmacy Specialists gain additional experience and greater job prospects. **TABLE 14.1** shows some projection data provided by the U.S. Department of Labor.

Earnings

The median annual wage and salary of pharmacists in May 2020 was $128,710. The lowest 10% earned less than $85,210, and the highest 10% earned more than $164,980 per year.

Related Occupations

Pharmacy technicians and pharmacy aides also work in pharmacies. Persons in other professions who may work with pharmaceutical compounds include biological scientists, medical scientists, chemists, and materials scientists. Increasingly, pharmacists are involved in patient care and therapy, work that they have in common with physicians and surgeons.

Additional Information

For information on pharmacy as a career, preprofessional and professional requirements, programs offered by colleges of pharmacy, and student financial aid, contact:

- American Association of Colleges of Pharmacy, 1400 Crystal Dr., Suite 300, Alexandria, VA 22202. https://www.aacp.org
- Accreditation Council for Pharmacy Education, 135 S. LaSalle Street, Suite 2850, Chicago, IL 60603-4810. https://www.acpe-accredit.org

TABLE 14.1 Projections Data for Pharmacists, 2019–2029

Occupational Title	Employment, 2019	Projected Employment, 2029	Change, 2019–2029	
			Number	Percentage
Pharmacists	321,700	311.200	-10,500	-3%

Data from Bureau of Labor Statistics. *Occupational Outlook Handbook.* U.S. Department of Labor; 2020.

General information on careers in pharmacy is available from:

- American Society of Health-System Pharmacists, 4500 East-West Highway, Suite 900, Bethesda, MD 20814. https://www.ashp.org
- National Association of Chain Drug Stores, 1776 Wilson Blvd., Suite 200, Arlington, VA 22209. https://www.nacds.org
- Academy of Managed Care Pharmacy, 675 North Washington St., Suite 220, Alexandria, VA 22314. https://www.amcp.org
- American Pharmacists Association, 2215 Constitution Ave., NW, Washington, DC 20037. https://www.pharmacist.com

Information on the North American Pharmacist Licensure Exam (NAPLEX) and the Multistate Pharmacy Jurisprudence Exam (MPJE) is available from:

- National Association of Boards of Pharmacy, 1600 Feehanville Dr., Mount Prospect, IL 60056. https://www.nabp.net

State licensure requirements are available from each state's board of pharmacy. Information on specific college entrance requirements, curricula, and financial aid is available from any college of pharmacy.

PHARMACY TECHNICIANS AND AIDES
Significant Points

- Job opportunities are expected to be good, especially for those with certification or previous work experience.
- Many technicians and aides work evenings, weekends, and holidays.
- About 51% of jobs are in a retail setting.

Work Description

Pharmacy technicians and aides help licensed pharmacists prepare prescription medications, provide customer service, and perform administrative duties within a pharmacy setting. **Pharmacy technicians** generally are responsible for receiving prescription requests, counting tablets, and labeling bottles, while **pharmacy aides** perform administrative functions such as answering phones, stocking shelves, and operating cash registers. In organizations that do not have aides, however, pharmacy technicians may be responsible for these clerical duties.

Pharmacy technicians who work in retail or mail-order pharmacies have various responsibilities, depending on state rules and regulations. Technicians receive written prescription requests from patients. They also may receive prescriptions sent electronically from doctors' offices, and in some states they are permitted to process requests by phone. They must verify that the information on the prescription is complete and accurate. To prepare the prescription, technicians retrieve, count, pour, weigh, measure, and sometimes mix the medication. Then they prepare the prescription labels, select the type of container, and affix the prescription and auxiliary labels to the container. Once the prescription is filled, technicians price and file the prescription, which must be checked by a pharmacist before it is given to the patient. Technicians may establish and maintain patient profiles as well as prepare insurance claim forms. They may organize inventory and alert the pharmacist to the need to restock medications or supplies. Technicians always refer any questions regarding prescriptions, drug information, or health matters to a pharmacist.

In hospitals, nursing homes, and assisted-living facilities, technicians have added responsibilities, including preparing sterile solutions and delivering medications to nurses or physicians. Technicians may also record the information about the prescribed medication in the patient's profile.

Pharmacy aides work closely with pharmacy technicians. They primarily perform administrative duties such as answering telephones, stocking shelves, and operating cash registers. They also may prepare insurance forms and maintain patient profiles. They may organize inventory and alert pharmacists to shortages in medications or supplies. Unlike pharmacy technicians, pharmacy aides do not prepare prescriptions or mix medications.

Work Environment

Pharmacy technicians and aides work in clean, organized, well-lit, and well-ventilated areas. Most of their workday is spent on their feet. They may be required to lift heavy boxes or to use stepladders to retrieve supplies from high shelves.

Technicians and aides often have varying schedules that include nights, weekends, and holidays. In facilities that are open 24 hours a day, such as hospital pharmacies, technicians and aides may be required to work nights. Many technicians and aides work part time.

Employment Opportunities

Pharmacy technicians and aides held about 461,200 jobs in 2019. Of these, about 422,300 were pharmacy technicians and about 38,900 were pharmacy aides. About 51% of jobs were in a retail setting, and about 17% were in hospitals.

Educational and Legal Requirements

There is no national training standard for pharmacy technicians, but employers favor applicants who have formal training, certification, or previous experience. There also are no formal training requirements for pharmacy aides, but a high school diploma may increase an applicant's prospects for employment.

Education and Training

There are no standard training requirements for pharmacy technicians, but some states require a high school diploma or its equivalent. Although most pharmacy technicians receive informal on-the-job training, employers favor those who have completed formal training and certification. On-the-job training generally ranges between 3 and 12 months. An example of on-the-job training is shown in **FIGURE 14.3**.

Formal technician education programs are available through a variety of organizations, including community colleges, vocational schools, hospitals, and the military. These programs range from six months to two years and include classroom and laboratory work. They cover a variety of subject areas, such as medical and pharmaceutical terminology, pharmaceutical calculations, pharmacy record keeping, pharmaceutical techniques, and pharmacy law and ethics. Technicians also are required to learn the names, actions, uses, and doses of the medications with which they work. Many training programs include **internships**, in which students gain hands-on experience in actual pharmacies. After completion, students receive a diploma, a certificate, or an associate's degree, depending on the program. The American Society of Health-System Pharmacists accredits pharmacy technician programs.[8]

There are no formal education requirements for pharmacy aides, but employers may favor applicants with a high school diploma or its equivalent. Experience operating a cash register, interacting with customers, managing inventory, and using computers may be helpful. Pharmacy aides also receive informal on-the-job training that generally lasts less than three months.

Certification and Other Qualifications

In most states, pharmacy technicians must be registered with the state board of pharmacy. Eligibility requirements vary, but in some states applicants must possess a high school diploma or its equivalent and pay an application fee.

Most states do not require technicians to be certified, but voluntary certification is available through several private organizations. The Pharmacy Technician Certification Board (PTCB)[9] and the National Healthcareer Association[10] administer national certification examinations. Certification through such programs may enhance an applicant's prospects for employment and is required by some states and employers. To be eligible for either exam, candidates must have a high school diploma or its equivalent and no felony convictions of any kind. In addition, applicants for the PTCB exam must not have had any drug-related or pharmacy-related convictions, including misdemeanors. Many employers will reimburse the cost of the exams.

Under these programs, technicians must be recertified every two years. Recertification requires 20 hours of continuing education within the two-year certification period. Continuing education hours can be earned from several different sources, including colleges, pharmacy associations, and pharmacy technician training programs. Up to 10 hours of continuing education also can be earned on the job under the direct supervision and instruction of a pharmacist.

Good customer service and communication skills are needed because pharmacy technicians and aides interact with patients, coworkers, and healthcare professionals. Basic mathematics, spelling, and reading skills also are important, as technicians must interpret prescription orders and verify drug doses. Technicians also must be precise: Details are sometimes a matter of life and death.

Advancement

Advancement opportunities generally are limited, but in large pharmacies and health systems, pharmacy technicians and aides with significant training or experience can be promoted to supervisory positions. Some may advance into specialty positions such as chemotherapy technician or nuclear pharmacy technician. Others may move into sales. With a substantial amount of formal training, some technicians and aides go on to become pharmacists.

Employment Trends

Employment is expected to grow about as fast as other occupations, and job opportunities are expected to be good.

Employment Change

Employment of pharmacy technicians and aides is expected to increase by 4% from 2019 to 2029, which is about as fast as the average for all occupations. The increased number of middle-aged and elderly people—who use more prescription drugs than younger people—will spur demand for pharmacy workers throughout the projection period. In addition, as scientific advances lead to new drugs and as more people obtain prescription drug coverage, pharmacy workers will be needed in growing numbers. Prescription drug coverage will continue to rise following the introduction of federally mandated health insurance.

Employment of pharmacy technicians is expected to increase by 4%. As cost-conscious insurers begin to use

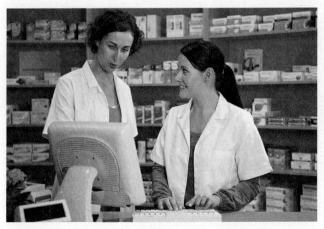

FIGURE 14.3 Pharmacist training a pharmacy technician.
© Robert Kneschke/Shutterstock.

TABLE 14.2 Projected Employment Data for Pharmacy Technicians, 2019–2029

Occupational Title	Employment, 2019	Projected Employment, 2029	Change, 2019–2029	
			Number	**Percentage**
Pharmacy technicians	422,300	437,600	15,200	9%

Data from Bureau of Labor Statistics. *Occupational Outlook Handbook*. U.S. Department of Labor; 2020.

pharmacies as patient-care centers and pharmacists become more involved in patient care, pharmacy technicians will continue to see an expansion of their role in the pharmacy. In addition, they will increasingly adopt some of the administrative duties that were previously performed by pharmacy aides, such as answering phones and stocking shelves. As a result of this development, demand for pharmacy aides should decrease.

Job Prospects

Job opportunities for pharmacy technicians are expected to be good, especially for those with previous experience, formal training, or certification. Job openings will result from employment growth as well as the need to replace workers who transfer to other occupations or leave the labor force.

Despite declining employment, job prospects for pharmacy aides also are expected to be good. As people leave this occupation, new applicants will be needed to fill the positions that remain (see **TABLE 14.2**).

Earnings

Median annual wages of pharmacy technicians in May 2020 were $35,100. The lowest 10% earned less than $25,400, and the highest 10% earned more than $50,430.

Median hourly wages of wage and salary pharmacy aides were $15.15 in May 2020. The middle 50% earned $29,280 annually. The lowest 10% earned less than $20.960 and the highest 10% earned more than $50,390 annually.

Certified technicians may earn more than noncertified technicians. Some technicians and aides belong to unions representing hospital or grocery store workers.

Related Occupations

Other occupations related to health care include dental assistants, medical assistants, medical records and health information technicians, medical transcriptionists, and pharmacists.

Additional Information

For information on pharmacy technician certification programs, contact:

- Pharmacy Technician Certification Board, 2215 Constitution Ave. NW, Suite 101, Washington DC 20037-2985. https://www.ptcb.org
- National Healthcareer Association, 11161 Overbrook Rd., Leawood, KS 66211. https://www.nhanow.com
- American Society of Health-System Pharmacists, 4500 East-West Highway, Suite 900, Bethesda, MD 20814. https://www.ashp.org

For pharmacy technician career information, contact:

- National Pharmacy Technician Association, P.O. Box 683148, Houston, TX 77268. https://www.pharmacytechnician.org

LEARNING PORTFOLIO

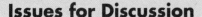

Issues for Discussion

1. Medications are sometimes expensive; for this reason, consumers sometimes look to online, out-of-country retailers to purchase medications at a lower price. Discuss what dangers may be present when buying medications from an online, out-of-country retailer. At minimum, address issues such as the possibility of purchasing counterfeit medications or whether the retailer possesses a legitimate license or certification.

2. Medications are accompanied by instructions on their use. Adhering to these instructions is sometimes problematic. Brainstorm reasons why patients might not adhere to these instructions and the effect failure to adhere to these instructions might have.

3. Which of the jobs discussed in this chapter would you be most likely to recommend to a friend or acquaintance interested in working in the healthcare field? Explain your selection and rationale.

Enrichment Activities

1. Using medicines to treat and prevent human disease has existed since ancient times. Search the Internet for examples of remedies that in today's time might seem odd or inappropriate for use. Prepare a list of such remedies and what the remedies were designed to treat, cure, or prevent. Share that list with your instructor and/or class.

2. Interest in using medicines to treat and prevent human disease has spanned many centuries. Create a timeline (as a written narrative piece, a poster, or an infographic) tracing the progression of pharmacy as a science and include the influence of the ancient Greeks and Romans, the Arabs, and those in the Renaissance. Name key players in the development of this field.

3. View the career videos titled "Inspiring Journeys" at https://www.careeronestop.org/videos/careeronestop -videos.aspx?videocode=29105100 and https://www .careeronestop.org/Toolkit/Careers/Occupations /occupation-profile.aspx?keyword=Pharmacy%20 Aides&onetcode=31909500&location=Arkansas& lang=en. Discuss your impressions of the variety of opportunities within the pharmacy profession with your instructor and classmates.

CASE STUDY: A PHARMACY CAREER

You are working as a pharmacy technician at a major drugstore chain. You have worked closely with the pharmacists over the past few years and studied hard for your pharmacy certification, which you earned last year. Your responsibilities have increased, and you are now able to take on an additional administrative duty. You enjoy the work and have decided to pursue a degree as a pharmacist once you have finished your first two years in college.

Based on the information you have read about pharmacists and pharmacy technicians as well as the case study, answer the following questions:

1. Identify the new administrative responsibility you have as a pharmacy technician.
   A. Consulting with a customer about a new prescription
   B. Completing the final review of the medication before dispensing it to the customer
   C. Taking inventory of the pharmacy stock in preparation for placing a drug order with the manufacturer
   D. Administering and documenting a flu shot given to a customer

2. Which national exam did you sit for to obtain your pharmacy technician credential?
   A. PTCE
   B. NAPLEX
   C. MPJE
   D. PCAT

3. Determine the undergraduate course that would best support your goal of becoming a pharmacist.
   A. History 101
   B. Geography 101
   C. Statistics 101
   D. Art Appreciation 101

4. Along with completing an application for pharmacy school, the next steps you will need to complete are to ____.
   A. prepare for an interview and sign up for classes
   B. take an entrance exam and choose your housing
   C. take an entrance exam and prepare for an interview
   D. call to see if you were accepted and sign up for classes

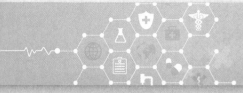

LEARNING PORTFOLIO

References

1. Get to Know Your Pharmacist, Centers for Disease Control and Prevention. https://www.cdc.gov/heartdisease/pharmacist.htm Accessed August 1, 2021.

2. Accreditation Council for Pharmacy Education. Pre-accredited and Accredited Professional Programs of Colleges and Schools of Pharmacy. https://www.acpe-accredit.org/pharmd-program-accreditation/ Accessed August 1, 2021.

3. Pharmacy College Admission Test. https://www.pearsonassessments.com/graduate-admissions/pcata/about.html Accessed August 1, 2021.

4. North American Pharmacist Licensure Examination. National Association of Boards of Pharmacy. https://www.napb.pharmacy/programs/examinations/naplex Accessed August 1, 2021.

5. Certification Board for Diabetes Care and Education. https://www.cbdce.org/ Accessed August 1, 2021.

6. Board of Pharmacy Specialties. https://www.bpsweb.org Accessed August 1. 2021.

7. Foreign Pharmacy Graduate Examination Committee. National Association of Boards of Pharmacy. https://nabp.pharmacy/programs/foreign-pharmacy/ Accessed August 1, 2021.

8. American Society of Health-Systems Pharmacists. Technician Program Accreditation. https://accreditation.ashp.org/directory/#/program/technician Accessed August 1, 2021.

9. Pharmacy Technician Certification Board. https://www.ptcb.org Accessed August 1, 2021.

10. National Healthcareer Association. Pharmacy Technician Certification. https://www.nhanow.com/nha-certifications/certified-pharmacy-technician-(cpht) Accessed August 1, 2021.

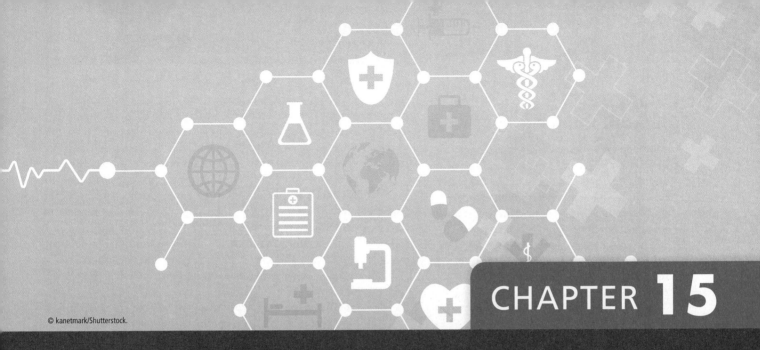

CHAPTER 15

Optometry*

KEY TERMS

Apprenticeship programs
Corrective lenses
Dispensing optician
Doctor of Optometry
Franchises
Health and visual sciences

Laser surgery
Lensometer
Low-vision rehabilitation
Ocular disease
Ophthalmic laboratory technician
Ophthalmologists

Optics
Optometrists
Optometry Admissions Test (OAT)
Vision therapy

* All information in this chapter, unless otherwise indicated, was obtained from Bureau of Labor Statistics. *Occupational Outlook Handbook 2020–2021 Edition.* Washington, DC: U.S. Department of Labor; 2021.

OPTOMETRISTS
Significant Points

- Admission to optometry school is competitive.
- Graduation from an accredited college of optometry and a state license administered by the National Board of Examiners in Optometry are required.
- Employment is expected to grow as fast as the average for all occupations.
- Because vision care needs attention for a growing and aging population, it is anticipated that the demand for optometrists will increase.
- Job opportunities are likely to be excellent.

WORK DESCRIPTION

Optometrists, also known as doctors of optometry, or ODs, are the main providers of vision care. They examine people's eyes to diagnose vision problems, such as nearsightedness and farsightedness, and they test patients' depth and color perception and ability to focus and coordinate the eyes (**FIGURE 15.1**). Optometrists may prescribe eyeglasses or contact lenses, or they may provide other treatments, such as **vision therapy** or **low-vision rehabilitation**.

Optometrists also test for glaucoma and other eye diseases and diagnose conditions caused by systemic diseases such as diabetes and high blood pressure, referring patients to other health practitioners as needed. They prescribe medication to treat vision problems or eye diseases, and some provide preoperative and postoperative care to cataract patients as well as to patients who have had corrective **laser surgery**. Like other physicians, optometrists encourage preventive measures by promoting nutrition and hygiene education to their patients to minimize the risk of eye disease and may refer patients to other healthcare practitioners when other diseases or disorders are present, such as diabetes or hypertension.

Although most work in a general practice as a primary care optometrist, some optometrists prefer to specialize in a particular field, such as contact lenses, geriatrics, pediatrics, or vision therapy. As a result, an increasing number of optometrists are forming group practices in which each group member specializes in a specific area while still remaining a full-scope practitioner. For example, an expert in low-vision rehabilitation may help legally blind patients by custom fitting them with a magnifying device that will enable them to read. Some may specialize in occupational vision, developing ways to protect workers' eyes from on-the-job strain or injury. Others may focus on sports vision, head trauma, or **ocular disease** and special testing. A few optometrists teach optometry, perform research, or consult.

Most optometrists are private practitioners who also handle the business aspects of running an office, such as developing a patient base, hiring employees, keeping paper and electronic records, and ordering equipment and supplies. Optometrists who operate franchise optical stores also may have some of these duties.

Optometrists should not be confused with **ophthalmologists** or **dispensing opticians**. Ophthalmologists are physicians who perform eye surgery as well as diagnose and treat eye diseases and injuries. Like optometrists, they also examine eyes and prescribe eyeglasses and contact lenses (**FIGURE 15.2**).

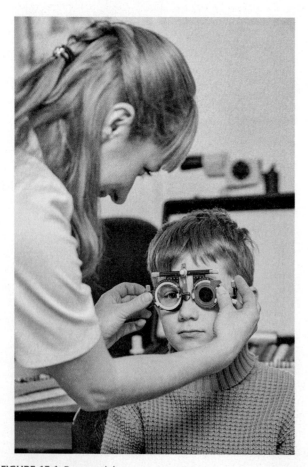

FIGURE 15.1 Boy receiving an eye exam.
© Dmitry Kalinovsky/Shutterstock.

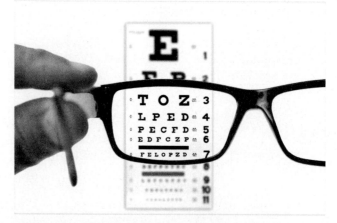

FIGURE 15.2 Optometrists, ophthalmologists, and dispensing opticians may all fit patients for contact lenses or glasses.
© CASTALDOstudio.com/Shutterstock.

Dispensing opticians fit and adjust eyeglasses and, in some states, may fit contact lenses according to prescriptions written by ophthalmologists or optometrists.

Work Environment

Optometrists usually work in their own offices, which are clean, well lit, and comfortable. Although most full-time optometrists work standard business hours, some work weekends and evenings to suit the needs of patients. Emergency calls, once uncommon, have increased with the passage of therapeutic-drug laws expanding optometrists' ability to prescribe medications.

Employment Opportunities

Optometrists held about 44,400 jobs in 2019. Salaried jobs for optometrists were primarily in offices of optometrists; offices of physicians, including ophthalmologists; and health and personal care stores, including optical goods stores. A few salaried jobs for optometrists were in hospitals, the federal government, or outpatient care centers, including health maintenance organizations. About 11% of optometrists are self-employed. A small number worked for optical chains or **franchises** or as independent contractors. According to the American Optometric Association, two-thirds of primary eye care in the United States is provided by optometrists.[1]

Educational and Legal Requirements

The **Doctor of Optometry** degree requires the completion of a four-year program at an accredited school of optometry, preceded by at least three years of pre-optometric study at an accredited college or university. All states require optometrists to be licensed.

Education and Training

Optometrists need a Doctor of Optometry degree, which requires the completion of a four-year program at an accredited school of optometry. In 2021, there were 25 colleges of optometry in the United States and one in Puerto Rico that offered programs accredited by the Accreditation Council on Optometric Education of the American Optometric Association.[2] Requirements for admission to optometry schools include college courses in English, mathematics, physics, chemistry, and biology. Because a strong background in science is important, many applicants to optometry school major in a science, such as biology or chemistry, as undergraduates. Other applicants major in another subject and take many science courses offering laboratory experience.

Admission to optometry school is competitive. All applicants must take the **Optometry Admissions Test (OAT)**, a standardized exam that measures academic ability and scientific comprehension.[3] The OAT consists of four tests: survey

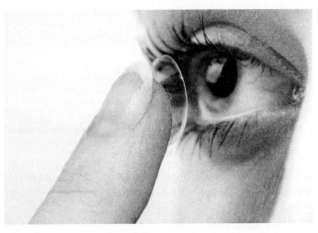

FIGURE 15.3 Postgraduate clinical residencies are available for optometrists wishing to specialize in one of several areas, such as cornea and contact lens care.
© abd/Shutterstock.

of the natural sciences, such as biology, general chemistry, and organic chemistry; reading comprehension; physics; and quantitative reasoning. As a result, most applicants take the test after their sophomore or junior year in college, allowing them an opportunity to take the test again and raise their score. A few applicants are accepted to optometry school after three years of college and complete their bachelor's degree while attending optometry school. Most students, however, have completed an undergraduate degree when accepted by a school or college of optometry. Each institution has its own undergraduate prerequisites, so applicants should contact the school or college of their choice for specific requirements.

Optometry programs include classroom and laboratory study of **health and visual sciences** and clinical training in the diagnosis and treatment of eye disorders. Courses in pharmacology, **optics**, vision science, biochemistry, and systemic diseases are included.

One-year postgraduate clinical residency programs are available for optometrists who wish to obtain advanced clinical competence within a particular area of optometry (**FIGURE 15.3**). Specialty areas for residency programs include family practice optometry, pediatric optometry, geriatric optometry, vision therapy and rehabilitation, low-vision rehabilitation, cornea and contact lenses, refractive and ocular surgery, primary eye care optometry, and ocular disease.

Licensure

All states and the District of Columbia require that optometrists be licensed. Applicants for a license must have a Doctor of Optometry degree from an accredited optometry school and must pass both a written national board examination and a national, regional, or state clinical examination. The written and clinical examinations of the National Board of Examiners in Optometry usually are taken during the student's academic career. Many states also require applicants to pass an additional clinical examination and an examination on relevant state laws. Licenses must be renewed every one to three years, and in all states, continuing education credits

TABLE 15.1 Projections Data for Optometrists, 2019–2029

Occupational Title	Employment, 2019	Projected Employment, 2029	Change, 2019–2029	
			Number	Percentage
Optometrists	44,400	46,300	1,900	4%

Data from Bureau of Labor Statistics. *Occupational Outlook Handbook.* U.S. Department of Labor; 2020.

are needed for renewal. Some optometrists decide to become board certified through the American Board of Optometry.

Other Qualifications

Business acumen, self-discipline, and the ability to deal tactfully with patients are important for success. The work of optometrists also requires attention to detail, manual dexterity, and decision-making skills.

Advancement

Optometrists who wish to teach or conduct research may study for a master's degree or PhD in visual science, physiological optics, neurophysiology, public health, health administration, health information and communication, or health education.

Employment Trends

Employment of optometrists is expected to grow as fast as average for all occupations through 2029 in response to the vision care needs of a growing and aging population. Excellent job opportunities are expected.

Employment Change

Employment of optometrists is projected to grow 4% between 2019 and 2029. A growing population that recognizes the importance of good eye care will increase demand for optometrists. Also, an increasing number of health insurance plans that include vision care should generate more job growth.

As the population ages, there will likely be more visits to optometrists and ophthalmologists because of the onset of vision problems that occur at older ages, such as cataracts, glaucoma, and macular degeneration. In addition, increased incidences of diabetes and hypertension in the general population as well as in the elderly will generate greater demand for optometric services as these diseases often affect eyesight.

Employment of optometrists would grow more rapidly if not for productivity gains that are expected to allow each optometrist to see more patients. These expected gains stem from the greater use of optometric assistants and other support personnel, who can reduce the amount of time optometrists need with each patient.

The increasing popularity of laser surgery to correct some vision problems was previously thought to have an adverse effect on the demand for optometrists as patients often do not require eyeglasses afterward. Optometrists will still be needed, however, to provide preoperative and postoperative care for laser surgery patients; therefore, laser eye surgery will likely have little to no impact on the employment of optometrists.

Job Prospects

Excellent job opportunities are expected over the next decade because there are only 26 schools of optometry in the United States, including Puerto Rico, resulting in a limited number of graduates each year. The number of graduates is not expected to keep pace with demand. Admission to optometry school is competitive.

In addition to job growth, the need to replace optometrists who retire will also create many employment opportunities. As these optometrists begin to retire, many opportunities will arise, particularly in individual and group practices. **TABLE 15.1** shows some projection for job growth for optometrists.

Earnings

Median annual wages of salaried optometrists were $118,050 in May 2020. The lowest 10% earned less than $60,750, and the highest 10% earned more than $195,810.

Benefits differ by employment setting. Self-employed optometrists must provide their own benefits. Practitioners associated with optical chains typically enjoy paid vacation, sick leave, and pension contributions.

Median annual wages in the industries employing the largest numbers of optometrists in May 2020 are shown in **TABLE 15.2**.

Related Occupations

Other workers who apply scientific knowledge to prevent, diagnose, and treat disorders and injuries include chiropractors, dentists, physicians and surgeons, podiatrists, psychologists, and veterinarians.

Additional Information

For information on optometry as a career and a list of accredited optometric institutions of education, contact:

- Association of Schools and Colleges of Optometry, 6110 Executive Blvd., Suite 420, Rockville, MD 20852. https://optometriceducation.org/

TABLE 15.2 Median Annual Earnings in the Industries Employing the Largest Numbers of Optometrists, May 2020	
Health and personal care stores	$120,060
Offices of physicians	$124,600
Offices of optometrists	$112,190

Data from Bureau of Labor Statistics. *Occupational Outlook Handbook.* U.S. Department of Labor; 2020.

Additional career information is available from:

- American Optometric Association, Educational Services, 243 N. Lindbergh Blvd., St. Louis, MO 63141. http://www.aoa.org

Additional information on becoming board certified is available from:

- American Board of Optometry, 243 N. Lindbergh Blvd., St. Louis, MO 63141. https://americanboardofoptometry.org/

The board of optometry in each state can supply information on licensing requirements. For information on specific admission requirements and sources of financial aid, contact the admissions officers of individual optometry schools.

OPTICIAN, DISPENSING
Significant Points

- Employers increasingly prefer dispensing opticians to complete certification or graduate from an accredited two-year associate's degree program in opticianry; some large employers may provide an apprenticeship.
- About half of states require a license to practice.
- Employment growth is projected to be as fast as the average for all occupations and reflect the steady demand for corrective lenses and fashionable eyeglass frames.
- Job opportunities are likely to be very good.

Work Description

Helping people see better and look good at the same time is the job of a dispensing optician. Dispensing opticians help select and fit eyeglasses and contact lenses for people with eye problems, following prescriptions written by ophthalmologists or optometrists. These selections are made to meet customer expectations, whether for a special need such as sports or an occupation or for routine vision needs. Dispensing opticians recommend eyeglass frames, lenses, and lens coatings after considering the prescription and the customer's occupation, habits, and facial features (**FIGURE 15.4**). When fitting new eyeglasses, opticians use sophisticated diagnostic instruments to measure various characteristics of a client's eyes, including the thickness, width, curvature,

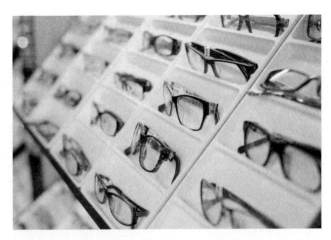

FIGURE 15.4 Dispensing opticians assist people with corrective lenses and frames.
© Ikonoklast Fotografie/Shutterstock.

and surface topography of the cornea. They also obtain a customer's prescription history to remake eyeglasses or contact lenses, or they may verify a prescription with the examining optometrist or ophthalmologist.

Dispensing opticians prepare work orders that give ophthalmic laboratory technicians the information they need to grind and insert lenses into a frame. The work order includes prescriptions for lenses and information on their size, material, color, and style. Some dispensing opticians grind and insert lenses themselves. They may also apply tint to lenses. After the glasses are made, dispensing opticians verify that the lenses meet the specifications, and then they may reshape or bend the frames with pliers for a custom fit.

Many opticians also spend time fixing and refitting broken frames as well as instructing clients about wearing or caring for eyeglasses. Additionally, administrative duties have become a major part of their work, including keeping records on customers' prescriptions, work orders, and payments and tracking inventory and sales.

Some dispensing opticians, after additional education and training, specialize in fitting contacts, artificial eyes, or cosmetic shells to cover blemished eyes. To fit contact lenses, dispensing opticians measure the shape and size of the eye, select the type of contact lens material, and prepare work orders specifying the prescription and lens size. Dispensing opticians observe customers' eyes, corneas, lids, and contact lenses with sophisticated instruments and microscopes. During several follow-up visits, opticians teach the proper insertion, removal, and care of contact lenses.

Work Environment

Dispensing opticians work indoors, mainly in medical offices, optical stores, or large department or club stores. Opticians spend a fair amount of time on their feet. If they prepare lenses, they need to take precautions against the hazards of glass cutting, chemicals, and machinery. Although most dispensing opticians work during regular business hours, those in retail stores may work evenings and weekends. Some work part time.

Employment Opportunities

Dispensing opticians held about 73,800 jobs in 2019. About 41% worked in optometrists' offices. Another 29% worked in health and personal care stores, including optical goods stores. Many of these stores offer one-stop shopping where customers can have their eyes examined, choose frames, and have glasses made on the spot. Some opticians work in optical departments of department stores or other general merchandise stores, such as warehouse clubs and superstores. About 10% worked in offices of physicians, primarily ophthalmologists, who sell glasses directly to patients; 3% were self-employed and ran their own businesses.

Educational and Legal Requirements

Many employers increasingly prefer dispensing opticians to complete certification or graduate from an accredited two-year associate's degree program in opticianry; some large employers may provide an apprenticeship that may last two years or longer.

Education and Training

Although a high school diploma is all that is required to enter this occupation, most workers have completed at least some college courses or a degree. Classes in physics, basic anatomy, algebra, and trigonometry as well as experience with computers are particularly valuable. These classes prepare dispensing opticians to learn job skills, including optical mathematics, optical physics, and the use of precision measuring instruments and other machinery and tools.

Structured **apprenticeship programs** are more commonly available in states where licensing is not mandatory, and these programs are usually offered by large employers. Apprentices receive technical instruction along with training in office management and sales. Under the supervision of an experienced optician, optometrist, or ophthalmologist, apprentices work directly with patients, fitting eyeglasses and contact lenses.

Formal training in the field is offered in community colleges and in a few four-year colleges and universities. As of 2021, the Commission on Opticianry Accreditation accredited 18 associate's degree and certificate programs in 13 states.[4] Graduation from an accredited program in opticianry can be advantageous as it provides a nationally recognized credential.

Licensure

As of 2021, about half of the states require dispensing opticians to be licensed. States may require individuals to pass one or more of the following for licensure: a state practical examination, a state written examination, and certification examinations offered by the American Board of Opticianry (ABO) and the National Contact Lens Examiners (NCLE). To qualify for the examinations, states often require applicants to complete postsecondary training or work as apprentices for two to four years.

Another avenue to licensure is to complete an apprenticeship program. As of 2021, 12 states have recognized the Ophthalmic Career Progression Program (OCPP), operated by the National Academy of Opticianry.[5] These apprentice programs are designed for individuals who are already working in the field.

Some states allow graduates of opticianry programs to take the licensure exam immediately upon graduation; others require a few months to a year of experience. Continuing education is commonly required for licensure renewal. Information about specific licensing requirements is available from the state board of occupational licensing.

Certification

Any optician can apply to the ABO and the NCLE for certification of their skills. Certification signifies to customers and employers that an optician has a certain level of expertise. Certification must be renewed every three years through continuing education.

Other Qualifications

Dispensing opticians deal directly with the public, so they should be tactful, pleasant, and able to communicate well. Fitting contact lenses requires considerable skill, care, and patience, so manual dexterity and the ability to do precision work are essential.

Advancement

Some experienced dispensing opticians open their own optical stores. Others become managers of optical stores or sales representatives for wholesalers or manufacturers of eyeglasses or lenses.

Employment Trends

Employment of dispensing opticians is expected to grow as fast as the average for all occupations through 2029, as the population ages and demand for **corrective lenses** increases. Very good job prospects are expected.

Employment Change

Employment in this occupation is expected to rise 4% over the 2019–2029 decade. Middle age is a time when many individuals use corrective lenses for the first time, and elderly people generally require more vision care than others. As the share of the population in these older age groups increases and as people live longer, more opticians will be needed to provide service to them. In addition, awareness of the importance of regular eye exams is increasing across all age groups, especially children and those older than

TABLE 15.3 Projections Data for Dispensing Opticians, 2019–2029

Occupational Title	Employment, 2019	Projected Employment, 2029	Change, 2019–2029	
			Number	Percentage
Opticians, dispensing	73,800	76,800	3,000	4%

Data from Bureau of Labor Statistics. *Occupational Outlook Handbook*. U.S. Department of Labor; 2020.

65 years of age. Recent trends indicate a movement toward a "low-vision" society, where a growing number of people view things that are closer in distance, such as computer monitors, over the course of an average day. This trend is expected to increase the need for eye care services. Fashion also influences demand. Frames come in a growing variety of styles, colors, and sizes, encouraging people to buy more than one pair.

Somewhat moderating the need for optician services is the increasing use of laser surgery to correct vision problems. Although the surgery remains relatively more expensive than eyewear, patients who successfully undergo this surgery may not require glasses or contact lenses for several years. Also, new technology is allowing workers to make the measurements needed to fit glasses, therefore allowing dispensing opticians to work faster and limiting the need for more workers.

Job Prospects

Overall, the need to replace dispensing opticians who retire or leave the occupation will result in very good job prospects. Employment opportunities for opticians in offices of ophthalmologists—the largest employer—will be particularly good as an increasing number of ophthalmologists are expected to utilize better-trained opticians to handle more tasks, allowing ophthalmologists to see more patients.

Job opportunities also will be good at general merchandise stores because this segment is expected to experience much faster than average growth as well as high turnover because of less favorable working conditions, such as long hours and mandatory weekend shifts.

Nonetheless, the number of job openings overall will be somewhat limited because the occupation is small. Also, dispensing opticians are vulnerable to changes in the business cycle because eyewear purchases often can be deferred for a time. Job prospects will be best for those who have certification and those who have completed a formal opticianry program. Job candidates with extensive knowledge of new technology, including new refraction systems, framing materials, and edging techniques, should also experience favorable conditions. **TABLE 15.3** shows some projections for employment.

Earnings

Median annual wages of dispensing opticians were $38,530 in May 2020. The lowest 10% earned less than $26,080, and the highest 10% earned more than $62,180. Median annual

TABLE 15.4 Median Annual Earnings in the Industries Employing the Largest Numbers of Dispensing Opticians, May 2020

Health and personal care stores	$37,360
Offices of physicians	$43,180
Offices of optometrists	$36,800

Data from Bureau of Labor Statistics. *Occupational Outlook Handbook*. U.S. Department of Labor; 2020.

wages in the industries employing the largest numbers of dispensing opticians in May 2020 are shown in **TABLE 15.4**.

Benefits for opticians are generally determined by the industries in which they are employed. In general, those who work part time or in small retail shops have fewer benefits than those who may work for large optical chains or department stores. Self-employed opticians must provide their own benefits.

Related Occupations

Other workers who deal with customers and perform delicate work include jewelers and precious stone and metal workers, ophthalmic laboratory technicians, and orthotists and prosthetists.

Additional Information

To learn about apprenticeship programs and state licensing requirements, contact:

- Opticians Association of America, 4064 E. Fir Hill Dr., Lakeland, TN 38002. https://www.oaa.org
- National Academy of Opticianry, 8401 Corporate Dr., Suite 605, Landover, MD 20785. https://www.nao.org

To learn about voluntary certification for opticians who fit eyeglasses as well as a list of state licensing boards for opticians, contact:

- American Board of Opticianry, 217 North Upper St., Suite 201, Lexington, KY 40507. https://www.abo-ncle .org/

For information on voluntary certification for dispensing opticians who fit contact lenses, contact:

- National Contact Lens Examiners, 217 North Upper St., Suite 201, Lexington, KY 40507. https://www .abo-ncle.org

For a list of associate's degree and certificate programs accredited by the Commission on Opticianry Accreditation, contact:

- National Federation of Opticianry Schools, 236 East Main St. #183, Sevierville, TN 37862. https://www.nfos.org
- Commission on Opticianry Accreditation, One Dupont Circle NW, Suite 510, Washington, DC 20036-1135. http://www.coaccreditation.com

OPHTHALMIC LABORATORY TECHNICIANS
Significant Points

- Most technicians learn their craft on the job, but many employers prefer to hire those with formal training.
- Job opportunities should be favorable because few people seek these positions.

Work Description

When patients require a medical device to help them see clearly, their healthcare providers send requests for such devices to **ophthalmic laboratory technicians**. These technicians produce a variety of implements to help patients.

Ophthalmic laboratory technicians—also known as manufacturing opticians, optical mechanics, or optical goods workers—make prescription eyeglasses or contact lenses. Prescription lenses are curved in such a way that light is correctly focused onto the retina of the patient's eye, improving vision. Some ophthalmic laboratory technicians manufacture lenses for other optical instruments, such as telescopes and binoculars. Ophthalmic laboratory technicians cut, grind, edge, and finish lenses according to specifications provided by dispensing opticians, optometrists, or ophthalmologists and may insert lenses into frames to produce finished glasses. Although some lenses still are produced by hand, technicians are increasingly using automated equipment to make lenses.

Ophthalmic laboratory technicians should not be confused with workers in other vision care occupations. Ophthalmologists and optometrists are "eye doctors" who examine eyes, diagnose and treat vision problems, and prescribe corrective lenses. Ophthalmologists are physicians who also perform eye surgery. Dispensing opticians assist customers in selecting eyewear and prepare work orders for ophthalmic laboratory technicians.

Ophthalmic laboratory technicians read prescription specifications, select standard glass or plastic lens blanks, and then mark them to indicate where the curves specified on the prescription should be ground. They place the lens in the lens grinder, set the dials for the prescribed curvature, and start the machine. After a minute or so, the lens is ready to be "finished" by a machine that rotates it against a fine abrasive to grind it and smooth out rough edges. The lens is then placed in a polishing machine with an even finer abrasive to polish it to a smooth, bright finish.

Next, the technician examines the lens through a **lensometer**, an instrument similar in shape to a microscope, to make certain the degree and placement of the curve are correct. The technician then cuts the lenses and bevels the edges to fit the frame, dips each lens into dye if the prescription calls for tinted or coated lenses, polishes the edges, and assembles the lenses and frame parts into a finished pair of glasses.

In small laboratories, technicians usually handle every phase of the operation. In large ones, in which virtually every phase of the operation is automated, technicians may be responsible for operating computerized equipment. Technicians also inspect the final product for quality and accuracy.

Work Environment

Ophthalmic laboratory technicians generally work in clean, well-lit, and well-ventilated laboratories. They have limited contact with the public. Salaried laboratory technicians usually work 40 hours a week, but some work part time. At times, technicians wear goggles to protect their eyes, gloves to handle hot objects, or masks to avoid inhaling dust. They may spend a great deal of time standing.

Employment Opportunities

Ophthalmic laboratory technicians held about 30,200 jobs in 2019. Many of the salaried jobs were in medical equipment and supply manufacturing laboratories, which usually are small, privately owned businesses with fewer than five employees. Some laboratories, however, are large; a few employ more than 1,000 workers. Others worked in health and personal care stores, optometrists' offices, and professional and commercial equipment and supplies merchant wholesalers.

Educational and Legal Requirements

Most ophthalmic laboratory technicians learn their craft on the job; many employers, however, prefer to hire those with formal training or at least a high school diploma.

Education and Training

High school students interested in becoming ophthalmic laboratory technicians should take courses in science, mathematics, computer programming, and art. Ophthalmic laboratory technicians usually begin as helpers and gradually learn new skills as they gain experience.

TABLE 15.5 Projection Data for Ophthalmic Laboratory Technicians, 2019–2020

Occupational Title	Employment, 2019	Projected Employment, 2029	Change, 2019–2029	
			Number	Percentage
Ophthalmic laboratory technicians	30,200	32,500	2.300	8%

Data from Bureau of Labor Statistics. *Occupational Outlook Handbook.* U.S. Department of Labor; 2020.

Ophthalmic laboratory technicians start on simple tasks if they are training to produce lenses by hand. They may begin with marking or blocking lenses for grinding and progress to grinding, cutting, edging, and beveling lenses and finally to assembling the eyeglasses. Depending on individual aptitude, it may take up to six months to become proficient in all phases of the work.

Employers filling trainee jobs prefer applicants who are high school graduates. Courses in science, mathematics, and computer science are valuable; manual dexterity and the ability to do precision work are essential. Technicians using automated systems will find computer skills valuable.

A few ophthalmic laboratory technicians learn their trade in the armed forces or in the few programs in optical technology offered by vocational-technical institutes or trade schools. In 2021, there were five programs in ophthalmic technology accredited by the Commission on Opticianry Accreditation (COA).[6]

Other Qualifications

Ophthalmic laboratory technicians need a high degree of manual dexterity, good vision, and the ability to recognize very fine color shadings and variations in shape. An artistic aptitude for detailed and precise work also is important.

Certification and Advancement

In large ophthalmic laboratories, technicians may become supervisors or managers. Some become dispensing opticians, although further education or training generally is required in that occupation.

Employment Trends

Overall, faster-than-average growth is expected for employment of ophthalmic laboratory technicians but varies by detailed occupation. Job opportunities should be favorable because few people seek these positions.

Employment Change

Ophthalmic laboratory technicians are expected to experience employment growth of 8%, faster than the average for all occupations. Demographic trends make it likely that many more Americans will need vision care in the years ahead. Not only will the population grow, but also the proportion of middle-aged and older adults is projected to increase rapidly. Middle age is a time when many people use corrective lenses for the first time, and elderly people usually require more vision care than others. The increasing use of automated machinery, however, will temper job growth for ophthalmic laboratory technicians.

Job Prospects

Job opportunities for ophthalmic laboratory technicians should be favorable due to expected faster-than-average growth. Those with formal training in an ophthalmic laboratory technology program will have the best job prospects. In addition to openings from job growth, many job openings also will arise from the need to replace technicians who transfer to other occupations or who leave the labor force. **TABLE 15.5** shows some projection data provided by the U.S. Department of Labor.

Earnings

Median annual earnings of wage and salary ophthalmic laboratory technicians were $34,440 in May 2020. The lowest 10% earned less than $25,770, and the highest 10% earned more than $63,910. The annual mean wage was $39,300 in medical equipment and supplies manufacturing, $32,730 in optometrist offices, and $32,880 in health care and personal stores, the three industries that employ the most ophthalmic laboratory technicians.

Related Occupations

Ophthalmic laboratory technicians manufacture and work with the same devices that are used by dispensing opticians, orthotists, prosthetists, and medical and ophthalmic laboratory technicians. Other occupations that work with or manufacture goods using similar tools and skills are precision instrument and equipment repair, and textile, apparel, and furnishings occupations.

Additional Information

For information on an accredited programs in ophthalmic laboratory technology, contact:

- Commission on Opticianry Accreditation, One Dupont Circle NW, Suite 510, Washington, DC 20036-1135. http://www.coaccreditation.com

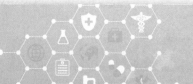

LEARNING PORTFOLIO

Issues for Discussion

1. Many schools offer vision screenings to their students as a way to identify previously undetected vision problems. By contrast, comprehensive eye exams fully evaluate eye health and vision. Review the content found in the American Optometry Association website on this subject (https://www.aoa.org/patients-and-public/caring-for-your-vision/comprehensive-eye-and-vision-examination/limitations-of-vision-screening-programs?sso=y), and discuss the differences and similarities between a vision screening and a comprehensive eye exam.

2. In your opinion, what is the most important responsibility of an optometrist? Explain why you feel this is most important.

3. Many individuals needing to correct vision acuity problems must decide between contact lenses and eyeglasses. Review the content found at https://www.allaboutvision.com/contacts/faq/contacts-vs-glasses.htm, which discusses the pros and cons of contact lenses and eyeglasses. If money was not an issue, decide whether you would want contact lenses or eyeglasses.

4. Lasik surgery is used to correct vision in people so that they no longer need to wear eyeglasses or contact lenses. More information about Lasik surgery can be found at https://www.webmd.com/eye-health/lasik-laser-eye-surgery. Do you think Lasik technology is a good thing for the optometry field? Why or why not?

Enrichment Activities

1. Lions Club International sponsors collection drives to recycle eyeglasses and send them to those in need in developing countries. Visit the Lions Club website on this subject: https://www.lionsclubs.org/en/resources-for-members/resource-center/recycle-eyeglasses. On your own or as part of a team of students, set up an eyeglass recycling program at your school. Report on the success of your program to your instructor and class.

2. Write a short skit that documents a professional interaction between an optometrist and another person. The other person can be a client or another employee. Use the skit to document your knowledge about some aspect of this profession.

3. Read the blog post titled "Optometry: An Inspired Career Choice" at https://optometriceducation.org/2015/09/24/optometry-an-inspired-career-choice/. Discuss with your instructor and classmates whether the content of the blog is helpful to someone deciding on a career as an optometrist.

CASE STUDY: EYE CARE PROFESSIONALS

Sorina has an appointment scheduled for today with a new eye care provider. She has questions regarding "who is who" in the office.

Based on the information you have read about optometry, answer the following questions:

1. The _____ performs Sorina's complete eye exam.

2. The _____ tests Sorina for glaucoma and other eye diseases.

3. The _____ writes Sorina's prescription for glasses.

4. The _____ helps Sorina find glasses that are stylish and comfortable and help her to see better.

5. The _____ helps Sorina select and fit her eyeglasses.

6. True or False? If Sorina needs to have surgery on her eyes to improve her vision, it will most likely be performed by the optometrist.

7. True or False? Sorina needs her glasses adjusted because they slide down her nose and are not comfortable. The receptionist tells her she needs to see the dispensing optician to make the needed adjustments.

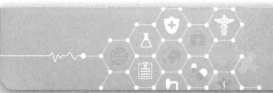

LEARNING PORTFOLIO

References

1. American Optometric Association. About the AOA. https://www.aoa.org/about-the-aoa?sso=y Accessed August 1, 2021.

2. Council on Optometric Education of the American Optometric Association. Accredited Professional Optometric Degree Programs. https://www.aoa.org/AOA/Documents/Education/ACOE/od_directory_%202020_12_01.pdf Accessed August 1, 2021.

3. Association of Schools and College of Optometry. Optometry Admission Test. https://www.ada.org/en/oat Accessed August 1, 2021.

4. Commission on Opticianry Accreditation. Degree Programs. http://coaccreditation.com/directory-of-programs/ Accessed August 1, 2021.

5. National Academy of Opticianry, Ophthalmic Career Progression Program. https://www.nao.org Accessed August 1, 2021.

6. National Academy of Opticianry, Ophthalmic Career Progression Program. https://www.nao.org Accessed August 1, 2021.

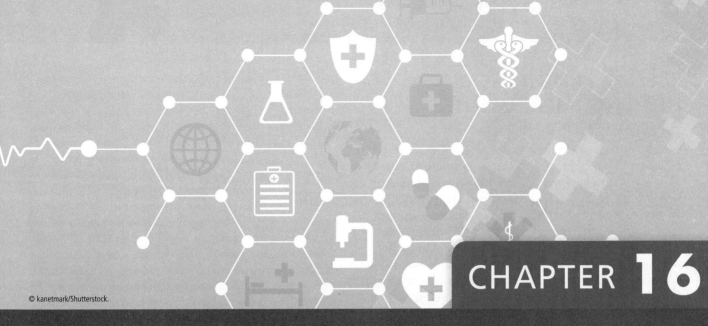
© kanetmark/Shutterstock.

CHAPTER 16

Communication Impairment Professionals*

KEY TERMS

American Speech-Language Hearing Association (ASHA)
Audiologist
Board Certified Specialist in Audiology (BCS-A)
Board Certified Specialist in Child Language and Language Disorders (BCS-CL)
Board Certified Specialist in Fluency (BCS-F)
Board Certified Specialist in Intraoperative Monitoring (BCS-IOM)
Board Certified Specialist in Swallowing and Swallowing Disorders (BCS-S)

Certificate of Clinical Competence in Audiology (CCC-A)
Certificate of Clinical Competence in Speech-Language Pathology (CCC-SLP)
Certified Audiology Assistant (C-AA)
Certified Speech-Language Pathology Assistant (C-SLPA)
Cochlear Implant
Cochlear Implant Specialty Certification (CISC)
Communication disorder
Doctor of Audiology (AuD)

Grammatical patterns
Hearing aid dispenser
Hearing impairment
Interprofessional Practice (IPP)
Interprofessional Collaborative Practice (ICP)
Language disorder
Pediatric Audiology Specialty Certification (PASC)
Ménière's disease
Speech disorder
Speech-Language Pathologist (SLP)
Telepractice
Tinnitus
Vertigo

* information in this chapter, unless otherwise indicated, was obtained from Bureau of Labor Statistics. *Occupational Outlook Handbook 2020–2021 Edition.* Washington, DC: U.S. Department of Labor; 2021.

SPEECH, LANGUAGE, AND HEARING IMPAIRMENTS: AN OVERVIEW

Speech, language, and hearing impairments hinder communication and can cause problems throughout life. Children who have difficulty speaking, hearing, or understanding language, for instance, cannot participate fully with others in play or classroom activities. Sometimes these children are thought to have mental or emotional problems when in fact the problem is one of language or hearing. Adults with speech, language, or hearing impairments may have problems on the job and may withdraw socially to avoid frustration and embarrassment. The aging process almost invariably brings some degree of hearing loss. Severe loss, if not treated, can result in diminished pleasure in everyday activities, social isolation, and, even worse, wrongful labeling of elderly people as demented or "confused."

A **language disorder** is defined as an inability to use the symbols of language through appropriate **grammatical patterns**, proper use of words and their meanings, and the correct use of speech sounds. A **speech disorder** is identified by difficulty in producing speech sounds, controlling voice production, and maintaining speech rhythm. Individuals with speech and language disorders also include those with physical conditions such as a stroke or head injury, cleft palate, or cerebral palsy. Other causes of speech and language disorders are hearing loss, viral diseases, certain drugs, poor speech and language models in the home, or a short attention span. Speech-language pathologists are trained to treat individuals with a variety of speech and language disorders.

Hearing impairment can take many forms. It can be an (1) inability to hear speech and other sounds clearly, even though the sounds are sufficiently loud; (2) inability to understand and use speech in communication, although speech is sufficiently loud and can be heard clearly; or (3) inability to hear speech and other sounds loudly enough, which is considered a loss of hearing sensitivity. A person can experience these three types of hearing impairments in combination. Thus, hearing impairment is more complex than simply the inability to hear speech or other sounds well enough. Some hearing impairments can be subtle and difficult to recognize. Hearing impairment can be a serious problem because the ability to communicate is our most human characteristic. Many individuals with hearing impairments experience social, emotional, and educational isolation, and untreated hearing loss in infants interferes with normal development.

Over 95% of newborn infants are screened for hearing loss (**FIGURE 16.1**); however, of those infants identified as having permanent hearing loss, one-third do not receive appropriate follow-up or intervention.

Infants identified as having a hearing impairment are referred to an **audiologist**, who does further testing to determine the appropriate treatment. Intervention may include hearing aids or a surgically placed cochlear implant. Hearing aids make sounds louder, whereas **cochlear implants** send sound signals directly to the hearing nerve.[1] A team of healthcare professionals works with the child and family during both diagnosis and treatment.

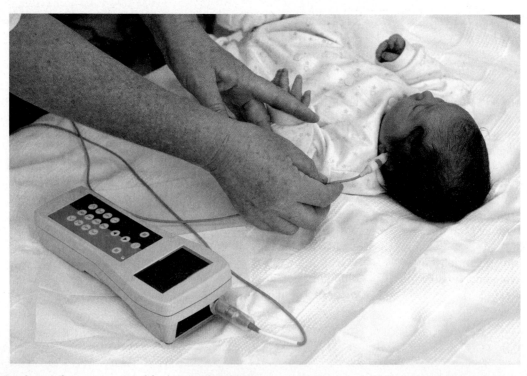

FIGURE 16.1 Newborn infants are screened for hearing impairments.
© ChameleonsEye/Shutterstock.

Causes of hearing loss are viral infections, head injuries, birth defects, exposure to excessively loud noises, drugs, tumors, heredity, and the aging process. In adults, balance disorders can be caused by various problems in the inner ear and are a reason for falls in older adults. An example is **Ménière's disease**, associated with hearing loss and **tinnitus** as well as **vertigo**.[2]

Hearing impairment is the disorder most frequently reported to physicians. Less than 1% of Americans younger than 20 years of age have a hearing disability. However, close to 9% of those between 65 and 74 years of age and 22% of those 75 years and older have hearing loss.[3] Since the cost of hearing aids is not covered by Medicare and because hearing aids are quite expensive, many older adults do not purchase hearing aids and suffer from the effects of hearing loss, which often include isolation and depression.

Speech-language pathologists and audiologists often work together with clients who have disorders in either speech or hearing, since a loss of hearing is most often a cause for speech and language disorders. These professionals often work together with other professionals in both healthcare and educational settings described as **interprofessional practice (IPP)** or **interprofessional collaborative practice (ICP)**. IPP occurs when multiple service providers from different professional backgrounds provide comprehensive services by working with individuals and their families, caregivers, and communities to deliver the highest quality of care across settings.[4] An excellent example of IPP is when professionals work together with a pediatric client receiving a cochlear implant. In addition to the client and their family, professionals who provide comprehensive services are the pediatric otolaryngologist, audiologist, speech pathologist, child life specialist, geneticist, developmental pediatrician, and psychologist. Each member evaluates different aspects of the client and family; working together ensures that the client receives the most comprehensive care. Another example of IPP is Early Intervention, a program for babies and young children with developmental delays and disabilities and their families. Health professionals who often are part of the team are speech-language pathologists, occupational therapists, physical therapists, dietitians, and social workers.

SPEECH-LANGUAGE PATHOLOGISTS
Significant Points

- A master's degree in speech-language pathology is the standard educational requirement; almost all states regulate these workers, and licensing requirements vary.
- In 2019, about 40% worked in educational services, and 23% worked in offices of other healthcare practitioners; others worked in hospitals and long-term care.
- Favorable job opportunities are expected especially in elementary and secondary schools.

Work Description

Speech-Language Pathologists (SLPs), sometimes called speech therapists, assess, diagnose, treat, and help prevent disorders related to speech, language, cognitive communication, voice, swallowing, and fluency.

SLPs work with people who cannot produce speech sounds or cannot produce them clearly; those with speech rhythm and fluency problems, such as stuttering; people with voice disorders, such as inappropriate pitch or harsh voice; those with problems understanding and producing language; those who wish to improve their communication skills by modifying an accent; and those with cognitive communication impairments, such as attention, memory, and problem-solving disorders. They also work with people who have swallowing difficulties.

Speech, language, and swallowing difficulties can result from a variety of causes, including stroke, brain injury, hearing loss, developmental delay, learning disabilities, cerebral palsy, cleft palate, Parkinson's disease, autism, voice pathology, or emotional problems. Problems can be congenital, developmental, or acquired. SLPs use special instruments and qualitative and quantitative assessment methods, including standardized tests, to analyze and diagnose the nature and extent of impairments.

SLPs evaluate the extent of communication problems in individuals by having a patient complete basic reading and vocalizing tasks or completing standardized tests. The SLP then develops an individualized plan of care tailored to each patient's needs. For individuals with little or no speech capability, SLPs may select augmentative or alternative communication methods, including automated devices and sign language, and teach their use. They teach patients how to make sounds, improve their voices, or increase their oral or written language skills by improving vocabulary and sentence structure to communicate more effectively. SLPs may work with people who are unable to understand language or with those who have voice disorders, such as inappropriate pitch or a harsh voice. Some specialize in working with those who rely on their voice for employment—professional singers, actors, teachers, or lawyers—or those with voice disorders because of asthma or allergies. They also teach individuals how to strengthen muscles or use compensatory strategies to swallow without choking or inhaling food or liquid. SLPs help patients develop or recover reliable communication and swallowing skills so patients can fulfill their educational, vocational, and social roles (**FIGURE 16.2**).

SLPs keep records on the initial evaluation, progress, changes in the client's condition or treatment plans, and final evaluation on discharge of clients. This helps pinpoint problems, tracks client progress, and justifies the cost of treatment when applying for reimbursement. They counsel individuals and their families concerning **communication disorders** and how to cope with the stress and

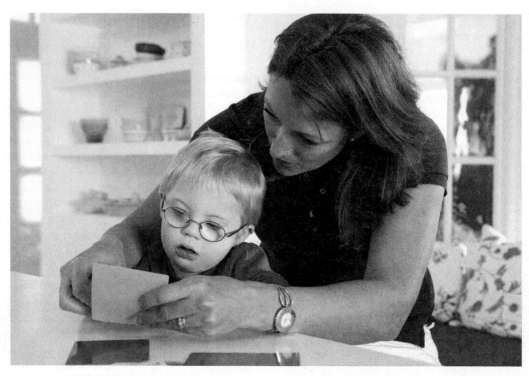

FIGURE 16.2 Speech-Language Pathologists (SLPs) assess, diagnose, and treat children with disorders of language development.
© Monkey Business Images/Shutterstock.

misunderstanding that often accompany these disorders. They also work with family members to recognize and change behavior patterns that impede communication and treatment and demonstrate communication-enhancing techniques to use at home.

Most SLPs provide direct clinical services to individuals with communication or swallowing disorders. In medical facilities, they may perform their job in conjunction with physicians, social workers, psychologists, dietitians, and other therapists. SLPs in schools collaborate with teachers from preschool through high school, special educators, interpreters, other school personnel, and parents to develop and implement individual or group programs, provide counseling, and support classroom activities. Some SLPs specialize in working with specific age groups, such as children or older adults. Others focus on treatment programs for specific communication or swallowing problems, such as those resulting from strokes or cleft palate.

Some SLPs conduct research on how people communicate. Others design and develop equipment or techniques for diagnosing and treating speech problems.

Work Environment

In medical facilities, SLPs work with physicians and surgeons, social workers, audiologists, psychologists, and other healthcare workers. In schools, they work with teachers, other school personnel, and parents to develop and carry out individual or group programs, provide counseling, and support classroom activities.

SLPs usually work at a desk or table in clean, comfortable surroundings. In medical settings, they may work at the patient's bedside and assist in positioning the patient. In schools, they may work with students in an office or classroom. Some work in clients' homes.

Although the work is not physically demanding, it requires attention to detail and intense concentration. The emotional needs of clients and their families may be demanding. Most full-time SLPs work 40 hours per week. Others work remotely using **telepractice**, the use of telecommunication technology to deliver professional services at a distance by linking a clinician to a client for assessment, intervention, and/or consultation.[5]

Those who work on a contract basis may spend a substantial amount of time traveling between facilities.

Employment Opportunities

Speech-language pathologists held about 162,600 jobs in 2019, and about half were employed in educational services (**FIGURE 16.3**).

Others were employed in hospitals, offices of other health practitioners, and nursing care and assisted-living facilities. SLPs provide services to all ages—from premature infants in neonatal intensive care units to veterans who have experienced a brain injury in a military hospital to an elderly resident in an assisted-living facility.

Some speech-language pathologists are self-employed and contract to provide services in schools, physicians' offices, hospitals, or nursing care facilities or work as consultants to industry (**TABLE 16.1**).

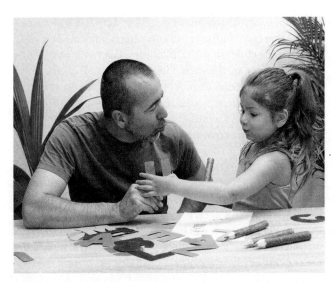

FIGURE 16.3 The majority of speech-language pathologists work in schools.
© Tibanna79/Shutterstock.

TABLE 16.1 Distribution of Speech-Language Pathologists by Industry, 2019

Industry	Percentage
Educational services	38%
Offices of health practitioners	23%
Hospitals	14%
Nursing and residential care facilities	5%
Self-employed	4%

Data from Bureau of Labor Statistics. Occupational Outlook Handbook. U.S. Department of Labor; 2020.

Educational and Legal Requirements

A master's degree is the most common level of education among SLPs. Licensure or certification requirements also exist but vary by state.

Education and Training

Most SLP jobs require a master's degree. The Council on Academic Accreditation is an entity of the **American Speech-Language-Hearing Association (ASHA)**; it accredits postsecondary academic programs in speech-language pathology. In 2020, there were 289 graduate programs in speech-language pathology accredited by the Council on Academic Accreditation.[6] Although master's programs do not specify a particular undergraduate degree for admission, certain courses must be taken before entering the program. Required courses vary by institution. Undergraduate courses in biology, physiology and anatomy, medical terminology, and communication are desirable. Typical graduate courses are statistics, physics,

chemistry, human anatomy and physiology, neuroanatomy and neurophysiology, and human genetics; courses in social/behavioral sciences may include psychology, sociology, anthropology, and public health. Graduate students may also learn the nature of speech, language and swallowing disorders, principles of acoustics, and psychological aspects of communication. During the supervised clinical practicum and fellowship, students learn to evaluate and treat speech, language, and swallowing disorders. Students enrolled in a graduate speech-language pathology program can expect to participate in IPE, when two or more professionals learn about, from, and with each other to enable effective collaboration and improve outcomes for individuals and families.[4]

Licensure

Typical licensing requirements are a master's degree from an accredited college or university, supervised clinical experience, and successful completion of the Praxis Examination in Speech-Language Pathology. Most states that require licensure for clinical practice or teacher credentialing require successful completion of the Praxis exam. Most states have continuing education requirements for licensure renewal. Medicaid, Medicare, and private health insurers generally require a practitioner to be licensed to qualify for reimbursement. Services through telepractice are increasingly being reimbursed. For specific regulation and eligibility requirements, contact your state's regulatory board.

State regulation of SLPs may differ for pathologists practicing in schools. For information on the state regulation of SLPs in public schools, contact your state's Department of Education.

Certification and Other Qualifications

The **Certificate of Clinical Competence in Speech-Language Pathology (CCC-SLP)** credential offered by the ASHA is a voluntary credential; however, the CCC-SLP meets some or all of the requirements for licensure in some states and may be required by some employers.

To earn a CCC, a person must have a graduate degree from an accredited university, which typically includes a supervised clinical practicum; complete a 36-week, full-time postgraduate clinical fellowship; and pass the Praxis Series examination in Speech-Language Pathology administered by the Educational Testing Service. Maintaining certification requires 30 professional development hours over a three-year period.[7] SLPs with CCC-SLP certification can apply for additional specialty certification as a **Board Certified Specialist (BCS)** in **Child Language and Language Disorders (BCS-CL)**, **Fluency (BCS-F)**, or **Swallowing and Swallowing Disorders (BCS-S)**.[8] More details about specialty certification are available under Additional Information at the end of the chapter.

Desirable qualities of SLPs are to be able to effectively communicate diagnostic test results, diagnoses, and proposed treatment in a manner easily understood by clients and their families. They must be able to approach problems objectively and be supportive of clients and their families. SLPs must have critical-thinking skills and be detail oriented in order to recognize small changes in articulation and voice quality and to modify treatment plans as needed to achieve treatment goals. Because a patient's progress may be slow, patience, compassion, and good listening skills are necessary.

Advancement

As SLPs gain clinical experience and engage in continuing professional education, many develop expertise with certain populations, such as preschoolers and adolescents, or disorders, such as aphasia and learning disabilities. Board recognition in a specialty area, such as child language, fluency or feeding and swallowing, can increase the number of referrals for those in private practice. Experienced clinicians may become mentors or supervisors of other therapists or be promoted to administrative positions.

Employment Trends

Faster-than-average employment growth is projected. Job opportunities are expected to be favorable.

Employment Change

Employment of SLPs is expected to grow by 25% from 2019 to 2029, much faster than the average for all occupations. As the members of the Baby Boom generation continue to age, the possibility of neurological disorders and associated speech, language, and swallowing impairments increases. Medical advances also are improving the survival rate of premature infants and trauma and stroke victims, who then need assessment and sometimes treatment. Technological advances in cochlear implants for infants with impaired hearing require the services of both an audiologist and speech therapist to develop language skills after the implant is placed.

Increased awareness of speech and language disorders, such as stuttering, in younger children should also lead to a need for more speech-language pathologists who specialize in treating that age group. In addition, medical advances are improving the survival rate of premature infants and victims of trauma and strokes, many of whom need help from SLPs.

Employment in educational services will increase with the growth in elementary and secondary school enrollments, including enrollment of special education students. The 2004

Individuals with Disabilities Education Act (IDEA) is a federal law that guarantees special education and related services to all eligible children with disabilities. Greater awareness of the importance of the early identification and diagnosis of speech and language disorders in young children will also increase employment.

In healthcare facilities, restrictions on reimbursement for therapy services may limit the growth of speech-language pathologist jobs in the near term. However, the long-run demand for therapists should continue to rise as growth in the number of individuals with disabilities or limited function spurs demand for therapy services.

The number of speech-language pathologists in private practice should increase because hospitals, schools, and nursing care facilities will contain costs by increasingly contracting out for these services.

Job Prospects

In addition to job growth, a number of job openings in speech-language pathology will be a result of retirements. Opportunities should be favorable, particularly for those with the ability to speak a second language, such as Spanish. Demand for SLPs can be regional, so job prospects are expected to be favorable for those who are willing to relocate, particularly to areas experiencing difficulty in attracting and hiring speech-language pathologists, especially in medically underserved areas such as urban centers and rural communities. Schools often have openings for speech pathologists, especially in the Mountain and Pacific states.[9] **TABLE 16.2** shows some projection data provided by the U.S. Department of Labor.

Earnings

Median annual wages of speech-language pathologists were $80,480 in May 2020. Median annual wages in the industries employing the largest numbers of speech-language pathologists in 2020 are shown in **TABLE 16.3**.

Related Occupations

Speech-language pathologists specialize in the prevention, diagnosis, and treatment of speech and language problems. Workers who treat other physical and mental health problems include audiologists, occupational therapists, physical therapists, psychologists, and recreational therapists.

TABLE 16.2 Projection Data for Speech-Language Pathologists, 2019–2029

Occupational Title	Employment, 2019	Projected Employment, 2029	Change, 2019–2029	
			Number	Percentage
Speech-language pathologists	162,600	203,100	40,500	25%

Data from Bureau of Labor Statistics. Occupational Outlook Handbook. U.S. Department of Labor; 2020.

TABLE 16.3 Median Annual Wages in the Industries Employing the Largest Numbers of Speech-Language Pathologists in May 2020	
Nursing care facilities	$95,010
Hospitals	$87,110
Office of health professionals	$83,250
Educational services	$71,410

Data from Bureau of Labor Statistics. Occupational Outlook Handbook. U.S. Department of Labor; 2020.

AUDIOLOGISTS
Significant Points

- A doctoral degree in audiology (hearing) is the standard level of required education.
- In 2019, about 51% worked in offices of physicians or offices of other healthcare workers—physical therapists, occupational therapists, speech therapists, and other audiologists. Others worked in hospitals or educational settings.
- All states regulate licensure of audiologists; requirements vary by state.

Work Description

Audiologists work with people who have hearing, balance, and related ear problems. They examine individuals of all ages and identify those with the symptoms of hearing loss and other auditory, balance, and related sensory and neural problems. They then assess the nature and extent of the problems including the psychological impact of hearing loss and help the individuals manage them. Using audiometers, computers, and other testing devices, they measure the loudness at which a person begins to hear sounds, the ability to distinguish between sounds, and the impact of hearing loss on daily life. In addition, audiologists use computer equipment to evaluate and diagnose balance disorders. Audiologists interpret these results and may coordinate results with medical, educational, and psychological information to make a diagnosis to determine a course of treatment. Audiologists work with physicians to fit a patient with **cochlear implants**—tiny devices placed under the skin near the ear that deliver electrical impulses directly to the auditory nerve in the brain. This allows a person with certain types of deafness to be able to hear. Hearing disorders can result from a variety of causes including trauma at birth, viral or bacterial infections, genetic disorders, multiple sclerosis, brain and auditory nerve tumors, exposure to loud noise, certain medications, or aging (**FIGURE 16.4**).

Treatment may include examining and cleaning the ear canal, fitting and dispensing hearing aids, and fitting and programming cochlear implants. Treatment also includes counseling on adjusting to hearing loss, training on the use

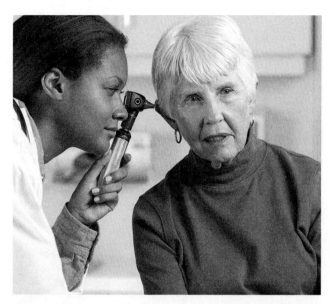

FIGURE 16.4 Audiologist examining the ear canal of an elderly client.
© Monkey Business Images/Shutterstock.

of hearing devices, and teaching communication strategies for use in a variety of environments. For example, they may provide instruction in listening strategies or communication techniques for those with profound hearing loss such as lip reading or the use of technology. Audiologists also may recommend, fit, and dispense personal or large-area amplification systems and alerting devices.

In audiology clinics, audiologists may independently develop and carry out treatment programs. They keep records on the initial evaluation, progress, and discharge of patients. In other settings, audiologists may work with other health and education providers as part of a team in planning and implementing services for children and adults. Audiologists who diagnose and treat balance disorders often work in collaboration with physicians as well as physical and occupational therapists. For cochlear implants, audiologists work with physicians, SLPs, social workers, and occupational therapists to assist the patient to learn to communicate effectively.

Some audiologists specialize in working with older adults, children, or hearing-impaired individuals who need special treatment programs. Others develop and implement ways to protect workers' hearing from on-the-job injuries. They measure noise levels in workplaces and conduct hearing protection programs in factories, schools, and communities.

Audiologists hold jobs in the military and public health settings and in the hearing device manufacturing industry. In addition, audiologists make recommendations to protect hearing for workers in the military, the music industry—especially performers exposed to loud music—and those exposed to loud noises in industries such as mining, construction, and other industrial settings. Some audiologists research new treatments for hearing, balance, and related disorders. Others design

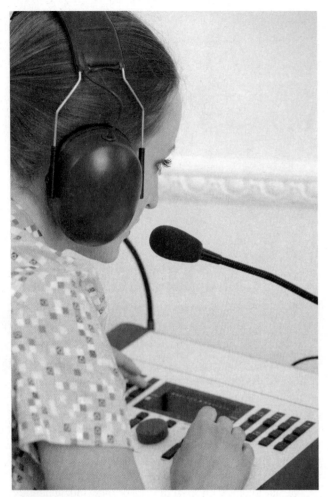

FIGURE 16.5 Audiologists conduct hearing protection programs in work settings with excessive noise.
© Capifrutta/Shutterstock.

TABLE 16.4 Employment of Audiologists by Industry, 2019	
Industry	Percentage
Offices of physicians	27%
Offices of other health professionals	24%
Hospitals	16%
Educational services	10%

Data from Bureau of Labor Statistics. Occupational Outlook Handbook. U.S. Department of Labor; 2020.

and develop equipment or techniques for diagnosing and treating these disorders (**FIGURE 16.5**).

Work Environment

Most audiologists work in healthcare facilities, such as hospitals, physicians' offices, and audiology clinics, and some have a private practice or work as consultants to such facilities. Others work in schools or school districts and travel between facilities. Audiologists work closely with registered nurses, audiology assistants, speech-language pathologists, and other healthcare professionals.

Most audiologists work full time. Some work weekends and evenings to meet patients' needs. Those who work on a contract basis may spend a lot of time traveling between facilities. For example, an audiologist who is contracted by a school system may have to travel between different schools to provide services.

Audiologists usually work at a desk or table in clean, comfortable surroundings. The job is not physically demanding but does require attention to detail and intense concentration. The emotional needs of patients and their families can be demanding. Most full-time audiologists work about 40 hours per week.

Audiologists who work in private practice also manage the business aspects of running an office, such as developing a patient base, hiring employees, keeping records, and ordering equipment and supplies.

Employment Opportunities

Audiologists held about 13,800 jobs in 2019. About 51% of all jobs were in offices of physicians or other health practitioners, including other audiologists. About 10% of jobs were in educational services (**TABLE 16.4**).

Educational and Legal Requirements

All states regulate the licensure of audiologists; requirements vary by state. A **Doctor of Audiology (AuD)** from a program accredited by the Council on Academic Accreditation is the requirement for licensure for entry-level audiologists. A bachelor's degree in any field is needed to enter one of these programs.

Education and Training

Individuals pursuing a career will need to earn a doctoral degree. The doctoral degree in audiology is a graduate program typically lasting four years and resulting in the AuD designation. The Council on Academic Accreditation (CAA) is an entity of the ASHA that accredits education programs in audiology. In 2020, the CAA accredited 78 doctoral programs in audiology.[6]

Requirements for admission to programs in audiology include courses in English, mathematics, physics, chemistry, biology, psychology, and communication. Graduate coursework in audiology includes anatomy; physiology; physics; genetics; normal and abnormal communication development; auditory, balance, and neural systems assessment and treatment; diagnosis and treatment; pharmacology; and ethics. Graduate curriculums also include supervised clinical practice and externships.

Licensure

Audiologists are regulated by licensure in all 50 states. Although some states may accept a master's degree in audiology for licensure, graduate programs have transitioned to an AuD, so those considering a career in audiology will be required to complete a doctorate. Some states regulate the practice of audiology and the dispensing of hearing aids separately, meaning some states will require an additional license as a hearing aid dispenser. Many states require that audiologists complete continuing education for license renewal. Eligibility requirements, hearing aid dispensing requirements, and continuing education requirements vary from state to state. Some audiologists become licensed to dispense hearing aids; however, **hearing aid dispensers** can be licensed to fit hearing aids without training as an audiologist. For specific requirements, contact your state's medical or health board. ASHA lists licensure requirements for audiologists and states that allow audiologists to dispense hearing aids.[10]

Certification and Other Requirements

Audiologists can earn the **Certificate of Clinical Competence in Audiology (CCC-A)** offered by ASHA. Since 2012, a doctoral degree is required for applicants for the CCC-A credential.[10] Audiologists with CCC-A certification can apply to become a **Board Certified Specialist in Intraoperative Monitoring (BCS-IOM)** from the American Audiology Board of Intraoperative Monitoring.[11] In addition, audiologists can apply for certification from the American Board of Audiology: **Board Certified Specialist in Audiology (BCS-A), Cochlear Implant Specialty Certification (CISC)**, and **Pediatric Audiology Specialty Certification (PASC)**. The CISC was developed to standardize training and knowledge of CISC audiologists and recognize those professionals who have acquired specialized knowledge in the field of cochlear implants, including expectations, surgical considerations, device operation, and rehabilitation. The PASC signifies expertise in pediatric audiology and demonstrates to colleagues, other healthcare providers, patients, and employers that the recipient has acquired a high level of knowledge in the field of pediatric audiology and is the best option for treating children with hearing and balance disorders and hearing loss. Board certification can improve career opportunities and advancement.[12] Professional credentialing may satisfy some or all of the requirements for state licensure.

Desirable characteristics for students interested in becoming an audiologist are the ability to effectively communicate diagnostic test results, diagnoses, and proposed treatments in a manner easily understood by their patients. They must be able to approach problems objectively and provide emotional support to patients and their families. Critical-thinking and problem-solving skills are necessary to be able to analyze the cause of hearing loss or balance problems and develop appropriate treatment to address these problems.

Because a patient's progress may be slow, patience, compassion, and good listening skills are necessary.

It is important for audiologists to be aware of new diagnostic and treatment technologies. Most audiologists participate in continuing education courses to learn new methods and technologies. In addition, many audiologists conduct research or participate in research to evaluate methods for evaluating and treating hearing loss.

Advancement

With experience, audiologists can advance to open a private practice. Audiologists working in hospitals and clinics can advance to management or supervisory positions.

Employment Trends

Employment growth is expected to be faster than average; however, because of the small size of the occupation, only about 1,800 new jobs are projected through 2029. Job prospects will be favorable for those possessing an AuD degree.

Employment Change

Employment of audiologists is expected to grow 13% from 2019 to 2029, much faster than the average for all occupations. Hearing loss is strongly associated with aging, so the growth of older population groups will cause the number of people with hearing and balance impairments to increase markedly.

Medical advances also are improving the survival rate of premature infants and trauma victims, who then need assessment and sometimes treatment for hearing loss. Greater awareness of the importance of the early identification and diagnosis of hearing disorders in infants also will increase employment. In addition to medical advances, technological advances in hearing aids may drive demand. Digital hearing aids have become smaller in size and also have quality-improving technologies like reducing feedback. Demand may be spurred by those who switch from analog to digital hearing aids as well as those who will desire new or first-time hearing aids. Also, those with a hearing impairment are more likely to wear them since newer hearing aids are less visible and can be worn longer.

Employment in educational services will increase along with growth in elementary and secondary school enrollments, including the enrollment of special education students. Growth in the employment of audiologists will be moderated by limitations on reimbursements made by third-party payers for the tests and services they provide.

Job Prospects

Job prospects will be favorable for audiologists because of the retirement of Baby Boomers. Only a few job openings for audiologists will arise from the need to replace those who leave the occupation because the occupation is relatively

TABLE 16.5 Projection Data for Audiologists, 2019–2020

Occupational Title	Employment, 2019	Projected Employment, 2020	Change, 2019–2020	
			Number	Percentage
Audiologists	13,800	15,600	1,800	13%

Data from Bureau of Labor Statistics. Occupational Outlook Handbook. U.S. Department of Labor; 2020.

small and workers tend to stay in this occupation until they retire. Demand may be greater in areas with large numbers of retirees, so audiologists who are willing to relocate may have the best job prospects. Greater awareness of the importance of early identification and diagnosis of hearing disorders in infants will increase employment. The number of audiologists in private practice will rise due to the increasing demand for direct services to individuals as well as the use of contract services by hospitals, schools, and nursing care facilities. Even though Medicare doesn't cover the cost of hearing aids, active older adults with adequate financial resources are likely to seek services of audiologists to be fitted for hearing aids to maintain an active lifestyle. Advances in hearing aid design, such as smaller size and the reduction of feedback, may make such devices more appealing as a means to minimize the effects of hearing loss. This may lead to more demand for audiologists. **TABLE 16.5** shows some projection data from the U.S. Department of Labor.

Earnings

Median annual wages of audiologists were $81,030 in May 2020. Salaries for audiologists working in different settings are shown in **TABLE 16.6**.

Related Occupations

Audiologists specialize in the prevention, diagnosis, and treatment of hearing problems. Workers who treat other problems related to physical or mental health include optometrists, physical therapists, psychologists, physicians and surgeons, and speech-language pathologists.

TABLE 16.6 Median Annual Wages in the Industries Employing the Largest Numbers of Audiologists, May 2020

Hospitals	$86,940
Educational services	$83,500
Offices of other health professionals	$80,230
Offices of physicians	$78,680

Data from Bureau of Labor Statistics. Occupational Outlook Handbook. U.S. Department of Labor; 2020.

SPEECH-LANGUAGE PATHOLOGY AND AUDIOLOGY ASSISTANTS

Speech-Language Pathology Assistants (SLPAs) and Audiology Assistants (AAs) have been employed with varying degrees of regulation and success in the field of communication sciences and disorders since the 1960s. Assistants improve access to patient care by increasing the availability of SLP and audiology services, increasing productivity by reducing wait times and enhancing patient satisfaction, and reducing costs by performing tasks that do not require the professional skills of a certified and/or licensed SLP or audiologist.[13]

Significant Points

- Speech-Language Pathology Assistants (SLPAs) and Audiology Assistants (AAs) work under the direct supervision of licensed SLPAs and AuDs to improve access to patient care.
- Assistants are required to be certified; educational pathways to certification include an associate's degree, bachelor's degree, or training in the military.

Work Description

In general, SLPAs work under the supervision of a licensed speech-language pathologist and audiology assistants work under the guidance and supervision of a licensed audiologist. SLPs and audiologists conduct assessments of clients and develop treatment plans and then assign tasks to their assistants. Assistants perform a variety of duties that may include cleaning and preparation of equipment, limited documentation, routine therapeutic activities as deemed appropriate by the licensed clinician, and other duties not otherwise limited by the scope of practice, education, or aptitude of the individual.[14] Both assistants perform hearing screening tests for infants and adults and document the results. SLPAs may also conduct speech, language, and developmental screening. Audiology assistants troubleshoot and perform minor repairs and cleaning of hearing aids and other amplification devices. They also instruct patients on the proper use and care of hearing aids.[15]

Professional Profiles

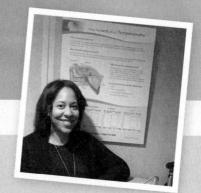

Name: Jasmine
Job Title: Audiology Assistant
Education: BS in Communication Disorders

Q: Describe your job and organization.

A: I work as an audiology assistant in a children's hospital in an urban setting. I assist with a range of clinical services for pediatric patients with a variety of hearing problems. I conduct universal newborn hearing screening and assist the audiologist in behavioral hearing tests. I also perform electroacoustic analysis of hearing aids and other amplification devices.

Q: Describe a typical workday.

A: At the beginning of the day, I check the function of the equipment and set up the testing booths. About 80% of my day, I provide direct patient care doing newborn hearing screening and assisting with behavior hearing tests. The rest of the day I troubleshoot problems and repair hearing aids and amplification devices. I also communicate with manufacturers and suppliers regarding the status of orders or repairs.

Q: Why did you choose this profession?

A: I chose this profession because it is related to my undergraduate degree in communication disorders. I like the direct patient contact with children, since each child is different, which offers new learning experiences.

Q: What challenges you most about this profession?

A: Each child is very different, which is difficult, since my job is to understand what each child needs in order to successfully complete an accurate hearing test.

Q: Name and explain what part of your academic training most prepared you for this profession.

A: There was no academic training required for this position; however, a two-week training through the hospital was required. The audiology courses that I completed for my undergraduate degree prepared me for this position and gave me background knowledge about hearing loss and the anatomy of the hearing mechanisms.

Q: Did you face obstacles in pursuing your goals? If so, describe them and how you overcame them.

A: An obstacle that I faced was allowing money to be a driving force of choosing a career in the health field. I overcame the obstacle by realizing that I get satisfaction from going to work and helping children every day.

Q: What do you wish you had known in high school or college about pursuing this career?

A: I wish I would have known that a doctorate degree is required to reach the next level of advancement in audiology.

Q: What advice would you give someone who is considering this career?

A: The advice that I would give someone considering this career is that having a passion and love for children is important. People skills are essential for being effective in this career in order to relate to the patients and their caregivers.

Q: What personal characteristics are needed for this work?

A: People skills are essential for being effective in this career in order to relate to the patients and their caregivers. Personality characteristics important for this work are compassion, enthusiasm, and motivation.

Work Environment

Since both SLPAs and audiology assistants work directly under the supervision of certified SLPs (CCC-SLP) or certified audiologists (CCC-A), assistants will work in the same settings. Assistants provide different levels of support unique to each work setting. Only two assistants are allowed to work under the supervision of one CCC-SLP or one CCC-A to ensure that the assistant has adequate supervision.

The majority of SLPAs can expect to work in educational settings across the life span from preschool and day care centers, elementary and secondary schools, and college and university clinics. Some SLPAs may work in homecare settings in Early Intervention, a program for young children, or treat older adults receiving therapy after a stroke. Some may work in hospitals and skilled nursing facilities. The majority of audiology assistants can expect to work in the offices of physicians and other health professionals; some may work in educational, industrial, or hospital settings.

Employment Opportunities

Opportunities for employment are expected to increase with certification, greater demands for services and productivity, and efforts to control the cost of delivering speech-language pathology and audiology services.

Educational and Legal Requirements

SLPAs or SLP-Assistants is the title used by individuals who have completed academic coursework, a clinical experience, and credentialing. Many states require assistants to register, fewer states require licensure to practice. However, the supervising audiologist is responsible for determining the applicable requirements in his or her state and work setting.

Education and Training

Minimum education requirements for assistants vary by state; some require an associate's degree while others require a bachelor's degree. There are a variety of training options for SLPAs, ranging from certificate programs to associate to bachelor degree programs. There are over 297 undergraduate programs in communication sciences and disorders in the United States, one of the options for becoming certified as either a SLPA or audiology assistant.[6] There are over 20 training programs specifically for SLPAs in the United States and seven in Canada. Being relatively new as a recognized profession, the first SLPA-specific educational programs did not graduate its first class until 2002.[16]

The three educational pathways to become certified as an SLPA require a minimum of 100 hours of both direct and indirect clinical services under the supervision of a CCC-SLP. The first educational option is a two-year associate's degree or certificate program in SLPA. The second educational option is a bachelor's degree in communication sciences and disorders from an accredited institution. The third educational option is an associate's or bachelor's degree—but not in the communication sciences—plus successfully completing several required courses from a speech-language pathology degree program—for example, normal anatomy and physiology related to speech and swallowing, phonetics, language development, language disorders, and communication disorders.[17] Audiology assistants have fewer options in terms of formal training specific for audiology assistants. Many start with on-the-job training under the supervision of a CCC-A or obtain training in the military. The three pathways to becoming an audiology assistant are similar to becoming a SLPA. All require clinical experience under the direct supervision of a CCC-A. The first option is to obtain a bachelor's degree in communication sciences and disorders; the second option is a college degree, high school diploma, or GED, together with the completion of an associate's degree or certificate program as an audiology assistant. The third option is documentation of a military job awarding certificate in audiology/ENT (ear, nose and throat) for active military personnel or veterans.[18]

Licensure

Assistants must be registered or licensed depending on state requirements; services delegated to an assistant are those permitted by state law. Regulations and laws for assistants in educational and other practice settings vary from state to state. Requirements differ among states regarding allowed titles, education, supervision, and continuing education.[19]

Certification and Other Requirements

The Assistants Certification Program—implemented by ASHA in 2020—standardizes training requirements and ensures competency for licensure/certification of assistants. Certification requires successful completion of a qualifying exam. In the past, the education and training requirements, certification/licensure, and scope and complexity of practice for assistants varied greatly by state. Once certified, assistants can use the title **Certified Audiology Assistant (C-AA)** for certified audiology assistants or **Certified Speech-Language Pathology Assistant (C-SLPA)** for certified SLPA.[20]

Advancement

Some SLPAs or audiologist assistants may see their role as a pathway to acceptance into a communication sciences and disorders (CSD) graduate program that leads to the SLP or audiology credential. Often, an individual with an undergraduate CSD degree will be able to work as an SLPA or audiology assistant while waiting to be accepted to graduate school. There are even a few programs that allow SLPAs to get an undergraduate degree or certificate while attending a graduate program and at the same time gain valuable experience in the CSD field.[14] Both SLPA and audiology assistants fluent in languages in addition to spoken English who also have the necessary training and skills may serve as translators and interpreters.[21,22] Audiology assistants may seek additional training as a teleaudiology clinical technician to provide patient/equipment interface support under the supervision of a certified/licensed audiologist using audio/video technology to deliver audiology services from a site located at a distance from the actual patient testing site. However, currently only the Veterans Administration system utilizes this technology.[23] Audiology assistants can also obtain specialized training in occupational hearing conservation and perform audiometric testing in industrial work settings to measure noise levels that can result in hearing loss.[14]

Employment Trends

There is no data from the U.S. Bureau of Labor for assistants; data from the Occupational Information Network (O*NET) report an expected 5% to 7% increase in SLPAs between 2019 and 2029, faster than average.[24]

Employment Change

In 2019, the number of SLPAs was 96,900 with an expected increase of 11,300 for a total of 108,200 by 2029.[24]

Job Prospects

An increase in demand for assistants is expected because of the Assistants Certification Program and greater recognition of assistants by the healthcare community. The number of SLPAs is expected to increase because of the demand for speech therapy in educational settings and in the aging population because of strokes and other neurological disorders with aging. Audiology assistants can also expect to be in greater demand because of the aging population with hearing loss and the need for fitting and maintenance of hearing devices.

Earnings

Median salaries for SLPAs was $40,000 in 2020.[25] An audiology technician's median salary was also $40,000 in 2020.[26]

Related Occupations

Other occupations that are similar to SLPAs and audiology assistants are occupational therapy assistants and physical therapy assistants who work under the supervision of occupational therapists and physical therapists, respectively.

Additional Information

State licensing boards can provide information on licensure requirements. State departments of education can supply information on certification requirements for those who wish to work in public schools. The American Speech-Language-Hearing Association lists educational requirements for licensure by state.

Career information, educational programs, a description of the CCC-A and CCC-SLP credentials, and information on state licensure for speech-language pathologists and audiologists is available from:

- American Speech-Language-Hearing Association (ASHA), 2200 Research Blvd., Rockville, MD 20850. http://www.asha.org

For information on specialty certification for speech-language pathologists, contact:

- American Board of Child Language and Language Disorders, #212 709 Plaza Drive, Suite 2, Chesterton, IN 46304. https://www.childlanguagespecialist.org/applicants/
- American Board of Fluency and Fluency Disorders, #212 709 Plaza Drive, Suite 2 Chesterton, IN 46304. https://www.childlanguagespecialist.org/applicants/
- American Board of Swallowing and Swallowing Disorders, #212 709 Plaza Drive, Suite 2 Chesterton, IN 46304 https://www.childlanguagespecialist.org/applicants/

For information on accredited AuD programs, contact:

- American Academy of Audiology, 11480 Commerce Park Drive, Suite 220, Reston, VA 20191. https://www.audiology.org/

For information on specialty certification for audiologists, contact:

- American Board of Audiology, 11480 Commerce Park Drive, Suite 200, Reston, VA 20191. https://www.audiology.org/american-board-of-audiology/
- American Audiology Board of Intraoperative Monitoring, 563 Carter Court, Kimberly, WI 54136. https://www.aabiom.com/

For more information on the career of audiology, contact:

- American Academy of Audiology Foundation, 11480 Commerce Park Drive, Suite 220, Reston, VA 20191. https://www.audiology.org/foundation/

For information on becoming an Occupational Hearing Conservationist (OHC), contact:

- Council for Accreditation in Occupational Hearing Conservation 555 E. Wells St., Suite 1100, Milwaukee, WI 53202. https://www.caohc.org/training-and-certifications/occupational-hearing-conservationist

For information on requirements for SLPAs or audiology assistants, contact:

- American Speech-Language-Hearing Association (ASHA), 2200 Research Blvd., Rockville, MD 20850. https://www.asha.org/assistants-certification-program/slpa-faqs/

For a list of educational programs for SLPAs, contact:

- American Speech-Language Association (ASHA), 2200 Research Blvd., Rockville, MD 20850. https://www.asha.org/assistants-certification-program/slpa-technical-training-programs/

LEARNING PORTFOLIO

Issues for Discussion

1. View videos of audiologists and speech pathologists describing their work. Based on the videos, describe some of the tasks of the professionals and where they work. Describe the educational or health problem of clients in each video.

   - View the two-minute video "Your Career Is Calling: David Alexander, Audiologist." https://www.you tube.com/watch?list=RDCMUC-RlNcHZEuc IevdNBeR-KPw&v=ekFK94uXnnM&feature=emb _rel_end
   - View the one-minute video "Audiologists Changing Lives. Dr. Julie Martinez Verhoff." http://www.asha .org/Careers/Julie-Martinez-Verhoff
   - View the two-minute video "Speech-Language Pathologists Make a Difference: Davetrina Seles Gadson." http://www.asha.org/Careers/Davetrina -Gadson
   - View the two-minute video "Speech-Language Pathologists Make a Difference: James Brinton". https://www.asha.org/Careers/James-Brinton

2. View the six-minute video "Telepractice" to learn how a speech pathologist delivers services using the internet. Describe the two settings shown in the video. Describe the benefits of telepractice for both the speech pathologist and the client. https://www .asha.org/Practice-Portal/Professional-Issues /Telepractice

3. Review the eight-minute video that describes inter-professional practice (IPP). List the service providers and how the team communicates with the parents or caregivers and other service providers. Discuss the benefits of IPP. https://www.scsha.net/asha-ipp-early -intervention-services

4. Review information about an associate's degree for speech-language-pathology assistants (SLPAs) at the College of DuPage, Glen Ellyn, Illinois. Review this website to determine the academic and clinical practicum requirements to obtain a degree in this program. List the names of several required courses as well as the usual cites for clinical experiences. https://www.cod.edu/academics/programs/slpa /faq.aspx

Enrichment Activities

1. Review an article written by a speech pathologist specializing in adult neurological disorders with dysphagia. The author reflects on her experiences as a patient with a brain tumor. McCoy Y. The Other Side of the Spoon. *The ASHA Leader*, October 2015, 20:80. doi:10.1044/leader.FPLP.20102015.80. https://leader.pubs.asha.org/doi/full/10.1044/leader .FPLP.20102015.80 Accessed August 5, 2021.

2. Review the speech pathologist's discussion of a client who was a preschool child with a tongue-tie who demonstrated behavioral problems including being a picky eater and unclear speech patterns. Archambault Besson N. The Tongue Was Involved but What Was the Trouble? *The ASHA Leader*. September 2015, 20 (9): doi:10.1044/leader.CP.20092015.np. https://leader.pubs.asha.org/doi/10.1044/leader .CP.20092015.np

3. Read the article "Remarkable Woman: Dana Suskind," *Chicago Tribune*, February 10, 2013. Dr. Suskind is a pediatric surgeon with a primary practice of cochlear implants for children born without the ability to hear. What is involved in teaching a child language skills after a cochlear implant? https://www .chicagotribune.com/lifestyles/ct-xpm-2013-02-10- ct-tribu-remarkable-suskind-20130210-story.html

4. Review the documentary video "Swallow: A Documentary—Dysphagia" from the patient's and patient's family's points of view for those with swallowing difficulties. https://www.youtube.com /watch?v=MrbEUDO6S5U

LEARNING PORTFOLIO

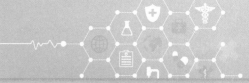

CASE STUDY: COMMUNICATION

Jeff is interested in a career in speech and language pathology for personal reasons. When he was a small child, he experienced severe difficulty developing his communication skills. He was almost five years old before he could even say his own name. The specialist explained to his parents the reason for the delay was probably due to a brain injury he received as a result of a traumatic birth. Now that Jeff is doing well and is ready to begin his career search, he would like to give back to the field of medicine that helped him overcome his disability.

The following questions relate to communication, speech, and language pathology. Please help Jeff answer them based on what you have learned in this chapter.

1. Jeff would like to work with children due to his own experience as a child. What type of job opportunities in this field should he expect?
   A. There may be some areas where there are jobs working with young children in the future.
   B. None because this is usually a disability that affects only older adults.
   C. There are favorable opportunities in elementary and secondary schools.
   D. There are no statistics to support the future job market for SLPs.

2. In addition to working with children who have speech disorders, what other types of disorders can Jeff expect to learn to work with if he becomes a speech-language pathologist?
   A. People with speech rhythm and fluency problems
   B. People who stutter
   C. People with inappropriate voice pitch or harsh voices
   D. People with swallowing difficulties
   E. All of these are correct.

3. Jeff is planning to begin his career in a different state than the one in which he will be attending to college. He also realizes that states often have different regulations for SLPs practicing in schools. Because Jeff's goal is to practice in a school with children, where can he get information regarding state regulations of SLPs in public schools?
   A. The college registrar
   B. The state department of education
   C. The phone book
   D. Social media

References

1. Centers for Disease Control and Prevention. *Hearing Loss in Children*. http://www.cdc.gov/ncbddd/hearingloss/research.html Accessed July 2, 2020.

2. National Institute on Aging. NIH. *Balance Problems and Disorders*. https://www.nia.nih.gov/health/balance-problems-and-disorders Updated May 1, 2017. Accessed August 5, 2021.

3. Erickson W, Lee C, von Schrader S. (2019). *2017 Disability Status Report: United States*. Ithaca, NY: Cornell University Yang-Tan Institute on Employment and Disability (YTI).

4. American Speech-Language-Hearing Association. *Interprofessional Education/ Interprofessional Practice (IPE/IPP)*. https://www.asha.org/Practice/Interprofessional-Education-Practice/ Accessed July 2, 2020.

5. American Speech-Language-Hearing Association. *Telepractice*. http://www.asha.org/Practice-Portal/Professional-Issues/Telepractice/ Accessed July 2, 2020.

6. American Speech-Language-Hearing Association. *EdFind*. https://find.asha.org/ed/#sort=relevancy Accessed August 5, 2021.

7. American Speech-Language-Hearing Association. *Maintaining Your Certification*. https://www.asha.org/certification/maintain-ccc/ Accessed July 2, 2020.

8. American Speech-Language-Hearing Association. *Clinical Specialty Certification*. https://www.asha.org/certification/specialty/ Accessed July 2, 2020.

9. American Speech-Language-Hearing Association. *Workforce Reports*. https://www.asha.org/research/memberdata/workforcereports/ Accessed August 5, 2021.

10. Council for Clinical Certification in Audiology and Speech-Language Pathology of the American Speech-Language-Hearing Association. (2018). *2020 Standards for the Certificate of Clinical Competence in Audiology*. https://www.asha.org/certification/2020-audiology-certification-standards/

11. American Audiology Board of Intraoperative Monitoring. *What is the Value of Specialty Board Certification in IOM for an Audiologist?* http://www.aabiom.com/ Accessed July 2, 2020.

12. American Board of Audiology. *Why get Certified?* https://www.audiology.org/american-board-of-audiology/about-the-aba/why-get-certified/ Accessed August 5, 2021.

13. American Speech-Language-Hearing Association. *ASHA Assistants Program*. https://www.ashaassistants.org/ Accessed August 5, 2021.

14. American Speech-Language-Hearing Association. *Career Pathway for Assistants*. https://www.asha.org/assistants

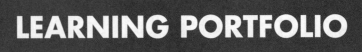

-certification-program/career-pathway-for-assistants / Accessed July 2, 2020.

15. American Speech-Language-Hearing Association. *Audiology Assistants.* https://www.asha.org/practice-portal/professional-issues/audiology-assistants/ Accessed August 5, 2021.

16. Douglas J. A Glimpse into the World of Speech-Language Pathology Assistants (SLPAs) in the Health Care Setting. *Associates Insight.* https://www.asha.org/articles/a-glimpse-into-the-world-of-speech-language-pathology-assistants-in-the-health-care-setting/ Accessed August 5, 2021.

17. American Speech-Language-Hearing Association. *Become a Certified Speech-Language Pathology Assistant (SLPA).* https://www.ashaassistants.org/pathways-speech-language-pathology-assistant/

18. American Speech-Language-Hearing Association. *Become a Certified Audiology Assistant.* https://www.ashaassistants.org/pathways-audiology-assistant/ Accessed August 5, 2021.

19. American Speech-Language-Hearing Association. *State Licensure Trends.* https://www.asha.org/advocacy/state/statelicensuretrends/ Accessed August 9, 2021.

20. Association of Speech-Language-Hearing Association. *About Assistant's Certification.* https://www.asha.org/certification/about-assistants-certification/ Accessed August 9, 2021.

21. American Speech-Language-Hearing Association. *Audiology Assistants.* https://www.asha.org/practice-portal/professional-issues/audiology-assistants/ Accessed August 6, 2021.

22. American Speech-Language-Hearing Association. *Speech-Language Pathology Assistant Scope of Practice.* https://www.asha.org/policy/SP2013-00337/#sec1.6.2 Accessed August 5, 2021.

23. American Speech-Language Hearing Association. *Tele-audiology Clinical Technicians.* https://www.asha.org/Practice-Portal/Professional-Issues/Audiology-Assistants/Teleaudiology-Clinical-Assistants/ Accessed July 2, 2020.

24. National Center for O*NET Development. *31-9099.01— Speech-Language Pathology Assistants. O*NET OnLine.* https://www.onetonline.org/link/summary/31-9099.01 Accessed August 5, 2021.

25. Payscale. *Average Speech-Language Pathology Assistant (SLPA) Hourly Pay.* https://www.payscale.com/research/US/Job=Speech-Language_Pathology_Assistant_(SLPA)/Hourly_Rate Accessed July 2, 2020.

26. Payscale. *Average Audiology Technician Hourly Pay.* https://www.payscale.com/research/US/Job=Audiology_Technician/Hourly_Rate Accessed July 2, 2020.

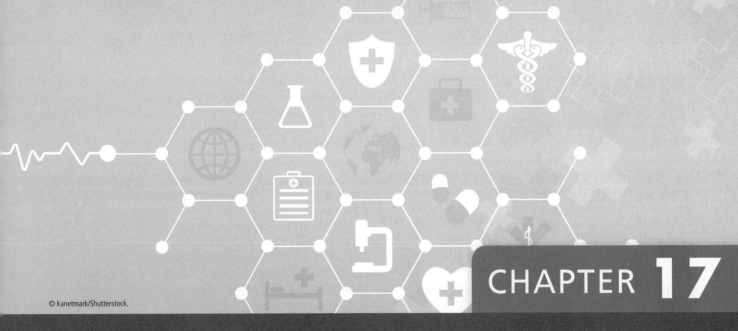
© kanetmark/Shutterstock.

CHAPTER 17

Physical Therapy, Orthotists, and Prosthetists*

KEY TERMS

Assistive device
Deep tissue massage
Electrical stimulation
Evidence-based practice
Orthotic and prosthetic technician
Orthotics and prosthetics (O&P)
Orthotist

Outcomes assessment
Paraffin bath
Pedorthist
Photosensitivity
Physical therapist
Physical therapist aide
Physical therapist assistant
Physical therapy

Prosthetist
Rehabilitation
Research
Soft tissue mobilization
Sports medicine
Tests and measurements
Therapeutic exercise

* All information in this chapter, unless otherwise indicated, was obtained from Bureau of Labor Statistics. *Occupational Outlook Handbook 2020–2021 Edition*. Washington, DC: U.S. Department of Labor; 2021.

PHYSICAL THERAPY AND OUR HEALTH

Physical therapy is a health profession in which the primary purpose is the promotion of optimal human health and functioning through the application of scientific principles to prevent, identify, assess, correct, or alleviate acute or prolonged movement dysfunction. Physical therapy encompasses areas of specialized competence and includes the development of new principles and applications to effectively meet existing and emerging health needs. **Physical therapists** restore, maintain, and promote overall fitness and health. Their patients include accident victims and individuals with disabling conditions such as lower-back pain, arthritis, heart disease, fractures, head injuries, and cerebral palsy. Other professional activities in which physical therapists engage are **research**, education, consultation, and administration.

PHYSICAL THERAPISTS
Significant Points

- Employment is projected to grow much faster than average, and job opportunities should be good, especially for therapists treating older adults.
- Physical therapists must possess a post-baccalaureate degree from an accredited program to work in this field.
- Physical therapists are regulated in all 50 states; requirements vary by state.
- Most jobs are in offices of other health practitioners and in hospitals.

Work Description

Physical therapists provide services that help individuals who have suffered injuries or illness to manage their pain and improve their movement. Conditions they treat are wide-ranging, including problems resulting from back and neck injuries; sprains, strains, and fractures; arthritis; amputations; neurological disorders, such as stroke or cerebral palsy; injuries related to work and sports; and other conditions. Physical therapists restore function, improve mobility, relieve pain, and prevent or limit permanent physical disabilities. They focus on preventive care, rehabilitation, and treatment for patients suffering from chronic conditions, illnesses, or injuries.

Therapists examine patients' medical histories and then use **tests and measurements** to evaluate and measure the patients' strength, range of motion, balance and coordination, posture, muscle performance, respiration, and motor function. Specific tests may evaluate muscle strength, force, endurance, and tone; joint motion, mobility, and stability; reflexes and automatic reactions; movement skill and accuracy; sensations and perception; peripheral nerve integrity; locomotor skill, stability, and endurance; activities of daily living; cardiac, pulmonary, and vascular functions; fit, function, and comfort of prosthetic, orthotic, and other assistive devices; posture and body mechanics; limb length, circumference, and volume; thoracic excursion and breathing patterns; vital signs; **photosensitivity**; and home and work physical environments. Next, physical therapists develop plans describing a treatment strategy and its anticipated outcome.

Treatment often includes exercise, especially for patients who have been immobilized or who lack flexibility, strength, or endurance. Physical therapists encourage patients to use their muscles to increase their flexibility and range of motion. More advanced exercises focus on improving strength, balance, coordination, and endurance. The goal is to improve how an individual functions at work and at home.

Physical therapists also use **electrical stimulation**, hot packs or cold compresses, and ultrasound to relieve pain and reduce swelling. They may use traction or **deep tissue massage** to relieve pain and improve circulation and flexibility. Therapists also teach patients to use **assistive devices**, such as crutches, prostheses, and wheelchairs. They demonstrate **therapeutic exercises** and perform **soft tissue mobilization**, neuromuscular reeducation, bronchopulmonary hygiene, and ambulation or gait training. An example of an assistive device is seen in **FIGURE 17.1**. They also may show patients how to do exercises at home to expedite their recovery. As treatment continues, they continue to evaluate their patients' progress and make modifications based upon observations and patient reports. They may institute new treatments as necessary. They communicate with patients and their families about what to expect from therapy and how to cope with the recovery process. Physical therapists document patients' progress on a regular basis. With the increased use of electronic health records (EHRs), physical therapists must understand the computer software the EHR uses when documenting patients' progress.

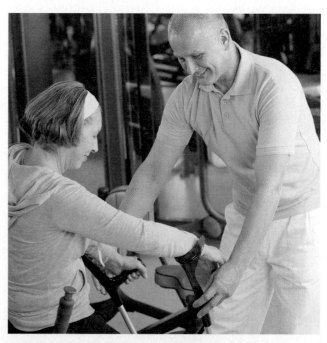

FIGURE 17.1 Woman using assistive device to walk.
© CandyBox Images/Shutterstock.

Professional Profiles

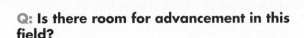

Name: Rachel, DPT, CSCS, MSC, USN
Job Title: Physical Therapist
Education: PhD in Physical Therapy, BS in Exercise Science,
Fellow-in-Training in the Army–Baylor Doctoral Fellowship
of Orthopedic Manual Physical Therapy

Q: Describe your job and organization.

A: As a physical therapist in the U.S. Navy, I work in an academic setting with a mix of both inpatients and outpatients while earning a Doctor of Science degree through a fellowship in Orthopedic Manual Physical Therapy. The settings are very similar to civilian practice with a variety of ages—for example, in a hospital-based setting with young active-duty service members recovering from orthopedic injuries or older veterans recovering from neurologic or orthopedic injuries. I have also worked in a forward deployed setting as the primary musculoskeletal provider, where I was able to see patients without a physician referral.

Q: Describe a typical workday.

A: I usually see 12 patients a day, which includes four to six initial evaluations and six to eight reevaluations or follow-up treatments. I see patients half of the day, and I'm either in class or conducting research the rest of the day. Each patient visit requires a note in the medical record that includes a physical therapy diagnosis, treatment plan, and prognosis.

Q: Why did you choose this profession?

A: I was very active in sports as a kid and required physical therapy to recover from sports injuries. I have always been interested in serving others, so serving those in the Navy as a physical therapist was a bonus! I have been able to help patients learn to walk again after a stroke or amputation and return to sport after an acute ankle sprain. Each day is different, which keeps me engaged and excited.

Q: What challenges you most about this profession?

A: Keeping up with the most recent evidenced-based research can be challenging. Physical therapy is a rapidly growing profession with research to support or refute evaluation or treatment techniques, and the profession requires a commitment to continuous learning in order to provide the best possible outcomes for patients.

Q: Is there room for advancement in this field?

A: A new graduate from a physical therapy program can take a residency in a specialty area such as orthopedics, neurology, or pediatrics and obtain specialty certification. Further training in a fellowship and obtaining a Doctor of Science or PhD are also options. Advancement is also possible as a clinic manager or director of rehabilitation services.

Q: Explain what part of your academic training most prepared you for this profession.

A: There was a significant emphasis on patient-friendly communication, which I consider essential to be an effective physical therapist. As a professional, I ask my patients to engage in a treatment plan that will help them recover, but this requires work and participation on their part. If they don't understand why they need to do what I am instructing them to do, I won't get patient compliance and might not be successful in helping them get better.

Q: What obstacles have you had in pursuing your goals, and how did you overcome them?

A: I was never particularly good in general science classes, so that was a challenge for me as an undergraduate. I was able to overcome obstacles through study groups and tutors. As a newly licensed physical therapist, it was challenging to apply what I learned in classes to certain patients who didn't fit a specific diagnosis. Talking through clinical scenarios with clinical mentors has been very helpful.

Q: What advice would you give someone who is considering this career?

A: I would recommend observing or shadowing a licensed physical therapist in a variety of settings to learn about the many different areas where physical therapists can be employed. Good hands-on skills are important as is being personable, kind, patient, and a good communicator.

Physical therapists often consult and practice with a variety of other professionals, such as physicians, dentists, nurses, educators, social workers, occupational therapists, speech-language pathologists, and audiologists. Because of their close interaction with patients, physical therapists must observe strict confidentiality requirements and only discuss patients' confidential information with those medical personnel who are involved in treating the patients.

Some physical therapists treat a wide range of ailments; others specialize in areas such as pediatrics, geriatrics, orthopedics, **sports medicine**, neurology, and cardiopulmonary physical therapy. Some therapists work to prevent injury and loss of mobility, developing fitness and wellness programs to obtain and maintain a healthy and active lifestyle.

Work Environment

Physical therapists practice in hospitals, clinics, and private offices that have specially equipped facilities. They also treat patients in hospital rooms, homes, or schools. These jobs can be physically demanding because therapists often have to stoop, kneel, crouch, lift, and stand for long periods. In addition, physical therapists move heavy equipment and lift patients or help them turn, stand, or walk.

In 2021, most full-time physical therapists worked a 40-hour week; some worked evenings and weekends to fit their patients' schedules. Part-time work is common for physical therapists.

Employment Opportunities

Physical therapists held about 258,200 jobs in 2019. The number of jobs is greater than the number of practicing physical therapists because some physical therapists hold two or more jobs. For example, some may work in a private practice but also work part time in another healthcare facility.

About 60% of physical therapists worked in hospitals or in offices of other physical therapists. Additional jobs were in the home healthcare services industry, nursing care facilities, outpatient care centers, and offices of physicians. Some self-employed physical therapists in private practice saw individual patients and contracted to provide services in hospitals, **rehabilitation** centers, nursing care facilities, home healthcare agencies, adult day care programs, and schools. Physical therapists also teach in academic institutions and conduct research.

Educational and Legal Requirements

Today's entrants to this profession need a post-baccalaureate degree from an accredited physical therapy program. All states regulate the practice of physical therapy, which usually requires passing scores on national and state examinations.

Education and Training

The American Physical Therapy Association's (APTA) accrediting body, the Commission on Accreditation of Physical Therapy Education (CAPTE), accredits entry-level academic programs in physical therapy. In 2021, there were 260 physical therapist education programs, all of which awarded doctoral degrees.[1] Doctoral degree programs typically last three years, with most programs requiring a bachelor's degree and completion of prerequisites. Most accredited programs require applicants to use the Physical Therapist Centralized Application Service (PTCAS).[2]

Physical therapist education programs include foundational science courses, such as biology, anatomy, physiology, cellular histology, exercise physiology, neuroscience, biomechanics, pharmacology, pathology, and radiology/imaging, as well as behavioral science courses, such as **evidence-based practice** and clinical reasoning. Some of the clinically based courses include medical screening, examination tests and measures, diagnostic process, therapeutic interventions, **outcomes assessment**, and practice management. In addition to classroom and laboratory instruction, students receive supervised clinical experience.

Physical therapists may also pursue a clinical residency in a specialized area after graduation, and some physical therapists go further and pursue a fellowship after completing their clinical residency. The American Board of Physical Therapy Residency and Fellowship Education maintains a directory of residency and fellowship programs.[3]

Among the undergraduate courses that are useful when one applies to a physical therapist education program are anatomy, biology, chemistry, physics, social science, mathematics, and statistics. Before granting admission, many programs require volunteer experience in the physical therapy department of a hospital or clinic.

Licensure

All states regulate the practice of physical therapy. Eligibility requirements vary by state. Typical requirements for physical therapists include graduation from an accredited physical therapy education program, passing the National Physical Therapy Examination, and fulfilling state requirements such as jurisprudence exams. A number of states require continuing education as a condition of maintaining licensure.

Certification and Other Qualifications

Physical therapists may obtain certification in 10 specialty areas through the American Board of Physical Therapy Specialists. Certification is offered in the following areas: cardiovascular and pulmonary care, clinical electrophysiology, geriatrics, neurology, oncology, orthopedics, pediatrics, sports, women's health, and wound management. Requirements include completion of at least 2,000 hours of clinical work or completion of an APTA-accredited program in a specialty area and passing an examination.

TABLE 17.1 Projections Data for Physical Therapists, 2019–2029

Occupational Title	Employment, 2019	Projected Employment, 2029	Change, 2019–2029	
			Number	Percentage
Physical therapists	258,200	305,200	47,000	18%

Data from Bureau of Labor Statistics. Occupational Outlook Handbook 2019–2020 Edition. U.S. Department of Labor; 2020.

Physical therapists should have strong interpersonal and communication skills so they can educate patients about their condition and physical therapy treatments and communicate with patients' families. Physical therapists also should be compassionate and possess a desire to help patients. Manual dexterity is important because of the need to provide therapeutic exercises and manual therapy.

Advancement

Physical therapists are expected to continue their professional development by participating in continuing education courses and workshops. Some physical therapists become board-certified in a clinical specialty. Opportunities for physical therapists exist in academia and research. Some become self-employed, providing contract services or opening a private practice.

Employment Trends

Employment of physical therapists is expected to grow much faster than average. Job opportunities will be good, especially in acute hospital, rehabilitation, and orthopedic settings.

Employment Change

Employment of physical therapists is expected to grow 18% from 2019 to 2029, much faster than the average for all occupations. The demand for physical therapists should continue to rise as new treatments and techniques expand the scope of physical therapy practices. Moreover, the increasing numbers of individuals with disabilities or limited function will spur demand.

The increasing population of older adults will drive growth in the demand for physical therapy services. The older adult population is particularly vulnerable to chronic and debilitating conditions that require therapeutic services. Also, the Baby Boom generation is entering the prime age for heart attacks and strokes, increasing the demand for cardiac and physical rehabilitation. And increasing numbers of children will need physical therapy as technological advances save the lives of a larger proportion of newborns with severe birth defects.

Future medical developments also should permit a higher percentage of trauma victims to survive, creating additional demand for rehabilitative care. In addition, growth may result from advances in medical technology that could permit the treatment of an increasing number of disabling conditions that were untreatable in the past. Physical therapists will play a role in assisting these patients to health.

Widespread interest in health promotion also should increase demand for physical therapy services. A growing number of employers are using physical therapists to evaluate work sites, develop exercise programs, and teach safe work habits to employees.

Job Prospects

Job opportunities will be good for licensed physical therapists in all settings. Job opportunities should be particularly good in acute hospital, rehabilitation, and orthopedic settings, where older adults are most often treated. Physical therapists with specialized knowledge of particular types of treatment also will have excellent job prospects. Physical therapists willing to work in rural areas will be at an advantage because most physical therapists reside in highly populated urban and suburban areas. **TABLE 17.1** shows some projection data provided by the U.S. Department of Labor.

Earnings

Median annual wages of physical therapists were $91,010 in May 2020. The lowest 10% earned less than $63,530, and the highest 10% earned more than $126,780. Median annual wages in the industries employing the largest numbers of physical therapists in May 2020 are shown in **TABLE 17.2**.

Related Occupations

Physical therapists rehabilitate people with physical disabilities. Others who work in the rehabilitation field include audiologists, chiropractors, occupational therapists, recreational therapists, rehabilitation counselors, respiratory therapists, and speech-language pathologists.

TABLE 17.2 Median Annual Wages in the Industries Employing the Largest Numbers of Physical Therapists, May 2020

Home healthcare services	$95,320
Nursing care facilities	$97,610
Hospitals: state, local, and private	$93,060
Offices of physical, occupational, and speech therapists and audiologists	$85,680

Data from Bureau of Labor Statistics. Occupational Outlook Handbook 2019–2020 Edition. U.S. Department of Labor; 2020.

Additional Information

Career information on physical therapy and a list of schools offering accredited programs can be obtained from:

- The American Physical Therapy Association, 3030 Potomac Ave, Suite 100, VA 22305-3085. https://www.apta.org
- Commission on Accreditation in Physical Therapy Education, 3030 Potomac Ave, Suite 100 Alexandria, VA 22305-3085. https://www.capteonline.org/home.aspx

For information about specialty certification, contact:

- American Board of Physical Therapy Specialists, 3030 Potomac Ave, Suite 100, Alexandria, VA 22305-3085. https://www.abpts.org/home.aspx

For information about licensure, contact:

- The Federation of State Boards of Physical Therapy, 124 West St. South, Alexandria, VA 22314. https://www.fsbpt.org

PHYSICAL THERAPIST ASSISTANTS AND AIDES
Significant Points

- Employment is projected to grow much faster than average.
- Physical therapist assistants should have very good job prospects; on the other hand, aides may face keen competition from the large pool of qualified applicants.
- Aides usually learn skills on the job, while physical therapist assistants have an associate's degree; most states require licensing for assistants.
- Most jobs are in offices of other health practitioners and in hospitals.

Work Description

Physical therapist assistants and aides help physical therapists provide treatment that improves patient mobility, relieves pain, and prevents or lessens physical disabilities of patients. A physical therapist might ask an assistant to help patients exercise or learn to use crutches, for example, or an aide to gather and prepare therapy equipment. Patients include accident victims and individuals with disabling conditions such as lower-back pain, arthritis, heart disease, fractures, head injuries, and cerebral palsy.

Physical therapist assistants perform a variety of tasks. Under the direction and supervision of physical therapists, they provide part of a patient's treatment. This might involve exercises, massages, electrical stimulation, **paraffin baths**, hot and cold packs, traction, and ultrasound. Physical therapist assistants record the patient's responses to treatment and report the outcome of each treatment to the physical therapist. An example of a physical therapist assistant helping a patient is seen in **FIGURE 17.2**.

Physical therapist aides help make therapy sessions productive under the direct supervision of a physical therapist or physical therapist assistant. They usually are responsible for keeping the treatment area clean and organized and for preparing for each patient's therapy. When patients need assistance moving to or from a treatment area, aides push them in a wheelchair or provide them with a shoulder to lean on. Physical therapist aides are not licensed and do not perform the clinical tasks of a physical therapist assistant in states where licensure is required.

The duties of aides include some clerical tasks, such as ordering depleted supplies, answering the phone, and filling out insurance forms and other paperwork. The extent to which an aide or an assistant performs clerical tasks depends on the size and location of the facility.

Work Environment

Physical therapist assistants and aides need a moderate degree of strength because of the physical exertion required in assisting patients with their treatment. In some cases, assistants and aides need to lift patients. Frequent kneeling, stooping, and standing for long periods also are part of the job.

The hours and days that physical therapist assistants and aides work vary with the facility. Part-time work is common for physical therapist assistants and aides. Many outpatient physical therapy offices and clinics keep evening and weekend hours to accommodate patients' personal schedules.

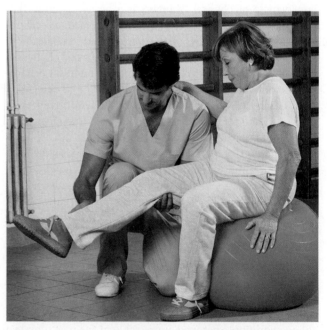

FIGURE 17.2 A physical therapist assistant helping a patient exercise.
© Tyler Olson/Shutterstock.

Employment Opportunities

Physical therapist assistants and aides held about 149,300 jobs in 2019. Physical therapist assistants held about 98,700 jobs; physical therapist aides held approximately 50,600. Both work with physical therapists in a variety of settings. About three-quarters of jobs were in offices of physical therapists or in hospitals. Others worked primarily in nursing care facilities, offices of physicians, home healthcare services, and outpatient care centers.

Educational and Legal Requirements

Most physical therapist aides are trained on the job, but most physical therapist assistants earn an associate's degree from an accredited physical therapist assistant program. Some states require licensing for physical therapist assistants.

Education and Training

Employers typically require physical therapist aides to have a high school diploma. They are trained on the job, and most employers provide clinical on-the-job training.

In most states, physical therapist assistants are required by law to hold an associate's degree. The American Physical Therapy Association's Commission on Accreditation in Physical Therapy Education (CAPTE) accredits postsecondary physical therapy assistant programs. In 2021, there were 376 accredited programs, which usually last two years and culminate in an associate's degree.[4]

Programs are divided into academic study and hands-on clinical experience. Academic course work includes algebra, anatomy and physiology, biology, chemistry, and psychology. Clinical work includes certifications in cardiopulmonary resuscitation (CPR) and other first aid as well as field experience in treatment centers. Both educators and prospective employers view clinical experience as essential to ensuring that students understand the responsibilities of a physical therapist assistant.

Licensure

Licensing is not required to practice as a physical therapist aide. However, most states require licensure or registration in order to work as a physical therapist assistant. States that require licensure stipulate specific educational and examination criteria, such as graduation from an accredited program and passing the National Physical Therapy Exam administered by the Federation of State Boards of Physical Therapy. Additional requirements may include certification in CPR and other first aid and a minimum number of hours of clinical experience. Complete information on regulations can be obtained from state licensing boards.

Other Qualifications

Physical therapist assistants and aides should be well organized, detail oriented, and caring. They usually have strong interpersonal skills and a desire to help people in need. They need physical stamina and should enjoy physical activity.

Advancement

Some physical therapist aides advance to become therapist assistants after gaining experience and, often, additional education. Sometimes, this education is required by law. Some physical therapist assistants advance by specializing in a clinical area. They gain expertise in treating a certain type of patient, such as geriatric or pediatric, or a type of ailment, such as sports injuries. Many physical therapist assistants advance to administrative positions. These positions might include organizing all the assistants in a large physical therapy organization or acting as the director for a specific department such as sports medicine. Other assistants go on to teach in accredited physical therapist assistant academic programs, lead health risk-reduction classes for older adults, or organize community activities related to fitness and risk reduction.

Employment Trends

Employment is expected to grow much faster than average because of increasing consumer demand for physical therapy services. Job prospects for physical therapist assistants are expected to be very good. Aides should experience keen competition for jobs.

Employment Change

Employment of physical therapist assistants is expected to grow by 33% over the 2019 to 2029 decade, much faster than the average for all occupations. Employment of physical therapist aides is expected to grow by 21% over the 2019 to 2029 decade, much faster than the average for all occupations. Long-term demand for physical therapist assistants and aides will continue to rise, as the number of individuals with disabilities or limited function grows.

The increasing number of people who need therapy reflects, in part, the increasing elderly population. The older adult population is particularly vulnerable to chronic and debilitating conditions that require therapeutic services. These patients often need additional assistance in their treatment, making the roles of assistants and aides vital. In addition, the large Baby Boom generation is entering the prime age for heart attacks and strokes, further increasing the demand for cardiac and physical rehabilitation. Moreover, future medical developments should permit an increased percentage of trauma victims to survive, creating added demand for therapy services.

Physical therapists are expected to increasingly use assistants to reduce the cost of physical therapy services. Once a patient is evaluated and a treatment plan is designed by the

TABLE 17.3 Projections Data Physical Therapist Assistants and Aides, 2019–2029

Occupational Title	Employment, 2019	Project Employment, 2029	Change, 2019–2029	
			Number	Percentage
Physical therapist assistants and aides	149,200	192,300	43,000	29%
Physical therapist assistants	98,700	130,900	32,200	33%
Physical therapist aides	50,600	61,300	10,800	21%

Data from Bureau of Labor Statistics. Occupational Outlook Handbook 2019–2020 Edition. U.S. Department of Labor; 2020.

physical therapist, the physical therapist assistant can provide many parts of the treatment, as approved by the therapist.

Job Prospects

Opportunities for individuals interested in becoming physical therapist assistants are expected to be very good. Physical therapist aides may face keen competition from the large pool of qualified individuals. In addition to employment growth, job openings will result from the need to replace workers who leave the occupation permanently. Physical therapist assistants and aides with prior experience working in a physical therapy office or other healthcare setting will have the best job opportunities. **TABLE 17.3** shows some projection data provided by the Department of Labor.

Earnings

Median annual wages of physical therapist assistants were $59,770 in May 2020. The lowest 10% earned less than $33,840, and the highest 10% earned more than $82,470. Median annual wages in the industries employing the largest numbers of physical therapist assistants in May 2020 are included in **TABLE 17.4**.

Median annual wages of physical therapist aides were $28,450 in May 2020. The lowest 10% earned less than $20,500, and the highest 10% earned more than $40,580. Median annual wages in the industries employing the largest numbers of physical therapist aides in May 2020 are shown in **TABLE 17.5**.

Related Occupations

Physical therapist assistants and aides work under the supervision of physical therapists. Other workers in the healthcare field who work under similar supervision include dental assistants; medical assistants; occupational therapist assistants and aides; pharmacy aides; pharmacy technicians; nursing, psychiatric, and home health aides; personal and home care aides; and social and human service assistants.

Additional Information

Career information on physical therapy and a list of schools offering accredited programs can be obtained from:

- The American Physical Therapy Association, 3030 Potomac Ave, Suite 100, Alexandria, VA 22305-3085. https://www.apta.org
- Commission on Accreditation in Physical Therapy Education, 3030 Potomac Ave., Suite 100, Alexandria, VA 22305-3085. https://www.capteonline.org /home.aspx

For information about licensure, contact:

- The Federation of State Boards of Physical Therapy, 124 West St. South, Alexandria, VA 22314. https://www .fsbpt.org

TABLE 17.4 Median Annual Earnings in the Industries Employing the Largest Numbers of Physical Therapist Assistants, May 2020

Home healthcare services	$64,700
Nursing care facilities	$67,120
Hospitals: state, local, and private	$58,460
Offices of physical, occupational, and speech therapists, and audiologists	$58,050
Offices of physicians	$56,730

Data from Bureau of Labor Statistics. Occupational Outlook Handbook 2019–2020 Edition. U.S. Department of Labor; 2020.

TABLE 17.5 Median Annual Earnings in the Industries Employing the Largest Numbers of Physical Therapist Aides, May 2020

Nursing care facilities	$34,800
Hospitals: state, local, and private	$30,620
Government	$28,360
Offices of physicians	$29,760
Offices of physical, occupational, and speech therapists, and audiologists	$27,080

Data from Bureau of Labor Statistics. Occupational Outlook Handbook 2019–2020 Edition. U.S. Department of Labor; 2020.

ORTHOTISTS AND PROSTHETISTS
Significant Points

- Employment is projected to grow much faster than average.
- Orthotists and prosthetists should have very good job prospects.
- A master's degree, certification, and a residency are required for a practitioner.
- Most jobs are in ambulatory care services or medical equipment and supplies manufacturing.

Work Description

Orthotics and prosthetics (O&P) refers to the evaluation, fabrication, and custom fitting of artificial limbs and orthopedic braces. Examples of artificial limbs are seen in **FIGURE 17.3**. An **orthotist** designs and fits corrective braces, inserts, and supports for body parts that need straightening or other curative functions. A **prosthetist** designs, measures, fits, and adjusts artificial limbs for amputees and devices for people with musculoskeletal or neurological conditions. An **orthotic and prosthetic technician** assists a credentialed individual by providing technical support. All of these professionals combine knowledge of cutting-edge technology and hands-on patient care. These individuals are sometimes referred to as O&P professionals.

O&P professionals evaluate and interview patients to determine their needs. They measure patients so that their medical devices are properly designed and will fit well. An example using technology to measure a patient's foot for an orthotic is seen in **FIGURE 17.4**. These professionals may create a mold of the patient's body part that will be fitted with a brace or artificial limb and select the materials to be used in fabricating the device. After fitting, testing, and adjusting the device on a patient, they will provide instructions on how to use and care for the devices. As needed, they will repair or update a patient's orthotic or prosthetic device.

O&P professionals document the patient's progress on a regular basis. With the increased use of electronic health records (EHRs), they must understand the computer software the EHR uses when documenting the patient's progress. Because of their close interaction with patients, orthotists and prosthetists must observe strict confidentiality requirements and only discuss patient confidential information with those medical personnel who are involved in treating the patient.

Some individuals work as **pedorthists**. A pedorthist selects, modifies, or creates footwear to help people maintain or regain as much mobility as possible. Pedorthists combine knowledge of human anatomy and biomechanical evaluation to treat painful and disabling conditions of the foot and ankle.

Work Environment

Orthotists and prosthetists practice in a variety of places including patient care facilities, hospitals, clinics, and private offices. Most orthotists and prosthetists work in ambulatory care services or medical equipment and supplies

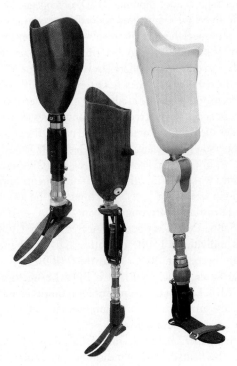

FIGURE 17.3 Artificial limbs.
© Vereshchagin Dmitry/Shutterstock.

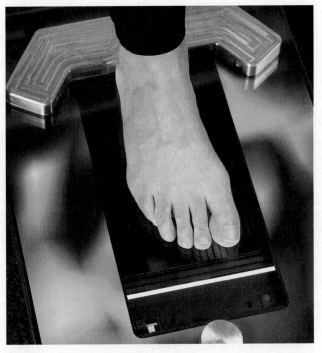

FIGURE 17.4 A foot on a 3D scanner for orthotics.
© Rainer Plendl/Shutterstock.

manufacturing, including the shops where the orthotics and prosthetics are created. They may also work in Veterans Administration (VA) facilities, rehabilitation facilities, long-term care facilities, and patients' homes. Most work is performed in private offices where they meet with patients and then design orthotic and prosthetic devices. Pedorthists work in settings such as specialty shoe stores, orthotic and prosthetic patient care facilities, VA facilities, and rehabilitation facilities.

Because O&P professionals may be exposed to health and safety hazards when working with certain materials, they must be follow proper procedures and use safety devices such as goggles, gloves, and masks. Doing so minimizes the risk of illness or injury.

Employment Opportunities

Orthotists and prosthetists held about 10,000 jobs in 2019. More than 50% of these jobs were held in companies involving medical equipment and supplies manufacturing or in ambulatory healthcare services. Most O&P professionals work full time.

Educational and Legal Requirements

Orthotists and prosthetists require a master's degree and certification before beginning work in the field. A one-year residency is required before obtaining certification. Technicians frequently graduate from a two-year associate's program.

Education and Training

Orthotist and prosthetist practitioners must receive a master's degree in orthotics and prosthetics. These programs generally take two years to complete and involve courses in upper- and lower-extremity orthotics and prosthetics, spinal orthotics, and plastics and other materials. A bachelor's degree is required for admission and can be in any discipline as long as certain prerequisites are met. Those prerequisites included courses in science and mathematics.

A clinical residency is required as part of the master's program. At least 500 hours of clinical experience are required, split evenly between orthotics and prosthetics.

Orthotic and prosthetic technicians may either graduate from an associate's degree program or possess a high school diploma, GED, or college degree and complete two years of technical experience under the supervision of a credentialed individual.

Two organizations accredit academic programs in orthotics and prosthetics. The Commission on Accreditation of Allied Health Education Programs (CAAHEP) has accredited a total of 19 programs: 13 programs at the master's degree level and six programs at the technician level.[5] The National Commission on Orthotic and Prosthetic Education (NCOPE) accredits academic programs in orthotics and prosthetics [6] Most accredited programs require applicants to use the

Orthotics and Prosthetics Residency Centralized Application Service (OPRESCAS).[7]

Licensure

Some states require licensure. For those that do, becoming certified through the American Board for Certification in Orthotics, Prosthetics, and Pedorthics (ABC) is also a requirement.[8] Eligibility requirements vary by state.

Certification and Other Qualifications

The American Board for Certification in Orthotics, Prosthetics, and Pedorthics (ABC) is the oldest established governing body that issues credentials in this field. Orthotists who complete a master's degree program and clinical residency may sit for a three-part examination and receive the Certified Orthotist (CO) credential. Prosthetists who complete a master's degree program and clinical residency may sit for a three-part examination and receive the Certified Prosthetist (CP) credential. Individuals who meet the requirements and pass the examinations of both disciplines may receive the Certified Prosthetist Orthotist (CPO) credential.

Orthotic and prosthetic technicians who complete an associate's degree program or possess a high school diploma, GED, or college degree and two years of clinical experience may sit for an examination and receive the Certified Orthotic Technician (CTO) or Certified Prosthetic Technician (CTP) credential. Individuals who meet the requirements and pass the examinations of both disciplines may receive the Certified Prosthetic-Orthotic Technician (CTPO) credential.

Those individuals seeking to work as pedorthists must possess a high school diploma, GED, or college degree and complete an NCOPE-approved pedorthic precertification program. If they meet these requirements and pass an examination, they can receive the Certified Pedorthist (C.Ped.) credential.

Other credentials are offered by the ABC. One may obtain the Certified Fitter-orthotics (CFo) credential, the Certified Fitter-mastectomy (CFm) credential, or the Certified Fitter-therapeutic shoes (CFts) credential. If one serves in an assistant role, meets the ABC requirements, and passes the certification exam, a person may be awarded the Certified Orthotic Assistant (COA) or Certified Prosthetic Assistant (CPA) credential. Candidates who have met the ABC requirements and passed certification exams for both disciplines will be awarded the Certified Prosthetic-Orthotic Assistant (CPOA) credential.

The Board of Certification/Accreditation (BOC) also certifies individuals in the orthotics and prosthetics field. One can become a BOC Pedorthist (BOCPD), a BOC Orthotic Fitter (BOC COF), or a BOC Mastectomy Fitter (BOC CMF). Each of these credentials requires an individual to complete an education program specific to the identified role and pass an examination.[9]

Both interpersonal and technical skills are needed to be successful in this field. Recording measurements requires attention to detail, and designing orthotics or prosthetics requires manual dexterity. Creativity and problem-solving skills are necessary to address complex patient situations. Communication skills

TABLE 17.6 Projections Data for Orthotists and Prosthetists, 2019–2029

Occupational Title	Employment, 2019	Project Employment, 2029	Change, 2019–2029	
			Number	Percentage
Orthotists and prosthetists	10,000	11,700	1,700	17%

Data from Bureau of Labor Statistics. Occupational Outlook Handbook 2019–2020 Edition. U.S. Department of Labor; 2020.

are crucial in order to obtain information from patients and instruct them on the use and care of devices.

Employment Trends

Employment is expected to grow much faster than average because of increasing consumer demand for orthotic and prosthetic services.

Employment Change

Employment of orthotists and prosthetists is expected to grow by 17% over the 2019 to 2029 decade, much faster than the average for all occupations. Because of the small numbers of persons in the profession, the total increase over the next decade is only expected to be 1,700.

The increasing number of people who need therapy reflects, in part, the increasing elderly population. Two of the leading reasons for limb loss, diabetes and cardiovascular diseases, are common among older adults. Technological advances that result in an increase in natural movement while using an artificial device may spur demand. Braces and other orthopedic footwear will also be needed by older adults. Advances in medicine now permit many people to survive traumatic events. Those persons surviving these events will need the assistance of orthotists and prosthetists to regain or improve mobility and functionality.

Job Prospects

Opportunities for individuals interested in becoming orthotists and prosthetists are expected to be very good. In addition to employment growth, job openings will result from the need to replace workers who leave the occupation permanently. Those individuals possessing professional certification will have the best job opportunities. **TABLE 17.6** shows some projection data provided by the U.S. Department of Labor.

Earnings

Median annual wages of orthotists and prosthetists were $70,190 in May 2020. The lowest 10% earned less than $41,790, and the highest 10% earned more than $110,130. Median annual wages in the industries employing the largest numbers of orthotists and prosthetists in May 2020 are shown in **TABLE 17.7**.

According to a 2013 study by the American Orthotic and Prosthetic Association of compensation and benefits, O&P practitioners received average compensation of $75,300, assistants received $43,000, technicians received $45,630, pedorthists received $52,065, and fitters received $39,000.

Related Occupations

Orthotists and prosthetists work both independently and with team members. Other workers in the healthcare field who work under similar circumstances include dental and ophthalmic laboratory technicians, medical appliance technicians, physicians and surgeons, physical therapists, and respiratory therapists.

Additional Information

For more information about orthotists and prosthetists, visit:

- American Academy of Orthotists and Prosthetists, 7910 Woodmont Ave., Suite 760, Bethesda, MD 20814. https://www.oandp.org
- American Orthotic & Prosthetic Association, 330 John Carlyle St., Suite 200, Alexandria, VA 22314. https://www.aopanet.org

For information on accredited programs, visit:

- National Commission on Orthotic and Prosthetic Education, 330 John Carlyle St., Suite 200, Alexandria, VA 22314. https://www.ncope.org

For information about certification, contact:

- American Board for Certification in Orthotics, Prosthetics, and Pedorthics, 330 John Carlyle St., Suite 210, Alexandria, VA 22314. https://www.abcop.org
- Board of Certification/Accreditation, 10451 Mill Run Circle, Suite 200, Owings Mill, MD 21117-5575. https://www.bocusa.org

TABLE 17.7 Median Annual Wages in the Industries Employing the Largest Numbers of Orthotists and Prosthetists, May 2020

Medical equipment and supplies manufacturing	$74,330
Health and personal care stores	$63,980
Hospitals: state, local, and private	$59,340
Ambulatory healthcare services	$72,760
Federal executive branch	$76,030

Data from Bureau of Labor Statistics. Occupational Outlook Handbook 2019–2020 Edition. U.S. Department of Labor; 2020.

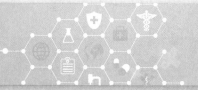

LEARNING PORTFOLIO

Issues for Discussion

1. Many individuals have experienced the assistance of physical therapists directly. Discuss with your instructor and classmates the experiences you have had with a physical therapist and the effect physical therapy had upon the problem for which you received treatment.

2. Watch the career video about physical therapy at https://www.careeronestop.org/Toolkit/Careers/Occupations/occupation-profile.aspx?keyword=Physical%20Therapists&onetcode=29112300&location=UNITED%20STATES and view the materials on Becoming a PT at https://www.apta.org/your-career/careers-in-physical-therapy/becoming-a-pt. Decide what about this video or these materials strikes you as explaining the essence of working as a physical therapist. Discuss with your instructor and classmates.

3. Watch the video about a career as an orthotist or prosthetist at https://www.careeronestop.org/videos/careeronestop-videos.aspx?videocode=29209100. Discuss with your instructor and classmates what impressions this video gives you and decide whether you would suggest any of the careers in the video to your friends or acquaintances.

Enrichment Activities

1. Artificial limbs have a long history. Research this history and create a timeline (whether a narrative piece, a PowerPoint presentation, or an infographic) that describes the types of prosthetics created, the materials used, and the types of assistance these prosthetics have offered.

2. Interview a physical therapist, physical therapist assistant or aide, or O&P professional. Create and submit to your instructor a list of questions and answers from your interview and identify which answer, if any, was the most surprising.

CASE STUDY: A CAREER IN PHYSICAL THERAPY

Priti was a student athlete in high school who received help from a physical therapist to return to sports after suffering an injury. This experience prompted Priti to consider physical therapy as a future occupation. Priti has decided to shadow the professionals working at a physical therapy clinic to gain more understanding of what is involved in the day-to-day work of the profession. Based on the information you have read about physical therapists and physical therapy assistants and aides and the preceding case study, answer the following questions.

1. Which activity would Priti not see during the shadow visit at the physical therapy clinic?
   A. Range of motion exercises
   B. Prescribing medications
   C. Deep tissue massage
   D. Tests of motor function

2. Which certifications may be held by the physical therapy professionals Priti is shadowing?
   A. Sports specialty

   B. Cardiopulmonary resuscitation (CPR)
   C. Orthopedics specialty
   D. Any of the above

3. Determine the undergraduate course that would best support Priti's goal of becoming a physical therapist.
   A. Music Appreciation 100
   B. Biology 100
   C. History 100
   D. Anthropology 100

4. Priti realizes that _____ stamina is important because physical therapists spend much of their days on their feet and stooping, kneeling, and crouching are part of their duties when working with patients.
   A. mental
   B. emotional
   C. physical
   D. financial

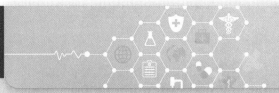

LEARNING PORTFOLIO

References

1. Commission on Accreditation in Physical Therapy Education (CAPTE). Accredited PT Programs. https: aptaapps .apta.org/accreditedschoolsdirectory/AllPrograms.aspx Accessed August 8, 2021.

2. Physical Therapist Centralized Application Service. https: //www.ptcas.org/home.aspx Accessed August 8, 2021.

3. The American Board of Physical Therapy Residency and Fellowship Education. https://abptrfe.apta.org/ Accessed August 8, 2021.

4. Commission on Accreditation in Physical Therapy Education. Accredited PTA Programs. https:aptaapps.apta.org /accreditedschoolsdirectory/AllPrograms.aspx Accessed 8, 2021.

5. The Commission on Accreditation of Allied Health Education Programs. https://www.caahep.org/Students/Find-a -Program.aspx Accessed August 8, 2021.

6. National Commission on Orthotic and Prosthetic Education. List of Schools. https://ncope.org/index.php/home -page-v2/academic-programs/ Accessed August 8, 2021.

7. Orthotics and Prosthetics Residency Centralized Application Service. https://ncope.org/index.php/home-page-v2 /residency-and-professional-experiences/oprescas-candidate -information/ Accessed August 8, 2021.

8. American Board for Certification in Orthotics, Prosthetics, and Pedorthics. https://www.abcop.org/ Accessed August 8, 2021.

9. Board of Certification/Accreditation. https://www.bocusa .org/ Accessed August 8, 2021.

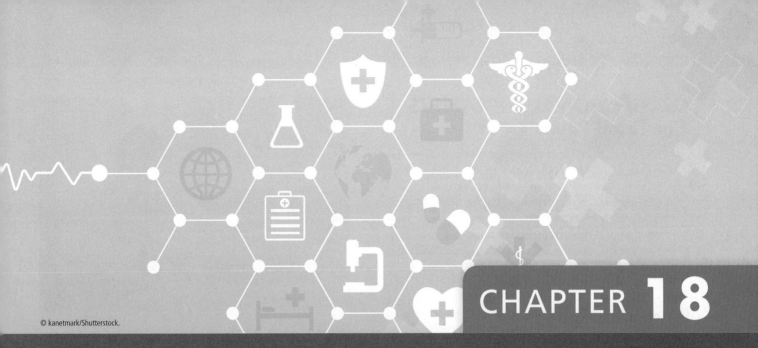
© kanetmark/Shutterstock.

CHAPTER 18

Occupational Therapy*

KEY TERMS

Adaptive equipment	Multidisciplinary team	Perceptual skills
Cognitive skills	Occupational therapist	Physical disabilities
Emotional disorders	Occupational therapy	Rehabilitation center
Home health care	Occupational therapy aide	Wellness and health
Mental health	Occupational therapy assistant	promotion

* All information in this chapter, unless otherwise indicated, was obtained from Bureau of Labor Statistics. *Occupational Outlook Handbook 2020–2021 Edition*. Washington, DC: U.S. Department of Labor; 2021.

OCCUPATIONAL THERAPISTS
Significant Points

- Employment is expected to grow much faster than average, and job opportunities should be good, especially for therapists treating older adults.
- Occupational therapists are regulated in all 50 states; requirements vary by state.
- Occupational therapists are increasingly taking on supervisory roles, allowing assistants and aides to work more closely with clients under the guidance of a therapist.

Work Description

Occupational therapy refers to therapy provided to those who are recovering from illness or injury that encourages rehabilitation by performing the activities of daily life. **Occupational therapists** treat people with mental, physical, developmental, or emotional disabilities so that they may participate in the things they want and need to do through therapeutic use of daily activities. They employ a variety of techniques designed to help individuals develop or maintain daily living skills and cope with the physical and emotional effects of disability. With support and direction from the therapist, patients learn (or relearn) many of the "ordinary" tasks that are performed every day at home, at work, at school, and in the community. The therapist's goal is to help clients establish a lifestyle that is as independent, productive, and satisfying as possible.

Like other health professionals, occupational therapists often work as members of a **multidisciplinary team** whose members may include a physician, nurse, physical therapist, psychologist, rehabilitation counselor, and social worker. Team members evaluate the patient in terms of their individual specialties and work together to develop goals that meet the patient's needs. During the course of treatment, team meetings are held to evaluate progress and to modify the treatment plan, if necessary.

Activities of various kinds can be used for treatment purposes. When working with children, for example, occupational therapists often use toys, an example of which is seen in **FIGURE 18.1**. For adults, therapy may include anything from activities that strengthen muscles to using a computer. Although some treatments may give the appearance of recreation, all have a serious purpose. Working in the kitchen may produce a cake, but the skills practiced include memory, sequencing, coordination, and safety precautions, which are important for independent living at home. "Word find" games can help improve visual acuity and the ability to discern patterns. Specially designed computer programs help patients improve **cognitive skills**, including decision making, abstract reasoning, and problem solving, along with **perceptual skills**, such as peripheral vision and discrimination of letters, colors, and shapes. All of these treatments are designed to foster independence at home and at work.

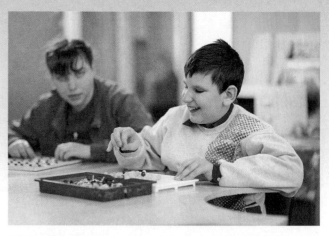

FIGURE 18.1 Use of a toy to develop cognitive ability.
© Olesia Bilkei/Shutterstock.

During each therapy session, the therapist assesses the patient to determine treatment effectiveness and progress made toward meeting the treatment's goals. These assessments serve as the basis for modifying goals and therapeutic procedures. A person with short-term memory loss, for instance, might be encouraged to make lists to aid recall. One with coordination problems might be given tasks to improve eye–hand coordination.

In addition to helping individuals strengthen basic motor functions and reasoning abilities, occupational therapists help them master daily living skills. Helping individuals with severe disabilities learn to cope with seemingly ordinary tasks such as getting dressed, using a bathroom, or driving a car requires sensitivity as well as skill. A disability may be recently acquired, such as a spinal cord injury resulting from a traffic accident, or a chronic condition present at birth, such as cerebral palsy. Therapists provide individuals with **adaptive equipment** such as wheelchairs, splints, and aids for eating and dressing. They may design and make special equipment and recommend changes in the home or work environment to facilitate functioning. An example of adaptive equipment used in walking is seen in **FIGURE 18.2**.

Computer-aided adaptive equipment offers the prospect of independence to some people with severe disabilities. Occupational therapists often work with rehabilitation engineers to develop such special equipment. Examples include microprocessing devices that permit individuals with paraplegia and quadriplegia to operate wheelchairs and household switches for appliances such as telephones, television sets, and radios. As such devices move out of the research and development stage, occupational therapists become involved in helping patients learn to use them.

An occupational therapist tends to work with a particular disability or age group. Many therapists work principally with persons who have **physical disabilities**, while others work with those who have psychological, emotional, or developmental problems. Some therapists provide early intervention to infants and toddlers who have or are at risk of having developmental delays. A growing number of

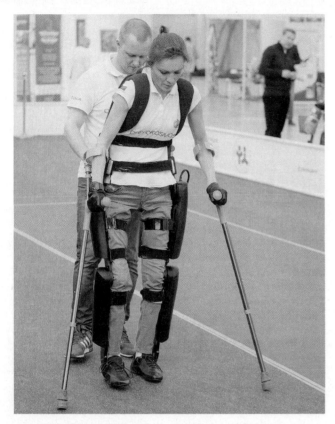

FIGURE 18.2 Adaptive equipment used for walking.
© Vereshchagin Dmitry/Shutterstock.

therapists are working in the **wellness and health promotion** areas. Often, the practice setting determines the age level and treatment needs of a therapist's patients. In **home health care**, for instance, a growing number of referrals involve older individuals with conditions such as arthritis, cardiac problems, and hip and other fractures. Therapists may recommend changes in the home environment after identifying potential hazards their patients may encounter.

The goals of occupational therapy in public schools focus not on treatment or rehabilitation but on the resources that an individual child needs to participate effectively in the educational program. This may involve making an initial evaluation of a child's abilities and the implications for learning; recommending special therapeutic activities; consulting with parents and teachers; modifying classroom equipment or school facilities; and developing the functional, motor, and perceptual skills necessary for learning. Like teachers, these occupational therapists work regular school hours and participate in teachers' meetings and other activities.

Occupational therapists in **mental health** settings treat individuals with mental illness or emotional problems. Among the disorders and diseases often treated mainly as **emotional disorders**, occupational therapists encounter alcoholism, drug abuse, depression, eating disorders, and stress-related disorders. Therapists provide individual and group activities that simulate real-life experiences to help people learn to cope with the daily stresses of life and

to manage their work and leisure more effectively. These activities include tasks that require planning and time-management skills, budgeting, shopping, meal preparation and homemaking, self-care, and using community resources such as public transportation and service agencies.

Keeping notes is an important part of an occupational therapist's job. Some of the records for which an occupational therapist may be responsible include an initial evaluation, progress notes, written reports to the physician, special internal staff notes, Medicare records, and discharge notes. Careful and complete documentation is required for reimbursement by insurance companies and Medicare. With the increased use of electronic health records (EHRs), occupational therapists must understand the computer software the EHR uses. Because of their close interaction with patients, occupational therapists must observe strict confidentiality requirements and only discuss a patient's confidential information with those medical personnel who are involved in treating the patient.

Besides working with patients, occupational therapists may supervise student therapists, occupational therapy assistants, volunteers, and auxiliary nursing workers. Chief occupational therapists in a hospital may teach medical and nursing students the principles of occupational therapy. Many therapists supervise occupational therapy departments, coordinate patients' activities, or act as consultants to public health departments and mental health agencies. Some teach or conduct research in colleges and universities.

Work Environment

Although occupational therapists generally work a standard 40-hour week, they may occasionally have to work evenings or weekends to accommodate patient schedules. Their work environment varies according to the setting and available facilities. In a large **rehabilitation center**, for example, the therapist may work in a spacious room with a variety of equipment. In a nursing home, the therapist may work in a kitchen when using food preparation as therapy. Wherever they work and whatever equipment they use, they generally have adequate lighting and ventilation. The job can be physically tiring because therapists are on their feet much of the time. Those providing home health care may spend several hours a day driving from appointment to appointment. Therapists also face hazards such as back strain from lifting and moving patients and equipment.

Therapists are increasingly taking on supervisory roles. In an effort to curtail rising healthcare costs, third-party payers are beginning to encourage occupational therapy assistants and aides to take more hands-on responsibility. Having assistants and aides work more closely with clients under the guidance of a therapist should reduce the cost of therapy. Part-time work is available in the field.

Employment Opportunities

Occupational therapists held about 143,300 jobs in 2019. The largest number of jobs were in offices of other health

Professional Profiles

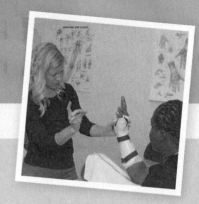

Name: Erica, OTR, CHT
Job Title: Occupational Therapist, Certified Hand Therapist
Education: MS in Occupational Therapy, BS in Occupational Science

Q: Describe your job and organization.

A: I work in an outpatient orthopedic private practice setting as an occupational therapist with certification in hand therapy. The clinic is staffed with eight physical therapists and two other occupational therapists specializing in hand therapy. Our practice is in two different locations in a very active urban area close to the beach.

Q: Describe a typical workday.

A: On a typical workday, I see 12 patients who are scheduled for a 30-minute session, except for new evaluations, which take an hour. The length of the patient sessions ranges from 45 to 60 minutes. I spend four to five minutes documenting each visit except for new evaluations, which takes 15 minutes. Therapists document in electronic medical records and fax reports to the offices of the patient's physician.

Q: Why did you choose this profession?

A: I chose occupational therapy because I love to work with people. I originally wanted to work with children with disabilities. However, I fell in love with the complexity of therapy of the hand and upper extremity through my mentorship program. Motivating people to return to a previous level of functioning is the most gratifying part of my job.

Q: What challenges you the most about this profession?

A: Staying up to date with all of the changes in health insurance is challenging! If documentation is incomplete or incorrect, the patient's health insurance may not cover the cost of therapy—ultimately delaying therapy and delaying the patient's return to normal functioning.

Q: Is there room for advancement in this field?

A: We must stay up to date with the times, keeping ourselves and clients educated. From the orthopedic world, I feel that we could better educate the public on how to prevent injuries and how to manage our bodies as we age. Occupational therapists can advance in their field through specialization in pediatrics, orthopedics, mental health, physical disabilities, or older adults and other areas. Certification in hand therapy requires working in a hand clinic for five years before sitting for the exam to become a Certified Hand Therapist (CHT).

Q: Name and explain what part of your academic training most prepared you for this profession.

A: Clinical rotations best prepared me for my profession. Combining classes with clinical rotations assisted in the application of knowledge. Courses that provided the foundation for my profession were gross anatomy and physical disabilities. The course in physical disabilities was beneficial because eventually a therapist will see patients with those unconventional injuries, diseases, and disabilities.

Q: What do you wish you would have known in high school or college about pursuing this career?

A: I would have spent more time observing occupational therapists in different work settings before selecting clinical rotations. Once in graduate school, you must quickly decide which areas to choose for fieldwork, and fieldwork prepares you to work in specific areas such as orthopedics or mental health.

Q: What advice would you give someone who is considering this career?

A: Observe occupational therapists in multiple work settings—each setting is dynamic in its own way. The more information you have about the different specialty areas, the easier it is to choose fieldwork sites and specialty areas as a professional. The outpatient setting is very fast paced, and skills most essential for success in this setting are the ability to multitask, problem-solve and set priorities throughout the day. You need to be confident in what you have learned and to continue learning. Desirable personality characteristics are to be outgoing, empathetic, and nonjudgmental.

practitioners (including offices of other occupational therapists), which employed about 26% of occupational therapists, and hospitals, which employed about 26% of occupational therapists. Other major employers included home healthcare services, public and private educational services, and nursing care facilities. Some occupational therapists were employed by home healthcare services, outpatient care centers, physicians' offices, individual and family services, community care facilities for older adults, and government agencies.

A small number of occupational therapists are self-employed in private practice. These practitioners treated clients referred by other health professionals. They also provide contract or consulting services to nursing care facilities, schools, adult day care programs, and home healthcare agencies.

Educational and Legal Requirements

Occupational therapists must be licensed, requiring a master's degree in occupational therapy, six months of supervised fieldwork, and passing scores on national and state examinations.

Education and Training

A master's degree or higher in occupational therapy is the minimum requirement for entry into the field. In addition, occupational therapists must attend an academic program accredited by the Accreditation Council for Occupational Therapy Education (ACOTE) in order to sit for the national certifying exam. In 2021, there were over 400 accredited programs or, with 194 of those programs at the doctoral degree level.[1] Some schools offer dual degree programs, allowing a student to earn both a bachelor's and a master's degree in five years.

Most schools have full-time programs, although a growing number are offering weekend or part-time programs as well. Coursework in occupational therapy programs includes the physical, biological, and behavioral sciences as well as applied occupational therapy theory and skills. Programs also require the completion of at least 24 weeks of supervised fieldwork as part of the academic curriculum.

People considering the profession of occupational therapy should take high school courses in biology, chemistry, physics, health, art, and the social sciences. College admissions offices also look favorably on paid or volunteer experience in the healthcare field. Relevant undergraduate majors include biology, psychology, sociology, anthropology, liberal arts, and anatomy.

Licensure

All 50 states, Puerto Rico, Guam, and the District of Columbia regulate the practice of occupational therapy. To obtain a license, applicants must graduate from an accredited educational program and pass a national certification examination. Those who pass the exam are awarded the title Occupational Therapist, Registered (OTR). Some states have additional requirements for therapists who work in schools or early intervention programs. These requirements may include education-related classes, an education practice certificate, or an early intervention certification.

Certification and Other Qualifications

Certification is voluntary. The National Board for Certification in Occupational Therapy certifies occupational therapists through a national certifying exam.[2] In some states the requirements may vary, but all states recognize the national certifying exam as meeting the requirements for regulation.

Some occupational therapists obtain certification in a particular specialty. Board certifications currently recognized by the American Occupational Therapy Association include gerontology, mental health, pediatrics, and physical rehabilitation. Specialty certifications include driving and community mobility; environmental modification; feeding, eating, and swallowing; and low vision.

Occupational therapists need patience and strong interpersonal skills to inspire trust and respect in their clients. Patience is necessary because many clients may not show rapid improvement. Ingenuity and imagination in adapting activities to individual needs are assets. Writing skills are important because an occupational therapist must be able to explain the patient's treatment plan to the patient and record the patient's progress. Occupational therapists working in home healthcare services also must be able to adapt to a variety of settings.

Advancement

Occupational therapists are expected to continue their professional development by participating in continuing education courses and workshops. In fact, a number of states require continuing education as a condition of maintaining licensure.

Therapists are increasingly taking on supervisory roles. Because of rising healthcare costs, third-party payers are encouraging occupational therapy assistants and aides to take more hands-on responsibility for clients. Occupational therapists can choose to advance their careers by taking on administrative duties and supervising assistants and aides.

Occupational therapists also can advance by specializing in a clinical area and gaining expertise in treating a particular type of patient or ailment. Therapists have specialized in gerontology, mental health, pediatrics, and physical rehabilitation. In addition, some occupational therapists choose to teach classes in accredited occupational therapy educational programs.

Employment Trends

Employment of occupational therapists is expected to grow much faster than the average for all occupations. Job opportunities should be good, especially for occupational therapists treating older adults.

TABLE 18.1 Projections Data for Occupational Therapists, 2019–2029				
			Change, 2019–2029	
Occupational Title	**Employment, 2019**	**Projected Employment, 2029**	**Number**	**Percentage**
Occupational therapists	144,300	166,000	22,700	16%

Data from Bureau of Labor Statistics. Occupational Outlook Handbook 2019–2020 Edition. U.S. Department of Labor; 2020.

Employment Change

Employment of occupational therapists is expected to increase 16% between 2019 and 2029, much faster than the average for all occupations. The increasing older adult population will drive growth in the demand for occupational therapy services. Over the long term, the demand for occupational therapists should continue to rise as a result of the increasing number of individuals with disabilities or limited function who require therapy services. The Baby Boom generation's movement past middle age, a period when the incidence of heart attack and stroke increases, will spur demand for therapeutic services. Growth in the population of those 75 years and older—an age group that suffers from high incidences of disabling conditions—also will increase demand for therapeutic services. In addition, medical advances now enable more patients with critical problems such as birth defects or limb amputations to survive—patients who ultimately may need extensive therapy.

Hospitals will continue to employ a large number of occupational therapists to provide therapy services to acutely ill inpatients. Hospitals also will need occupational therapists to staff their outpatient rehabilitation programs.

Employment growth in schools will result from the expansion of the school-age population, the extension of services for disabled students, and an increasing prevalence of sensory disorders in children. Increased insurance coverage for therapy related to autism spectrum disorder will further spur the demand for services. Therapists will be needed to help children with disabilities prepare to enter special education programs.

Job Prospects

Job opportunities should be good for licensed occupational therapists in all settings, particularly in acute hospital, rehabilitation, and orthopedic settings because older adults receive most of their treatment in these settings. Occupational therapists with specialized knowledge in a treatment area also will have increased job prospects. Driver rehabilitation and fall-prevention training for older adults are emerging practice areas for occupational therapy. **TABLE 18.1** shows some projection data provided by the U.S. Department of Labor.

Earnings

Median annual earnings of occupational therapists were $86,280 in May 2020. The lowest 10% earned less than $57,330, and the highest 10% earned more than $122,670.

Median annual earnings in the industries employing the largest numbers of occupational therapist in May 2020 are shown in **TABLE 18.2**.

Related Occupations

Occupational therapists use specialized knowledge to help individuals perform daily living skills and achieve maximum independence. Other workers performing similar duties include athletic trainers, audiologists, chiropractors, physical therapists, recreational therapists, rehabilitation counselors, respiratory therapists, and speech-language pathologists.

Additional Information

For information on a career in occupational therapy and a list of accredited programs, contact:

- American Occupational Therapy Association, 6116 Executive Blvd., Suite 200, North Bethesda, MD 20852-4929. https://www.aota.org
- Accreditation Council for Occupational Therapy Education, 6116 Executive Blvd., Suite 200, North Bethesda, MD 20852-4929. https://acoteonline.org

For information about becoming certified as an occupational therapist, contact:

- National Board for Certification in Occupational Therapy, 12 South Summit Ave., Suite 100, Gaithersburg, MD 20877. https://www.nbcot.org

TABLE 18.2 Median Annual Earnings in the Industries Employing the Largest Numbers of Occupational Therapists, May 2020	
Home healthcare services	$91,830
Nursing care facilities	$92,260
Offices of other health practitioners	$86,830
Hospitals: state, local and private	$86,910
Education services: state, local, and private	$76,560

Data from Bureau of Labor Statistics. Occupational Outlook Handbook 2019–2020 Edition. U.S. Department of Labor; 2020.

OCCUPATIONAL THERAPY ASSISTANTS AND AIDES
Significant Points

- Typical entry-level education for occupational therapy assistants is an associate's degree; in contrast, occupational therapy aides usually receive their training on the job.
- Many states regulate the practice of occupational therapy assistants either by licensing, registration, or certification; requirements vary by state.
- Employment is projected to grow much faster than average as demand for occupational therapist services rises and as occupational therapists increasingly use assistants and aides.
- Job prospects should be very good for occupational therapy assistants; job seekers holding only a high school diploma might face keen competition for occupational therapy aide jobs.

Work Description

Occupational therapy assistants and aides work under the direction of occupational therapists to provide rehabilitative services to patients suffering from mental, physical, emotional, or developmental impairments. They help patients develop, recover, and improve as well as maintain the skills needed for daily living and working. The ultimate goal is to improve clients' quality of life by helping them compensate for limitations. For example, occupational therapy assistants help injured workers reenter the labor force by helping them improve their motor skills; alternatively, they may help persons with learning disabilities increase their independence by teaching them to prepare meals or use public transportation.

Occupational therapy assistants help clients with the rehabilitative activities and exercises that are outlined in the treatment plan devised by the occupational therapist. The activities range from teaching the patient the proper method of moving from a bed into a wheelchair to the best way to stretch and limber the muscles of the hand. An example of demonstrating the manner in which to stretch as hand is seen in **FIGURE 18.3**. Assistants monitor the individual to ensure that the client is performing the activities correctly and to provide encouragement. They may teach patients how to use special equipment to ease difficulties with life activities. They also record their observations with regard to the patient's progress for use by the occupational therapist. If the treatment is not having the intended effect or if the client is not improving as expected, the treatment program may be altered to obtain better results. Assistants also document billing submitted to the patient's health insurance provider.

Occupational therapy aides typically prepare materials and assemble equipment used during treatment, transport patients, and clean treatment areas and equipment. They are responsible for performing a range of clerical tasks. Their duties may include scheduling appointments, answering the

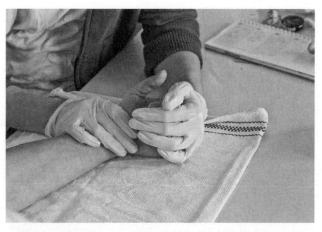

FIGURE 18.3 Stretching of a hand.
© Meinzahn/iStockPhoto.

telephone, restocking or ordering depleted supplies, and filling out insurance forms or other paperwork. Aides are not licensed, so by law they are not allowed to perform as wide a range of tasks as occupational therapy assistants do.

Work Environment

Occupational therapy assistants and aides need to have a moderate degree of strength because of the physical exertion required to assist patients. For example, assistants and aides may need to lift patients. Constant kneeling, stooping, and standing for long periods also are part of the job. Because of the physical demands placed upon them, occupational therapy assistants have one of the highest rate of injuries and illnesses of all occupations.

The work schedules of occupational therapy assistants and aides vary by facility and whether they are full or part time. For example, many outpatient therapy offices and clinics have evening and weekend hours to accommodate patients' schedules.

Employment Opportunities

Occupational therapy assistants and aides held about 55,100 jobs in 2019. Occupational therapy assistants held about 47,100, and occupational therapy aides held approximately 8,000. About 47% of jobs for assistants were in offices of other health practitioners, 15% were in hospitals, and 16% were in nursing care facilities. About 47% of jobs for aides were in offices of other health practitioners, 23% were in hospitals, and 12% were in nursing care facilities. The rest were primarily in community care facilities for older adults, home healthcare services, individual and family services, educational services, and state government agencies.

Educational and Legal Requirements

An associate's degree or a certificate from an accredited community college or technical school is generally required to qualify for occupational therapy assistant jobs. In contrast, occupational therapy aides usually receive most of their training on the job.

Education and Training

There were over 260 accredited occupational therapy assistant programs in 2021.[3] The first year of study typically involves an introduction to health care, basic medical terminology, anatomy, and physiology. In the second year, courses are more rigorous and usually include occupational therapy courses in areas such as mental health, adult physical disabilities, gerontology, and pediatrics. Students also must complete 16 weeks of supervised fieldwork in a clinic or community setting.

Applicants to occupational therapy assistant programs can improve their chances of admission by taking high school courses in biology and health and by performing volunteer work in nursing care facilities, occupational or physical therapists' offices, or other healthcare settings.

Occupational therapy aides usually receive most of their training on the job. Qualified applicants must have a high school diploma, strong interpersonal skills, and a desire to help people in need. Applicants may increase their chances of getting a job by volunteering their services, thus displaying initiative and aptitude to the employer.

Licensure

In most states, occupational therapy assistants are regulated and must pass a national certification examination after they graduate. Those who pass the test are awarded the title Certified Occupational Therapy Assistant.

Certification and Other Qualifications

Certification is voluntary. The National Board for Certifying Occupational Therapy certifies occupational therapy assistants through a national certifying exam.[4] Those who pass the test are awarded the title Certified Occupational Therapy Assistant (COTA). In some states, the national certifying exam meets requirements for regulation, but other states have their own requirements beyond the licensing exam.

Occupational therapy assistants are expected to continue their professional development by participating in continuing education courses and workshops in order to maintain certification. A number of states require continuing education as a condition of maintaining licensure.

Assistants and aides must be responsible, patient, and willing to take directions and work as part of a team. They must possess moderate strength so that they can assist patients. Furthermore, they should be caring and want to help people who are not able to help themselves.

Advancement

Occupational therapy assistants may advance into administration positions. They might organize all the assistants in a large occupational therapy department or act as the director for a specific department such as sports medicine. Some assistants go on to teach classes in accredited occupational therapy assistant academic programs or lead health risk reduction classes for older adults.

Employment Trends

Employment is expected to grow much faster than average as demand for occupational therapy services rises and as occupational therapists increasingly use assistants and aides. Job prospects should be very good for occupational therapy assistants. Job seekers holding only a high school diploma might face keen competition for occupational therapy aide jobs.

Employment Change

Employment of occupational therapy assistants and aides is expected to grow 35% and 20% respectively from 2019 to 2029, much faster than the average for all occupations. The ability of patients to pay for services will impact the demand for therapy services offered by occupational therapy assistants and aides. Over the long term, demand for services will continue to rise because of the increasing number of individuals with disabilities or limited function.

The growing older adult population is particularly vulnerable to chronic and debilitating conditions that require therapeutic services. These patients often need additional assistance in their treatment, making the role of assistants and aides vital. As the large Baby Boom generation ages, it enters the prime age bracket for heart attacks and strokes, further increasing the demand for cardiac and physical rehabilitation. In addition, future medical developments should permit an increasing percentage of trauma victims to survive, creating added demand for therapy services. An increase of sensory disorders in children will also spur demand for occupational therapy services.

Occupational therapists are expected to increase their utilization of assistants and aides to reduce the cost of occupational therapy services. Once a patient is evaluated and the therapist designs a treatment plan, the occupational therapy assistant can provide many aspects of treatment, as prescribed by the therapist.

Job Prospects

Opportunities for individuals interested in becoming occupational therapy assistants are expected to be very good. In addition to employment growth, job openings will result from the need to replace occupational therapy assistants and aides who leave the occupation permanently between 2019

TABLE 18.3 Projections Data for Occupational Therapy Assistants and Aides, Occupational Therapy Assistants, and Occupational Therapy Aides, 2019–2029

Occupational Title	Employment, 2019	Projected Employment, 2029	Change, 2019–2029	
			Number	Percentage
Occupational therapy assistants and aides	55,100	73,000	17,900	32%
Occupational therapy assistants	47,100	63,500	16,300	35%
Occupational therapy aides	8,000	9,500	1,600	20%

Data from Bureau of Labor Statistics. Occupational Outlook Handbook 2019–2020 Edition. U.S. Department of Labor; 2020.

and 2029. Occupational therapy assistants and aides with prior experience working in an occupational therapy office or other healthcare setting will have the best job opportunities. However, individuals with only a high school diploma may face keen competition for occupational therapy aide jobs. **TABLE 18.3** shows some projection data provided by the U.S. Department of Labor.

Earnings

Median annual earnings of occupational therapy assistants were $62,940 in May 2020. The lowest 10% earned less than $43,180, and the highest 10% earned more than $84,090. Median annual earnings in the industries employing the largest numbers of occupational therapy assistants in May 2020 are included in **TABLE 18.4**.

Median annual earnings of occupational therapy aides were $30,180 in May 2020. The lowest 10% earned less than $20,010, and the highest 10% earned more than $58,800. Median annual earnings in the industries employing the largest numbers of occupational therapy aides in May 2020 are shown in **TABLE 18.5**.

Related Occupations

Occupational therapy assistants and aides work under the supervision and direction of occupational therapists. Other workers in the healthcare field who work under similar supervision include dental assistants; medical assistants; nursing, psychiatric, and home health aides; personal and home care aides; pharmacy aides; pharmacy technicians; and physical therapist assistants and aides.

Additional Information

For information on a career in occupational therapy and a list of accredited programs, contact:

- American Occupational Therapy Association, 6116 Executive Blvd., Suite 200, North Bethesda, MD 20852-4929. https://www.aota.org

For information about becoming certified as an occupational therapy assistant, contact

- National Board for Certification in Occupational Therapy, One Bank St., Suite 300, Gaithersburg, MD 20878. https://www.nbcot.org

TABLE 18.4 Median Annual Earnings in the Industries Employing the Largest Numbers of Occupational Therapy Assistants, May 2020

Home healthcare services	$67,760
Offices of other health practitioners	$63,250
Nursing care facilities	$67,460
Hospitals: state, local, and private	$59,040
Educational services: state, local, and private	$51,520

Data from Bureau of Labor Statistics. Occupational Outlook Handbook 2019–2020 Edition. U.S. Department of Labor; 2020.

TABLE 18.5 Median Annual Earnings in the Industries Employing the Largest Numbers of Occupational Therapy Aides, May 2020

Specialty (except psychiatric and substance abuse) hospitals	$29,020
Hospitals: state, local, and private	$32,710
Offices of physical, occupational and speech therapists, and audiologists	$24,410
Social assistance	$33,530
Nursing care facilities	$33,840

Data from Bureau of Labor Statistics. Occupational Outlook Handbook 2019–2020 Edition. U.S. Department of Labor; 2020.

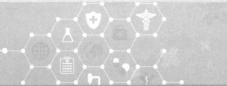

LEARNING PORTFOLIO

Issues for Discussion

1. Occupational therapists work with a wide variety of patients and need to know many areas within their discipline in order to assist those patients. Brainstorm with your classmates what those areas are and decide which area in particular might be most advantageous to know.

2. This chapter addresses three related roles within the occupational therapy profession. Discuss with your instructor and classmates which of these roles you would recommend to a friend or acquaintance to pursue and why.

Enrichment Activities

1. View videos of occupational therapy students found at https://www.youtube.com/watch?v=jwwOXlLYQ4Q and https://www.aota.org/Education-Careers/Considering-OT-Career/CareerStories.aspx. Choose which video resonates with you and discuss the reason(s) behind that choice.

2. Many people assume the discipline of occupational therapy is rather new. Research the history and development of occupational therapy as a discipline. Create a timeline (whether a narrative piece, a poster, or an infographic) that describes the different stages of development and name significant individuals and organizations in the discipline.

CASE STUDY: OT CAREER OPPORTUNITY

Luke has always enjoyed being around people. You would be inclined to call him a "people person." He has been working as a restaurant manager for the past two years since graduating from high school. Lately he has been feeling unsatisfied with his job. Luke has been looking into going to college and changing his career. He has been looking into the field of occupational therapy. Occupational therapy really interests Luke. He remembers when his uncle was in a vehicle accident and worked with an occupational therapist to regain the strength in his badly injured hand. Luke would like to learn more about the field of occupational therapy.

The following questions relate to occupational therapy. Please help Luke answer them based on what you have learned in this chapter.

1. Luke is hoping he will be eligible for financial aid to offset the cost of his education. He would like to enter the workforce with the minimum entry-level degree for occupational therapists. Which of the following is the minimum entry-level degree for an occupational therapist (OT)?

   A. Master's degree
   B. Bachelor's degree
   C. Doctorate degree
   D. Associate's degree in applied sciences

2. Luke is self-supporting and has car, mortgage, and furniture payments he makes on a monthly basis. He is concerned about the availability of jobs for occupational therapists. Which of the following statements is most accurate as a predictor of the future job market for OTs?

A. The job market will remain the same for the next five to 10 years.
B. The job market will show a decline in the need for OTs during the next five to 10 years.
C. The job market should show an increase of approximately 16% for OTs between 2019 and 2029.
D. There is no accurate way to project what the job market will be like in years to come.

3. Luke is thinking he may be able to start working in the field of occupational therapy as an aide or assistant to gain experience while earning money to further his education and become an occupational therapist. What is the projection for employment for occupational therapy assistants and aides?

A. Employment is projected to grow much faster than average as demand for occupational therapist services rises and as OTs increasingly use assistants and aides.
B. Employment is projected to decline much faster than average as demand for occupational therapist services decreases.
C. Employment is projected to stay about the same as demand for occupational therapist services level out and as occupational therapists do not use as many assistants and aides.
D. Employment will be shifted from occupational to physical therapy needs. Physical therapy assistants will be much more employable.

LEARNING PORTFOLIO

References

1. Accreditation Council for Occupational Therapy Education. Accredited Programs. https://www.aota.org/Education-Careers/Find-School.aspx Accessed August 25, 2021.

2. National Board for Certification in Occupational Therapy. https://www.nbcot.org Accessed August 25, 2021.

3. Accreditation Council for Occupational Therapy Education. OTA Programs. https://www.aota.org/Education-Careers/Find-School.aspx Accessed August 25, 2021.

4. National Board for Certification in Occupational Therapy. https://www.nbcot.org Accessed August 25, 2021.

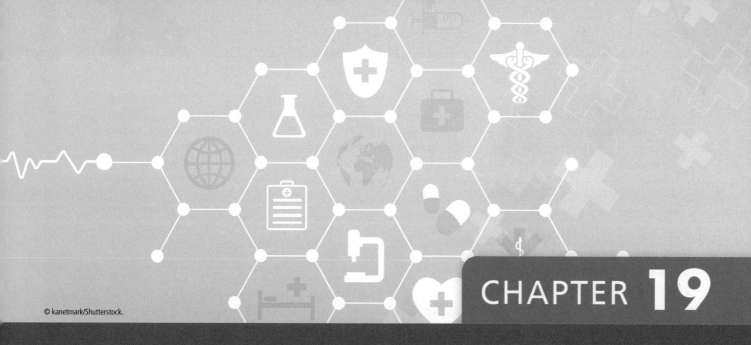

© kanetmark/Shutterstock.

CHAPTER **19**

Athletic Trainers, Exercise Physiologists, and Kinesiotherapists*

* All information in this chapter, unless otherwise indicated, was obtained from Bureau of Labor Statistics. *Occupational Outlook Handbook 2020–2021 Edition*. Washington, DC: U.S. Department of Labor; 2021.

National Collegiate Athletic
  Association (NCAA)
Physician practice manager
Recreational sports

Registered Clinical Exercise
  Physiologist (RCEP)
Registered Kinesiotherapist (RKT)
Repetitive stress injuries

Sports centers
Teacher's certificate, license
Third-party reimbursement
Work-related injuries

SPORTS MEDICINE—AN INTRODUCTION

Sports medicine is a broad discipline and an area of practice for many health professionals from a personal fitness trainer to a cardiac rehabilitation specialist.[1] Requirements to become a **ASCM Certified Personal Trainer (ASCM-CPT)** through the **American College of Sports Medicine (ACSM)** are a high school diploma and certification in **cardiac pulmonary resuscitation (CPR)** and the use of **automated external defibrillators (AEDs)**. Those meeting these requirements can sit for the CPT certification exam. In contrast, a master's degree is the minimum requirement to become a **Certified Athletic Trainer (ATC)**.[2]

Health professionals in sports medicine work with individuals of all ages who participate in physical activity as part of a healthy lifestyle or as a professional athlete. Athletic trainers focus on improving athletic performance or treating **muscle** or **bone injuries**. Clinical exercise physiologists develop and supervise exercise programs to improve functioning in individuals with heart, lung, orthopedic, or neuromuscular disease.[1] Kinesiotherapists use rehabilitative exercises, reconditioning, and physical education to treat patients who have problems moving in any way. Sports medicine physicians may work for an athletic team or a university sports team or consult with athletic directors, coaches, and athletic trainers on **injury prevention** and treatment as well as enhancing performance.[1]

Physicians, nurses, dietitians, exercise physiologists, and physical therapists are examples of health professionals who specialize in sports medicine by working in cardiac or pulmonary rehabilitation. Athletic trainers, physicians, and dietitians often work for a college or professional sports team.

For students interested in sports medicine, there are many possibilities for a career depending on the preferred work environment and educational goals. The focus of this chapter is the athletic trainer, exercise physiologist, and kinesiotherapist.

ATHLETIC TRAINERS
Significant Points

- Although a bachelor's degree has been the minimum requirement for Athletic Trainers, beginning in 2022 only master's-level programs can admit new students in an athletic training program.
- Long hours, sometimes including nights and weekends, are common.
- Job prospects should be good in the healthcare industry and in high schools, but competition is expected for positions with professional and college sports teams.

Work Description

Athletic trainers (AT) help prevent and treat injuries for people of all ages and all skill levels. Their patients and clients include everyone from professional athletes to industrial workers. Recognized by the American Medical Association as allied health professionals, ATs specialize in the prevention, diagnosis, assessment, treatment, and rehabilitation of muscle or bone injuries (**FIGURE 19.1**). ATs, as one of the first healthcare providers on the scene when injuries occur, must be able to recognize, evaluate, and assess injuries and provide immediate care when needed.

ATs should not be confused with fitness or personal trainers, who are not healthcare workers but rather train people to become physically fit. Athletic trainers try to prevent injuries by educating people on how to reduce their risk for injuries and advising them on the proper use of equipment. ATs instruct athletes in exercises to improve balance and strength by using in-home exercises and therapy programs. They also help apply protective or

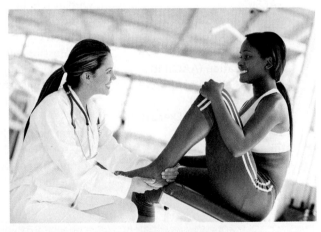

FIGURE 19.1 Athletic Trainers (AT) specialize in treatment of bone and muscle injuries.
© Andresr/Shutterstock.

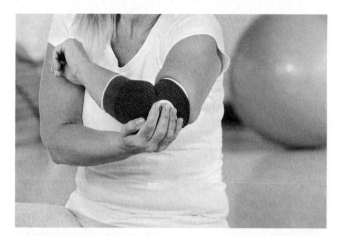

FIGURE 19.2 Athletic Trainers (ATs) use devices to prevent elbow injury.
© Robert Kneschke/Shutterstock.

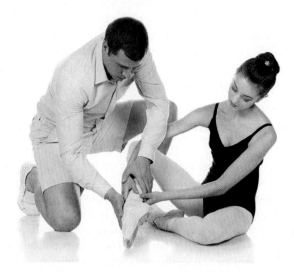

FIGURE 19.3 Athletic Trainer (AT) evaluating an injury of a ballet dancer.
© Nanette Grebe/Shutterstock.

injury-preventive devices such as tape, bandages, and braces (**FIGURE 19.2**).

ATs may work under the direction of a licensed physician and in cooperation with other healthcare providers. The extent of the direction ranges from discussing specific injuries and treatment options with a physician to performing evaluations and treatments as directed by a physician. Some athletic trainers meet with the team physician or consulting physician once or twice a week; others interact with a physician every day. ATs often have administrative responsibilities including keeping records and writing reports on injuries and treatment programs for athletes and other clients. Other duties may include regular meetings with an athletic director, **physician practice manager**, or other administrative officer to deal with budgets, purchasing, policy implementation, and other business-related issues.

Work Environment

Many ATs work in educational facilities, such as secondary schools or colleges. Others may work in physicians' offices or for a wide variety of professional sports teams including baseball, football, basketball, and ice hockey. Some work in rehabilitation and therapy clinics, in the military, or with performing artists such as ballet dancers or figure skaters (**FIGURE 19.3**).

The industry and individual employer are significant in determining the work environment of athletic trainers. Many AT work indoors most of the time; others, especially those in some sports-related jobs, spend much of their time working outdoors. The job also might require standing for long periods, working with **medical equipment**, and being able to walk, run, kneel, stoop, or crawl. Travel out of town for competitive events is often required.

Schedules vary by work setting. AT in non-sports settings generally have an established schedule—usually about 40 to 50 hours per week—with nights and weekends off. AT working in hospitals and clinics may spend part of their time working at other locations doing outreach services. The most common outreach programs include conducting athletic training services and speaking at high schools, colleges, and commercial businesses.

Athletic trainers in sports settings have schedules that are longer and more variable. These AT must be present for team practices and competitions, which often are on evenings and weekends, and their schedules can change on short notice when games and practices have to be rescheduled. In high schools, AT who also teach may work 60 to 70 hours a week or more. In **National Collegiate Athletic Association (NCAA)** Division I colleges and universities, athletic trainers generally work with one team; when that team's sport is in season, working at least 50 to 60 hours a week is common. AT in Division II or III, representing smaller colleges and universities, often work with several teams and have teaching responsibilities. During the off-season, a 40- to 50-hour workweek may be normal in most settings. AT for professional sports teams generally work the most hours per week. During training camps, practices, and competitions, they may be required to work up to 12 hours a day.

There is some stress involved with being an athletic trainer. The work of athletic trainers requires frequent interaction with others. ATs consult with physicians as well as have frequent contact with athletes and patients to discuss and administer treatments, rehabilitation programs, injury prevention practices, and other health-related issues. AT are responsible for their clients' health and sometimes have to make quick decisions that could affect the health or career of their clients. AT also can be affected by the pressure to win, which is typical of competitive sports teams.

Employment Opportunities

Athletic trainers held about 32,100 jobs in 2019 and are found in every part of the country. Most AT jobs are related to sports, although an increasing number also work in non-sports settings. The majority of AT work either in educational settings including colleges, universities, and middle and high schools or in hospitals and offices of other health professionals. About 6% work in fitness and **recreational sports** centers. Others work with the military, law enforcement, professional sports teams, or performing artists.

Education and Legal Requirements

Students applying to an athletic training program can expect to enroll in a master's degree program since new students will not be accepted into a bachelor's program beginning in 2022.[2] The degree program includes both classroom and clinical components, including science and health-related courses. Many AT hold a master's or doctoral degree. In 2020, 49 states and the District of Columbia required athletic trainers to be licensed or hold some form of registration.[3]

Education and Training

Students in these programs are educated both in the classroom and in clinical settings. Formal education includes many science and health-related courses, such as human anatomy, physiology, nutrition, and biomechanics. The **Commission on Accreditation of Athletic Training Education (CAATE)** accredits athletic trainer programs as well as post-professional and residency athletic trainer programs. Athletic trainers will need a higher degree to be eligible for some positions, especially those in colleges and universities, and to increase their advancement opportunities. Because some positions in high schools involve teaching along with athletic trainer responsibilities, a **teaching certificate or license** could be required.

Licensure and Certification

Athletic trainers must be licensed or certified in the majority of states. In 2020, 49 states and the District of Columbia required AT to be licensed or registered; this requires certification from the **Board of Certification, Inc. (BOC)**.[3] For BOC certification, athletic trainers need a master's degree from a CAATE-accredited program and must pass the rigorous BOC examination. To retain certification, credential holders must continue taking medical-related courses and adhere to the BOC standards of practice. In California, where licensure is not required, certification is voluntary but may be helpful for those seeking jobs and advancement.[3] The **National Athletic Trainer's Association (NATA)** offers continuing education programming and other membership benefits.

Other Qualifications

Because all AT deal directly with a variety of people, they need good social and **communication skills**. They should be able to manage difficult situations and the stress associated with them, such as when disagreements arise with coaches, patients, clients, or parents regarding suggested treatment.

Athletic trainers also should be organized, be able to manage time wisely, be inquisitive, and have a strong desire to help people.

Advancement

There are a few ways for ATs to advance. ATs may choose a post-professional residency program in one of eight specialty areas to demonstrate advanced knowledge and skills—for example, in pediatrics, orthopedics, or rehabilitation.[4] Some athletic trainers advance by switching teams or sports to gain additional responsibility or pay. Assistant athletic trainers may become head athletic trainers and, eventually, athletic directors or physician, hospital, or clinic practice administrators, where they assume a management role. Some AT move into sales and marketing positions, using their expertise to sell medical and athletic equipment. ATs working in colleges and universities may pursue an advanced degree to increase their advancement opportunities.

Employment Trends

Employment is projected to grow much faster than average. Job prospects should be good in the healthcare industry and in high schools, but competition should be expected for positions with professional and college sports teams.

Employment Change

Employment of AT is projected to grow 16% from 2019 to 2029, much faster than the average for all occupations, because of their role in preventing injuries and reducing healthcare costs. However, because it is a small occupation, the fast growth will result in only about 5,200 new jobs over the 10-year period. In 2019, the majority of ATs worked for colleges and university sports teams and in hospitals and offices of other health practitioners. (**TABLE 19.1**).

As people become more aware of sports-related injuries at a young age, demand for AT is expected to increase. Recent research reveals that the effects of concussions are particularly severe and long-lasting in child athletes. Although concussions are dangerous to athletes at any age, children's brains are still developing and are at risk for permanent complications.

TABLE 19.1 Industries Employing the Largest Numbers of Athletic Trainers, 2019

Educational services	36%
Hospitals	19%
Ambulatory health care	14%
Fitness and recreational centers	6%
Self-employed	4%

Professional Profiles

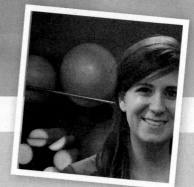

Name: Cat, MS, ATC, LAT
Job Title: Athletic Trainer
Education: MS in Athletic Training, BS in Exercise Science

Q: Describe your job and organization.

A: I work as a clinical athletic trainer in a busy outpatient sports medicine and orthopedic physical therapy clinic in an urban setting. The clinic has about 400 patient visits per week, ranging from children to professional athletes to the geriatric population. Also, I provide medical coverage for sporting events in the city for another employer.

Q: Describe a typical workday.

A: At the beginning of the day, I meet with the physical therapist overseeing the care of patients and athletes to discuss any updates and new treatment options. I check in with each patient as they are doing their exercises to ensure that they are following the correct form and to maximize the effectiveness of their therapeutic program. I provide 15 to 25 minutes of manual therapy for each patient to ensure that they understand which exercises to do at home and to evaluate their ability to complete activities of daily living.

Q: Why did you choose this profession?

A: I was drawn to this profession being a former athlete. I enjoy working with those who are active and motivated and can't get enough of the fast-paced nature of sports medicine. There is constantly something new to learn and integrate into my practice. I enjoy interacting with the wide variety of athletes and patients and learning from physicians and orthopedic surgeons. I also value the reflection and growth required of me as a professional.

Q: Is there room for advancement in this field?

A: There is plenty of room for advancement for athletic trainers. Most entry-level positions are for an assistant athletic trainer. Advancement can be to specialize in a specific age group, sport, or athletic team or as the head athletic trainer.

Q: Name and explain what part of your academic training most prepared you for this profession.

A: Students take part clinical rotations in various settings under the supervision, guidance, and mentorship of certified athletic trainers. Realistic and hands-on practice helps solidify techniques and critical-thinking skills before entering the professional world. The real-world practice builds the confidence to perform the job correctly and safely.

Q: What do you wish you would have known in high school or college about pursuing this career?

A: I wish I had known all of the possible work settings for athletic trainers in addition to the well-known team-based or school setting. I would have gained experience in as many settings as possible and avoided becoming discouraged about not working in what I thought were the most desired settings.

Q: What advice would you give someone who is considering this career?

A: I would recommend researching all health fields before making a decision, especially within the field of sports medicine. To be effective in this field, athletic trainers must be able to remain calm and think on their feet during emergency treatments, be creative and able to tailor unique rehab programs for patients, and be able to prioritize time and responsibilities. It is also critical to communicate the needs of the athlete to the family, physician, and physical therapist as well as the athlete. Desirable qualities for athletic trainers are to be outgoing, adaptable, hardworking, and empathetic with a genuine concern for people and to have a desire to continue learning.

Parents and coaches are becoming educated about these greater risks through community health efforts. Because ATs are usually onsite with athletes and are often the first responders when injuries occur, the demand for trainers should continue to increase. Additionally, advances in injury prevention and detection and more sophisticated treatments are projected to increase the demand for athletic trainers. Growth in an increasingly active middle-aged and older adult population will likely lead to an increased incidence of athletic-related injuries, such as sprains. Sports programs at all ages and for all experience levels will continue to create demand for athletic trainers.

Insurance and workers' compensation costs have become a concern for many employers and insurance companies, especially in areas where employees are often injured on the job. For example, military bases hire AT to help train and rehabilitate injured military personnel. These trainers also create programs aimed at keeping injury rates down. Depending on the state, some insurance companies recognize athletic trainers as healthcare providers and reimburse the cost of an AT's services.

Job Prospects

Future job growth will be concentrated in the healthcare industry, including hospitals and offices of health practitioners. Fitness and recreation **sports centers** also will provide new jobs, as these establishments grow and continue to need additional athletic trainers to provide support for their clients. Growth in positions with sports teams will be somewhat slower, however, as most professional sports clubs and colleges and universities already have the needed staff. TABLE 19.2 shows some projection data from the National Employment Matrix.

In some states, efforts are underway to have an AT in every high school to work with student-athletes, which may lead to growth in the number of athletic trainers employed in high schools. In addition, as more young athletes specialize in certain sports, there is increasing demand for ATs to deal with **repetitive stress injuries**.

The demand for health care, with an emphasis on preventive care, should grow as the population ages and as a way to reduce healthcare costs. Increased licensure requirements and regulation have led to a greater acceptance of athletic trainers as qualified healthcare providers. As a result, **third-party reimbursement** is expected to continue to grow for athletic training services. ATs will benefit from this expansion because they provide a cost-effective way to increase the number of health professionals in an office or other setting.

As ATs continue to expand their services, more employers are expected to use these workers to reduce healthcare costs by preventing **work-related injuries**. ATs can help prevent injuries and provide immediate treatment for many injuries that do occur. For example, some may be hired to increase the fitness and performance of police officers and firefighters.

Job prospects should be good for ATs in the healthcare industry and in high schools. Those looking for a position with a professional or college sports team may face competition. Because of relatively low turnover, the settings with the best job prospects will be the ones that are expected to have the most job growth, primarily positions in the healthcare and fitness and recreational sports centers industries. Additional job opportunities may arise in elementary and secondary schools as more positions are created. Some of these positions also will require teaching responsibilities.

There are relatively few positions for professional and collegiate sports teams in comparison to the number of applicants. Turnover among professional sports teams' athletic trainers is also limited. Many ATs prefer to continue to work with the same coaches, administrators, and players when a good working relationship already exists.

There also are opportunities for ATs to join the military, although they would not be classified as athletic trainers. Instead, the U.S. Department of Veterans Affairs (VA) facilities hire kinesiotherapists (described later in this chapter) in physical reconditioning units for current and former military personnel with physical injuries.[5] Enlisted soldiers and officers who are athletic trainers are usually placed in another program, such as health educator or training specialist, in which their skills are useful.

This occupation is expected to continue to change over the next decade since entry to the profession requires a master's degree. Athletic trainers can expect to be required to assume more administrative responsibilities, adapt to new technology, and work with larger populations; job seekers must be prepared to adapt to these changes.

Earnings

The median annual wage was $49,860 for ATs in May 2020. Most athletic trainers work in full-time positions and typically receive benefits. The salary of an AT depends on experience and job responsibilities and varies by job setting. Many employers pay for some of the continuing education

Occupational Title	Employment, 2019	Projected Employment, 2029	Change, 2019–2029	
			Number	Percentage
Athletic trainers	32,100	37,300	5,200	16%

TABLE 19.2 Projections Data for Athletic Trainers, 2019–2029

required to remain certified, although the amount covered varies from employer to employer.

Related Occupations

Other allied health professionals with job duties similar to athletic trainers include athletic coaches, chiropractors, emergency medical technicians (EMTs) and paramedics, massage therapists, occupational therapists, physical therapists, recreational therapists, and respiratory therapists.

EXERCISE PHYSIOLOGISTS
Significant Points

- A bachelor's degree is the minimum requirement for a certified exercise physiologist.
- Since exercise physiology is a small and relatively new profession, there is strong competition for jobs.
- About 62% of exercise physiologists are self-employed; others work in hospitals or offices of other health professionals.
- Greater emphasis on exercise as part of preventing and treating chronic diseases, especially cardiovascular and pulmonary disease, diabetes, and obesity, is expected to increase the demand for exercise physiologists.

Work Description

ACSM Certified Exercise Physiologist (ACSM-CEP) develop fitness and exercise programs that help patients recover from chronic diseases and improve cardiovascular and pulmonary function, body composition, and flexibility. Many of their patients suffer from health problems such as diabetes, cardiovascular disease, and pulmonary disease or are obese. For patients with these conditions, exercise is medical treatment much the same as surgery and prescription drugs are medical treatment for other diseases. These professionals provide health education and develop exercise plans to reduce risk for disease by improving key health indicators such as body weight, blood pressure, blood cholesterol, and blood glucose. Exercise physiologists develop fitness and exercise programs to prevent, maintain, or restore health status for people of all ages and health conditions—from orthopedic, musculoskeletal, and neuromuscular conditions to recovery from cancer treatments.

Exercise physiologists review the patient's medical history, perform fitness tests, and monitor body fat, blood pressure, heart rhythm, and oxygen usage to determine the best exercise and fitness program. Those exercise physiologists working in a **cardiac rehabilitation program** will monitor patients during testing and during exercise to ensure patient safety (**FIGURE 19.4**).

Exercise physiologists work closely with primary physicians who may prescribe exercise regimens for their patients and refer them to exercise physiologists. The exercise physiologist then works with patients to achieve goals for improving their health status.

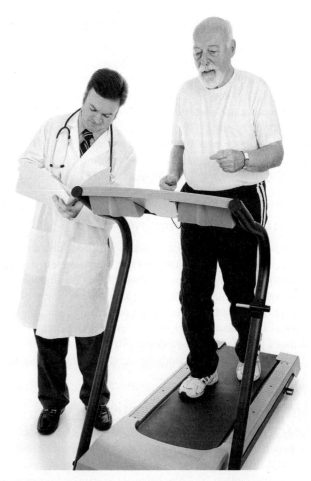

FIGURE 19.4 Exercise physiologists monitor patients during testing.
© Lisa F. Young/Shutterstock.

Work Environment

About 62% of exercise physiologists are self-employed; others work in hospitals and offices of other healthcare professionals and outpatient clinics. They also work in athletic training settings in colleges and universities, fitness facilities, corporate wellness programs, military training centers, and rehabilitation clinics and hospitals. Some may be employed as sports directors, coaches, trainers for athletic programs, corporate wellness directors, program coordinators, exercise managers in fitness facilities, or rehabilitation specialists. Exercise physiologists are hired to assist in the development of athletic equipment and gear. Others may work as sports or athletic performance consultants. Most physiologists work full time.

Employment Opportunities

Exercise physiologists held about 19,800 jobs in 2019. This is a small occupation; compared to athletic trainers, licensure for exercise physiologists is less common, and therefore there are fewer recognized standards of practice for exercise physiologists.

Education and Legal Requirements

The **Committee on Accreditation for the Exercise Sciences (CoAES)**, a subcommittee of the **Commission on Accreditation of Allied Health Education Programs (CAAHEP)**, guides educational programs in ensuring that accreditation requirements are met. CAAHEP accredits both bachelor's- and master's-level programs; there are 66 bachelor's-level exercise science and 13 master's-level exercise physiology programs in the United States.[5] In addition, the **American Society of Exercise Physiologists (ASEP)** accredits programs in exercise physiology.

Education and Training

Exercise physiologists need at least a bachelor's degree from an accredited college or university in exercise science, exercise physiology, or kinesiology. Master's degree programs are also common, and over 50% of exercise physiologists have a master's degree. Degree programs have classroom and clinical components, including science and health-related courses, such as biology, anatomy, physiology, and nutrition. An internship provides hands-on experience developing and monitoring exercise programs.

Licensure and Certification

Only Louisiana requires exercise physiologists to be licensed, although many states have pending legislation to create formal licensure requirements. Certification requires graduation with a bachelor's degree in exercise science or exercise physiology and successfully completing the certification exam. The exam includes academic knowledge as well as hands-on laboratory and practical skills. Maintaining certification requires continuing education courses every five years. The ACSM offers certification for exercise physiologists, the **ACSM Certified Clinical Exercise Physiologist (ACSM-CEP)** credential for candidates with a bachelor's degree in exercise science, 1,200 hours of clinical experience, and successful completion of the certification exam. Those with a master's degree in exercise physiology and 600 hours of clinical experience are also eligible to sit for the exam.[6] After certification, exercise physiologists can become registered through the CEPA. An application requires three years of clinical experience for those with a bachelor's degree and one year of clinical experience for those with a master's or doctorate in exercise physiology. Registration entitles exercise physiologists to use the title, **Registered Clinical Exercise Physiologist (RCEP)**. The Registry is a way to promote the profession of exercise physiology and is a central location for employers to locate Clinical Exercise Physiologists.[7] Exercise physiologists with a goal of working for college or university athletic departments are advised to obtain certification through ACSM, recognized by NCAA.

Exercise physiologists can sit for an exam to become a **Certified Cardiac Rehabilitation Professional (CCRP)** through the **American Association of Cardiovascular and**

Cardiopulmonary Rehabilitation (AACVPR). The requirements are a minimum of a bachelor's degree in a health-related field and 1,200 hours of clinical experience in cardiac rehabilitation.[8]

Other Qualifications

Exercise physiologists need to feel comfortable working with people who have a variety of chronic health problems as well as those who are healthy with a goal of achieving maximum physical performance. Good listening skills are important to be able to assess a client's motivation and response to an exercise program. Being able to present clear instructions on an exercise program to individual clients and in a group setting is necessary. Since many exercise physiologists are managers of wellness and rehabilitation programs, they must be organized and detail oriented in order to maintain detailed clinical records of clients and to provide reports to the client's physician.

Advancement

Exercise physiologists with some business training have better opportunities to advance into management positions, such as the director of a rehabilitation program or manager of a wellness program.

Employment Trends

Employment opportunities in exercise physiology are expanding as doctors, patients, and society learn of the value of exercise as an important healthcare treatment. Certifications by both the American Society of Exercise Physiologists and the American Society for Sports Medicine increase the credibility of exercise physiologists as part of the healthcare team.

Employment Change

Employment of exercise physiologists is projected to grow 11% from 2019 to 2029, much faster than average for all occupations. Demand may rise with greater emphasis on preventive health and as health insurance coverage includes exercise and other preventive measure to reduce the incidence of chronic diseases. There are few available exercise physiologist positions, so competition for work remains high. The majority of exercise physiologists are self-employed; others work in hospitals or in the offices of other health professionals (**TABLE 19.3**).

TABLE 19.3 Place of Employment for Exercise Physiologists, 2019	
Self-employed	62%
Hospitals	22%
Ambulatory health care	6%
Government	2%

Data from Bureau of Labor Statistics. Occupational Employment and Wage Statistics. U.S. Department of Labor; May 2018. http://www.bls.gov/oes/#data

Job Prospects

Demand for exercise physiologists may rise as hospitals emphasize exercise and preventive care as part of their treatment for chronic diseases and long-term rehabilitation. The need for exercise physiologists in residential housing for seniors offers new job opportunities because older adults frequently have diseases that would benefit from a structured exercise program. A master's degree is usually required for exercise physiologists to work in cardiac rehabilitation programs. There are few available exercise physiologist positions, so competition for work remains high. **TABLE 19.4** shows some projection data from the National Employment Matrix.

Earnings

The median annual wage for exercise physiologists was $50,280 in May 2020. The median wage for those in government jobs was $75,740, while the median salary for those working in a hospital was $50,390. Managers or coordinators of wellness programs or rehabilitation specialists with a master's degree can expect higher salaries.

Related Occupations

Health professionals that require similar education and training and those who do similar work are chiropractors, EMTs and paramedics, occupational therapists, physical therapists, physician's assistants, podiatrists, registered nurses, and respiratory therapists.

KINESIOTHERAPIST

A health career similar to that of an athletic trainer is a **kinesiotherapist**. Formerly called corrective therapy, kinesiotherapy is the study of body-movement mechanics. This career started in 1946 after World War II in response to the needs of soldiers returning to active duty after injury or illness. The goal of corrective therapy was to restore function so that soldiers could return to active duty as soon as possible.[9]

Significant Points

- A career in kinesiotherapy began after World War II as corrective therapy to rehabilitate injured service members.
- Most kinesiotherapists are employed by Veterans Administration hospitals and clinics.

- Eligibility for registration requires graduation from an accredited bachelor's program in kinesiotherapy or a master's degree in exercise science to be qualified to take the registration exam.

Work Description

The **Registered Kinesiotherapist (RKT)** is a healthcare professional who, under the direction of a physician, treats the effects of disease, injury, and congenital disorders through the use of therapeutic exercise and education. Their practice includes a wide spectrum of health conditions—neurologic, orthopedic, medical, surgical, and mental health—for patients who have had a stroke, spinal cord injury, traumatic brain injury (TBI), or limb amputation.[10]

RKTs are competent in administering musculoskeletal, neurological, ergonomic, biomechanical, psychosocial, and task-specific functional tests and measures. After evaluating the results of the tests, RKTs use rehabilitative exercise, reconditioning, and physical education to treat patients who have problems moving in any way. They apply tools, techniques, and psychology to help those with physical and mental conditions meet their treatment goals. They instruct patients in proper exercise techniques and use of equipment to meet specified objectives such as improvement of walking gait, joint flexibility, endurance, strength, and emotional self-confidence and security. For the physically handicapped, the exercise routines are aimed at developing strength, dexterity, and muscle coordination. Therapists teach exercise routines to patients who use wheelchairs, instruct amputees or partially paralyzed patients how to walk and move around, and sometimes give driving lessons using specially equipped automobiles. They also advise patients on the use of braces, artificial limbs, and other devices. For the emotionally ill or developmentally disabled, therapists use exercises to relieve frustration or tension or to bring about social involvement.[11] Kinesiotherapists often work as part of a team with other health professions—for example, a dietitian, social worker, and nurse.[10]

Work Environment

Kinesiotherapists are trained to work wherever people with disabilities need treatment. For example, rehabilitation or long-term care facilities, group homes for the developmentally disabled, the Department of Defense,

TABLE 19.4 Projections Data for Exercise Physiologists, 2019–2029				
			Change, 2019–2029	
Occupational Title	Employment, 2019	Projected Employment, 2029	Number	Percentage
Exercise physiologists	19,800	22,100	2,200	11%

Data from Bureau of Labor Statistics. Occupational Outlook Handbook. U.S. Department of Labor; 2020. https://www.bls.gov/ooh/healthcare/exercise-physiologists.htm#tab-6

and workers' compensation programs. The work setting depends on the type of care; for example, aquatic therapy takes place in pools, and therapy for patients receiving psychiatric care is often provided in hospitals. RKTs work in Veterans Affairs medical centers and in private and public hospitals and may be employed in clinics for cardiac patients or special schools and camps for children with disabilities.[13] Those who work in home-care travel to visit their patients instead of working in a fixed location.[10] Physical reconditioning units for military or veterans are primarily in VA hospitals; 323 kinesiotherapists were employed in the VA system in 2017.[12]

In clinics, hospitals, and other settings, they may have standard 9-to-5 hours and work entirely onsite. They work a 40-hour week, usually in an indoor setting, although outdoor recreation areas and pools are also used. A variety of physical demands are involved in being a kinesiotherapist, including demonstrating exercises and equipment use, lifting and balancing patients, and handling and adjusting therapeutic exercise equipment.

Educational and Legal Requirements

Entry-level positions in kinesiotherapy require a bachelor's degree in kinesiology plus an internship with 1,000 hours of clinical experience. Typical course requirements are anatomy, physiology, physiological basis of exercise, clinical aspects of ageing, and therapeutic exercise and sports.[13]

Education and Training

There are only two undergraduate programs accredited by CAAHEP, although a master's degree in exercise science is another route to becoming a kinesiotherapist. Registration with the American Kinesiotherapy Association requires a minimum of a bachelor's degree with an internship and successful completion of a qualifying exam.[5] An internship may include rotations in neurology, orthopedics, pediatrics, geriatrics, and cardiac rehabilitation and wellness programs. The majority of internships are located in VA hospitals and clinics.[12]

Certification and Other Qualifications

Registration is usually required to be employed as a kinesiotherapist. For those with work experience, the **Council on Professional Standards for Kinesiotherapy (COPSKT)** administers specialty certification for Registered Kinesiotherapist (RKTs). There are 19 specialty areas for RKTs having experience and skills in an area of kinesiotherapy—for example, driver rehabilitation, ergonomic evaluation, functional capacity evaluation, adaptive sports, amputee, and geriatrics. Eligibility requirements are three-year registration status and documentation of 2,000 hours of clinical experience in the specialty area.[14]

Other Qualifications

Kinesiotherapists need to have good communication and interpersonal skills, enjoy people, and be comfortable working with people from a variety of backgrounds with a variety of health problems. Other qualities needed to be successful as a kinesiotherapist are judgment, honesty, patience, a sense of humor, and the ability to respond to emergencies in a calm manner.

Employment Trends

A 2017 survey by the American Kinesiotherapy Association reported that 68% of RKTs were employed by the VA system with 8% each employed in education and private practice.[15] One of the frustrations for kinesiotherapists is that the profession is not fully recognized except in the VA system, which limits employment opportunities.[10] State licensure and recognition as a profession would improve the ability for RKTs to receive third-party reimbursement and expand work opprotunities.[16]

Earnings

Since RKTs work primarily in VA facilities, most are federal employees. They generally work at the GS-7 to GS-12 level, which had base pay of $34,319 and $60,877, respectively, in 2014.[10] A 2017 survey reported the average salary to be $67,000.[15]

Related Occupations

Health professionals who do similar work are chiropractors, occupational therapists, physical therapists, occupational therapy assistants, physical therapy assistants, and registered nurses.

Additional Information

For more information about careers in sports medicine:

- ExploreHealthCareers.org. *Sports Medicine Overview.* https://explorehealthcareers.org/field/sports-medicine

For information about ensuring the health and safety of college athletes:

- National Collegiate Athletic Association, 700 W. Washington St., P.O. Box 6222, Indianapolis, IN 46206. http://www.ncaa.org/health-and-safety

For information on accredited programs in athletic training, contact:

- Commission on Accreditation of Athletic Trainers Education (CAATE), 2001 K Street NW, 3rd Floor North, Washington, DC 20006. https://caate.net/search-for-accredited-program
- National Athletic Trainers' Association (NATA), 1620 Valwood Pkwy., Suite 115, Carrollton, TX 75006. http://www.nata.org

For information on certification of athletic trainers, contact:

- Board of Certification, Inc., 1415 Harney St., Suite 200, Omaha, NE 68102. http://bocatc.org

For further information on accredited programs in exercise physiology:

- American Society for Exercise Physiologists. https://www.asep.org
- Commission on Accreditation of Allied Health Education Programs, 9355 - 113th St. N, #7709, Seminole, FL 33775. https://www.caahep.org

For further information on certification and registration as an exercise physiologist:

- American College of Sports Medicine, 401 West Michigan St., Indianapolis, IN 46202. http://www.acsm.org

For information on certification in cardiac rehabilitation:

- American Association of Cardiovascular and Pulmonary Rehabilitation, 330 N. Wabash Ave., Suite 2000, Chicago, IL 60611. https://www.aacvpr.org/Certification

For information on kinesiotherapy:

- American Kinesiotherapy Association, P.O. Box 24822, Richmond, VA 23224. http://akta.org
- ExploreHealthCareers.org. *Kinesiotherapist.* https://explorehealthcareers.org/career/sports-medicine/kinesiotherapist
- Commission on Accreditation of Allied Health Education Programs. *Find a Program.* https://www.caahep.org/Students/Find-a-Program.aspx

LEARNING PORTFOLIO

Issues for Discussion

1. Compare the educational requirements and usual work settings of a certified personal trainer, certified athletic trainer, and registered clinical exercise physiologist. Which of these career paths is most appealing to you, and why?

2. View the five-minute video clip "What Is a Clinical Exercise Physiologist?" Describe the health problems that led Matt (shown in the video) into the care of the ACSM Certified Clinical Exercise Physiologist (ACSM-CEP). What goals did the CEP have for Matt, and how were these goals achieved?

3. https://www.youtube.com/watch?v=L_8_w2kBJ -8View the nine-minute video "AACVPR and LSI Featured on Discovery Channel!" Learn more about the role of cardiac rehabilitation. Which patients are referred to a cardiac rehab program? What are the benefits for patients who participate in a cardiac rehab program? https://www.youtube.com/watch?v=40RZtEFeCgo

4. Discuss the role of the National Collegiate Athletic Association in ensuring the safety of college and university athletes. http://www.ncaa.org

Enrichment Activities

1. View the five-minute video from the National Athletic Trainers' Association titled "Advocacy Video: Unsung Heroes of Sports Medicine." How do physicians work with athletic trainers? https://vimeo.com/47686550

2. Go to the webpage for the American College of Sports Medicine and identify different certifications available. What are the advantages of becoming certified in a specialty area? https://www.acsm.org/get-stay -certified/get-certified

CASE STUDY: ATHLETIC TRAINERS AND EXERCISE PHYSIOLOGISTS

Amelia has a dream of becoming an exercise physiologist. She has been working with her guidance counselor at school to research some of the specifics regarding this profession. The following questions relate to exercise physiologists. Please help Amelia answer them based on what you have learned in this chapter.

1. In order for Amelia to become a ACSM Certified Clinical Exercise Physiologist (ACSM-CEP), she must meet the minimum requirement of a(n):
   A. high school diploma.
   B. associate's degree.
   C. bachelor's degree.
   D. master's degree.

2. Based on employment statistics for exercise physiologists in 2019, Amelia should expect to work for:
   A. hospitals.
   B. offices of physicians.
   C. offices of other health professionals.
   D. herself.

3. As an exercise physiologist, Amelia will:
   A. develop physical exercise routines for physically disabled patients.
   B. provide health education and develop exercise plans to reduce risk for disease.
   C. perform surgical procedures for physically disabled patients.
   D. demonstrate exercise routines for professional athletes.

4. Which of the following job duties would Amelia expect to do in her role as an exercise physiologist?
   A. Perform fitness tests
   B. Monitor body fat
   C. Assess blood pressure
   D. All of these are correct.

5. If Amelia works as an exercise physiologist in a hospital environment, she can expect to earn a median annual wage of:
   A. $30,000 to $39,000.
   B. $40,000 to $49,000.
   C. $50,000 to $59,000.
   D. $60,000 to $69,000.

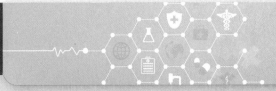

LEARNING PORTFOLIO

References

1. ExploreHealthCareers.org. *Sports Medicine Overview*. https://explorehealthcareers.org/field/sports-medicine Accessed July 2, 2020.

2. Commission on Accreditation of Athletic Training Education. *Becoming an Athletic Trainer*. https://caate.net/becoming-an-athletic-trainer Accessed July 2, 2020.

3. Board of Certification for the Athletic Trainer. *State Regulators*. https://www.bocatc.org/state-regulation Accessed July 2, 2020.

4. Commission on Accreditation of Athletic Training Education. *Residency Programs*. https://caate.net/residency-programs Accessed July 2, 2020.

5. Commission on Accreditation of Allied Health Education Programs. *CAAHEP Accredited Program Search*. http://www.caahep.org/Find-An-Accredited-Program Accessed July 2, 2020.

6. American College of Sports Medicine. *Become Your Passion. Become an ACSM Certified Clinical Exercise Physiologist*. https://www.acsm.org/get-stay-certified/get-certified/cep Accessed July 2, 2020.

7. Clinical Exercise Physiology Association. *What Is a Registered Exercise Physiologist?* https://cepa.clubexpress.com/content.aspx?page_id=22&club_id=324409&module_id=319786 Accessed August 10, 2021.

8. American Association of Cardiovascular and Cardiopulmonary Rehabilitation. *Certified Cardiac Rehabilitation Professional (CCRP)*. https://www.aacvpr.org/Certified-Cardiac-Rehabilitation-Professional Accessed August 9, 2021.

9. American Kinesiotherapy Association. *Our History*. https://akta.org/about Accessed August 9, 2021.

10. Green K. You're a What? Kinesiotherapist. *Career Outlook*. December 2014. U.S. Department of Labor.

11. ExploreHealthCareers.org. *Kinesiotherapist*. https://explorehealthcareers.org/career/sports-medicine/kinesiotherapist Accessed August 7, 2021.

12. Rehabilitation and Prosthetics Services. *Kinesiotherapy* https://www.rehab.va.gov/PROSTHETICS/factsheet/KT-FactSheet.pdf Updated November 2020. Accessed August 7, 2021.

13. Norfolk State University. *Kinesiotherapy*. https://www.nsu.edu/Academics/Faculty-and-Academic-Divisions/Schools-and-Colleges/School-of-Education/Departments/Health-Physical-Education-Exercise-Science/Programs Accessed May 23, 2020.

14. American Kinesiotherapy Association. *Become Recognized for your Area of Expertise*. https://akta.org/professional-development/available-specializations Accessed July 2, 2020.

15. American Kinesiotherapy Association. *Employment Statistics*. https://akta.org/employment-opportunities/careers/employment-statistics Accessed July 2, 2020.

16. Purvis JW. *Kinesiotherapy, Past, Present, and Future*. American Kinesiotherapy Association. https://akta.org/about/kinesiotherapy-past-present-and-future Accessed July 2, 2020.

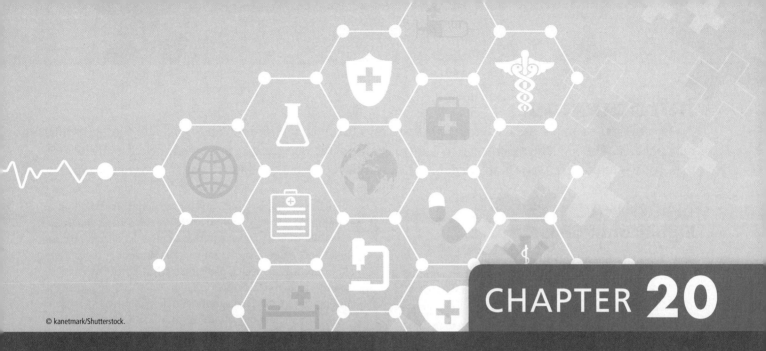

© kanetmark/Shutterstock.

CHAPTER 20

Chiropractors*

KEY TERMS

Alignment	Group practice	Nervous system
Chiropractor	Manipulation	Spinal adjustments
Complementary medicine	Musculoskeletal system	Solo practice

* All information in this chapter, unless otherwise indicated, was obtained from Bureau of Labor Statistics. *Occupational Outlook Handbook 2020–2021 Edition*. Washington, DC: U.S. Department of Labor; 2021.

Introduction

Perhaps the most familiar use of chiropractic services is the treatment of back and neck pain through spinal manipulation. Although this treatment remains a major use of that service, the chiropractic field goes far beyond that. Today, chiropractic services are used not only to address pain but to address a patient's overall health.

CHIROPRACTORS
Significant Points

- Job opportunities should be favorable.
- Employment will grow as interest in integrative or complementary medicine to treat pain increases.
- Chiropractic offices employ about 63% of all chiropractors.

Work Description

Chiropractors are primary care professionals who focus on patients' overall health and work to relieve pain, increase mobility, and improve performance. They are sometimes referred to as Doctors of Chiropractic or chiropractic physicians. The chiropractic profession concentrates on disorders of the **musculoskeletal and nervous systems**, focusing on how these systems affect an individual's general health. Examples of the musculoskeletal and nervous systems are seen in **FIGURES 20.1** and **20.2**. Chiropractors believe that malfunctioning spinal joints and other somatic tissues can affect a person's neuromuscular system, resulting in poor health. Said simply, a person's structure affects their ability to function properly. As such, chiropractors pay special attention to a patient's nerves, bones, muscles, ligaments, and tendons.

Chiropractors assess patients by performing a physical examination, taking a medical history of the patient, and listening to the patient's concerns. They analyze a patient's posture, spine, and reflexes and conduct tests, including X-rays and ultrasounds. They create a patient record, in either paper or electronic form, to record this information. These actions permit the chiropractor to make a diagnosis and develop a treatment plan.

Chiropractors rely on nonsurgical methods of treatment and do not use drugs as a treatment method. This is an alternative approach to pain relief, as conventional methods most often involve surgery and medication. Chiropractors perform neuromusculoskeletal therapy, including **spinal adjustments** and **manipulations** of other joints to treat numerous types of pain, including tension headaches, frozen shoulder syndrome, and sciatic nerve pain. An example of chiropractic spinal adjustment is shown in **FIGURE 20.3**. The concept is that different techniques are used to adjust ("manipulate") a patient's spine or other parts of the patient's body so that the spine or other body part can be in proper form, or **alignment**. Chiropractors may employ massage therapy and rehabilitative exercises and apply heat and cold therapy to injured areas. Some patients require support to treat and relieve pain, with the chiropractor providing braces and shoe inserts for that support. Due to the focus on overall health, they may provide patients

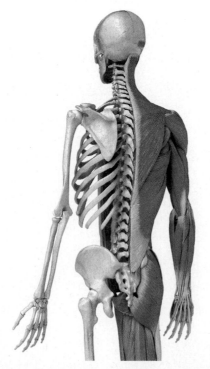
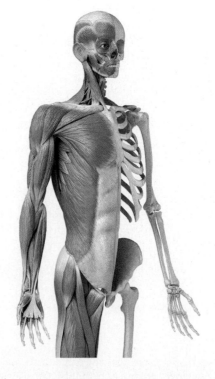

FIGURE 20.1 The human musculoskeletal system.

HUMAN NERVOUS SYSTEM

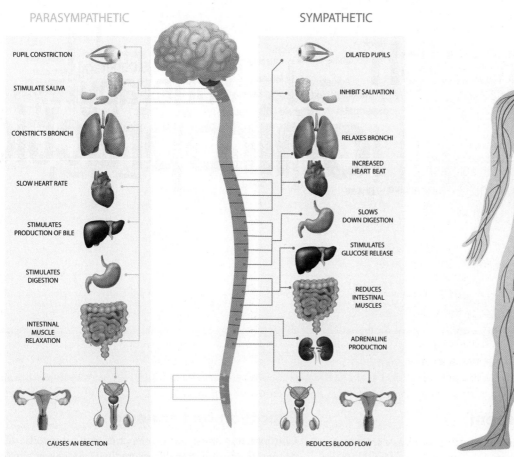

PARASYMPATHETIC

- PUPIL CONSTRICTION
- STIMULATE SALIVA
- CONSTRICTS BRONCHI
- SLOW HEART RATE
- STIMULATES PRODUCTION OF BILE
- STIMULATES DIGESTION
- INTESTINAL MUSCLE RELAXATION
- CAUSES AN ERECTION

SYMPATHETIC

- DILATED PUPILS
- INHIBIT SALIVATION
- RELAXES BRONCHI
- INCREASED HEART BEAT
- SLOWS DOWN DIGESTION
- STIMULATES GLUCOSE RELEASE
- REDUCES INTESTINAL MUSCLES
- ADRENALINE PRODUCTION
- REDUCES BLOOD FLOW

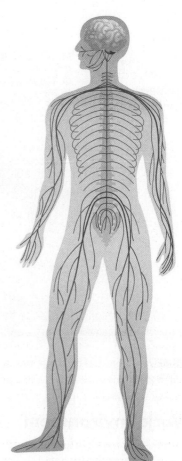

FIGURE 20.2 The human nervous system.
© Macrovector/Shutterstock.

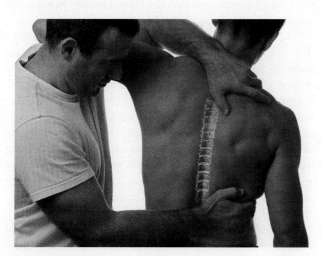

FIGURE 20.3 Chiropractic adjustment.
© Albina Gavrilovic/Shutterstock.

nutritional, lifestyle, and dietary counseling as well. Many of the concepts included in the chiropractic field are listed in **FIGURE 20.4**.

Chiropractors may refer patients to other health-care professionals if medical circumstances warrant a referral. For example, chiropractors typically do not treat patients with traumatic injuries, such as bone fractures, but refer them to other medical professionals for treatment. It is not uncommon for patients to be cared for by both a medical and a chiropractic physician simultaneously. Being cared for through both traditional medical approaches and chiropractic approaches is a form of **complementary medicine**.

Some chiropractors specialize in areas requiring advanced expertise and training. These specialized areas include but are not limited to sports, neurology, orthopedics, pediatrics, and nutrition. For example, a chiropractor specializing in sports may work with athletes to improve balance and coordination, thereby improving their performance, preventing injuries, and reducing recovery time for those injuries that do occur. Improving balance and coordination also benefits senior citizens, who are at an increased risk of falling due to decreased balance ability. Chiropractors may specialize their practice to aid seniors, not only in improving their balance but also in increasing range of motion, easing arthritis symptoms, and decreasing pain. The goal is to allow seniors to stay in their homes safely and live longer lives.

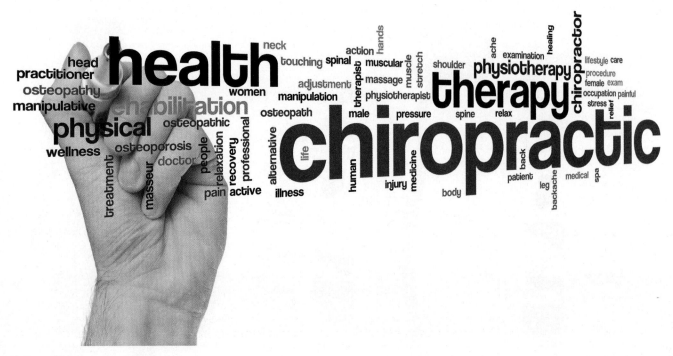

FIGURE 20.4 Concepts in chiropractic care.
© ibreakstock/Shutterstock.

Work Environment

Chiropractors work in an office setting, often as a **solo practice** or a **group practice** with other chiropractors. In fact, the largest employer of chiropractors is offices of chiropractors, which employ 63% of all chiropractors. About 31% of chiropractors are self-employed, and 3% are employed in physician offices. Most chiropractors work full time, and some offer evening and weekend hours to accommodate the needs of their patients. Some chiropractors offer home visits to clients to provide treatment. Chiropractors who own their practice may spend time on business-related matters, such as hiring employees, keeping records, marketing, and managing inventory. They must be able to stand on their feet for long periods of time when examining and treating patients.

Employment Opportunities

Chiropractors held 51,100 jobs in 2019. Chiropractors face favorable opportunities as a career due to the increased interest of people across all age groups in integrative or complementary health care as a way to treat pain and improve overall wellness.

Educational and Legal Requirements

Chiropractors must earn a Doctor of Chiropractic (DC) degree at an accredited school before becoming licensed.

Education and Training

Chiropractors must earn a Doctor of Chiropractic (DC) degree from a nationally accredited, four-year doctoral graduate school program.[1] In 2021, there were 16 nationally accredited chiropractic doctoral graduate education programs at 19 locations across the United States.[2] Schools are accredited by the Council on Chiropractic Education.

Admission to chiropractic programs requires completion of the equivalent of three academic years of undergraduate study (90 semester hours) at an institution(s) accredited by an agency recognized by the U.S. Department of Education or an equivalent foreign agency. Students should hold a GPA for these 90 hours of not less than 3.0 on a 4.0 scale to be considered for admission. At least 24 semester hours of the 90 hours must be in life and physical science courses.[3] An increasing number of programs require an applicant to hold a bachelor's degree. Students interested in attending a chiropractic program should check with individual schools for specific coursework requirements needed prior to admission to the program.

Characteristics of a chiropractic curriculum include training in a classroom, a laboratory, and a clinical internship. Typically, chiropractic students spend at least a year of their training working with patients, although this is not a formal residency program. Additional classwork may address business practice concerns such as the finance, billing, and management aspects of running a business. Many chiropractic programs offer a dual-degree option, allowing a student to obtain a bachelor's degree or a master's degree in a separate field while simultaneously studying for a chiropractic degree.

Professional Profiles

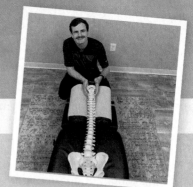

Name: Rosario, MS, CSCS, DC
Job Title: Doctor of Chiropractic
Education: BS in Biopsychology, Cognition, and Neuroscience; MS in Exercise Physiology; DC

Q: Tell us about your job and the type of organization you work in.

A: I work in a private chiropractic practice. We have two chiropractors (myself included), one chiropractic assistant, one employee in charge of billing, and a front desk receptionist.

My job as a chiropractor includes much more than just manipulating/adjusting joints. Every new patient visit begins with a detailed history of the patient's chief complaint, a review of their past medical history, family history, and finally the patient's social history. After a thorough history, we begin the physical examination where we begin to narrow down the list of potential diagnoses. Sometimes the list of diagnoses includes disorders involving body systems outside of what can be treated by manual therapy/chiropractic manipulation. In these instances, chiropractors are well versed in making the appropriate referrals to other medical professionals. The number one rule of all musculoskeletal examinations is to RULE OUT RED FLAGS! This means that the chiropractor needs to make sure that the source of the patient's pain is not something more sinister like malignancy, infection, fracture, neurological disease, etc.

When a reasonable musculoskeletal diagnosis has been reached, we explain the diagnosis to the patient in what is termed the "report of findings." If the patient consents to treatment, we offer a multitude of treatment modalities. Some procedures are more gentle, such as flexion/distraction therapy. Other therapies are what we term "high velocity, low amplitude" (HVLA) manipulation, which is what most people envision when thinking about chiropractors. HVLA manipulation can be performed on most joints in the human body, not just the spine! Still, this is not all we offer at our clinic. Dry needling, instrument-assisted soft tissue massage, movement therapy, and various rehabilitation techniques are all implemented when appropriate.

Q: Describe a typical workday.

A: A typical day involves several new patient exams, but the vast majority of patient encounters are with established patients. Visits with established patients usually consist of a brief conversation about how the patient is doing on that particular day and how they have been doing in the days/weeks since their last treatment. Assuming no new complaints are reported by the patient, a typical treatment takes between 15 and 30 minutes. During these treatments, we utilize spinal manipulation the most, but we will also provide patients with interventions such as dry needling, cupping therapy, rehabilitation exercises, patient education, as well as others when appropriate.

Accurate note taking also takes up a significant amount of time on a daily basis. Every patient visit needs to be documented properly. For every single patient visit, the note must follow a specific outline. We jot down the patient's subjective information (anything the patient directly reports during the visit), objective information (any findings found directly by the clinician, i.e., areas of joint restriction or pain), the assessment (pertaining to the patient's prognosis), and lastly the plan (if any changes need to be made to the treatment plan).

Between treating patients and taking accurate notes, a typical chiropractor stays busy the entire day with not much down time. Depending on the structure of the practice, chiropractors can see anywhere from just a handful of patients to 50 to 100 patients per day. The wide scope of practice for chiropractors in most states is very beneficial for creating a practice model that fits your own personality. It is a very rewarding profession in that respect!

Q: Why did you choose this profession?

A: I have always wanted to serve individuals who are looking for a solution to a problem. Additionally, as a lifelong athlete, I have always been fascinated with developing mastery in a physical skillset. Chiropractic was the perfect mix of the two. It allows me to be an expert in musculoskeletal health care within my community, and it allows me to solve these musculoskeletal problems using my own two hands when appropriate.

Q: What do you like most about this profession, and what challenges you?

A: Obviously, getting patients back to pre-injury status is what makes being a chiropractor so rewarding. It's what makes getting to the office every morning a joy rather than a dread. Musculoskeletal disorders can be debilitating, and seeing the progress that certain patients make throughout treatment is astounding. The greatest challenge is mastering the art of joint manipulation. It is an athletic endeavor, just the same as learning how to throw a perfect spiral football or a curve ball in baseball. It can be very frustrating in the beginning, but it is important to stay focused and remind yourself that you're doing it for all those patients who trust you with their health and wellness.

Q: Is there room for advancement in this field?

A: "Advancement" may not be the right word, but there is certainly room for growth. Chiropractors are becoming more mainstream in hospital systems, in interdisciplinary private clinics, within amateur and professional sports teams, and even in corporate America. Clinical research has continually demonstrated the efficacy of chiropractic co-management in cases of chronic back pain, and it is likely this body of research will continue to grow in the future, opening up new opportunities.

Q: What kind of academic training is required in this field, and how long does it take?

A: A bachelor's degree is needed in order to apply to chiropractic school, although some schools have an agreement with local universities that allow for college students who have the necessary prerequisite coursework to enroll in the chiropractic program early. These students will earn both their bachelor's degree and their Doctor of Chiropractic degree all within the 3.5 years (10 trimesters) it takes to go through chiropractic school. As far as prerequisite coursework, this includes all your general education classes offered at most four-year universities: biology, chemistry, physics, anatomy, physiology, psychology, English, etc.

Q: Name and explain what part of your academic training most prepared you for this profession.

A: My master's degree in exercise physiology was highly relevant due to the detail that was covered on topics such as cardiovascular physiology, renal physiology, endocrinology, and sports psychology.

Q: Did you face obstacles in pursuing your goals? If so, describe them and how you overcame them.

A: One of my biggest obstacles was that I had not taken physics in undergrad, so I had to spend tons of time studying functional anatomy/biomechanics. It was well worth it, though, because now I have become a biomechanics nerd, and it really helps with both assessing and treating patients.

Q: What do you wish you had known in high school/college about pursuing this career?

A: The fact that some chiropractic programs offer early enrollment to undergraduate students who have not yet obtained their bachelor's degree is something I wish I would have known. You can save tons of money by bypassing two full years of undergrad, and you will likely be a practicing clinician by the time you are 24 or 25. Education is expensive, so it would have saved me a ton of time and money.

Q: What advice would you give someone who is considering this career?

A: Do *not* expect to go through school doing the bare minimum and be successful the day after you graduate. IT DOES NOT WORK LIKE THAT! Join clubs and take seminars outside what is offered at school. It may seem like a waste of time to go to that club meeting a day before a big exam… GO ANYWAYS. It may seem like a waste of money to go to that weekend seminar everyone is talking about… IT ISN'T. All those extracurricular activities provide opportunities to expose yourself to new ideas and to fill in the holes in your knowledge base. Furthermore, you must get out and network with practicing doctors before you start school *and* while you are in school. Find local clinicians who will allow you to shadow them and go back if you enjoyed it. Build these relationships and you may even have a job waiting for you after graduation.

Licensing and Certification

Doctors of Chiropractic must be licensed in all 50 states and the District of Columbia. After graduation, they must pass a series of four national board exams[4] in order to obtain a license to practice. And they must meet continuing education requirements every year to keep their licenses.

Some chiropractors choose to obtain specialty credentials, referred to as diplomate credentials. These credentials are offered through the American Board of Chiropractic Specialties as board certifications and fellowship credentials. As of 2021, eight board credentials were offered through the American Board of Chiropractic Specialties.[5] Additional board certifications may be available through independent organizations.

Advancement

Chiropractors advance by obtaining diplomate credentials or by choosing to educate future chiropractors in graduate programs.

Employment Trends

Employment is expected to grow about as fast as the average for all occupations. Job opportunities should be good, particularly as the population ages and older adults require care to manage joint problems.

Employment Change

Employment of chiropractors is projected to grow 4% from 2019 to 2029, about as fast as the average for all occupations (**TABLE 20.1**). Job growth will occur due to longer lives of the elderly population, requiring care to remain active over time. Insurance coverage is increasing prevalent for chiropractic services, addressing the ability of patients to pay for services. Nonsurgical methods to treat pain without medications appeal to many people and will drive patients to chiropractors for this care. Finally, the increased acceptance of complementary medicine and research supporting chiropractic techniques will result in additional referrals to chiropractors.

Earnings

The median annual wage for chiropractors was $70,720 in May 2020. The lowest 10% earned less than $35,390, and the highest 10% earned more than $137,950.

Earnings for chiropractors vary due to several factors, including geographic region of practice, the number of years of practice experience, and the number of hours worked. The number of years of practice experience correlates with increased earnings, with the establishment of a client base, and ownership in a chiropractic practice.

Related Occupations

Other workers who treat problems of the musculoskeletal and nervous systems include physicians and surgeons, podiatrists, optometrists, athletic trainers, exercise physiologists, physical therapists, massage therapists, and occupational therapists.

Additional Information

For career information on becoming a chiropractor, contact:

- American Chiropractic Association, 1701 Clarendon Blvd. Suite 200, Arlington, VA 22209. https://www.acatoday.org
- International Chiropractic Association, 6400 Arlington Blvd., Falls Church, VA 22042. https://www.chiropractic.org

For educational information on becoming a chiropractor, contact:

- Association of Chiropractic Colleges, 4424 Montgomery Ave., Suite 202, Bethesda, MD 20814. https://www.chirocolleges.org
- Council on Chiropractic Education, 10105 E Via Linda Suite 103 PMB 3642, Scottsdale, AZ 85258. https://www.cce-usa.org

For state education and licensure requirements, contact:

- Federation of Chiropractic Licensing Boards, 5401 W. 10th St., Suite 101, Greeley, CO 80634. https://www.fclb.org

For information about licensing exams, contact:

- National Board of Chiropractic Examiners, 901 54th Ave., Greeley, CO 80634. https://www.nbce.org

TABLE 20.1 Projections Data for Chiropractors, 2019–2029				
			Change, 2019–2029	
Occupational Title	Employment, 2019	Projected Employment, 2029	Number	Percentage
Chiropractors	51,100	53,400	2,300	4%

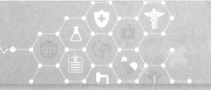

LEARNING PORTFOLIO

Issues for Discussion

1. Review the videos found at https://www.spine-health.com/treatment/chiropractic/videos to understand the techniques chiropractors commonly use to address back pain. After reviewing these videos, do you feel more or less comfortable considering chiropractic care? Explain why you reached this conclusion.

2. In your opinion, what is the most important responsibility of a chiropractor? Explain why you feel this is most important.

3. Some patients receive chiropractic care for years after initially receiving treatment. If you were such a patient, how would you evaluate the progress of the care you received, and what questions would you ask the chiropractor about assessing the root cause of your pain and your progress as a patient in relieving that pain?

Enrichment Activities

1. Write a short skit that documents a professional interaction between a chiropractor and another person. The other person can be a client or another employee. Use the skit to document your knowledge about some aspect of this profession.

2. Using the Internet, research the history and development of the chiropractic profession. Identify the reason(s) why the profession was created and when and how the federal government and insurance companies decided to reimburse care provided by chiropractors. Prepare a written narrative or infographic of this information to your instructor.

3. Create a one-page infographic or flyer for students who are thinking of a career as a chiropractor. The pamphlet should inform students on what a chiropractor is, what a chiropractor does, and both the benefits and drawbacks of this occupation.

CASE STUDY: CAREER SHADOW

Kenji has been a student athlete all his life, having benefited from both training in his sport and methods to prevent injury. Kenji plans to pursue a chiropractic career so that he can assist fellow athletes to perform better and prevent injuries. Kenji has decided to shadow a chiropractor in his area.

Based on the information you have learned in this chapter, answer the following questions.

1. Identify which goals a chiropractor may assist an athlete to attain.
   A. Improved balance and coordination
   B. Injury prevention
   C. Reduced recovery time from injury
   D. All of the above

2. Identify which underlying condition a chiropractor would not perform service for a patient.
   A. Tension headaches
   B. Frozen shoulder syndrome
   C. Fractured bone
   D. Sciatic nerve pain

3. If Kenji were to not finish his bachelor's degree after completing 90 course hours but instead enroll directly into a graduate chiropractic program, what degrees would he receive at the end of the graduate program?
   A. A bachelor's degree and a doctor of osteopathy degree
   B. An associate's degree and a Doctor of Chiropractic degree
   C. A bachelor's degree and a doctor of medicine degree
   D. A bachelor's degree and a Doctor of Chiropractic degree

4. As part of the shadowing, Kenji will learn that chiropractors rely on these methods of treatment.
   A. Musculoskeletal therapy, pain medications, and massage therapy
   B. Musculoskeletal therapy, massage therapy, and surgery
   C. Musculoskeletal therapy, rehabilitation exercises, and radiation therapy
   D. Musculoskeletal therapy, rehabilitation exercises, and cold therapy

LEARNING PORTFOLIO

References

1. The Association of Chiropractic Colleges. Academic Requirements. https://www.chirocolleges.org/academic-requirements Accessed August 8, 2021.

2. Council on Chiropractic Education (CCE). Accredited Programs. https://www.cce-usa.org Accessed August 8, 2021.

3. The Association of Chiropractic Colleges. Academic Requirements. https://www.chirocolleges.org/academic-requirements Accessed August 8, 2021.

4. National Board of Chiropractic Examiners. https://www.nbce.org Accessed August 8, 2021.

5. American Board of Chiropractic Specialties. Recognized Board Certifications. https://www.acatoday.org/Communities-Related-Organizations-American-Board-of-Chiropractic-Specialties Accessed August 8, 2021.

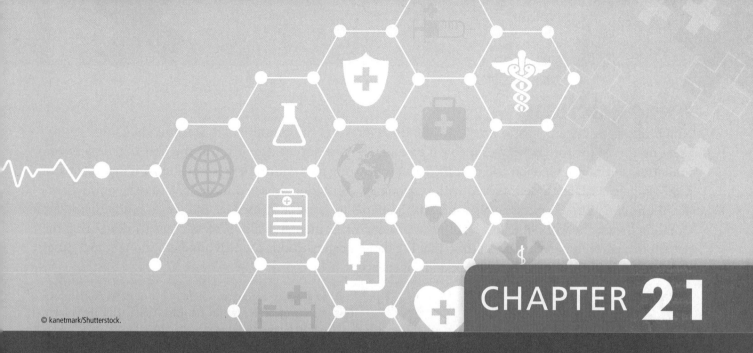
© kanetmark/Shutterstock.

CHAPTER **21**

Mental Health Professionals*

* All information in this chapter, unless otherwise indicated, was obtained from Bureau of Labor Statistics. *Occupational Outlook Handbook 2020–2021 Edition*. Washington, DC: U.S. Department of Labor; 2021.

Introduction

Numerous stressors are part of everyday life; these stressors sometimes affect an individual's well-being. Treating these stressors by way of medical care alone does not always result in the best outcome for an individual. Promoting mental and psychological well-being falls within the responsibility of mental health professionals, such as those involved with psychology, substance abuse counseling, and behavioral disorder counseling. These professionals work with patients to prevent, diagnose, and treat mental disorders. Combined with the work of fellow healthcare professionals, mental health professionals work to bring the patient to a place in life of total health so that the patient can use both cognitive and emotional capabilities to function in society and meet the demands of everyday life.

PSYCHOLOGISTS
Significant Points

- About 31% of psychologists are self-employed, mainly as private practitioners and independent consultants.
- Employment growth will vary by specialty—for example, clinical, counseling, and school psychologists will have 3% growth; industrial-organizational psychologists, 3% growth; and 2% growth is expected for all other psychologists.
- Acceptance to graduate psychology programs is highly competitive.
- Job opportunities should be the best for those with a doctoral degree in a subfield, such as health; those with a master's degree will have good prospects in industrial-organization psychology; bachelor's degree holders will have limited prospects.

Psychologists study the human mind and human behavior. Psychology examines both normal and abnormal aspects of human behavior. **Psychology** refers to a scientific approach to gathering, quantifying, analyzing, and interpreting data on why people act as they do, and it provides insight into varied forms of human behavior and related mental and physical processes. Through the application of highly developed skills and knowledge, psychologists seek to identify, prevent, and solve various problems of human behavior.

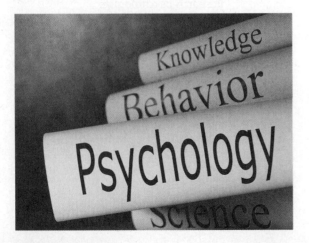

Psychology book titles.
© alejandro dans neergaard/Shutterstock.

As a health career, psychology is one of the allied professions devoted to **mental health**. Along with psychiatry, psychiatric nursing, and psychiatric social work, psychology contributes both to the prevention of mental illness and to its diagnosis and treatment. As distinguished from psychiatry, which is a branch of medicine, psychology is a nonmedical science. As distinguished from psychiatric social work, psychology looks first at the individual's reaction to his or her circumstances—family, job, and social relationships. The psychiatric social worker looks first at the individual's surrounding circumstances and relationships.

Work Description

Psychologists study the behavior of individuals or groups to ascertain and understand the fundamental processes of human behavior. They observe, interpret, and record how people relate to their environment. Some psychologists interview people and develop, administer, and score a variety of psychological tests. Others work in mental health and rehabilitation centers, hospitals, and private practice providing counseling and therapy to persons suffering emotional or adjustment problems. Because psychology is basically a science, the psychologist is often the most knowledgeable member among mental health team members regarding research. The science of psychology is one of the main sources of our increasing understanding of mental capacity and intelligence and of the effect of emotions on health. Psychological research contributes continuously to the improvement of diagnostic methods and to the treatment and prevention of mental and emotional disorders. Psychologists also work with disabled persons, either individually or in groups, to diagnose behavioral problems and to help correct or compensate for these impairments.

A psychologist may also design, develop, and evaluate materials and procedures in order to resolve problems in educational and training programs. In addition, psychologists employ scientific techniques to deal with problems of motivation and morale in work settings. Psychologists design and conduct experiments and analyze the results in an effort to improve understanding of human and animal behavior.

Some psychologists engage in private practice; others work in colleges and universities, where they train graduate and undergraduate students and engage in basic research. Increasingly, they work as administrators of psychology programs in hospitals, clinics, and community health agencies. Many psychologists practice in federal, state, and local agencies; a variety of business and industrial organizations; and various branches of the armed forces.

The field of psychology offers a number of specializations that an individual can consider when planning a career. These include clinical psychology, counseling psychology, developmental psychology, educational psychology, engineering psychology, personnel psychology, experimental psychology, industrial psychology, psychometric psychology, rehabilitation psychology, school psychology, and social psychology.

Clinical psychologists specialize in the assessment and treatment of persons with mental, behavioral, and emotional problems and illnesses. They apply experience and scientific knowledge of human behavior to diagnose and treat psychological problems ranging from the developmental crises of adolescence to extreme psychotic conditions. They may design behavior modification programs and assist patients in implementing those programs. Working in hospitals, clinics, or similar medical institutions, clinical psychologists design and conduct research either alone or in conjunction with physicians or other social scientists. Although the emphasis may differ considerably from one position to another, all clinical psychologists apply scientific knowledge of human behavior to the care and treatment of the handicapped and the disturbed. Their purpose is to help the individual who is maladjusted learn new and better habits of behavior so as to find a more satisfactory way of living.

Clinical psychologists work directly with the patient, or client, to uncover everything that will help in understanding his or her difficulties. They also talk with the patient's family, friends, physicians, and teachers to round out this background. At times they consult with the psychiatrist, social worker, and others concerned with diagnosis and treatment.

Areas of specialization within clinical psychology include health psychology, neuropsychology, and geropsychology. **Health psychologists** promote good health through health maintenance counseling programs designed to help people achieve health-oriented goals, such as to stop smoking or lose weight. **Neuropsychologists** study the relationship between the brain and behavior. They often work in stroke and head injury programs. **Geropsychologists** deal with the special problems faced by the elderly. The emergence and subsequent growth of these specialties reflect the increasing participation of psychologists in providing direct services to special patient populations.

Counseling psychologists help normal or moderately maladjusted persons, either individually or in groups, to gain self-understanding, recognize problems, and develop methods of coping with their difficulties. Counseling psychologists pay particular attention to the role of education and work in a person's behavior and to the interaction between individuals and the environments in which they live. This type of counseling primarily emphasizes preventing or forestalling the onset of mental illness. Growing public awareness of mental health problems has highlighted the importance of and need for the services that counseling psychologists provide.

Developmental psychologists specialize in investigating the development of individuals from prenatal origins through old age. In studying the changes involved in mental, physical, emotional, and social growth, psychologists seek to determine the origins of human behavior and the reasons for human growth and decline. For example, psychologists study how an infant's behavior and feelings are related to the biological growth of the body. Another example is the study of the influence of social learning and socialization on an infant's development into a socialized person.

Educational psychologists design, develop, and evaluate materials and procedures to resolve problems in educational and training programs. These psychologists analyze educational problems, develop instructional materials, determine the best conditions for instruction, and evaluate the effectiveness of educational programs. Educational psychologists are employed by school systems, the military, private research and development firms, and industrial concerns.

Engineering psychologists deal with the design and use of the systems and environments in which people live and work. Their main purpose is the development of efficient and acceptable interactions between individuals and the environments in which they function. These psychologists help to design equipment, work areas, and systems involving the direct interaction of humans with machines. In addition, they develop the aids, training devices, and requirements necessary to train personnel to operate such systems successfully.

Personnel psychologists apply their professional knowledge and skills to the hiring, assignment, and promotion of employees in order to increase productivity and job satisfaction. These psychologists place great emphasis on data gathered from tests and interviews, and apply the techniques of other psychological specialties, such as experimental, developmental, and psychometric, to normal work activities.

The **experimental psychologist** designs, conducts, and analyzes experiments to develop knowledge regarding human and animal behavior. Experimental psychology is a general term referring to the methods employed in studying behavioral processes. There are different types of experimental psychologists who are identified by their areas of specialization, such as comparative psychologists, learning psychologists, and physiological psychologists.

Industrial psychologists use scientific techniques to deal with problems of motivation and morale in the work setting. These psychologists study how work is organized and what working styles are employed and suggest improvements designed to increase quality, productivity, and worker satisfaction. They consult with all levels of management and present recommendations for developing better training programs and preretirement counseling services.

Psychometric psychologists directly measure human behavior, primarily through the use of tests. Typically well trained in mathematics, statistics, and the use of computers, they design, develop, and validate intelligence, aptitude, and personality tests; analyze complex statistical data; and design various types of research investigations. In addition, they conduct pilot studies of newly developed materials and devise and apply procedures for measuring the **psychological variables** affecting human behavior.

Rehabilitation psychologists work with disabled persons, either individually or in groups, to assess the degree of disability and develop ways to correct or compensate for these impairments. The primary concern of these psychologists is the restoration of the patient's emotional, physical, social, and **economic effectiveness**.

School psychologists are concerned with developing effective programs for improving the intellectual, social, and emotional development of children in an educational system or school. They diagnose the needs of gifted, handicapped, and disturbed children and plan and carry out corrective programs to enable them to do schoolwork at their highest potential and to adjust to everyday pressures. To determine a child's needs, limitations, and potential, school psychologists often observe the child in the classroom and at play, study school records, consult with teachers and parents, and administer and interpret various tests. They advise school administrators and parent–teacher groups in matters involving psychological services within the school system and serve as consultants in education for children who are handicapped, mentally disturbed, or have intellectual disabilities. School psychologists also engage in planning and developing special programs in the area of adult education.

Social psychologists study the effects of groups and individuals on the thoughts, feelings, attitudes, and behavior of the individual. They study, for example, the ways in which social attitudes develop and how members of families, neighborhoods, and communities influence each other.

Research psychologists work in university and private research centers and in business, nonprofit, and governmental organizations. They study the behavior of both human beings and animals such as rats, monkeys, and pigeons. Prominent areas of study in research psychology include motivation, thought, attention, learning and memory, sensory and perceptual processes, and the effects of substance abuse. Research psychologists also study genetic and neurological factors affecting behavior.

Forensic psychologists work in the criminal justice and legal fields. They assist judges, lawyers, and other legal specialists to understand the psychological aspects of a particular case. They may specialize in a particular area, such as family law, criminal law, or civil law, and often serve as expert witnesses in court cases.

Work Environment

A psychologist's specialty and place of employment determine his or her working conditions. Clinical and counseling psychologists in private practice have their own offices and set their own hours. They often offer evening and weekend hours to accommodate their clients. Psychologists employed in hospitals, nursing homes, and other health facilities may work shifts including evenings and weekends, whereas those who work in schools and clinics generally work regular hours.

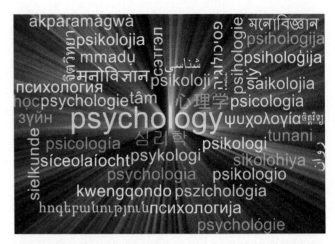

Psychology in multiple languages.
© Kheng Guan Toh/Shutterstock.

Psychologists employed as faculty by colleges and universities divide their time between teaching and research and may also have administrative responsibilities. Many have part-time consulting practices. Most psychologists in government and industry have well-structured schedules.

Increasingly, many psychologists work as part of a team and consult with other psychologists and various healthcare professionals to treat illnesses and promote overall wellness. Many experience pressures due to deadlines, tight schedules, and overtime work. Their routines may be interrupted frequently. Travel is required to attend conferences or conduct research.

Employment Opportunities

Psychologists held about 192,300 jobs in 2019. Educational institutions employed about 24% of psychologists in positions other than teaching, such as counseling, testing, research, and administration. About 18% were employed in ambulatory health care services, primarily in offices of mental health practitioners, hospitals, physicians' offices, and outpatient mental health and substance abuse centers. Government agencies at the state and local levels employed psychologists in correctional facilities, law enforcement, and other settings.

After several years of experience, some psychologists—usually those with doctoral degrees—enter private practice or set up private research or consulting firms. About one-third of psychologists were self-employed in 2019.

In addition to the previously mentioned jobs, many psychologists held faculty positions at colleges and universities and as high school psychology teachers.

Educational and Legal Requirements

A master's or doctoral degree and a license are required for most psychologists.

Education and Training

A doctoral degree usually is required for independent practice as a psychologist. Psychologists with a PhD or Doctor of Psychology (PsyD) qualify for a wide range of teaching, research, clinical, and counseling positions in universities, healthcare services, elementary and secondary schools, private industry, and government. Psychologists with a doctoral degree often work in clinical positions or in private practice, but they also sometimes teach, conduct research, or carry out administrative responsibilities.

A doctoral degree generally requires about five years of graduate study, culminating in a dissertation based on original research. Courses in quantitative research methods, which include the use of computer-based analysis, are an integral part of graduate study and are necessary to pass a comprehensive examination and complete the dissertation. The PsyD degree may be based on practical work and examinations rather than a dissertation. In clinical, counseling, and school psychology, the requirements for the doctoral degree include an internship of at least one year.

A specialist degree or its equivalent is required in most states for an individual to work as a school psychologist, although a few states still credential school psychologists with master's degrees. A specialist (EdS) degree in school psychology requires a minimum of two years of full-time graduate study (at least 60 graduate semester hours) and a one-year full-time internship during the third year. In professional practice, school psychologists address both the educational and the mental health components of students' development; as a consequence, their training includes coursework in both education and psychology.

People with a master's degree in psychology may work as industrial-organizational psychologists. They also may work as psychological assistants under the supervision of doctoral-level psychologists and may conduct research or psychological evaluations. A master's degree in psychology requires at least two years of full-time graduate study. Degree requirements usually include practical experience in an applied setting and a master's thesis based on an original research project.

Competition for admission to graduate psychology programs is keen. Some universities require applicants to have an undergraduate major in psychology. Others prefer only coursework in basic psychology with additional courses in statistics, mathematics, and the biological, physical, and social sciences.

A bachelor's degree in psychology qualifies a person to assist psychologists and other professionals in community mental health centers, vocational rehabilitation offices, and correctional programs. Bachelor's degree holders may also work as research or administrative assistants for psychologists. Some work as technicians in related fields, such as marketing research. Many find employment in other areas, such as sales, service, or business management.

In the federal government, candidates having at least 24 semester hours in psychology and one course in statistics qualify for entry-level positions. However, competition for these jobs is keen because this is one of the few ways in which one can work as a psychologist without an advanced degree.

The American Psychological Association (APA) presently accredits doctoral training programs in clinical, counseling, and school psychology as well as institutions that provide internships for doctoral students in school, clinical, and counseling psychology.[1] The National Association of School Psychologists, with the assistance of the National Council for Accreditation of Teacher Education, helps approve advanced degree programs in school psychology.[2]

Licensure

Psychologists in independent practice or those who offer any type of patient care—including clinical, counseling, and school psychologists—must meet certification or licensing requirements in all states and the District of Columbia. Licensing laws vary by state and by type of position but require licensed or certified psychologists to limit their practice to areas in which they have developed professional competence through training and experience. Clinical and counseling psychologists usually need a doctorate in psychology, an approved internship, and one to two years of professional experience. In addition, all states require that applicants pass an examination. Most state licensing boards administer a standardized test, and many supplement that with additional oral or essay questions. Some states require continuing education for renewal of the license. The Association of State and Provincial Psychology Boards provides specific licensing information by jurisdiction.[3]

The National Association of School Psychologists (NASP) awards the Nationally Certified School Psychologist (NCSP) designation, which recognizes professional competency in school psychology at a national level. Currently, 33 states recognize the NCSP and allow those with the certification to transfer credentials from one state to another without taking a new certification exam. In states that recognize the NCSP, the requirements for certification or licensure and those for the NCSP often are the same or similar. Requirements for the NCSP include the completion of 60 graduate semester hours in school psychology; a 1,200-hour internship, 600 hours of which must be completed in a school setting; and a passing score on the National School Psychology Examination.[4]

Other Qualifications

Aspiring psychologists who are interested in direct patient care must be emotionally stable, mature, and able to deal effectively with people. Sensitivity, compassion, good communication skills, and the ability to lead and inspire others are particularly important qualities for people wishing to do clinical work and counseling. Research psychologists should be able to do detailed work both independently and as part of a team. Patience and perseverance are vital qualities because achieving results in the psychological treatment of patients or in research may take a long time.

Certification and Advancement

The American Board of Professional Psychology (ABPP) recognizes professional achievement by awarding specialty certification in 15 different areas, such as psychoanalysis, rehabilitation, forensic, group, school, clinical health, and couple and family.[5] Candidates for ABPP certification must meet general criteria that consist of a doctorate in psychology as well as state licensure. Each candidate must then meet additional criteria of the specialty field, which is usually a combination of postdoctoral training in their specialty, several years of experience, and professional endorsements, as determined by the ABPP. Applicants are then required to pass the specialty board examination. The American Board of Clinical Neuropsychology provides a certificate in neuropsychology.[6] Psychologists can improve their advancement opportunities by earning an advanced degree and by participation in continuing education. Many psychologists opt to start their own practice after gaining experience working in the field.

Employment Trends

As-fast-as-average employment growth is expected for psychologists, including industrial-organizational psychologists, whose employment numbers are expected to rise by 3% through 2029. Job prospects should be best for people who have a doctoral degree from a leading university in an applied specialty, such as counseling or health, and people with a specialist or doctoral degree in school psychology. Master's degree holders in fields other than industrial-organizational psychology will face keen competition. Opportunities will be limited for bachelor's degree holders.

Employment Change

Employment of psychologists is expected to grow 3% from 2019 to 2029, about as fast as the average for all occupations. Employment will grow because of increased demand for psychological services in schools, hospitals, social service agencies, mental health centers, substance abuse treatment clinics, consulting firms, and private companies.

Employment growth will vary by specialty. Growing awareness of how students' mental health and behavioral problems, such as bullying, affect learning will increase demand for school psychologists to offer student counseling and mental health services.

The rise in healthcare costs associated with unhealthy lifestyles, such as smoking, alcoholism, and obesity, has made prevention and treatment more critical. An increase in the number of **employee assistance programs (EAPs)**, which help workers deal with personal problems, also should lead to employment growth for clinical and counseling specialties. Clinical and counseling psychologists also will be needed to help people deal with depression and other mental disorders, marriage and family problems, job stress, and addiction. The growing number of elderly will increase the demand for psychologists trained in geropsychology to help people deal with the mental and physical changes that occur as individuals grow older. There also will be an increased need for psychologists to work with military veterans returning from armed conflicts and for those who have survived other trauma.

Industrial-organizational psychologists also will be in demand to help to boost worker productivity and retention rates in a wide range of businesses. Industrial-organizational psychologists will help companies deal with issues such as workplace diversity and antidiscrimination policies. Companies also will use psychologists' expertise in survey design, analysis, and research to develop tools for marketing evaluation and statistical analysis.

Job Prospects

Job prospects should be the best for people who have a doctoral degree from a leading university in an applied specialty, such as counseling or health, and people with a specialty or doctoral degree in school psychology. Psychologists with extensive training in quantitative research methods and computer science may have a competitive edge over applicants without such a background.

Master's degree holders in fields other than industrial-organizational psychology will face keen competition for jobs because of the limited number of positions that require only a master's degree. Master's degree holders may find jobs as psychological assistants or counselors, providing mental health services under the direct supervision of a licensed psychologist. Still others may find jobs involving research and data collection and analysis in universities, government, or private companies.

Opportunities directly related to psychology will be limited for bachelor's degree holders. Some may find jobs as assistants in rehabilitation centers or other jobs involving data collection and analysis. Those who meet state certification requirements may become high school psychology teachers. **TABLE 21.1** shows some projection data provided by the U.S. Department of Labor.

Earnings

The median annual salary for psychologists as of May 2020 was $82,180. The lowest 10% of the occupation earned less than $46,270, while the top 10% earned more than $137,590. The Occupational Outlook Handbook separates psychologists into three categories. **TABLE 21.2** lists the median annual wage for each category as May 2020.

Related Occupations

Psychologists work with people, developing relationships and comforting them. Other occupations with similar duties include counselors, social workers, clergy, sociologists, special education teachers, funeral directors, market and survey researchers, recreation workers, and managers and specialists in human resources, training, and labor relations. Psychologists also sometimes diagnose and treat problems and assist patients in recovery. These duties are similar to those for physicians and surgeons, radiation therapists, audiologists, dentists, optometrists, and speech-language pathologists.

TABLE 21.1 Projections Data for Psychologists, 2019–2029

Occupational Title	Employment, 2019	Projected Employment, 2029	Change, 2019–2029	
			Number	Percentage
Psychologists	192,300	198,100	5,700	3%
Clinical, counseling, and school psychologists	171,500	176,700	5,300	3%
Industrial-organizational psychologists	1,100	1,100	0	3%
Psychologists, all other	19,800	20,200	400	2%

Data from Bureau of Labor Statistics. Occupational Outlook Handbook. U.S. Department of Labor; 2020. https://www.bls.gov/ooh/life-physical-and-social-science/psychologists.htm#tab-6

TABLE 21.2 Median Annual Earnings in the Industries Employing the Largest Number of Psychologists, May 2020

Industrial-organizational psychologists	$96,270
Clinical, counseling, and school psychologists	$79,820
All other psychologists	$105,780

Data from Bureau of Labor Statistics. Occupational Outlook Handbook. U.S. Department of Labor; 2020. https://www.bls.gov/ooh/life-physical-and-social-science/psychologists.htm#tab-5

Additional Information

For information on careers, educational requirements, financial assistance, and licensing in all fields of psychology, contact:

- American Psychological Association, Center for Psychology Workforce Analysis and Research and Education Directorate, 750 1st St. NE, Washington, DC 20002. https://www.apa.org/students

For information on careers, educational requirements, certification, and licensing of school psychologists, contact:

- National Association of School Psychologists, 4340 East West Hwy., Suite 402, Bethesda, MD 20814. https://www.nasponline.org

Information about state licensing requirements is available from:

- Association of State and Provincial Psychology Boards, P.O. Box 849, Tyrone, GA 30290. https://www.asppb.net

Information about psychology specialty certifications is available from:

- American Board of Professional Psychology, 600 Market St., Suite G3, Chapel Hill, NC 27516. https://www.abpp.org
- American Board of Clinical Psychology, 600 Market St., Suite G3, Chapel Hill, NC 27516. https://www.abpp.org

SUBSTANCE ABUSE, BEHAVIORAL DISORDER, AND MENTAL HEALTH COUNSELORS
Significant Points

- Most substance abuse, behavioral disorder, and mental health counselors work in outpatient mental health and substance abuse centers.
- Job prospects are expected to be favorable, particularly for those with specialized training or education.
- Educational requirements range from a high school diploma to a master's degree, depending on a variety of factors.

Work Description

Mental health refers to an individual's psychological and emotional well-being and the individual's ability to function in ordinary life. Two disciplines within the mental health field that deal with improving an individual's psychological and emotional well-being are substance abuse counselors, behavioral disorder counselors, and mental health counselors.

Substance abuse counselors, also called addiction counselors, advise individuals dealing with alcoholism, illegal drug addiction, and other addictions, such as those involving tobacco, gambling, and painkillers. They provide treatment and support to assist the individual's recovery by evaluating their client's mental and physical health, addictive behaviors, and openness to treatment. With the client's input, the counselor develops a treatment and recovery plan and assists the client with identifying and dealing with behaviors that interfere with both processes. The counselor also assists the client's family with developing strategies to deal with the client's addiction problems.

Behavioral disorder counselors advise individuals how to modify their behavior to deal with specific aspects of their life, often those associated with eating. Well-known eating disorders include **anorexia nervosa**, which is characterized

Professional Profiles

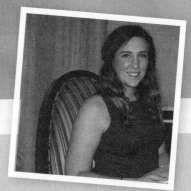

Name: Katie, BS, MEd, PLPC
Job Title: Clinical Mental Health Counselor
Education: BS Psychology; minor, Criminology, MEd, Clinical Mental Health Counseling

Q: Tell us about your job and the type of organization you work in.

A: I work for an outpatient behavioral health unit with clients who suffer from severe mental illness and who are typically in a lower socioeconomic status. My work is community-based, meaning I meet with clients in their homes or at public places like the library. Within my company, different locations are broken up into territories. My territory makeup is a suburban area ranging from low income to middle class.

Q: Why did you choose this profession?

A: I chose this profession due to always wanting to help people. I also chose this field due to knowing people who struggled with addiction and seeing how it took over them. Seeing someone struggle with addiction made me realize I wanted to be a counselor to help people who need someone to believe in them.

Q: What do you like most about this profession?

A: The aspect of being able to see the smile on a client's face when they recover their mental health or overcome their addiction. I have found that many clients lose their happiness and sense of their self due to a mental health diagnosis or an addiction, so seeing them get on the path to finding themselves again is rewarding.

Q: What challenges you most about this profession?

A: Seeing people struggle with suicidal thoughts. I have had many clients who feel their life is not worth living anymore, and I have to be there to support them and help them realize it is worth living. As a counselor, you are mandated to admit someone to the hospital to keep them safe if they have stated they have a suicidal plan or cannot keep themselves safe. It can be hard to feel like you are forcing someone to go somewhere they don't want to and also to make the judgment call of if they need to go, but it's worth a client's safety.

Q: Is there room for advancement in this field?

A: I think there is a huge chance for advancement in the field due to there being so many different aspects of counseling such as private practice, teaching, working for an agency, and doing research. Recently there has also been advancement in government focus on mental illness, so the field is expected to grow.

Q: Name and explain what part of your academic training most prepared you for this profession.

A: My academics prepared me for the hardships that come with the field. Dealing with clients who struggle with addiction or severe mental illness, it can be hard to understand their struggles. In my training I learned the biology behind an addiction and how mental illness affects the body. By knowing this information, I can educate my clients. My graduate program emphasized multicultural issues. This has helped me to be a better clinician and better able to understand members of different cultures.

Q: What advice would you give someone who is considering this career?

A: Find a way to shadow someone who works in the field or talk to a professional to see what they do every day. Look for seminars and speakers at your university who are talking about mental health topics.

Q: What personality characteristics are needed for this line of work?

A: Someone who is able to listen to people talk about the smallest or the biggest problems in their life and not judge them. Counseling also requires someone to remain calm in all situations, even under high stress. A counselor needs to be open-minded and not try to make a client fit into their picture of what should happen. It is the client's choice how to live their life, and a counselor should help them along the way.

as a refusal to eat; **bulimia nervosa**, which is characterized as involving cyclical binging and purging episodes; and **binge-eating disorder**, which involves periods of binge eating that are not followed by compensatory behaviors, such as purging, excessive exercise, or fasting. Binge-eating disorder often leads to **obesity**, a weight that is higher than what is considered a healthy weight for a given height. Behavioral disorder counselors provide treatment and support by evaluating the patient's mental and physical health to develop a treatment and recovery plan and assist the client with identifying and dealing with behaviors that interfere with the plans. Typical goals identified by behavioral disorder counselors include restoring adequate nutrition, bringing weight to a healthy level, reducing excessive exercise, and stopping binging and purging behaviors. Behavioral disorder counselors frequently assist the client's family with developing strategies to cope with the client's behavioral problems.

Both types of counselors work with clients individually and in group settings to teach patients how to cope with stress and life's problems in ways that will help them recover. Some counselors work with specific populations, such as teenagers, veterans, people with disabilities, or individuals who have been ordered by a judge to receive addiction treatment, They help their patients improve their professional relationships, reestablish their career, and/or improve their personal relationships and reconnect with family and friends.

Mental health counselors advise individuals, families, couples, and groups how to handle a variety of conditions. Those conditions may include anxiety, depression, grief, low self-esteem, stress, and suicidal impulses. They may assist with mental health issues and relationship problems. Some mental health counselors specialize by working with specific populations, such as the elderly, college students, or children.

Work Environment

Substance abuse behavioral disorder, and mental health counselors work in multiple settings. Some work in mental health or residential treatment facilities where clients live for a fixed period of time. With other health professionals, such as psychiatrists, social workers, physicians, and registered nurses, they develop treatment plans and coordinate care for patients. Other counselors work in private practice, either alone or with a group of other counselors or other professionals. Because they manage their private practices as a business, they engage in typical business activities such as recruiting new patients and billing insurance companies to receive payment for their services.

Some counselors work in nontraditional settings, including those involving persons who have violated the law in some way. These settings include prisons, halfway houses, juvenile detention facilities, and probation or parole agencies. Other counselors work in EAPs. These programs are provided by employers to help employees deal with personal problems.

Counselors who work with patients with addictive or behavioral disorders experience stressful situations. They may need to intervene in crisis situations or work with agitated clients, thereby increasing tension and stress. Their workloads are large, and they often do not have sufficient resources to meet the demand for their services. An example of the cravings of addiction is shown in **FIGURE 21.1**.

Employment Opportunities

Substance abuse, behavioral disorder, and mental health counselors held 319,400 jobs in 2019. About 29% of these counselors work in one of two settings: (1) outpatient mental health and substance abuse centers or (2) nursing and residential care facilities. The remaining work in hospitals, state and local government, and individual and family services settings.

Most substance abuse, behavioral disorder, and mental health counselors work full time. Because of the needs of an employment setting, these counselors may need to work evenings, nights, and weekends.

Education and Legal Requirements

Education requirements vary from the level of a high school diploma to the level of a master's degree.

Education and Training

The wide span of educational requirements is dependent upon the employment setting in which the counselor works, the range of responsibilities involved, the type of work, and state regulations. Those holding a high school diploma typically go through a period of on-the-job training. Such training addresses how to respond to crisis situations and deal with persons who

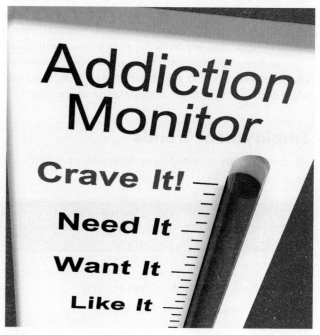

FIGURE 21.1 Addiction monitor showing cravings.
© Stuart Miles/Shutterstock.

suffer from addiction. Those with more education, such as those holding a master's degree, are able to provide more services to patients, including private one-on-one counseling sessions. Because of their higher level of education, they require less supervision than those possessing a high school diploma.

Licensure and Certification

Any substance abuse, behavioral disorder, or mental health counselor who wishes to work in a private practice setting must be licensed. All states require a license for this setting and also require the counselor to possess a master's degree and have engaged in 2,000 to 4,000 hours of supervised clinical experience. Additionally, counselors must pass a state-recognized exam and engage in continuing education on an annual basis. The National Board for Certified Counselors (NBCC) maintains information about each state's regulating board. The NBCC requires a master's degree or higher from an accredited program to become a certified counselor.[7] For those substance abuse, behavioral disorder, and mental health counselors who do not work in private practice, licensure and certification requirements vary by state. Some states specify the level of education required, while others require applicants to pass an exam. Additional information about licensing requirements for those not working in private practice can be found through the Addiction Transfer Technology Center.

Other Qualifications

Counselors should be sensitive and compassionate to patients' needs in light of difficult and stressful situations the patients undergo. Interpersonal skills are important because most of a counselor's time is spent working directly with a variety of clients or other professionals. Counselors need good listening skills so that they can understand their patient's concerns, problems, and values. Because of the need to deal with patients effectively, counselors need strong speaking skills. This will assist the patient in understanding ideas and concepts expressed by the counselor. Counselors also need patience and the ability to stay calm, especially when dealing with difficult, disgruntled, or angry patients.

Employment Trends

Job prospects are expected to be favorable, particularly for those with specialized training or education.

Employment Change

Employment of substance abuse, behavioral disorder, and mental health counselors is expected to grow by 25% from 2019 to 2029, much faster than average for all occupations. The increasing demand will result from more patients receiving coverage under existing health insurance plans and the increase in numbers of patients who possess health insurance as a result of the federal legislative mandate that individuals receive health insurance coverage.

Some states may see a need for more substance abuse, behavioral disorder, and mental health counselors as they move from a model of jail time for drug offenders to treatment and counseling services. States have dealt with budget issues and overcrowded prisons by changing who should go to prison and who should receive treatment instead, finding these choices to be cost-effective. States have also found that those addicted to drugs and other substances are less likely to participate in criminal activity if they receive treatment for their addiction.

Job Prospects

Job opportunities are expected to be good, especially for those with specialized education and training. Some counselors are forced to leave the occupation early because of the stress involved in their jobs, providing openings for new counselors. Some employers experience difficulty recruiting workers with the proper educational requirements and experience in working with addiction. These two points will result in favorable job prospects for those entering the field. TABLE 21.3 shows some projection data from the U.S. Department of Labor.

Earnings

The median annual salary for substance abuse, behavioral disorder, and mental health counselors as of May 2020 was $47,660. The middle 50% earned between $31,400 and $50,010. The lowest 10% of the occupation earned less than $30,590, while the top 10% earned more than $78,710. TABLE 21.4 shows the median annual earnings of industries employing the largest number of substance abuse, behavioral disorder, and mental health counselors.

Related Occupations

Other occupations with job duties similar to those of substance abuse, behavioral disorder, and mental health

TABLE 21.3 Projections Data for Substance Abuse, Behavioral Disorder, and Mental Health Counselors, 2019–2029

Occupational Title	Employment, 2019	Projected Employment, 2029	Change, 2019–2029 Number	Percentage
Substance abuse and behavioral disorder counselors	319,400	398,400	79,000	25%

Data from Bureau of Labor Statistics. Occupational Outlook Handbook. U.S. Department of Labor; 2020. https://www.bls.gov/ooh/community-and-social-service/substance-abuse-behavioral-disorder-and-mental-health-counselors.htm#tab-6

TABLE 21.4 Median Annual Earnings in the Industries Employing the Largest Number of Substance Abuse, Behavioral Disorder, and Mental Health Counselors, May 2020

Government	$54,070
Hospitals: state, local, and private	$50,460
Individual and family services	$47,580
Outpatient mental health and substance abuse centers	$45,960
Residential mental health and substance abuse centers	$40,560

Data from Bureau of Labor Statistics. Occupational Outlook Handbook. U.S. Department of Labor; 2020. https://www.bls.gov/ooh/community-and-social-service/substance-abuse-behavioral-disorder-and-mental-health-counselors.htm?utm_source=bisk.com&utm_medium=pdf&utm_campaign=ft_bisk_micropgae_corporate&campaignid=701610000008c18AAA#tab-5

counselors include marriage and family therapists; registered nurses, rehabilitation counselors; social workers; social and community service workers; and social and human service assistants. Because they diagnose and treat problems and assist patients in recovery, their duties are similar to those for physicians, surgeons, and psychologists.

Additional Information

For information on careers, educational requirements, licensing, and credentialing in the field of addiction counseling, contact:

- Addiction Technology Transfer Center Network, Network Coordinating Office, UMKC School of Nursing & Health Studies, 2464 Charlotte, HSB, Kansas City, MO 64108 https://attcnetwork.org/
- National Association for Addiction Professionals, 44 Canal Center Plaza, Suite 301, Alexandria, VA 22314. https://www.naadac.org

For more information about counseling and counseling specialties, visit:

- American Counseling Association, 6101 Stevenson Ave., Suite 600, Alexandria, VA 22304. https://www.counseling.org

For information on state regulating boards, contact:

- National Board for Certified Counselors, 3 Terrace Way, Greensboro, NC 27403. https://www.nbcc.org

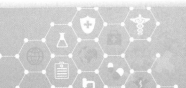

LEARNING PORTFOLIO

Issues for Discussion

1. The discipline of psychology is complex with multiple specialty areas. Review the specialty areas listed in this chapter and chose the specialty area in which you have the most interest or that you would recommend to a friend or acquaintance. Explain why you find the specialty area interesting and why you chose this specialty over other specialties.

2. In your opinion, what is the most important responsibility of a psychologist? Explain why you feel this is most important.

3. In your opinion, what is the most important personal attribute a substance abuse or behavioral disorder counselor must have? Explain why you feel this is most important.

Enrichment Activities

1. Use the internet to research the requirements of your state and two neighboring states to become licensed or certified as a psychologist. List the requirements that you find. Compare and contrast these licensing, certification, and/or registration requirements for this career with any other career you have already examined in this course.

2. Interest in psychology has spanned many centuries. Create a timeline (either as a narrative piece, a poster, or an infographic) tracing the progression of psychology as a science and include the names of key theorists and movements in the field.

3. Watch the career video titled "Imagine Who You Could Save" from the Addiction Technology Transfer Center Network (https://www.youtube.com /watch?v=Ny5tahISA5I). Discuss the role of an addiction counselor with your instructor and classmates.

4. Create a table comparing the duties, work environment, licensing requirements, and salary of psychologists and substance abuse/behavioral disorder counselors.

CASE STUDY: MENTAL HEALTH AWARENESS

Olivia is a senior in high school. She has always had a keen interest in the human brain and how it works. She is interested in the field of mental health and wants to learn more about it. Olivia is trying to decide which direction to take as she prepares for a career.

The following questions relate to mental health professionals. Please help Olivia answer them based on what you have learned in this chapter.

1. Which of the following best describes the difference between psychology and psychiatry?
   A. Psychology is a branch of medicine, and psychiatry is a nonmedical science.
   B. Psychology and psychiatry are basically the same with minor differences.
   C. Psychiatry is a branch of medicine, and psychology is a nonmedical science.
   D. Psychologists can perform surgery, and psychiatrists are not trained to do so.

2. Which of the following psychologists would most likely be involved in directly measuring human behavior through the use of tests, statistical data, and mathematics?
   A. Rehabilitation psychologists
   B. Psychometric psychologists
   C. Social psychologists
   D. Clinical psychologists

3. Olivia would like to be able to open a private practice in the future if she pursues her interest in psychology. What would the most likely educational requirement be for her to do this?
   A. A master's degree
   B. A bachelor's degree
   C. A doctorate degree
   D. A certificate or diploma from an accredited school

LEARNING PORTFOLIO

References

1. American Psychological Association. Office of Program Consultation and Accreditation. https://www.accreditation.apa.org/ Accessed August 8, 2021.

2. National Association of School Psychologists. Graduate Program Approval. https://www.nasponline.org/standards-and-certification/graduate-program-approval-and-accreditation Accessed August 8, 2021.

3. Association of State and Provincial Licensing Boards. https://www.asppb.net/ Accessed August 8, 2021.

4. National Association of School Psychologists. NCSP Eligibility. https://www.nasponline.org/standards-and-certification/national-certification Accessed August 8, 2021.

5. American Board of Professional Psychology. Specialty Boards. https://www.abpp.org/Applicant-Information/Specialty-Boards.aspx Accessed August 8, 2021.

6. American Board of Clinical Neuropsychology. Specialty Boards. https://www.abpp.org/Applicant-Information/Specialty-Boards.aspx Accessed August 8, 2021.

7. National Board for Certified Counselors. National Certified Counselor. https://nbcc.org/certification/ncc Accessed August 8, 2021.

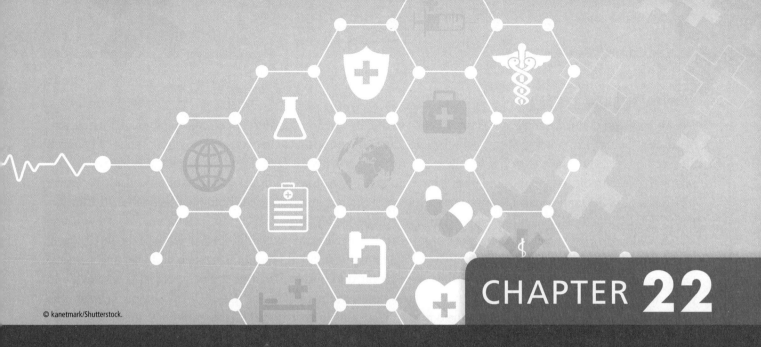
© kanetmark/Shutterstock.

CHAPTER 22

Social Workers*

KEY TERMS

American Board of Clinical
   Social Work (ABCSW)
Association of Social Work
   Boards (ASWB)
Board Certified Diplomate in
   Clinical Social Work (BCD)
Bachelor's Degree in Social
   Work (BSW)
Certified Community Behavioral
   Health Clinics (CCBHC)
Child and family social worker
Child or adult protective
   services social worker
Child welfare social worker
Clinical social worker (CSW)
Conflict resolution
Council on Social Work Education

Council for Standards in
   Human Services Education
   (CSHSE)
Doctorate in Clinical Social Work
   (DSW)
Emotional stress
Employee assistance programs
   (EAPs)
Environmental factors
Family services social worker
Geriatric social worker
Healthcare social worker
Hospice and palliative care
   social worker
Human Service Board-Certified
   Practitioner (HS-BCP)
Human service worker

Licensed Clinical Social Worker
   (LCSW)
Master's Degree in Social Work
   (MSW)
Meals on Wheels
Medical social worker
Mental health and substance
   abuse social worker
Psychological treatment
School social worker
Social and human service assistant
Social work administrator
Social work planners and
   policy makers
Social work researchers
Veterans
Vulnerable populations

* All information in this chapter, unless otherwise indicated, was obtained from Bureau of Labor Statistics. *Occupational Outlook Handbook 2020–2021 Edition*. Washington, DC: U.S. Department of Labor; 2021.

Introduction

Health has been defined not merely as the absence of disease but as a condition of complete physical, mental, and social well-being. The effect of social, economic, and **environmental factors** on an individual's state of health is an accepted fact, and studies reveal a definite relationship between these factors and occurrences of disease. Recognizing this, health officials are placing increasing emphasis on the **psychological treatment** as well as the clinical treatment of patients in health facilities. Very often a patient's restoration to and maintenance of health is influenced by many factors that can be dealt with by other professionals, including competently trained social workers.

Social work in the health field involves programs and services that meet the special needs of the ill, disabled, elderly, or otherwise handicapped. Social workers deal with the total emotional, social, cultural, and physical needs of patients in whom the effects of illness go far beyond bodily discomfort. Such problems usually lie in three areas—problems within the patient, problems between the patient and family, or problems between the patient and the patient's environment. Illness invariably results in **emotional stress** and often causes significant changes in the lives of patients and their families. Medical care alone, even if it is of the highest quality, is often not sufficient. Social workers help patients and members of the health team deal with these problems by providing a skilled appraisal of the source and significance of social, emotional, environmental, and economic factors affecting health. Their efforts with individual patients or groups of patients help bring about constructive and meaningful changes in terms of total health. Advocacy is an important aspect of social work. Social workers advocate or raise awareness on behalf of their clients and the social work profession on local, state, and national levels.

SOCIAL WORKERS
Significant Points

- Although a bachelor's degree is necessary for entry-level positions, a master's degree in social work is required for some positions.
- About one-half of social workers worked in child and family services or in schools and one-fourth worked in health care in 2019.
- Job prospects are expected to be favorable, particularly for social workers who specialize in the aging population or work in rural areas.

Work Description

Social work is a profession for those with a strong desire to help improve people's lives. Social workers assist people by helping them cope with and solve issues in their everyday lives, such as family and personal problems and dealing with relationships. Some social workers help clients who face a disability, life-threatening disease, or social problem, such as inadequate housing, unemployment, or substance abuse. Social workers also assist families that have serious domestic conflicts, sometimes involving child or spousal abuse.

Settings for social workers include schools, colleges and universities, military bases and hospitals, state and local governments, child welfare agencies, nursing and assisted-living facilities, correctional facilities, community mental health clinics, hospitals, and primary care centers, including clinics for veterans. Additionally, they may conduct research, advocate for improved services, or become involved in planning or policy development. Many social workers specialize in serving a particular population or working in a specific setting.

Child and family social workers provide social services and assistance to improve the social and psychological functioning of children and their families. Workers in this field assess their clients' needs and offer assistance to improve their situation. This often includes coordinating available services to assist a child or family. They may assist single parents in finding day care, arrange adoptions, or help find foster homes for neglected, abandoned, or abused children. These workers may specialize in working with a particular problem, population, or setting, such as child protective services, adoption, homelessness, domestic violence, or foster care. Clinical social workers provide mental health care to help children and families cope with changes in their lives, such as divorce or other family problems (**FIGURE 22.1**).

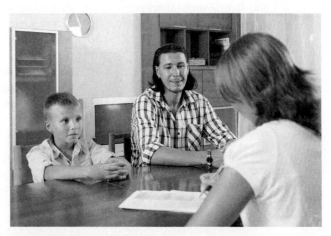

FIGURE 22.1 Child, family, and school social workers represent about half of all social workers.
© Iakov Filimonov/Shutterstock.

School social workers often serve as the link between students' families and the school, working with parents, guardians, teachers, and other school officials to ensure that students reach their academic and personal potential. They also assist students in dealing with stress or emotional problems. Many school social workers work directly with children with disabilities and their families. In addition, students and their families are often referred to social workers to deal with problems such as aggressive behavior, bullying, or frequent absences from school. School social workers may teach workshops to entire classes on topics like **conflict resolution**.

Child, family, and school social workers may be known as **child welfare social workers**, **family services social workers**, or **child or adult protective services social workers**. These workers often work for individual and family services agencies, schools, or state or local governments.

Healthcare social workers provide psychosocial support to individuals, families, or **vulnerable populations** so they can cope with chronic, acute, or terminal illnesses, such as Alzheimer's disease, cancer, or HIV/AIDS. They also advise family caregivers, counsel patients, and help plan for patients' needs after discharge from hospitals. They may arrange for at-home services, such as **Meals on Wheels** or home care. Some work on interdisciplinary teams that evaluate certain kinds of patients, such as geriatric, kidney dialysis, or organ-transplant patients. In addition, they may provide information on services, such as home health care or support groups, to help patients manage their illness or disease. Social workers help doctors and other healthcare professionals understand the effects that diseases and illnesses have on patients' mental and emotional health.

Some healthcare social workers specialize in geriatric social work, hospice and palliative care, or medical social work. **Geriatric social workers** help the elderly and their families find services for older adults such as Meals on Wheels or personal assistance in the home. In some cases, they provide information about other care options such as assisted-living or nursing care facilities or work with older adults in those settings. They help clients and their families make plans for possible health complications or where clients will live if they can no longer care for themselves (**FIGURE 22.2**).

Hospice and palliative care social workers help patients adjust to serious, chronic, or terminal illnesses. Palliative care focuses on relieving or preventing pain and other symptoms associated with serious illness. Hospice is a type of palliative care for people who are dying. Social workers in this setting provide and find services such as support groups or grief counselors to help patients and their families cope with the illness or disease.

Medical social workers in hospitals help patients and their families by linking patients with resources in the hospital and in their own community. They may work with medical staff to create discharge plans, make referrals to community agencies, facilitate support groups, or a conduct follow-up visits with patients once they have been discharged.

Clinical Social Workers (CSW)—also called **Licensed Clinical Social Workers (LCSWs)**—diagnose and treat mental, behavioral, and emotional disorders, including anxiety and depression. They provide individual, group, family, and couples therapy; they work with clients to develop strategies to change behavior or cope with difficult situations; and they refer clients to other resources or services, such as support groups or other mental health professionals. Clinical social workers can develop treatment plans with the client, doctors, and other healthcare professionals and may adjust the treatment plan if necessary based on their client's progress. Many clinical social workers also work with those with substance abuse.

Mental health and substance abuse social workers help clients with mental illnesses or addictions. They provide information on services, such as support groups or 12-step programs, to help clients cope with their illness (**FIGURE 22.3**). Some mental health/substance abuse social workers may

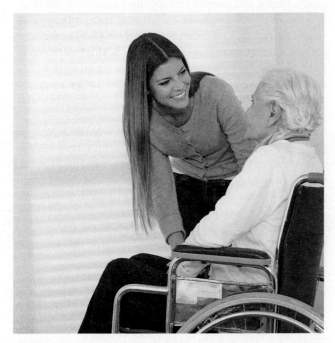

FIGURE 22.2 Healthcare social workers often specialize in geriatrics.
© Robert Kneschke/Shutterstock.

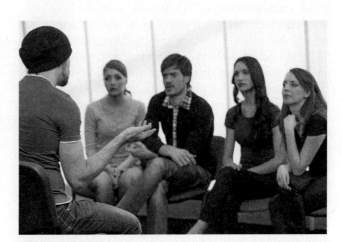

FIGURE 22.3 Some social workers specialize in mental health and substance abuse and do individual group therapy.
© BlueSkyImage/Shutterstock.

work in employee assistance programs (EAPs). In this setting, they may help people cope with job-related pressures or with personal problems that affect the quality of their work.

Many clinical social workers work in private practice. In these settings, clinical social workers have administrative and recordkeeping tasks such as working with insurance companies to receive payment for their services. Some work in a group practice with other social workers or mental health professionals. Other social workers are employed as **social work administrators**, **social work researchers**, and **social work planners and policy makers**. In these roles, the social worker develops and implements programs to address issues such as child abuse, homelessness, substance abuse, poverty, and violence. This may require research and analysis of policies, programs, and regulations; grant writing; and writing legislation to change policies. Some social workers become legislators at the state and federal level to influence policies not only for the profession of social work but also related to services for those with mental illness or substance abuse disorders.

Work Environment

Social workers usually spend most of their time in an office or residential facility, but they also may travel locally to visit clients, meet with service providers, or attend meetings. Some may meet with clients in one of several offices within a local area. Social work, although satisfying, can be challenging. Understaffing and large caseloads add to the pressure in some agencies. Full-time social workers usually work a standard 40-hour week, but some occasionally work evenings and weekends to meet with clients, attend community meetings, and handle emergencies. Some work part time, particularly in voluntary nonprofit agencies. Many clinical social workers work in private practice. In these settings, clinical social workers have administrative and recordkeeping tasks such as working with insurance companies to receive payment for their services.

Employment Opportunities

Social workers held about 713,200 jobs, in 2019. About one-half were child, family, and school social workers; one-fourth were healthcare social workers; and one-fifth worked in mental health and substance abuse. Although most social workers are employed in cities or suburbs, some work in rural areas. Employment for healthcare social workers and mental health and substance abuse social workers in 2019 is summarized in **TABLE 22.1**.

Educational and Legal Requirements

Although most social workers need a bachelor's degree in social work, clinical social workers must have a master's degree and two years of post-master's experience in a supervised clinical setting. Clinical social workers must also be licensed in the state in which they practice.

TABLE 22.1 Industries Employing the Largest Numbers of Social Workers, 2019

Industry	Percent
Individual and family services	18%
Local government, excluding education and hospitals	14%
State government, excluding education and hospitals	14%
Ambulatory healthcare services	13%

Data from Bureau of Labor Statistics. Occupational Outlook Handbook. U.S. Department of Labor; 2020. https://www.bls.gov/ooh/community-and-social-service/social-workers.htm#tab-3

Education and Training

A **Bachelor's Degree in Social Work (BSW)** is the most common minimum requirement to qualify for a job as a social worker; however, those who major in psychology, sociology, and related fields may qualify for some entry-level jobs, especially in small community agencies. These programs teach students about diverse populations, human behavior, social welfare policy, and ethics in social work. All programs require students to complete supervised fieldwork or an internship.

Although a bachelor's degree is sufficient for entry into the field, a Master of Social Work (MSW) is required for some positions. Social workers who are licensed to diagnose and treat mental, behavioral, and emotional disorders are called CSW . The majority of states require CSW to complete a **Master's Degree in Social Work (MSW)**—also described as Master of Social Work-- to be eligible for licensure. CSW who are licensed use the title LCSW. They provide individual, group, family, and couples therapy; they work with clients to develop strategies to change behavior or cope with difficult situations; and they refer clients to other resources or services, such as support groups or other mental health professionals. CSW can develop treatment plans with the client, doctors, and other healthcare professionals and may adjust the treatment plan if necessary based on their client's progress. They may work in a variety of specialties. CSW who have not completed two years of supervised practice use the title MSW. A MSW is typically required for positions in health and school settings and is required for clinical work as well. Some jobs in public and private agencies may require an advanced degree, such as an MSW with a concentration in social services policy or administration. Supervisory, administrative, and staff training positions usually require an advanced degree. College and university teaching positions and most research appointments normally require a doctorate in social work.

In 2020, the **Council on Social Work Education**, which accredits educational programs, listed 552 baccalaureate and 311 master's social work programs.[1] In 2016, the Group for the Advancement of Doctoral Education listed 82 doctoral programs (PhD) in social work in the United States, nine in Canada, and one in Israel[2] and 17 programs that offered the **Doctorate in Clinical Social Work (DSW)**. The DSW prepares social workers to assume advanced professional roles as a practitioner, administrator, or educator and is comparable to professional doctorates in nursing and physical therapy.[3] The PhD is a doctor of philosophy or research degree for those seeking an academic position.

Bachelor's degree programs prepare graduates for direct service positions, such as caseworker, mental health assistant, group home worker, and residential counselor. These programs include courses in social work values and ethics, dealing with a culturally diverse clientele and at-risk populations, the promotion of social and economic justice, human behavior and the social environment, social welfare policy and services, social work practice, social research methods, and field education. Accredited programs require a minimum of 400 hours of supervised field experience.

Master's degree programs prepare graduates for work in their chosen field of concentration and continue to develop the skills required to perform clinical assessments, manage large caseloads, take on supervisory roles, and explore new ways of drawing upon social services to meet the needs of clients. Master's degree programs usually last two years and include a minimum of 900 hours of supervised field instruction or internship. A part-time program may take four years. Entry into a master's degree program does not require a bachelor's degree in social work, but courses in psychology, biology, sociology, economics, political science, and social work are recommended. In addition, a second language can be very helpful. Most master's degree programs offer advanced standing for those with a bachelor's degree from an accredited social work program. Mental health and behavioral health professionals are eligible for loan repayment programs through the National Health Services Corps.[4]

Licensure

All 50 states, the District of Columbia, the U.S. Virgin Islands, and all 10 Canadian provinces regulate the practice of social work and the use of professional titles. Most states require two years or 3,000 hours of supervised clinical experience for the licensure of clinical social workers. In addition to educational requirements, licensure requires successful completion of the licensing exam prepared by the **Association of Social Work Boards (ASWB)**. Examinations are available for associate's, bachelor's, master's, advanced generalist, and clinical social workers based on education and practice experience. Because licensing requirements vary by state, those interested should contact their state board. Most states also have licenses for nonclinical social workers. For more information about regulatory licensure board by state, contact the ASWB.[5]

Certification and Other Qualifications

The National Association of Social Workers (NASW) offers advanced practice specialty credentials to members of NASW based on their area of practice and experience. Some specialty areas are military, case management, clinical, gerontology, hospice and palliative care, addictions, school, and youth and family.[6] Those with advanced clinical practice can

qualify as a **Board Certified Diplomate in Clinical Social Work (BCD)** in one of four areas of practice--advanced clinical generalist, clinical supervisor, children/families practitioner, and psychoanalyst. Certifications are administered by the American Board of Clinical Social Work (ABCSW).[7]

Social workers should be emotionally mature, objective, and sensitive to people and their problems. They must be able to handle responsibility, work independently, and maintain good working relationships with clients and coworkers. Volunteer or paid jobs as a social work aide can help people test their interest in this field.

Advancement

Social workers certified in a specialty area are recognized as having achievements beyond the minimum requirements in knowledge and experience. Employers may use specialty certification to fill certain positions, and certified employees can expect higher salaries. Credentials are especially important for social workers in private practice as insurance companies often require the necessary credentials for reimbursement for services.

Advancement to supervisor, program manager, assistant director, or executive director of a social service agency or department usually requires an advanced degree and related work experience. Other career options for social workers include teaching, research, and consulting. Some of these workers help formulate government policies by analyzing and advocating policy positions in government agencies, in research institutions, and on legislators' staffs.

Some social workers go into private practice. Most private practitioners are clinical social workers who provide psychotherapy, usually paid for through health insurance or by the clients themselves. Private practitioners must have at least a master's degree and a period of supervised work experience. A network of contacts for referrals also is essential.

Employment Trends

Employment for social workers is expected to grow 13% from 2019 to 2029, much faster than average for all occupations. Employment growth will be driven by increased demand for health care and social services but will vary by specialty.

Employment Change

Employment of child, family, and school social workers is expected to grow by about 12%, about average for all occupations. Demand for child and family social workers should continue, as these workers are needed to investigate child abuse cases and place children in foster care and with adoptive families. However, growth for these workers may be hampered by the budget constraints of state and local governments, who are among the largest employers of these workers. Furthermore, demand for school social workers will continue and lead to more jobs as efforts are expanded to respond to rising student enrollments as well as the continued emphasis on integrating children with disabilities into

TABLE 22.2 Projection Data for Social Workers, 2019–2029

Occupational Title	Employment, 2019	Projected Employment, 2029	Change, 2019–2029	
			Number	Percentage
All social workers	713,200	803,800	90,700	13%
Child, family, and school social workers	342,500	382,600	40,100	12%
Healthcare social workers	185,000	211,700	26,700	14%
Mental health and substance abuse social workers	123,200	143,800	20,700	17%

Data from Bureau of Labor Statistics. Occupational Outlook Handbook. U.S. Department of Labor; 2020. https://www.bls.gov/ooh/community-and-social-service/social-workers.htm#tab-6

the general school population. There could be competition for school social work jobs in some areas because of the limited number of openings. The availability of federal, state, and local funding will be a major factor in determining the actual job growth in schools.

Employment of mental health and substance abuse social workers will grow by almost 17%, which is much faster than the average. In particular, social workers specializing in substance abuse will experience strong demand. Substance abusers are increasingly being placed into treatment programs instead of being sentenced to prison. Also, growing numbers of the substance abusers sentenced to prison or probation are being required by correctional systems to have substance abuse treatment added as a condition to their sentence or probation. As this trend grows, demand will strengthen for treatment programs and social workers to assist abusers on the road to recovery. Furthermore, the passage of legislation that requires insurance plans offered by employers to cover mental health treatment and substance abuse disorders in a manner that is equal to the treatment of physical health may increase the demand for mental health treatment. The opioid crisis in the United States and recent funding to establish comprehensive **Certified Community Behavioral Health Clinics** are expected to increase the demand for LCSW specializing in addiction counseling.[8]

Growth of employment of healthcare social workers is expected to be about 17%, which is much faster than the average for all occupations. Because social workers tend to change positions or leave the profession, jobs should be plentiful for entry-level positions.[9] One of the major contributing factors is the rise in the elderly population. These social workers will be needed to assist in finding the best care and assistance for the aging as well as to support their families. Employment opportunities for social workers with backgrounds in gerontology should be excellent, particularly in the growing numbers of assisted-living and senior living communities. The expanding senior population also will spur demand for social workers in nursing and assisted-living facilities, homecare agencies, and hospices.

TABLE 22.3 Median Annual Wages in the Industries Employing the Largest Numbers of Social Workers, May 2020

Industry	Salary
Local government	$57,660
Ambulatory healthcare services	$52,850
State government	$49,860
Individual and family services	$43,820

Data from Bureau of Labor Statistics. Occupational Outlook Handbook. U.S. Department of Labor; 2020. https://www.bls.gov/ooh/community-and-social-service/social-workers.htm#tab-5

Job Prospects

Overall, job prospects should be very good, particularly for clinical social workers. The continuing growth of healthcare spending and treatment increases the opportunities for clinical social workers as compared to social workers who do not offer treatment services. Many job openings will stem from growth and the need to replace social workers who leave the occupation. However, competition for social worker jobs is expected in cities where training programs for social workers are prevalent. Opportunities should be good in rural areas, which often find it difficult to attract and retain qualified staff. By specialty, job prospects may be best for those social workers with a background in gerontology and substance abuse treatment. **TABLE 22.2** shows some job projections data from the U.S. Department of Labor.

Earnings

Median annual wages of social workers was $51,760 in May 2020. Median annual wages in the industries employing the largest numbers of social workers in May 2020 are shown in **TABLE 22.3**.

Median annual wages for social workers by specialty in May 2020 are shown in **TABLE 22.4**.

TABLE 22.4 Median Annual Wages for Social Workers by Specialization, May 2020

Specialty	Salary
Healthcare social workers	$57,630
Child, family, and school social workers	$48,720
Mental health and substance abuse social workers	$48,430

Reproduced from Bureau of Labor Statistics. Occupational Outlook Handbook. U.S. Department of Labor; 2019. http://web.archive.org/web/20210305013224/https://www.bls.gov/OOH/community-and-social-service/social-workers.htm#tab-5

Related Occupations

Through direct counseling or referral to other services, social workers help people solve a range of personal problems. Workers in occupations with similar duties include counselors, health educators, probation officers and correctional treatment specialists, psychologists, and social and human service assistants.

SOCIAL AND HUMAN SERVICE ASSISTANTS
Significant Points

- A high school diploma is the minimum educational requirement, but employers often seek individuals with relevant work experience or education beyond high school.
- Employment is projected to grow much faster than the average for all occupations.
- Job opportunities should be excellent, particularly for applicants with appropriate postsecondary education, but wages remain low.

Work Description

Social and human service assistants help people get through difficult times or get additional support. They help clients to identify and obtain benefits and services such as food stamps and Medicaid. In addition to initially connecting clients with benefits or services, social and human service assistants may follow up with clients to ensure that they are receiving the services and that the services are meeting their needs. They work under the direction of social workers, psychologists, or others who have more education or experience. Social and human service assistants have many job titles, including case work aide, clinical social work aide, family service assistant, social work assistant, addictions counselor assistant, and **human service worker**.

With children and families, assistants ensure that children live in safe homes and may help parents obtain resources such as food assistance programs or child care. With older adults, they help clients stay in their own homes whenever

possible by coordinating meal deliveries or finding personal care aides to help with their day-to-day needs, such as running errands or bathing (**FIGURE 22.4**).

In some cases, human service workers help look for residential care facilities, such as nursing care or assisted-living facilities. For people with disabilities, social and human service assistants help find rehabilitation services or work with employers to adapt the elements of a job to make it accessible to people with disabilities. Some workers find personal care services to help clients with daily living activities, such as bathing or making meals.

For people with addictions to alcohol, drugs, or gambling, assistants help people find support groups or 12-step programs. They help **veterans** who have been discharged from the military adjust to civilian life with practical needs such as finding housing and applying skills gained in the military to civilian jobs. With immigrants, workers help clients adjust to living in a new country. They help the clients locate jobs and housing. They also may help find programs that teach English, or they may find legal assistance for applying for resident status (**FIGURE 22.5**).

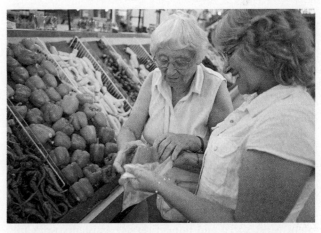

FIGURE 22.4 Social and human service assistants may help the elderly with grocery shopping.
© Paul Vasarhelyi/Shutterstock.

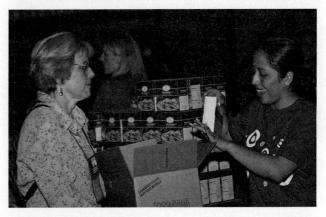

FIGURE 22.5 Social and human service assistants may help new immigrants find food and housing.
© lev radin/Shutterstock.

For people with mental illnesses, social and human service assistants help clients find resources such as self-help and support groups. In addition, they may find personal care services or group housing to help those with more severe mental illnesses. With the homeless, assistants help clients find temporary or permanent housing and locate soup kitchens or food pantries. With former prison inmates, assistants find housing and job training or placement programs to help clients reenter society.

Social and human service assistants play a variety of roles in the community. For example, they may organize and lead group activities, assist clients in need of counseling or crisis intervention, or administer food banks or emergency food programs. In halfway houses, group homes, and government-supported housing programs, they assist adults who need supervision with personal hygiene and daily living tasks. They review clients' records, ensure that clients take prescribed medication, talk with family members, and confer with medical personnel and other caregivers to provide insight into clients' needs. Assistants also give emotional support and help clients become involved in community recreation programs and other activities.

Work Environment

Social and human service assistants work for nonprofit organizations, private for-profit social service agencies, and state and local governments. They may work in offices, clinics, hospitals, group homes, and shelters. Some travel around their communities to see clients.

Working conditions of social and human service assistants vary. Some work in offices, clinics, and hospitals, while others work in group homes, shelters, and day programs. Traveling to see clients is required for some jobs. Sometimes working with clients can be dangerous, even though most agencies do everything they can to ensure their workers' safety. Most social and human service assistants work full time. Some work nights and weekends. Low pay and heavy workloads cause many workers to leave this occupation, creating opportunities for new workers entering the field.

Educational and Legal Requirements

The minimum requirement is a high school diploma or the equivalent, but some employers prefer to hire workers who have additional education or experience. Without additional education, advancement opportunities are limited.

Education and Training

Social and human service assistants without any postsecondary education usually undergo a period of on-the-job training. Because such workers often are dealing with multiple clients from a wide variety of backgrounds, on-the-job training in case management helps them respond to the different needs of their clients and to crises the clients sometimes undergo.

A certificate or an associate's degree in a subject such as human services, gerontology, or social or behavioral science is becoming more common for workers entering this occupation. Human services degree programs train students to observe and interview patients, carry out treatment plans, handle people who are undergoing a crisis, and use proper case management and referral procedures. Many programs include fieldwork to give students hands-on experience. The level of education completed often determines job responsibilities. Those with a high school diploma are likely to do lower-level work, such as helping clients fill out paperwork. However, assistants with some college education may coordinate program activities or manage a group home. Social and human service assistants with proven leadership ability, especially acquired from paid or volunteer experience in social services, often have greater autonomy in their work. Regardless of the academic or work background of employees, most employers provide some form of in-service training, such as seminars and workshops, to their employees.

Typical courses are general education courses in liberal arts, sciences, and the humanities. Most programs also offer specialized courses related to addictions, gerontology, child protection, and other areas. Many degree programs require the completion of a supervised internship. The **Council for Standards in Human Service Education (CSHSE)** lists 60 accredited programs in human services in 44 community colleges and universities; degrees listed are at the associate's and bachelor's degree level.[8]

Certification and Other Qualifications

A relatively new certification for those who work in human services, **Human Service Board-Certified Practitioner (HS-BCP)**, was designed for those who provide services to a variety of populations and who have educational backgrounds that range from certificates to graduate degrees. Those who become certified are recognized as having met educational and experience requirements to work in human services.[10]

The requirements for becoming board certified are education: an associate's, bachelor's or master's degree, documented hours of experience in the field, and successful completion of the certifying examination. Continuing education is required for maintaining certification. Applicants with degrees other than human services are required to complete courses in ethics, interviewing and intervention, and assessment and treatment as well as other courses.

Desirable qualities for social and human service assistants are a strong desire to help others, effective communication skills, a sense of responsibility, and the ability to manage time effectively. Excellent interpersonal skills are necessary for clients to feel comfortable working with assistants; these skills are also needed by assistants in building relationships with referral sources. Many human service jobs involve direct contact with people who are vulnerable to exploitation or mistreatment, so patience and understanding are also highly valued characteristics. It is becoming more common for employers to require a criminal background check, and in some settings, workers may be required to have a valid driver's license.

Advancement

Formal education is almost always necessary for advancement. In general, advancement to case management or social work jobs requires a bachelor's or master's degree in human services, counseling, rehabilitation, social work, or a related field.

Employment Opportunities

Social and human service assistants held about 425,600 jobs in 2019. The majority worked in individual and family services. (**TABLE 22.5**).

Employment Trends

Employment of social and human service assistants is expected to grow much faster than the average for all occupations. Job prospects are expected to be excellent, particularly for applicants with relevant postsecondary education.

Employment Change

The number of social and human service assistants is expected to grow by nearly 17% between 2019 to 2029, much faster than the average for all occupations. Growth will be

due to an increase in the older adult population and rising demand for health care and social services. The elderly population often needs services such as delivery of meals and adult day care. Social and human service assistants, who help find and provide these services, will be needed to meet this increased demand.

In addition, growth is expected as more people seek treatment for their addictions and more drug offenders are sent to treatment programs rather than to jail. The result will be an increase in demand for social and human service assistants who work in treatment programs or work with people with addictions. There also will be continued demand for child and family social and human service assistants. These workers will be needed to help others, such as social workers, investigate child abuse cases as well as place children in foster care and with adoptive families.

Job Prospects

Job prospects for social and human service assistants are expected to be excellent, particularly for individuals with appropriate education after high school. Job openings will come from job growth but also from the need to replace workers, who advance into new positions, retire, or leave the workforce for other reasons. There will be more competition for jobs in urban areas than in rural areas, but qualified applicants should have little difficulty finding employment. **TABLE 22.6** shows projections data from the U.S. Department of Labor.

Earnings

Median annual wages of social and human service assistants were $35,960 in May 2020. Mean annual wages in the industries employing the largest numbers of social and human service assistants in May 2020 are shown in **TABLE 22.7**.

Related Occupations

Workers in other occupations that require skills similar to those of social and human service assistants include childcare workers, correctional officers, counselors, health educators and community health workers, personal and home care aides, probation officers and correctional treatment specialists, rehabilitation counselors, and social workers.

TABLE 22.5 Distribution of Social and Human Service Assistants by Industry, 2019

Industry	Percentage
Individual and family services	30%
Local and state government	20%
Nursing and residential care facilities	12%
Community and vocational rehabilitation services	10%

Data from Bureau of Labor Statistics. Occupational Outlook Handbook. U.S. Department of Labor; 2020. https://www.bls.gov/ooh/community-and-social-service/social-workers.htm#tab-5

TABLE 22.6 Projection Data for Social and Human Service Assistants, 2019–2029

Occupational Title	Employment, 2019	Projected Employment, 2029	Change, 2019–2029	
			Number	Percentage
Social and human service assistants	425,600	497,100	71,500	17%

Data from Bureau of Labor Statistics. Occupational Outlook Handbook. U.S. Department of Labor; 2020. https://www.bls.gov/ooh/community-and-social-service/social-and-human-service-assistants.htm#tab-6

TABLE 22.7 Median Annual Wages in the Industries Employing the Largest Numbers of Social and Human Services Assistants, May 2020

Industry	Salary
Local government	$41,620
State government	$38,010
Individual and family services	$35,190
Community and vocational rehabilitation services	$32,640
Nursing and residential care facilities	$32,320

Data from Bureau of Labor Statistics. Occupational Outlook Handbook. U.S. Department of Labor; 2020. https://www.bls.gov/ooh/community-and-social-service/social-and-human-service-assistants .htm#tab-5

Additional Information

For information about career opportunities in social work and voluntary credentials for social workers, contact:

- National Association of Social Workers, 750 First St. NE, Suite 800, Washington, DC 20002-4241. http://www.socialworkers.org/

For a listing of accredited social work programs, contact:

- Council on Social Work Education, 333 John Carlyle Street, Suite 400, Alexandria, VA 22314. http://www.cswe.org

For information on becoming board certified in clinical social work contact:

American Board of Clinical Social Work. 19 Mantua Road, Mount Royal, NJ 08061

- https://www.abcsw.org/contact-us

Information on licensing requirements and testing procedures for each state may be obtained from state licensing authorities or from:

- Association of Social Work Boards, 17126 Mountain Run Vista Ct. Culpeper, Virginia 22701. http://www.aswb.org

For information on education programs and careers for social and human service assistants, contact:

- Council for Standards in Human Services Education, 3337 Duke St., Alexandria, VA 22314. https://cshse.org/
- National Organization for Human Services, 147 SE 102nd Ave., Portland, Oregon 97216. https://www.nationalhumanservices.org/
- Center for Credentialing & Education. 3 Terrace Way, Greensboro, NC 27403-3660 https://www.cce-global.org/credentialing/hsbcp

Information on job openings may be available from state employment service offices or directly from city, county, or state departments of health, mental health and mental retardation, and human resources.

LEARNING PORTFOLIO

Issues for Discussion

1. Read the article "Interview with a Social Worker" with Elizabeth Kelly, a caseworker and medical social worker in Washington, DC, written by Sara Royster from the *Career Outlook* section of the U.S. Bureau of Labor Statistics. Describe three different roles (or job responsibilities) for this medical social worker. Describe one aspect of her job that she especially likes and one obstacle that she experiences in her job as a social worker. What are her future goals? http://www.bls.gov/careeroutlook/2015/interview/social-worker.htm

2. Review the 1½-minute video that describes the role of a social worker employed in Child and Family Services. Based on the video clip, describe three typical tasks of a social worker in this setting. https://youtu.be/HvzxznYOhQM

3. Use the Association of Social Work Boards (ASWB) website to locate the licensing board for social workers in your state. Are there different categories for licensing social workers in your state? What are the educational requirements for each category? Are there different licensing exams for each category of social worker? https://www.aswb.org/licensees/about-licensing-and-regulation/social-work-regulation

4. Use the Social Work Career Center of the National Association of Social Workers website to review the job listings. Are there positions in your state? Which positions would be considered entry level, and which would require special certification or experience? https://joblink.socialworkers.org/jobs

5. Go to the College of DuPage Human Services webpage and review the certificate programs offered in human services. List the certificate programs, length of training, cost of training, and employment rate for graduates. What are the advantages of obtaining a certificate for those interested in working in human services? https://www.cod.edu/academics/programs/human_services

Enrichment Activities

1. View the six-minute video "This Could Be You: The Many Faces of Social Work." https://www.youtube.com/watch?v=77UGDj48oHs

2. Go to the National Association of Social Workers website and review specialty areas for certification for social workers. https://www.socialworkers.org/Careers/Credentials/Apply-for-NASW-Social-Work-Credentials

CASE STUDY: SOCIAL WORKERS

Meghan finished a bachelor's degree in psychology and worked for two years for AmeriCorps in a senior building. She plans to apply for a program that will prepare her to work as a licensed clinical social worker in a healthcare setting as part of a team of health professionals. Her mother has chronic kidney disease and is on dialysis. Meghan became interested in a career as a social worker through the experience of her mother, who participated in a support group for patients on dialysis. Her mother experienced a period of depression after her doctor told her that she needed chronic dialysis.

These questions are based on this case study.

1. Meghan is exploring different educational programs. Which degree program is the minimum educational requirement to become a Licensed Clinical Social Worker (LCSW)?
   A. Bachelor's Degree in Social Work (BSW)
   B. Master's Degree in Social Work (MSW)
   C. Doctorate in Clinical Social Work (DSW)
   D. Doctorate Degree in Social Work (PhD)

2. The title _____ designates a graduate of a master's degree program in social work without supervised work experience.

3. The title _____ designates a graduate of a master's degree program in social work with two years of supervised work experience.

4. According to 2020 Bureau of Labor Statistics data, social workers demanding the highest salaries specialize in:
   A. child, family, and school.
   B. health care.
   C. mental health and substance abuse.
   D. family services.

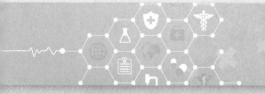

LEARNING PORTFOLIO

References

1. Council on Social Work Education. *Accreditation.* https://www.cswe.org/Accreditation/Directory-of-Accredited-Programs.aspx Accessed August 11, 2021.

2. Lightfoot E, Beltran R. *The GADE Guide: A Program Guide to Doctoral Study in Social Work.* St. Paul, MN: The Group for the Advancement of Doctoral Education in Social Work, 2016.

3. Group for the Advancement of Doctoral Education in Social Work. *DSW Programs.* https://www.gadephd.org/Membership/DSW-Programs Accessed August 11, 2021.

4. National Health Services Corps. *NHSC Loan Repayment Program.* Health Resources & Service Administration. U.S. Department of Health and Human Services. https://nhsc.hrsa.gov/loan-repayment/nhsc-loan-repayment-program.html Accessed August 11, 2021.

5. Association of Social Work Boards. *Licensing Board or College Websites, Statutes and Administrative Rules.* http://aswbsocialworkregulations.org/licensingWebsitesReportBuilder.jsp Accessed August 13, 2021

6. National Association of Social Workers. *Apply for NASW Social Work Credentials.* https://www.socialworkers.org/Careers/Credentials-Certifications/Apply-for-NASW-Social-Work-Credentials Accessed August 13, 2021.

7. American Board of Clinical Social Work. *Welcome to the ABCSW.* https://abcsw.memberclicks.net/overview-mission Accessed August 13, 2021.

8. National Council for Mental Health Wellbeing. CCBHC. Certified Community Behavioral Health Clinic. *Leading a Bold Shift in Mental Health & Substance Use Care. CCBHC Impact Report, 2021.* https://www.thenationalcouncil.org/wp-content/uploads/2021/08/2021-CCBHC-Impact-Report.pdf?daf=375ateTbd56 Accessed September 21, 2021.

9. Council for Standards in Human Service Education. *CSHSE Accredited Programs,* 2020. https://cshse.org/members-and-accredited-programs/cshse-accredited-programs/

10. Torpey E. Careers in Social Work: Outlook, pay, and more. *Career Outlook,* U.S. Bureau of Labor Statistics, March 2018.

11. Center for Credentialing & Education. *Credentialing Advance Your Journey.* https://www.cce-global.org/credentialing Accessed August 13, 2021.

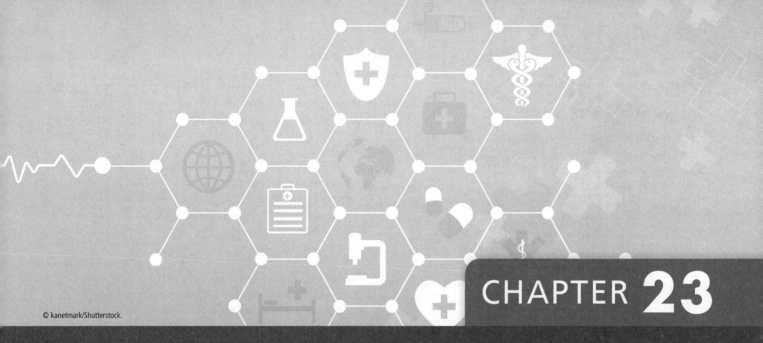
© kanetmark/Shutterstock.

CHAPTER 23

Genetic Counselors*

KEY TERMS

Accreditation Council for
  Genetic Counseling (ACGC)
American Board of Genetic
  Counseling (ABGC)
Carrier testing
Chromosomes

Genetic counselor
Human Genome Project
Mutations
National Society of Genetic
  Counselors (NSGC)
Newborn screening

Pedigree
Predictive genetic counseling
Prenatal screening
Psychiatric genetic
  counseling
Reproductive technology

* All information in this chapter, unless otherwise indicated, was obtained from Bureau of Labor Statistics. *Occupational Outlook Handbook 2020–2021 Edition*. Washington, DC: U.S. Department of Labor; 2021.

GENETIC COUNSELORS
Significant Points

- This is a relatively new health profession, with the first graduate program in genetic counseling offered in 1969.
- A master's degree from an accredited program in genetic counseling is required to be eligible for licensure and to take the certification exam.
- Genetic counselors interpret laboratory results and communicate findings related to genetic conditions to physicians and patients.
- Genetic counselors assist patients and families in making healthcare decisions based on risks for genetic disorders.
- Employment opportunities for genetic counselors are excellent because of advanced technology in DNA testing.
- Most jobs for genetic counselors are in hospitals and offices of physicians in urban areas and teaching hospitals.

Work Description

Genetic counselors provide information and advice to other healthcare providers and to individuals and families concerned with the risk of inherited conditions. A career as a genetic counselor combines a strong scientific background with counseling skills. Genetic counselors assess individual or family risk for a variety of inherited conditions, such as genetic disorders and birth defects. They provide information and advice to other healthcare providers and to individuals and families concerned with the risk of inherited conditions.

Genetic counseling is one of the fastest-growing health professions. The **Human Genome Project** has uncovered the genetic basis for many diseases, which has increased the demand for genetic counselors to assist individuals, families, and physicians in making decisions regarding health care and treatment.

Genetic counselors identify specific genetic disorders or syndromes that are inherited or passed down from parents to their children. For parents who are expecting children, counselors use genetic tests to predict whether a baby is likely to have hereditary disorders, such as Down syndrome or cystic fibrosis, among others (**FIGURE 23.1**).

Genetic counselors can also test whether an adult is likely to develop a chronic disease such as cardiovascular disease or ovarian cancer. Counselors identify the probability of developing certain diseases by studying patients' genes through DNA or chromosomal testing. Counselors often perform the lab tests themselves, although sometimes they have medical laboratory technologists perform the tests, which they then interpret and use for counseling. They share this information with other health professionals, such as physicians, and with patients and their families. Physicians use the results of lab tests to make decisions regarding treatment; for example, chemotherapy drugs to treat breast cancer are selected based on the cancer's genetic

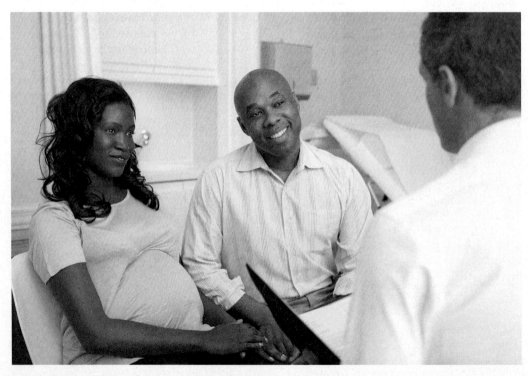

FIGURE 23.1 Genetic counselors discuss prenatal screening for genetic disorders with parents-to-be.
© Monkey Business Images/Shutterstock.

profile obtained via genetic testing. When a genetic disorder is diagnosed, the genetic counselor helps the individual and families understand the genetic disease and ways that the disease can be treated. Families can ask questions and express concerns about their health and options for treatment. As with other counseling, the genetic counselor will continue counseling until understanding and acceptance are achieved by individuals and/or families.

Genetic counselors are often consulted by a physician when a genetic disorder has been identified through prenatal or **newborn screening** or **carrier testing**. Individuals and families may also seek genetic counseling after an individual or family member has received a medical diagnosis for a disease or disorder that is genetically transmitted. Couples may seek genetic counseling in order to make a decision about having children. Examples of when couples may seek counseling are if there is a history of a miscarriage or stillbirth, the birth of a child with a genetic disorder or birth defect, or a family history of a genetic disease.[1] Genetic counselors usually schedule an hour for each session and will schedule a follow-up session to discuss the results of genetic tests. Additional follow-up sessions will be scheduled by the counselor to evaluate understanding and how well the individual and family are managing and accepting the genetic condition.

During an initial counseling session, the counselor will ask questions to obtain a more complete family and medical history to complete a **pedigree**, or specialized family tree that includes the health conditions and causes and the age of death of the biological family members. The family tree aids the genetic counselor in mapping genetic patterns. For example, genetic testing of a child with autism may confirm the cause as fragile X syndrome and identify that the mother is the carrier. Additional information about family members through completion of the pedigree confirms other conditions in the family that can be attributed to the fragile X gene—a maternal aunt has a child with special needs, another maternal aunt was treated for infertility, and the maternal grandfather died of Parkinson's disease.[3]

The counselor may recommend that specific tests be done in potential parents to determine whether either parent is a carrier for a genetic disease. Tests that are done are cytogenic tests, which evaluate for abnormalities in **chromosomes**; biochemical testing to evaluate for **mutations** in critical proteins, enzymes, hormones, and other regulatory proteins; and molecular testing for small mutations of DNA.[3] The counselor will conduct follow-up sessions with the family after testing to provide not only information but emotional support to reduce anxiety and to assist the family in adjusting to the test results. The genetic counselor can also assist the family in making decisions about communicating genetic testing results with extended family members that may be impacted by a diagnosis—for example, early-onset Alzheimer's disease, which has a genetic basis.[3]

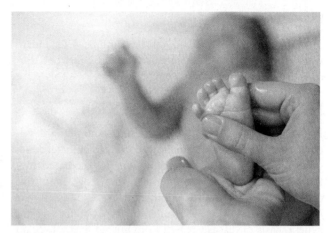

FIGURE 23.2 Genetic screening in newborns identifies genetic disorders and allows for early intervention.
© Pavel Ilyukhin/Shutterstock.

Prenatal screening is recommended for all pregnant women over 35 years of age because of a higher risk for the chromosomal abnormality responsible for Down syndrome. All state public health departments conduct newborn screening to identify inherited disorders such as phenylketonuria (PKU), which is treated with a diet restricted in the amino acid phenylalanine in the infant soon after birth to prevent an intellectual disability (**FIGURE 23.2**).

Carrier testing may be done for partners who are considering having a family to determine whether either partner carries the risks for genetic diseases known to be present in their family. For example, sickle cell anemia is transmitted to offspring if both parents are carriers for the disease. **Predictive genetic counseling** may be done when adult family members have been diagnosed with dementia, cardiovascular disease, or cancer at an early age. Adult women who have a strong family history of breast cancer may seek further information to evaluate for the presence of BRCA mutations that dramatically increase the risk for breast cancer.[3] **Psychiatric genetic counseling** is a newer area of genetic counseling that may be requested by individuals with a history of autism or a serious mental illness such as schizophrenia or bipolar disease in their family.[1] This information can be used when parents have concerns about the behavior of one of their children and to assist the physician or behavioral counselor in determining if there is a genetic basis for the child's behavior and to seek appropriate treatment.

Work Environment

Genetic counselors held about 2,600 jobs in 2019. Genetic counselors work in university medical centers, private and public hospitals, physicians' offices, and diagnostic laboratories. In 2019, 43% worked in hospitals, 11% worked in medical and diagnostic laboratories, and 13% worked in offices of physicians. They work with families, patients, and other medical professionals.

Work Schedules

Most genetic counselors work full time and have a standard work schedule. Counselors may also work evenings or Saturdays to meet the needs of working families.

Employment Opportunities

In the 1960s, when the career of genetic counseling developed, counselors spent the majority of time in prenatal counseling.[2] Demand for genetic counselors has increased over the past decade in response to more knowledge about diseases that are genetically transmitted because of the Human Genome Project. There is greater public awareness of the genetic basis of disease as well as improved technology for genetic testing for many diseases. In addition, there is greater demand for **reproductive technology** for couples who have been unsuccessful in having a biological child.[3]

Education and Legal Requirements

Genetic counselors typically need at least a master's degree in genetic counseling or genetics, and some earn a PhD. Certification is required by most employers.

Education and Training

A master's degree program in genetic counseling is required to be eligible for licensure and to take the certification exam. A bachelor's degree in one of the biological or social sciences is recommended for applicants. Often those with a degree in biology, genetics, psychology, or public health or those already employed in nursing or social work may choose to become a genetic counselor. Coursework in genetic counseling includes clinical genetics, population genetics, cytogenetics, and molecular genetics as well as psychosocial theory, ethics, and counseling techniques. Classes emphasize genetics, public health, and counseling techniques. Advanced courses focus on clinical observations, review of previous genetic research, and health communication strategies. Students must complete supervised clinical rotations where they work directly with patients and clients. Clinical rotations provide a variety of experiences in different work environments, such as prenatal diagnostic centers, pediatric hospitals, or cancer centers.

Master's degree programs in genetic counseling require clinical training in a medical genetics center approved by the **Accreditation Council for Genetic Counseling (ACGC)**. The website in the Additional Information section at the end of this chapter lists accredited programs in the United States and Canada.[4] An application requires a written personal statement and personal interview. Since the field of genetic counseling is relatively new and the number of education programs is relatively small, acceptance into a graduate program in genetic counseling is competitive. Learning as much as possible about a career as a genetics counselor by volunteering or working in a genetics clinic before applying would improve chances of being accepted in a master's degree program in genetic counseling. The **National Society of Genetic Counselors (NSGC)** website provides tips for preparing the application packet.[5]

Licensure and Certification

As of 2021, all except two states—Vermont and Wyoming—required licensure or were in the process of rulemaking to require licensure to practice genetic counseling. Certification is typically needed to get a license.[6]

Certification and Other Qualifications

The **American Board of Genetic Counseling (ABGC)** provides certification for genetic counselors. To become certified, a student must first complete a master's degree program that has been accredited by the Accreditation Council for Genetic Counseling. Students then must pass a comprehensive certification exam and continue to accrue continuing education units throughout their careers. As of 2021, there were 51 accredited programs in the United States and four in Canada.[4]

Genetic counselors need a strong science background and the ability to explain complex information in a way that can be understood by someone without a science background. Critical-thinking skills are necessary in interpreting lab results and medical information accurately (**FIGURE 23.3**).

Compassion and sensitivity are important in determining what information will be useful and how to deliver news to individuals and families that is potentially upsetting. Genetic information is rapidly expanding, which requires that genetic counselors participate in professional organizations or conferences to keep abreast of developments in genetics and genomics to provide the most up-to-date services to patients.

Advancement

Genetic counselors who work in industry generally earn higher salaries. Since the profession is small, the opportunities for advancement are limited. Supervisory positions or

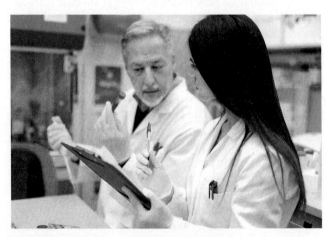

FIGURE 23.3 Genetic counselors discuss lab results with physicians.
© Minerva Studio/Shutterstock.

TABLE 23.1 Projections Data for Genetic Counselors, 2019–2029

Occupational Title	Employment, 2019	Projected Employment, 2029	Change, 2019–2029	
			Number	Percentage
Genetic counselor	2,600	3,200	600	21%

Data from Bureau of Labor Statistics. Occupational Outlook Handbook. U.S. Department of Labor; 2020. https://www.bls.gov/ooh/healthcare/genetic-counselors.htm#tab-6

training others to become genetic counselors may increase responsibilities and salaries.

Employment Trends

According to a 2016 survey from the National Society of Genetic Counselors, most genetic counselors specialize in traditional areas of genetic counseling: prenatal, cancer, and pediatrics. The survey noted that genetic counselors also may work in one or more specialty fields such as cardiovascular health, genomic medicine, neurogenetics, and psychiatry. Other job opportunities are in research and product development and marketing in the pharmaceutical industry.

Public awareness of the genetic basis for disease and scientific advances in reproductive technologies have increased the demand for genetic counselors. Work opportunities for genetic counselors are expanding to include not only clinical practice but public policy, public health, administration, research, teaching, and private practice.[7]

Ongoing technological innovations, including lab tests and developments in genomics, are giving counselors the opportunities to conduct more types of analyses. Cancer genomics, for example, can determine a patient's risk for specific types of cancer. The number and types of tests that genetic counselors can administer and interpret have increased over the past few years.

Most growth over the next 10 years for genetic counselors is expected to be in hospitals, and most jobs will be in teaching and research hospitals and in urban areas.

Employment Change

Employment of genetic counselors is projected to grow 21% from 2019 to 2029, much faster than the average for all occupations. However, because it is a small occupation, the fast growth will result in only about 600 new jobs over the 10-year period (**TABLE 23.1**).

Job Prospects

Genetic counselors can generally expect favorable job prospects. Ongoing innovations in genetic testing are likely to create demand for certified genetic counselors. Many types of genetic tests are covered by health insurance providers. Most opportunities will be in teaching and research hospitals or in physician's offices in large metropolitan areas.

Earnings

The median annual wage for genetic counselors was $85,700 in May 2020. The median annual wages for genetic counselors

TABLE 23.2 Median Annual Salaries for Genetic Counselors, May 2020

Medical and diagnostic laboratories	$87,400
Offices of physicians	$84,680
Hospitals	$82,900
Colleges, universities, and professional schools	$79,490

Data from Bureau of Labor Statistics. Occupational Outlook Handbook. U.S. Department of Labor; 2020. https://www.bls.gov/ooh/healthcare/genetic-counselors.htm#tab-5

in the top industries in which these counselors worked as of May 2020 are shown in **TABLE 23.2**.

Related Occupations

Occupations that require similar training and have similar job responsibilities are epidemiologists, health educators, medical scientists, physicians, mental health counselors, and marriage and family therapists.

Additional Information

For more information about a career in genetic counseling:

- *Genetic Counselor.* https://explorehealthcareers.org/career/allied-health-professions/genetic-counselor/
- Canadian Association of Genetic Counsellors. *FAQ for Students.* P.O. Box 52083, Oakville, Ontario, CA L6J 7N5 https://www.cagc-accg.ca/?page=314

For information about accreditation and schools offering education in genetic counseling in the United States and Canada visit:

- Accreditation Council for Genetic Counseling (ACGC), 7918 Jones Branch Dr., Suite 300, McLean, VA 22102. https://www.gceducation.org/program-directory

For information about genetic counselors, how to become a genetic counselor, and states that require licensure visit:

- National Society of Genetic Counselors (NSGC), 330 N. Wabash Ave., Suite 2000, Chicago, IL 60611. https://www.nsgc.org

For information on becoming certified as a genetic counselor in the U.S. and Canada contact:

- American Board of Genetic Counseling (ABGC), 4400 College Blvd., Suite 220, Overland Park, KS 66211. https://www.abgc.net

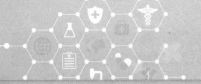

LEARNING PORTFOLIO

Issues for Discussion

1. Watch the two-minute video "I Am a Genetic Counselor." Describe the role of a genetic counselor based on information from the video. https://youtu.be/lItT3Vpnvhk

2. Discuss the advantages and disadvantages of communicating with extended family when a family member has been diagnosed with early-onset Alzheimer's disease, which has a genetic basis.

3. Discuss the pros and cons for parents deciding to bring a pregnancy to term, terminating the pregnancy, or putting up the child for adoption when prenatal testing determines that the fetus tests positive for Down syndrome.

4. Go to the National Society for Genetic Counselors website and review the steps for applying for a master's degree program in genetic counseling. List the steps beginning with choosing an undergraduate degree program through applying for a graduate program. https://www.aboutgeneticcounselors.org /Become-a-Genetic-Counselor/Applying-to-a -Training-Program5. Discuss the similarities and differences in the educational requirements and job responsibilities between a medical social worker and genetic counselor.

Enrichment Activities

1. Go to the National Society for Genetic Counselor's website to review the slideshow "NSGC Timeline," which reviews the role of genetics in human disease and the history of genetic counseling as a profession. https://www.nsgc.org/About/About-NSGC/Timeline

2. Go to the website *Baby's First Test* to find out the requirements for the state where you live for testing newborns for genetic conditions. https://www.babysfirsttest.org/newborn-screening/states

3. Go to the National Human Genome Research Institute to learn more about genetic counseling and testing for genetic diseases. https://www.genome.gov /FAQ/Genetic-Counseling

CASE STUDY: GENETIC COUNSELOR

Dan became interested in learning more about genetics and careers in genetics when his brother was diagnosed with schizophrenia at age 25 after graduating from college and teaching English in France. His parents were completely unprepared for this diagnosis. Dan is currently enrolled as a psychology undergraduate student at a state university.

The following questions are related to this case study and a career as a genetic counselor.

1. What college courses would you recommend for Dan to learn more about genetics?
   A. Genetics
   B. Physics
   C. Sociology
   D. History

2. What is the minimum educational requirement for application for a degree in genetic counseling?
   A. High school diploma
   B. Associate's degree
   C. Bachelor's degree
   D. Master's degree

3. A requirement to practice as a genetic counselor is:
   A. post-master's internship.
   B. degree in social work.
   C. certification.
   D. state licensure.

4. Currently the majority of genetic counselors work in the areas of _____, _____, or _____.

LEARNING PORTFOLIO

References

1. National Society of Genetic Counselors, Inc., *Making Sense of Your Genes. A Guide to Genetic Counseling*, 2008. Genetic Alliance. http://www.geneticalliance.org/publications/guide togeneticcounseling Accessed August 16, 2021.

2. Mullens J. You're a What? Genetic Counselor. *Occupational Outlook Quarterly*. June 2011. Bureau of Labor Statistics. U.S. Department of Labor. http://www.bls .gov/careeroutlook/2011/summer/yawhat.pdf Accessed August 16, 2021.

3. The New England Public Health Genetics Education Collaborative. *Understanding Genetics: A Guide for Patients and Health Professionals.* http://www.geneticalliance.org/sites /default/files/publicationsarchive/UnderstandingGenetics NewEngland.pdf Accessed August 16, 2021.

4. Accreditation Council for Genetic Counseling. *Program Directory.* https://www.gceducation.org/program-directory/ Accessed August 16, 2021.

5. National Society of Genetic Counselors (NSGC). *Genetic Counseling Training.* https://www.nsgc.org/page/genetic -counseling-training-page.

6. National Society of Genetic Counselors. *States Issuing Licenses for Genetic Counselors*, February 2020. https: //www.nsgc.org/Policy-Research-and-Publications/State -Licensure-for-Genetic-Counselors/States-Issuing-Licenses Updated July 2021. Accessed August 15, 2021.

7. ExploreHealthCareers.Org. *Genetic Counselor.* https: //explorehealthcareers.org/career/allied-health-professions /genetic-counselor/ Accessed August 16, 2021.

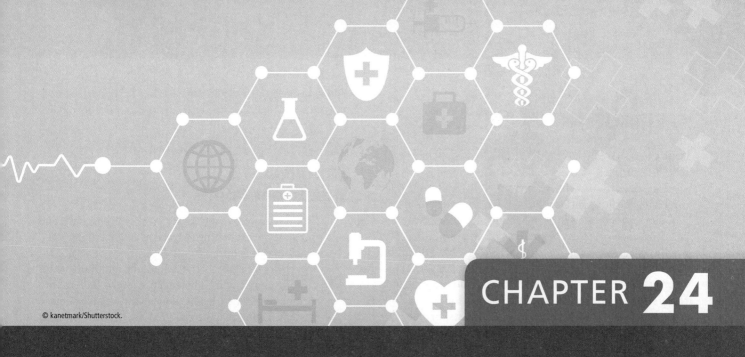

© kanetmark/Shutterstock.

CHAPTER **24**

Health Education*

KEY TERMS

Academy for Certification of
Vision Rehabilitation and
Education Professionals
(ACVREP)
Activities of daily living (ADLs)
Association for Education and
Rehabilitation of the
Blind and Visually Impaired
(AER)
Autism spectrum disorder (ASD)
Behavior analyst
Behavior Analyst Certification
Board (BACB)
Board-Certified Assistant
Behavior Analyst (BCaBA)

Board-Certified Behavior
Analyst (BCBA)
Certified Health Education
Specialist (CHES)
Certified Orientation and
Mobility Specialist (COMS)
Certified Vision Rehabilitation
Therapist (CVRT)
Community Health Worker
(CHW)
Council on Education for Public
Health (CEPH)
Health Education Specialist
Health educator
Independent activities of daily
living (IADLs)

Master Certified Health
Education Specialist
(MCHES)
Orientation and mobility
(O&M) specialist
National Commission for Health
Education Credentialing
(NCHEC)
Patient navigator
Registered Behavior
Technician (RBT)
School health educator
Vision Rehabilitation Therapist
(VRT)

* All information in this chapter, unless otherwise indicated, was obtained from Bureau of Labor Statistics. *Occupational Outlook Handbook 2020–2021 Edition*. Washington, DC: U.S. Department of Labor; 2021.

HEALTH CAREERS SPECIALIZING IN EDUCATION

The health field offers a variety of career opportunities for those interested in education: community health education, school health, and more specialized educational careers as a vision specialist or behavior analyst. This chapter includes careers for health educators, school health, orientation and mobility specialists, visual rehabilitation therapists, and behavior analysts. The *Occupational Outlook Handbook* is used as a resource for the sections on **Health Education Specialists** and **Community Health Workers (CHWs)** in this chapter. However, the handbook currently does not include careers for school health teachers, orientation and mobility instructors, vision rehabilitation therapists, or behavior analysts. Therefore, these sections will be briefer since less information is available. The U.S. Department of Labor collects salary data from employers across the United States, and professional organizations collect similar data from their members. However, limited salary data is available for newer careers or professional groups with smaller numbers of members. Therefore, salaries for these careers are based on figures from one recruiter listed under references.

Health education is an expanding field that emphasizes the importance of preventive health care. As professionals, **health educators** use educational skills and a sound knowledge of public health to educate the public about health and disease and what can be done to maintain good health, prevent disease, or secure treatment. Other work titles used to describe health educators are health education teachers, patient educators, health coaches, community organizers, public health educators, and health program managers. **CHWs** are support personnel who work together with health educators to provide outreach and to educate consumers on the importance and availability of healthcare services such as cancer screening.

While the health educator concentrates on the non-school community, **school health educators** are concerned with the school environment. Their main concerns are classroom teaching and the factors that influence the knowledge, behavior, attitudes, and practices that affect the health of students.

A significant branch of the health education field presents challenging career opportunities for work with individuals who have visual impairments. Professionals in this work provide essential services to persons with these conditions, enabling them to function successfully in a sighted world. The different types of specialists who work with those who have visual impairment include orientation and mobility specialists and vision rehabilitation therapists. The need for vision specialists is expected to increase with the aging population, especially for those over 75 years of age. In the United States, about 2% of adults 21 to 64 years of age have visual impairments compared to an estimated 9%, or nearly 2 million, in those 75 years of age and older.[1]

Another career that has recently gained recognition is **behavior analyst**, in response to the high number of children being diagnosed with **autism spectrum disorder**

(ASD). Behavior analysts provide services to clients who have problems with social, emotional, and communication skills.[2]

HEALTH EDUCATION SPECIALISTS
Significant Points

- Health education specialists work in hospitals and ambulatory care settings as well as in government and social service agencies.
- A bachelor's degree is the minimum requirement for entry-level jobs and to be eligible to take the exam to become a certified health education specialist, but a master's degree may be required for certain positions or advancement.
- Faster-than-average job growth is expected.

Work Description

Health education specialists teach people about behaviors that promote wellness and develop and implement strategies to improve the health of both individuals and communities. Health education specialists improve public health through community-wide education initiatives on health topics ranging from nutrition and fitness to injury and disease prevention. They help people make better use of available health services, adopt self-care practices, and become more active participants in their community's health system.[3] Community health workers also often have the task of educating legislators and other policymakers on the importance of considering consumer interests when planning and funding health programs.

With major changes taking place in the delivery of health care at local, regional, and national levels as a result of the Affordable Care Act, the participation of health education specialists is increasingly in demand. By seeking the involvement of all interested persons, health educators work toward the solution of a particular problem through a variety of avenues. They help define common goals and stimulate and guide a discussion to assist various groups in reaching their own decisions and determining implementation strategies. Whether helping a low-income neighborhood plan its own health center or helping representatives from state agencies agree on needed regional medical facilities, the health educator helps people help themselves by bringing needs and resources together to create new partnerships for health.

Health education specialists may work through a wide variety of intermediaries in the community—teachers, health officers, public health nurses, trade unions, program directors, scout leaders, and community group leaders. In this way, health education specialists can reach a much larger audience than they would otherwise. These various intermediaries have a personal relationship with those being educated and are therefore likely to have a greater influence.

Health education specialists also work with the mass media (newspapers, magazines, radio, and television) and social media (Facebook, Twitter, and blogs). They prepare or direct the preparation of appropriate articles, features, and photographs for use by the media or to post on social media. They may work directly with writers, editors, or program directors. As a result, their influence is extended to vast audiences that could not be reached otherwise.

The duties of health education specialists, vary with their work settings. Most work in healthcare facilities, colleges, public health departments, nonprofits, and private businesses or large corporations. Those who teach health classes in middle and high schools are considered teachers.

In healthcare facilities, health education specialists may work one-on-one with patients and their families. They teach patients about their diagnoses and about any necessary treatments or procedures (**FIGURE 24.1**).

They may be called **patient navigators** because they help consumers find out about their health insurance options and direct people to outside resources, such as support groups and home health agencies. Health education specialists in healthcare facilities also help organize health screenings, such as blood pressure checks, and health classes on topics such as installing an infant car seat correctly. They also create programs to train medical staff to interact better with patients. For example, they may teach doctors how to explain complicated procedures to patients in simple language.

In colleges, health education specialists create programs and materials on topics that affect young adults, such as smoking and alcohol use or preventing sexually transmitted diseases. They may train students to be peer educators and supervise the students' delivery of health information in person or through social media. They also advocate for campus-wide policies to promote health such as providing healthy food options in college food-service operations or work to change policies to make it easier for students to report incidences of rape.

In public health departments, health education specialists administer public health campaigns on topics such as emergency preparedness, immunizations, nutrition, or stress management. Those employed by state and local departments of public health administer state-mandated programs based on priorities and available funding. During weather emergencies such as hurricanes, they may provide safety information to the public and the media. Some work with other professionals to create public policies that support healthy behaviors and environments. They may also oversee grants and grant-funded programs to improve the health of the public. Some participate in statewide and local campaigns such as stopping the spread of sexually transmitted diseases such as herpes and HIV/AIDS, promoting breastfeeding, or developing smoke-free policies for large apartment buildings.

In nonprofits (including community health organizations), health education specialists create programs and materials about health issues for the community. They may form and lead community coalitions to address public health issues ranging from the availability of grocery stores or access to safe exercise areas in the community. They help organizations obtain funding and other resources. Many nonprofits focus on a particular disease or audience, so health education specialists in these organizations limit programs to that specific topic or audience. For example, a health education specialists may design a program to teach people with diabetes how to better manage their condition or a program for teaching teen mothers how to care for their newborns. In addition, they may educate policy makers about ways to improve public health and work on securing grant funding for programs to promote health and disease awareness.

In private businesses and corporations, health education specialists identify common health problems among employees and create programs to improve health. They work with management to develop incentives for employees to adopt healthy behaviors, such as participation in smoking-cessation or weight-management classes offered by the employer. Health education specialists recommend changes to improve employee health such as creating a smoke-free workplace, offering walking programs for employees, or changing menu items to healthier choices in the cafeteria and vending machines (**FIGURE 24.2**).

Health education specialists also conduct research and evaluate programs. An example is a young woman who completed a bachelor's degree in political science and a master's

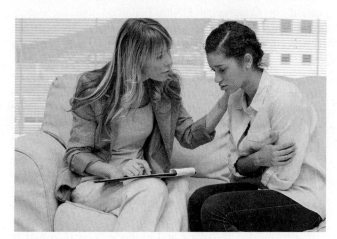

FIGURE 24.1 A health education specialist discusses a health diagnosis with a patient.
© wavebreakmedia/Shutterstock.

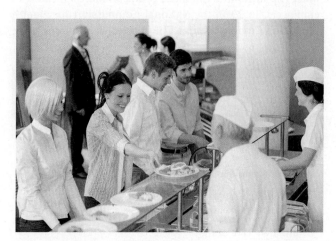

FIGURE 24.2 Health education specialists work with businesses to promote healthy menu items.
© CandyBox Images/Shutterstock.

degree in public health. She coordinates and directs projects related to cancer research and prevention. One of her projects is to evaluate a national colorectal cancer screening program to determine which programs are most successful in increasing colorectal cancer screening rates among different populations based on ethnicity, socioeconomic, and educational factors.[4]

Work Environment

Depending on the position, health education specialists work with other health professionals, community groups, state and local health departments, academic researchers, and the media. Although most work in an office, they may spend a lot of time away from the office to carry out programs or attend meetings and some positions require frequent travel. They also may need to work nights and weekends to attend programs or meetings. Most health education specialists work full time.

Employment Opportunities

Health education specialists held about 64,900 jobs in 2019. The industries that employed the most health educators in 2019 are shown in **TABLE 24.1**.

Educational and Legal Requirements

Entry-level health education specialists positions require a bachelor's degree in health education or public health.

Education and Training

Entry-level health education specialist positions require a bachelor's degree in health education, behavior health/health promotion, or public health. These programs teach theories and methods of health education and help students gain the knowledge and skills they need to develop health education materials and programs. Courses in psychology, human development, and a second language are helpful, and experience gained through an internship or other volunteer opportunities can make graduates more appealing to employers. In 2020, the **National Commission for Health Education Credentialing (NCHEC)** listed 47 programs at the

TABLE 24.1 Industries Employing the Largest Numbers of Health Education Specialists, 2019

Government	24%
Hospitals	22%
Individual and family services	8%
Religious, grantmaking, civic, and other professional organizations	7%
Outpatient care centers	7%

Data from Bureau of Labor Statistics. Occupational Outlook Handbook. U.S. Department of Labor; 2020. https://www.bls.gov/ooh/community-and-social-service/health-educators.htm#tab-3

undergraduate level, 31 programs at the master's level, and 8 programs at the doctoral level. The focus of these programs is health education, health behavior, and health promotion.[5] The **Council on Education for Public Health (CEPH)** listed under Additional Information at the end of this chapter lists accredited programs in public health.

Some positions require a master's or doctoral degree. Graduate programs are commonly in community health education, school health education, public health education, or health promotion. Entering a master's degree program requires a bachelor's degree, but a variety of undergraduate majors may be acceptable. Many students pursue their master's degree in health education after majoring or working in another related field, such as nursing or psychology. Those with doctoral degrees in this specialty will continue to be needed to meet the growing demand for research and evaluation skills in health education and for teaching in institutions of higher learning.

Licensure

In 2020, no states required licensure for health education specialists. Individual employers, however, may require certification. Since certification of health educators is relatively recent, contact your state's board of health, nursing, or human services to verify requirements for individual states.

Certification and Other Qualifications

Some employers require health educators to be a **Certified Health Education Specialist (CHES)**. CHES certification, offered by the NCHEC, is awarded after a candidate passes the qualifying exam. The exam is aimed at entry-level health education specialists who have completed a bachelor's degree or are within three months of completion. There is also a **Master Certified Health Education Specialist (MCHES)** credential for health educators with advanced education and experience; the requirements are experience working in the field for at least five years or a master's degree in Health Education, Public Health Education, School Health Education, or Community Health Education and successfully completing the MCHES competency exam. To maintain certification, health education specialists must complete 75 hours of continuing education every five years.[6]

Since health education specialists spend much of their time working with people, they must be comfortable working with both individuals and groups. They need to be good communicators and be comfortable speaking in public, as they may need to teach classes or give presentations. Health education specialists often work with diverse populations, so they must be sensitive to cultural differences and open to working with people of varied backgrounds. Health education specialists often create new programs or materials, so they should be creative and skilled writers. Analytical skills are also needed to collect and evaluate data since part of being a health education specialist is evaluating programs. An evaluation is useful in determining the needs of the

TABLE 24.2 Projections Data for Health Education Specialists, 2019–2029

Occupational Title	Employment, 2019	Projected Employment, 2029	Change, 2019–2029	
			Number	Percentage
Health educators	62,200	69,300	7,100	11%

Data from Bureau of Labor Statistics. Occupational Outlook Handbook. U.S. Department of Labor; 2020. https://www.bls.gov/ooh/community-and-social-service/health-educators.htm#tab-6

community as well as the effectiveness of programs. These specialists must be able to play a variety of roles successfully and adjust to the demands of different situations. At times, these educators work behind the scenes to help others start and carry out projects in the public interest.

Advancement

A graduate degree is usually required to advance to jobs such as executive director, supervisor, or senior health educator. Work in these positions may require more time on planning and evaluating programs than on implementation and require supervising other health education specialists who implement the programs. Health educators at this level may also work with administrators of related programs.

Employment Trends

As healthcare costs continue to rise, insurance companies, employers, and governments are trying to find ways to improve the quality of care and health outcomes while curbing costs. One of the challenges for health education specialists is that health educators focus on the prevention of disease while the healthcare system reimburses healthcare workers for treatment of disease.[7]

Employment Change

Employment of health education specialists is projected to grow 13% from 2019 to 2029, much faster than the average for all occupations. Growth will be driven by efforts to improve health outcomes and to reduce healthcare costs by teaching people about healthy habits and behaviors and utilization of available healthcare services.

One way to achieve these efforts is to employ health education specialists who teach people how to live healthy lives and how to avoid costly diseases and medical procedures. Lifestyle changes can reduce the probability of contracting a number of illnesses, such as lung cancer, HIV, heart disease, and skin cancer. Health educators also help people who already have a disease, such as asthma, understand how to manage their condition and avoid unnecessary trips to the emergency room. Health education specialists help people understand how what they do affects their health.

For many illnesses, such as breast cancer and testicular cancer, finding the disease early greatly increases the likelihood that treatment will be successful. Therefore, it is

important for people to know how to identify potential problems and when to seek medical help. The need to provide the public with this kind of information is expected to result in an increased demand for health education specialist.

Job Prospects

Job opportunities are expected to be excellent for health education specialist, especially for those who are certified and have a master's degree. As a result of federal health reform with greater access to medical care, health education specialist will be needed to direct patients in obtaining access to healthcare services. In addition, a number of state and local programs designed to manage conditions such as diabetes and obesity include health education specialists as part of intervention teams. **TABLE 24.2** lists projected new jobs between 2019 and 2029.

Earnings

The median annual wage for health educators was $56,500 in May 2020. The median annual wages for health education specialists in the top five industries in which these educators worked as of May 2020 are shown in **TABLE 24.3**.

Related Occupations

Other professions with similar educational requirements and job responsibilities include dietitians and nutritionists; epidemiologists; mental health counselors; social workers; substance abuse and behavior disorder counselors; elementary, secondary, and postsecondary teachers; training and development specialists; and patient representatives.

TABLE 24.3 Median Annual Wages in the Industries Employing the Largest Numbers of Health Education Specialists, May 2020

Hospitals	$65,530
Government	$59,070
Outpatient care centers	$57,850
Religious, grantmaking, civic, and professional organizations	$49,090
Individual and family services	$43,400

Data from Bureau of Labor Statistics. Occupational Outlook Handbook. U.S. Department of Labor; 2020. https://www.bls.gov/ooh/community-and-social-service/health-educators.htm#tab-6

SCHOOL HEALTH EDUCATORS
Work Description

School health educators help children, adolescents, and young adults develop the knowledge, attitudes, and skills they need to have a healthy life. They work closely with the school physician and nurse as well as other teachers, social workers, dietitians and/or food service directors, and administrators to develop a health education program for schools. Some health educators are responsible for coordinating and monitoring health screenings, especially for children in preschools or elementary schools. Health screening includes vision, hearing, height and weight, and immunizations. Referrals are made for students identified as needing other health services—for example, for children with impaired vision or hearing or a health condition requiring intervention.[8] Some health educators work in school-based health centers where health services are available for students and their families. Usually they also participate in community health activities as representatives of the school health education program. Health education has a place all the way from nursery school and kindergarten through high school and on into college because it deals with day-to-day living. It is health education when five-year-olds learn to eat new foods and when high school seniors make a field survey of the health services available in their community. Those who work in the college or university setting often combine roles of health educator and faculty in departments of public health, health education, or health promotion. The responsibilities can include directing wellness programs for students, faculty, and staff as well as teaching college courses in wellness.[9]

Depending on the school system and grade level for students in elementary or secondary schools, health courses may include such subject matter as family life education, first aid, safety education, choice and use of health services and products, nutrition, personal hygiene, air and water pollution, alcohol and drug abuse, and community health. Health courses include the principles of mental health and good human relations as well as marriage and family life. Comprehensive health education curricula include sex education where allowed; in some states, it is required.

School health educators may have even broader responsibilities as health coordinators. School health coordinators may work in a single school or in an entire school system; they furnish leadership in developing and maintaining an adequate, well-balanced health program and helping all groups interested in the health of schoolchildren work together effectively.

Work Environment

School health educators often work in a classroom setting but may travel between classrooms and to other schools in the district. Those responsible for health screening can expect to work with the school nurse. They also may be required to work evenings to conduct programs for parents and families.

Employment Opportunities

Employment for health education teachers may decrease in secondary schools. Many schools, facing budget cuts, ask teachers trained in other fields, such as science or physical education, to teach the subject of health education. In addition, few schools require students to take health classes.

Educational and Legal Requirements

The school health educator needs four years of college education leading to a bachelor's degree and to be licensed and/or certified to teach by the state where the educator is working.

Education and Training

Working as a school health educator requires a bachelor's degree with a background in the biological, behavioral, and social sciences and health education. Increasingly, a master's degree is required. States also require completing a teacher preparation program and supervised experience in teaching, typically gained through student teaching. Some states require a minimum grade point average. States typically require candidates to pass a general teaching certification test as well as a test that demonstrates their knowledge in the subject.

Licensure

All states require that public school teachers be licensed or certified. High school teachers typically are awarded a secondary or high school certification, which allows them to teach seventh through 12th grades. Requirements for certification vary by state; however, all states require at least a bachelor's degree in a teacher preparation program and supervised student teaching. States typically require successful completion of a certification exam.

Certification and Other Requirements

The school health educator must meet the regular certification standards for teachers in the state. Personal qualifications for this educational specialist are similar to those for a successful teacher in any field. It is important to like working with children and young people and to have patience, a sense of humor, good judgment, and emotional stability.

COMMUNITY HEALTH WORKERS
Significant Points

- About 50% of community health workers work for individual and family services; local governments; and religious, grantmaking, civic, and other professional organizations.

- Community health workers serve as a link between health educators and other health professionals and community members who need health or social services.
- An entry-level position as a community health worker requires a high school diploma; licensure or certification is not required. However, some states are considering certification, which would require completion of a one- to two-year approved training program.

Work Description

Community Health Workers (CHWs) provide a link between the community and health educators and other healthcare workers and develop and implement strategies to improve the health of individuals and communities. They collect data and discuss health concerns with members of specific populations or communities. Although the two occupations often work together, responsibilities of health educators and community health workers are distinct.

CHWs typically work in underprivileged and marginalized communities where people such as refugees or migrant workers have limited resources and lack access to quality health care. In addition, members of these communities are typically not fluent in English and have values and behaviors different from the dominant Western culture.[10] The role of CHWs is to serve as a bridge between the community and the healthcare, government, and social service systems.

CHWs have an in-depth knowledge of the communities they serve. They identify health-related issues that affect a community, collect data, and discuss health concerns with the people they serve. For example, they may help eligible residents of a neighborhood enroll in programs such as Medicaid, Medicare, or Women, Infants, and Children (WIC), explaining the benefits of these programs. CHWs address any barriers to care and provide referrals for such needs as food, housing, education, and mental health services. They also educate people about the importance and availability of healthcare services, such as cancer screenings or diabetes support groups. They also provide informal counseling and social support.

CHWs report their findings to health educators and healthcare providers so that the educators can create new programs or adjust existing programs or events to better suit the demands of their audience. Community health workers also advocate for the health needs of community members. In addition, they conduct outreach to engage community residents, assist residents with health system navigation, and to improve care coordination.

Work Environment

CHWs work in a variety of settings, including hospitals, nonprofit organizations, government, physicians' offices, private businesses and corporations, and colleges. Community health workers live and work in rural, urban, and metropolitan areas and Native American nations.[10] They may spend much of their time in the field, communicating with community members and holding events. Most community health workers work full time. They may need to work nights and weekends to attend programs or meetings.

TABLE 24.4 Industries Employing the Largest Numbers of Community Health Workers, 2019

Government	18%
Individual and family services	17%
Religious, grantmaking, civic, and other professional organizations	14%
Hospitals	8%
Outpatient care centers	8%

Data from Bureau of Labor Statistics. Occupational Outlook Handbook. U.S. Department of Labor; 2020. https://www.bls.gov/ooh/community-and-social-service/health-educators.htm#tab-3

Employment Opportunities

There were 64,900 jobs in 2019. The industries that employed the most CHWs in 2019 are shown in **TABLE 24.4**.

Education and Legal Requirements

Most entry-level jobs for CHWs require a high school diploma, although some employers may require a postsecondary certificate or an associate's degree. CHWs typically have a shared language or life experience and an understanding of the community that they serve.

Education and Training

CHWs typically have a high school diploma, although some jobs may require postsecondary education. Education programs may lead to a one-year certificate or a two-year associate's degree and cover topics such as wellness, ethics, and cultural awareness, among others. Education programs are based in colleges or in the community.

CHWs typically complete a brief period of on-the-job training. This training often covers core competencies such as communication or outreach skills as well as information about the specific health topics that they will be focusing on. For instance, CHWs who work with Alzheimer's patients may learn about how to communicate effectively with patients dealing with dementia.

Licensure

States do not require CHWs to be licensed. Since some states are considering certification, contact your state's board of health, nursing, or human services to verify requirements for individual states.

Certification and Other Qualifications

Most states do not require CHWs to become certified; however, voluntary certification exists or is being considered or developed in a number of states. Requirements vary but may include completing an approved training program. For more information, contact your state's board of health, nursing, or human services.

CHWs usually have some knowledge of a specific community, population, medical condition, or disability. The ability to speak a foreign language may be helpful. Since they interact with many people from a variety of backgrounds, CHWs must be good listeners and be culturally sensitive to respond to the needs of the people they serve.

Advancement

CHWs with advanced training and experience working with a specific population will have greater opportunities for advancement. In addition, opportunities may be better for candidates who speak a foreign language and understand the culture of the community that they intend to serve.

Employment Trends

As a result of federal health reform there is more emphasis on health prevention to reduce healthcare costs. Because of the emphasis on prevention, there is expected to be greater demands for both health educators and community health workers.

Employment Change

Employment of CHWs is expected to increase 15% between 2019 and 2029, much faster than other occupations. Job growth will come from expanded health coverage and efforts to prevent disease as a result of federal health reform.

Job Prospects

Community health workers who have completed a formal education program and those who have experience working with a specific population may enjoy favorable job prospects. In addition, opportunities may be better for candidates who speak a foreign language. **TABLE 24.5** lists projected new jobs between 2019 and 2029.

Earnings

The median annual wage for CHWs was $42,000 in May 2020. The lowest 10% earned less than $26,660, and the top 10% earned more than $70,790. In May 2020, the median annual wages for CHWs in the top five industries in which they worked are shown in **TABLE 24.6**.

TABLE 24.6 Median Annual Wages in the Industries Employing the Largest Numbers of Community Health Workers, May 2020	
Hospitals	$48,150
Government	$45,490
Outpatient care centers	$44,090
Religious, grantmaking, civic, and other professional organizations	$39,900
Individual and family services	$38,300

Data from Bureau of Labor Statistics. Occupational Outlook Handbook. U.S. Department of Labor; 2020. https://www.bls.gov/ooh/community-and-social-service/health-educators.htm#tab-5

Related Occupations

Other health professionals who have similar training requirements and job responsibilities are social and human service assistants.

ORIENTATION AND MOBILITY SPECIALISTS
Work Description

Orientation and mobility (O&M) specialists teach individuals with visual impairments to travel safely, confidently, and independently in their community. Specialists teach clients to become familiar with the physical space in which they live, work, and play so that they can move from place to place safely. For example, specialists often walk with the client in their neighborhood to teach them how to cross an intersection or to ride public transportation, often with the assistance of a white cane. They work with all ages from infants and children to adults usually on a one-to-one basis in the client's home or school, in a hospital, or in the community. O&M specialists are different from physical, occupational, and recreation therapists because they focus on people with vision loss.[11]

They also may work with those who have multiple disabilities to help them adjust psychologically and achieve maximum independence through specialized training. O&M specialists evaluate their clients to determine their level of adjustment, their degree of motivation, and the extent and safety of their indoor and outdoor mobility. Based on this information, they plan and provide individualized programs for instruction.[11]

Specialists assist clients in making the maximum use of their remaining senses, primarily auditory (sound) and

TABLE 24.5 Projections Data for Community Health Workers, 2019–2029				
			Change, 2019–2029	
Occupational Title	Employment, 2019	Projected Employment, 2029	Number	Percentage
Community health worker	64,900	74,800	9,900	15%

Data from Bureau of Labor Statistics. Occupational Outlook Handbook. U.S. Department of Labor; 2020. https://www.bls.gov/ooh/community-and-social-service/health-educators.htm#tab-6

tactile (touch). They train clients to orient themselves to physical surroundings and use a variety of actual or simulated travel situations to develop the client's ability to travel alone, with or without a cane. For example, the specialist may travel with a client to help them become comfortable and confident in traveling. This may include trips to the airport to become oriented to going through security, checking in before each flight, and locating ground transportation upon landing. For clients who live in a city with public transportation, the specialist would accompany a client to bus or train stops in the neighborhood, place of work, or shopping.[11]

Specialists train clients to use mobility devices and human or dog guides, electronic travel aids, and Global Positioning System (GPS) or other adaptive mobility devices. O&M specialists evaluate and prepare progress reports on each of their clients and work closely with other professionals such as physicians and social workers as well as volunteers and families of clients. They work with others to develop community resources within their area of expertise and attend various professional seminars, workshops, and conferences to keep abreast of the latest methods, techniques, and travel aids.[11]

An O&M specialist works with all ages, from encouraging a blind infant to move toward the sound of a musical toy to a grandmother so that she can navigate the airport to visit her grandchildren in another city. An instructor employed by a Veterans Administration (VA) clinic might orient a 30-year-old blinded veteran with a dog guide to a new job site. Another specialist employed by a university might orient an incoming freshman who is blind to locate classrooms, the library, the physical fitness center, and the cafeteria. In a school setting, the O&M instructor might counsel a high school junior who recently lost his vision about how to be independent despite knowing that he will not be able to obtain a driver's license. A specialist employed by a private agency that provides services for the blind teaches a young man to cross a busy intersection between his job and the nearby shopping center. As an advocate for the blind, the specialist consults with city planners and traffic engineers to design safe intersections for pedestrians who are visually impaired (**FIGURE 24.3**).[11]

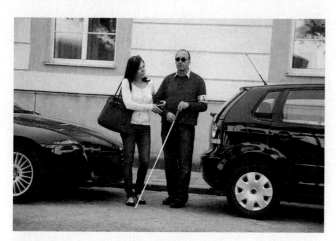

FIGURE 24.3 Orientation and mobility instructors teach the people who are blind to navigate city streets.
© Lisa S./Shutterstock.

Work Environment

O&M specialists are employed in a variety of settings. This could be in the client's home, residential schools for those who are blind, state rehabilitation agencies, assisted-living or nursing care facilities, or the client's place of employment. O&M specialists also work in public schools, colleges and universities, VA hospitals and clinics, public and private agencies for the blind, dog guide schools, and camps for those with disabilities. Some specialists in rural areas are responsible for clients over a large geographic area, requiring considerable travel time. Working conditions for specialists vary from client to client and from one facility to another.

O&M specialists can expect to work a 40-hour week, with hours from 8:00 a.m. to 4:30 p.m., working at one site and traveling to different sites during the day. Specialists may sometimes accompany their clients to recreational activities and social gatherings. Working conditions vary depending on where their client lives. O&M specialists need to be in good physical condition because they spend considerable time working outdoors in all kinds of weather and spend a lot of time walking. Some O&M specialists work as consultants and contract with agencies and private individuals.[11]

Employment Opportunities

Employment prospects for qualified O&M specialists are excellent; available openings far exceed the number of graduates entering the labor market each year. There is a national shortage of mobility instructors. However, vision rehabilitation services are not widely available, especially for older adults.

Except for the VA blind rehabilitation centers, visual impairment services have been available through public schools or social service agencies instead of through the healthcare system. Working adults with visual impairments may receive services through rehabilitation services. Since Medicare does not provide reimbursement for vision rehabilitation, services may be limited for the elderly unless the cost of the services are covered by individual states or by the individual. The medical model and the Centers for Medicare and Medicaid require research to demonstrate the effectiveness or cost-effectiveness of treatment, which is lacking for O&M specialists and vision rehabilitation therapists.[12]

Educational and Legal Requirements

The minimum requirement for entry-level O&M specialists is a bachelor's degree in orientation and mobility including a practicum and an internship.

Education and Training

Entry-level O&M specialists require a bachelor's degree. However, the majority of training programs are offered at the graduate level. For those with a bachelor's degree in another field, a master's degree or graduate certification in orientation and mobility is required. Some programs offer courses online. Successfully completing a certification examination is also required.[11] Degrees are offered in a variety of departments including education, special education, rehabilitation, or communication disorders. The **Association for Education and Rehabilitation of the Blind and Visually Impaired (AER)** lists accredited educational programs for O & M specialists. Academic programs for vision professionals are listed under Additional Information at the end of the chapter. Required courses include literary braille and rehabilitation counseling; core courses are orientation and mobility, communication and instructional methods for those with low vision, as well as a practicum and an internship. Financial aid is often available for students specializing in vision studies through scholarships, assistantships, or grants.[11]

Licensure

There are no nationwide uniform legal requirements for licensing, certification, or registration that serve as standards for employment. State or local licensing agencies should be contacted to determine relevant current standards.

Certification and Other Qualifications

The **Academy for Certification of Vision Rehabilitation (ACVREP)** provides certification for orientation and mobility specialists who meet specified education and experience standards and successfully complete the certification exam. Those who complete all requirements are designated as a **Certified Orientation and Mobility Specialist (COMS)**.[13]

Those considering a career in this area must enjoy working with people and have the capacity to learn from as well as teach clients. This work requires specialists to work closely with families, friends, and colleagues of clients. The work is also physically demanding and requires working outdoors in all kinds of weather. O&M specialists should possess mature judgment, emotional and social maturity, adaptability, resourcefulness, and leadership potential.

Advancement

O&M specialists can advance to supervisory, managerial, and administrative positions in this field. Generally, advancement is based on work experience and expertise, and the completion of advanced education courses.

Job Prospects

Job prospects are excellent for those who are certified as an O&M specialist. Most jobs will be located in large metropolitan areas and in cities that have public transportation. Less populated states may have only one or two O&M specialists that cover the entire state. The VA has 13 regional blind rehabilitation centers across the United States and Puerto Rico that offer O&M training for blind veterans.[14] Because there is a shortage of O&M specialists, training programs often have requests from prospective employers.

Earnings

The average annual salary for O&M specialists was $67,550 in 2020.[15]

Related Occupations

Other health professionals who have similar training requirements and job responsibilities are special education teachers, rehabilitation counselors, low-vision therapists, and vision rehabilitation therapists.

VISION REHABILITATION THERAPISTS
Work Description

Visual Rehabilitation Therapists (VRTs) provide instruction and guidance to clients who have visual impairments to use community resources and assistive technology to enable them to live safe and productive lives. VRTs, formerly called rehabilitation teachers, are specialists in independent living who teach people with limited vision to create new approaches to familiar routines. The VRT evaluates the ability of the client to perform **activities of daily living (ADLs)** and **independent acts of daily living (IADLs)** and psychosocial issues related to vision impairment. They provide specialized methods or adaptive techniques for communication and coping with the demands of daily living.[16]

The VRT may provide instruction to teach clients how to manage ADLs after the loss of sight—for example, personal hygiene, grooming, and table etiquette as well as IADLs (housekeeping, grocery shopping, meal preparation, minor home repairs, managing finances, and navigating the home environment and using public transportation). These therapists also help clients obtain specially designed equipment such as magnifying devices, braille clocks and watches, and various types of aides to compensate for loss of vision. The broad sphere of communication includes braille, the use of computer and recording technology, handwriting, and low-vision technology. They help those who are newly blind develop communication skills by providing instruction in the use of braille, large print, recorded materials, low-vision technology, keyboarding, and telephones. They also teach nonverbal communication skills, such as facial expressions, hand movements, and head nods for use in communication with sighted persons. An example of the VRT suggesting resources such as talking books, recording devices, and radio reading services is shown in **FIGURE 24.4**.[16]

VRTs work with clients of all ages to carry out daily activities; for example, a VRT might show a third grader how to use a magnifier to read directions for a board game, show a senior citizen to use a computer to send an email to a grandchild, teach a college student to read a braille menu when ordering carryout from a restaurant, and train an elderly man to organize and label medications.[16] Each client is unique; beyond the obvious fact that they have visual impairments, the most common attribute of clients is that they are individuals with their own needs and desires, levels

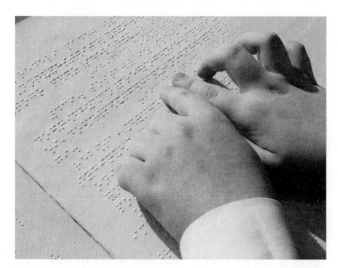

FIGURE 24.4 Visual rehabilitation therapists teach the people who are blind to use braille.
© Alsu/Shutterstock.

of functioning, and goals. These differences must be noted and respected by the therapist, whose role is to help the client reach the level of functioning he or she wishes rather than make the client fit a preconceived image.[16]

Work Environment

VRTs work with individuals or small groups in the home setting as well as in healthcare facilities, such as rehabilitation centers, hospitals and clinics, nursing homes and assisted-living facilities, or community centers. Some travel will be required for VRTs to go to the homes of clients to guide them in making changes to the home environment to make it easier to carry out daily activities. The VRT needs to be familiar with resources on both the local and national levels. They may work with other team members providing services to the client including occupational therapists, dietitians, and others.[16]

Employment Opportunities

The need for qualified VRTs is growing due to increases in the number of persons experiencing blindness or visual impairment, particularly among senior citizens. The elderly often do not receive the assistance needed to maintain independence with loss of vision because Medicare does not cover the cost of vision rehabilitation for nonworking individuals and because vision services for the blind have not been delivered through the healthcare system but instead by social service or educational agencies.[12] However, these individuals will need the professional specialized services that only a vision rehabilitation therapist can provide.

Educational and Legal Requirements

The minimum educational requirements for a VRT is a bachelor's degree plus a graduate certificate and completion of the certification exam for VRTs.

Education and Training

VRTs require a bachelor's degree in any field. Routes to become a VRT are to obtain a graduate certificate or a master's degree in vision rehabilitation therapy including an internship. Degrees are usually offered in education, special education, communication disorders, or rehabilitation programs. Some programs offer distance learning. Successfully completing a certification examination is also required.[16] AER, the professional organization for professionals employed to work with the visually impaired lists accredited programs in vision rehabilitee therapy. Academic programs for vision professionals are listed under Additional Information at the end of the chapter. Required courses include literary braille and rehabilitation counseling; core courses are orientation and mobility and communication and instructional methods for those with low vision.

Licensure

There are no requirements for VRTs to be licensed. However, most employers will require certification, which is not regulated by states.

Certification and Other Qualifications

The ACVREP provides certification for vision rehabilitation therapists. Those who meet specified education and experience standards and successfully complete the certification exam receive the title **Certified Vision Rehabilitation Therapist (CVRT)**.[13]

Advancement

Qualified VRTs can advance to supervisory or administrative positions in health agencies or to teaching positions in colleges or universities. Generally, advancement in this field is governed by experience, skill level, and the completion of advanced degree programs.

Job Prospects

Job prospects are excellent for those who are certified as a vision rehabilitation therapist, especially for those who are willing to go where the jobs are. Most jobs will be located in large metropolitan areas; in less densely populated states, there may only be one center that offers blind rehabilitation. Some jobs are available in schools for the blind and may require a bachelor's degree in special education. The VA has 13 regional blind rehabilitation centers across the United States and Puerto Rico and employ VRTs.[14]

Earnings

The average annual salary for VRTs was $77,337 in 2021.[17] VRTs employed as teachers of the blind in a public school setting can expect to receive a salary similar to other teachers with the same education and experience level.

Professional Profiles

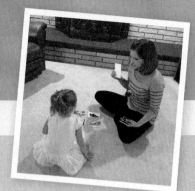

Name: Kristin, BCBA
Job Title: Board Certified Behavior Analyst
Education: BS in Psychology, MS in Psychology

Q: Describe your job and organization.

A: I work for an organization that provides in-home therapy based on the principles of applied behavior analysis to children and adults with autism spectrum disorder (ASD).

Q: Describe a typical workday.

A: Schedules are built around the client's availability, and sessions may occur for full days, before or after school, or weekends depending on the number of hours of therapy recommended by the Board-Certified Behavior Analyst (BCBA). Because every client presents with a different set of skills and skill deficits, each requires a highly individualized curriculum and plan for addressing maladaptive behavior. A BCBA will balance many responsibilities including the assessment of skills and behavior, treatment planning, collecting, graphing and analyzing data, leading meetings with families and staff, and staff training.

Q: Why did you choose this profession?

A: To help people achieve meaningful and socially significant change through the science of behavior analysis and personal qualities of curiosity, perseverance, diligence, ethics, and honesty.

Q: What challenges you most about this profession?

A: Behavior analysts work with clients who display challenging and sometimes dangerous behavior. This can be one of the more difficult aspects of the profession but also one of the most rewarding, particularly when these behaviors can be replaced with more appropriate and adaptive behavior that helps the individual function more effectively within their family unit and community.

Q: Is there room for advancement in this field?

A: Behavior analysts can advance to a clinical director role responsible for support and mentorship for newly certified BCBAs. A doctoral-level credential is also an option.

Q: Name and explain what part of your academic training most prepared you for this profession.

A: Graduate coursework helped to establish the foundation of basic concepts. Fieldwork in clinical settings under the direct supervision and mentorship of experienced behavior analysts was critical in learning to apply these concepts in systematic ways to understand human behavior in the natural world.

Q: What advice would you give someone who is considering this career?

A: Applied behavior analysis therapy with children with ASD is probably the most common and popular placement for a BCBA. However, behavior analysts also work with individuals in drug rehabilitation programs or with those at risk for overweight or obesity who need support in changing dietary or physical activity habits. In the field of organizational behavior management, BCBAs help modify environmental variables to improve work performance or in other settings requiring socially significant behavior change.

Related Occupations

Other health professionals who have similar training requirements job responsibilities are vocational rehabilitation counselor, rehabilitation teacher, orientation and mobility specialist, and occupational therapist.

BEHAVIOR ANALYSTS: AN OVERVIEW

Behavior analysts are in demand because of the high number of infants and children being diagnosed with ASD characterized by skill deficits in communication and adaptive behavior and problem behaviors.[2] All states require that health insurance cover services by behavior analysts. Because of a greater level of awareness of ASD and the effectiveness of behavior analysis in treating ASD, there is earlier diagnosis and intervention of children with ASD and a high demand for professionals able to provide these services. A greater awareness of autism and the need for services has accounted for a dramatic increase in the number of behavior analysts as well as state licensure over the past decade.[18]

There are three different levels of certification in the area of behavior analysis. The **Board-Certified Behavior Analyst (BCBA)** has graduate-level certification in behavior analysis and writes treatment plans and supervises implementation of behavior analysis plans by both the **Board-Certified Assistant Behavior Analyst (BCaBA)**, who has bachelor's level certification, and the **Registered Behavior Technician (RBT)**, a paraprofessional with 40 hours of postsecondary training. The role of the BCBA is to conduct assessments, develop treatment plans, supervise implementation of treatment plans by the BCaBA and RBT, and evaluate and document treatment and modify intervention as necessary. Successfully passing a certification exam administered by the **Behavior Analysis Certification Board (BACB)** is required by all three levels of professionals.[19]

Work Description

Behavior analysts work in schools, homes, and community settings and consult in the design and implementation of treatment plans for a variety of learners across a variety of skills. Behavior analysts are qualified to provide services to clients with a variety of needs and skill deficits—for example, communication and adaptive behavior and problem behavior (aggression, impulsivity, self-injurious behavior). Goals of behavior analysis and intervention are to improve language, motor, social, and reasoning skills. Services usually include conducting behavioral assessments, analyzing assessment data, writing and revising behavior-analytic treatment plans, training others to implement components of treatment plans, and supervising the implementation of treatment plans by others.[19]

Work Environment

Behavior analysts work in schools, hospitals, mental health centers, primary care centers, behavioral centers, residential facilities, and in the client's home. In addition to working with clients with autism who have skill deficits, behavior analysts work in educational settings in areas of curriculum design and evaluation to promote learning for all students (e.g., those in special education as well as the gifted). Work opportunities are expanding to include a variety of subspecialty areas—for example, in brain injury rehabilitation and behavioral gerontology; clients in both settings benefit from developing more appropriate behaviors. In mental health settings, behavior analysts work with those with a variety of symptoms (e.g., stress, chronic pain, anxiety, depression, substance misuse, and problems with relationships). There are new opportunities in corporations and industrial settings to teach job skills and promote work performance of employees. Behavior analysts supervise implementation of treatment plans and communicate with parents and employers.[20]

Employment Opportunities

Employment opportunities are expected to continue to be excellent for BCBA because research has demonstrated the benefits of early intervention and because all states require health insurance to cover the services of the BCBA. The majority (68%) work in the area of autism, 12% work in education, and 8% work in the area of developmental disabilities. Others work as consultants in centers that specialize in treatment of autism, in rehab centers, and in subspecialty areas.[21] Certified assistant behavior analysts and technicians can also expect excellent employment opportunities because these professionals are required to carry out treatment plans.

Education and Legal Requirements

The minimum requirement to become a certified behavior analyst is a master's degree in behavior analysis or certification for those with a master's degree in another field such as psychology, special education, speech pathology, or social work.

Education and Training

To be eligible for certification as a behavior analyst, a master's degree in behavior analysis is required plus 1,000 to 1,500 hours of fieldwork or a supervised internship. Students with a master's degree in a closely related field, such as special education or guidance and counseling, would need to complete a certification program to be eligible for board certification. Courses include behavior assessment, behavior change methods, behavior change systems, managing implementation, and supervision. Each program may have preferences for the educational or experience background of applicants. However, the BACB has specific course content and internship requirements. The Association for Behavior Analysis International lists accredited programs.[22] Programs are typically in departments of education, special education, or psychology. Many programs offer distance education and online courses.[22]

Licensure

In 2019, 31 states required licensure and one state required state certification of BCBA. For the BCaBA, 19 states require licensure, and four of the remaining states require certification or registration. The majority of RBTs are not regulated by the states with the exception of Oregon and Louisiana, which require registration, and Washington, which requires state certification.[23]

Certification and Other Requirements

The BCBA is a graduate-level certification in behavior analysis. Professionals who are certified at the BCBA level are independent practitioners who provide behavior-analytic services. In addition, BCBAs supervise the work of the BCaBA and the RBT, who implement behavior-analytic interventions.[19]

Employment Trends

There has been a rapid increase in the number of behavioral specialists in the United States as a result of licensure and third-party reimbursement for their services. For example, in 2021 there were about 48,000 BCBAs compared to 8,500 in 2011. The most dramatic increase has been for RBTs with about 300 in 2014 and nearly 103,000 in 2021.[21]

Earnings

The median salary for BCBA was $89,457 in August 2021 for those working full time.[24] Salary increases are expected with supervisory responsibilities such as a clinical director.

Additional Information

For more information about health educators, contact:

- ExploreHealthCareers.org. *Behavioral Science/Health Education.* http://explorehealthcareers.org/en/Career/46/Behavioral_ScienceHealth_Education

For more information about public health, visit:

- American Public Health Association, 800 I St. NW, Washington, DC. 20001. http://www.apha.org/what-is-public-health

For information about academic programs in health education, contact:

- Association of Schools and Programs of Public Health, 1615 L St. NW, Suite 510 Washington, DC 20036. http://www.aspph.org/

For accredited programs in public health including health promotion and health education, contact:

- Council on Education for Public Health, 1010 Wayne Ave., Suite 220, Silver Spring, MD 20910. https://ceph.org/about/org-info/who-we-accredit/accredited

For accredited programs in Health Education and Promotion and information on the requirements for CHES and MCHES credentials, contact:

- National Commission for Health Education Credentialing (NCHEC), 1541 Alta Dr., Suite 303, Whitehall, PA 18052-5642. http://www.nchec.org/resources

For information about school health programs, contact:

- American School Health Association, 501 N Morton St, Suite 110, Bloomington, IN 47404. http://www.ashaweb.org/

For academic programs in orientation and mobility and vision rehabilitation therapy, see:

- Texas School for the Blind and Visually Impaired Outreach Programs. *University Directory for Programs in Visual Impairments,* 2016. https://www.tsbvi.edu/images/outreach/Documents/UniversityDirectory-ProgramsVI2016.pdf
- Association for Education in Rehabilitation of the Blind and Visually Impaired (AER). 5680 King Centre Drive, Suite 600, Alexandria, VA 22315. https://aerbvi.org/the-national-accreditation-council/higher-education/

For further information on becoming certified in vision rehabilitation, contact:

- Academy for Certification of Vision Rehabilitation & Education Professionals (ACVREP), 4380 N. Campbell Ave, Suite #200, Tucson, AZ 85718. https://www.acvrep.org/

For more information about careers in vision therapy, contact:

- Association for Education and Rehabilitation of the Blind and Visually Impaired, 5680 King Centre Drive, Suite 600, Alexandria, VA 22315. https://aerbvi.org/

For a list of accredited academic programs offering degree programs that meet the requirements to apply for board certification as a behavior analyst, contact:

- Association for Behavior Analysis International. 550 W. Centre Avenue, Portage, MI 49024. https://accreditation.abainternational.org/accredited-programs.aspx

For information about state regulation of behavior analysts, contact:

- Association of Professional Behavior Analysts (APBA). 3435 Camino del Rio South, Suite 103, San Diego, CA 92108. https://www.apbahome.net

For more information about becoming certified as a behavior analyst, assistant behavior analyst, or behavior technician, contact:

- Behavior Analysis Certification Board. 7950 Shaffer Parkway, Littleton, CO 80127. https://www.bacb.com

LEARNING PORTFOLIO

Issues for Discussion

1. View the one-minute video about health educators from CareerOneStop.org. Based on the video, describe work settings, job responsibilities, and necessary personal qualities of health educators. https://www.careeronestop.org/videos/careeronestop-videos.aspx?videocode=21109100

2. Read the interview with a CHES who works as a Community Outreach Coordinator for a cancer program. https://www.nchec.org/news/posts/community-outreach-coordinator-profile from the National Commission for Health Educator Credentialing (NCHEC). What are the advantages to obtaining the CHES/MCHES credential? What are the requirements for each credential?

3. Go to the Rehabilitation and Prosthetic Services for the U.S. Department of Veterans Affairs website for fact sheets on blind rehabilitation and blind rehabilitation continuum of care. Identify blind rehabilitation specialists who provide service for the VA. http://www.prosthetics.va.gov/

4. Go to the Autism Speaks website to learn about insurance laws in your state for coverage of behavior analysts for treatment of ASD. Autism Speaks. *Health Insurance Coverage for Autism.* https://www.autismspeaks.org/health-insurance-coverage-autism Updated September 2019.

5. View the three-minute video "Behavior Analysis | An Overview" (June 28, 2018). Discuss at least three settings in which behavior analysis is used. https://www.youtube.com/watch?time_continue=31&v=HnyYwWlenJg

Enrichment Activities

1. Link to Careers on the National Commission for Health Education Credentialing website to review at least one work setting for health educators: community, school, worksite, academic, health department, or health care. Give a brief report during class discussion. Which of these settings appeals to you? https://www.nchec.org/

2. Go to the Behavior Analyst Certification Board website to learn more about newer work settings for behavior analysts to improve performance in wellness, sports, or organizational behavior management. https://www.bacb.com/about-behavior-analysis/#ABAFactSheets

3. Review the University Directory for Programs in Visual Impairments to locate a college or university in your state that offers a degree or certification in either orientation and mobility or visual rehabilitation therapy. What sources of financial aid are available for students pursuing either career? https://www.tsbvi.edu/images/outreach/Documents/UniversityDirectory-ProgramsVI2016.pdf

CASE STUDY: HEALTH EDUCATION #1

Trey has been working as a health educator for the D. L. Grove Medical Institute for the past six years. His most recent project centered on physician education and training and focused on a more positive interaction with the patient population that is served at the facility. He obtained his Certified Health Education Specialist (CHES) certification and is currently completing his master's degree in health promotion. Trey has plans to pursue his Master Certified Health Education Specialist (MCHES) within the next few weeks. Trey anticipates applying for a supervisor position with the institute after completing his advanced degree.

Based on the information you have read about health education, answer the following questions.

1. True or false? Trey's most recent project that centered on physician education and training would be considered a common job duty for a health educator in a healthcare facility.

2. True or false? In order for Trey to have obtained his CHES certification, he would have had to complete 180 hours of clinical externship as well as complete a basic diploma program prior to sitting for the qualifying examination.

3. Based on the known median annual wage for health education specialists in 2020, Trey can anticipate earning _____ after receiving his advanced degree.

A. $40,000 per year
B. $45,000 per year
C. $50,000 per year
D. less than $60,000 per year

4. Trey understands that in order to advance to a supervisory position, most facilities require:
A. a graduate degree.
B. at least 10 years of work experience at the facility.
C. specific supervisory training completed online.
D. All of these are correct.

5. Trey has plans to pursue his MCHES credentialing in the next few weeks. What are the requirements for this type of certification?
A. At least 3 years working in the healthcare field
B. Successfully completing the MCHES competency examination
C. Completing 180 hours of continuing education to maintain the certification
D. All of these are correct.

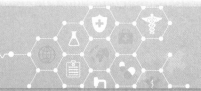

LEARNING PORTFOLIO

CASE STUDY: HEALTH EDUCATION #2

Peggy is preparing to return to the four-year institute where she will complete her bachelor's degree in health education this May. She has plans to complete a teacher preparation program through which she will gain experience through student teaching. Peggy has dreams of becoming a school health educator for the local school district. She anticipates that there will be an opening at the high school next fall and plans to have all of the requirements completed in order to apply. Peggy will also be scheduling her certification exam in May.

1. Peggy understands that most states typically require candidates to:
   A. complete a minimum number of observation hours.
   B. pass a general teaching certification test.
   C. have experience working with children.
   D. All of these are correct.

2. Peggy will meet the minimum requirement by completing:
   A. a bachelor's degree with a background in health education.
   B. a teacher preparation program.
   C. her certification examination.
   D. All of these are correct.

3. Although _____ work in a wide variety of settings these professionals have demonstrated their effectiveness in working with children with autism.

4. Vision specialists who teach their clients to learn skills needed to successfully navigate the community outside their home are _____, while those who teach their clients to function with limited sight in their home or place of employment are _____.

References

1. Erickson W, Lee C, von Schrader S. *2018 Disability Status Report: United States*. Ithaca, NY: Cornell University Yang-Tan Institute on Employment and Disability (YTI), 2020.

2. Centers for Disease Control and Prevention. *Autism Spectrum Disorder (ASD)*. National Center on Birth Defects and Developmental Disabilities. https://www.cdc.gov/ncbddd/autism/index.html Reviewed April 19, 2021. Accessed August 11, 2021.

3. ExploreHealthCareers.org. *Behavioral Science/Health Education*. https://explorehealthcareers.org/career/public-health/behavioral-science-health-education/ Accessed August 9, 2020.

4. Green K. My Career. Health Educator. *Occupational Outlook Quarterly*. Fall 2012. https://www.bls.gov/careeroutlook/2012/fall/mycareer.pdf Accessed August 10, 2021.

5. National Commission for Health Education Credentialing. 3 Ways to Use NCHEC's Health Education and Promotion Program Directory (HEPPD). *News*. June 24, 2020. https://www.nchec.org/news/posts/health-education-and-promotion-program-directory-heppd Accessed August 9, 2020.

6. National Commission for Health Education Credentialing *Exam Eligibility*. https://www.nchec.org/mches-exam-eligibility Accessed August 13, 2021.

7. Society for Public Health Education. *Affordable Care Act: Opportunities and Challenges for Health Education Specialists*. Vision and Leadership for Health Promotion. April 2013.

8. National Commission for Health Education Credentialing. *School Health Education*. https://www.nchec.org/career-profiles-school-health-education Accessed August 12, 2020

9. National Commission for Health Education Credentialing. *Academia & University Health Education*. https://www.nchec.org/career-profiles-academia-university-health-education Accessed August 12, 2020.

10. ExploreHealthCareers.org.. *Community Health Worker*. https://explorehealthcareers.org/career/allied-health-professions/community-health-worker/ Accessed August 9, 2020.

11. Association for Education and Rehabilitation of the Blind and Visually Impaired. *Orientation and Mobility Specialist (O & M): Let's Get Moving: Teaching Independent Travel Skills to Individuals with Vision Loss* https://aerbvi.org/wp-content/uploads/2019/11/OM20191.pdf

12. Agency for Healthcare Research and Quality. *Vision Rehabilitation: Care and Benefit Plan Models: Literature Review*. Rockville, MD: Agency for Healthcare Research and Quality; October 2002. https://www.ahrq.gov/prevention/resources/vision/index.html Accessed August 10, 2021.

13. Academy for Certification of Vision Rehabilitation and Education Professionals. *AVCREP Certifications*. https://www.acvrep.org/certifications/landing Accessed August 10, 2021

14. U.S. Department of Veteran Affairs. *Blind Rehabilitation Centers and Locations*. http://www.prosthetics.va.gov/blindrehab/locations.asp Accessed August 10, 2021.

LEARNING PORTFOLIO

15. ZipRecruiter. *Orientation and Mobility Specialist Salary.* https://www.ziprecruiter.com/Salaries/Orientation-and-Mobility-Specialist-Salary Accessed August 11, 2021.

16. Association for Education and Rehabilitation of the Blind and Visually Impaired. *Vision Rehabilitation Therapists (VRT): Restoring Independence for Individuals with Vision Loss.* https://aerbvi.org/wp-content/uploads/2019/11/VRT20191.pdf Accessed August 10, 2021.

17. ZipRecruiter. *Vision Rehabilitation Therapist Salary.* https://www.ziprecruiter.com/Salaries/Vision-Rehabilitation-Therapist-Salary Accessed August 11, 2021.

18. Johnston JM, Carr JE, Mellichamp FH. A History of the Professional Credentialing of Applied Behavior Analysts. *Behav Anal.* 2017; May 11. doi: 10.1007/s40614-017-0106-9.

19. Behavior Analysis Certification Board (BACB). *Credentials.* http://bacb.com/credentials/ Accessed August 10, 2021.

20. Behavior Analyst Certification Board. *Applied Behavior Analysis Subspecialty Areas.* May 2019. https://www.bacb.com/wp-content/uploads/2020/05/Executive-Summary_210125.pdf Accessed August 10, 2021.

21. Behavior Analyst Certification Board. *BACB Certificant Data.* https://www.bacb.com/BACB-certificant-data Accessed August 10, 2021.

22. The Association for Behavior Analysis International. *Accredited Programs.* https://accreditation.abainternational.org/accredited-programs.aspx Accessed August 10, 2021.

23. Association of Professional Behavior Analysts. *Overview of State Laws to Licensure or Otherwise Regulate Practitioners of Applied Behavior Analysis.* November 2019. https://cdn.ymaws.com/www.apbahome.net/resource/resmgr/State_Regulation_of_BA_Nov20.pdf Accessed August 10, 2021.

24. ZipRecruiter. *Behavioral Analyst Salary.* https://www.ziprecruiter.com/Salaries/Behavioral-Analyst-Salary Accessed August 10, 2021.

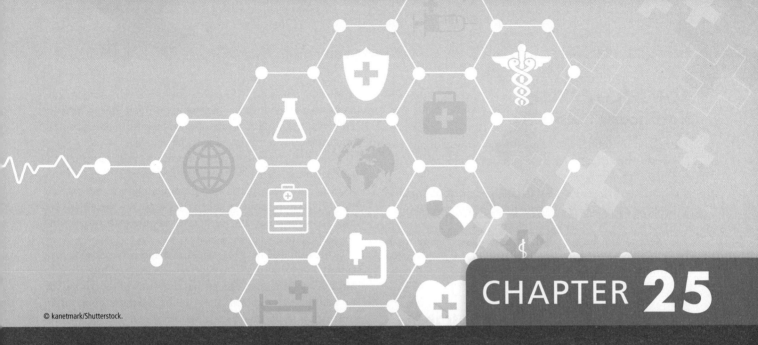
© kanetmark/Shutterstock.

CHAPTER 25

Health Services Administration*

KEY TERMS

Assistant administrators	Healthcare administrators	Philosophy
Associate administrator	Healthcare executives	Policies
Budgets	Marketing	Programs
Chief executive officer (CEO)	Medical and health services managers	Strategic planning
Coordinate	Negotiation	
Financial viability		

* All information in this chapter, unless otherwise indicated, was obtained from Bureau of Labor Statistics. *Occupational Outlook Handbook 2020–2021 Edition*. Washington, DC: U.S. Department of Labor; 2021.

ADMINISTRATION
Significant Points

- Job opportunities will be good, especially for applicants with work experience in health care and strong business and management skills.
- A master's degree is the standard credential, although a bachelor's degree is adequate for some entry-level positions.
- Medical and health services managers typically work long hours and may be called at all hours to deal with problems.

THE NEED FOR PROFESSIONAL MANAGEMENT

Health care is a business, and like every business, it needs good management to keep the business running smoothly. **Medical and health services managers**, also referred to as **healthcare executives** or **healthcare administrators**, plan, direct, coordinate, and supervise the delivery of health care. These workers are either specialists in charge of a specific clinical department, generalists who manage an entire facility or system, or managers of a physician group practice.

The structure and financing of health care are changing rapidly. Future medical and health services managers must be prepared to deal with the integration of healthcare delivery systems, technological innovations, an increasingly complex regulatory environment, restructuring of work, and an increased focus on preventive care. They will be called on to improve efficiency in healthcare facilities and the quality of the care provided.

Large facilities usually have several assistant administrators who aid the top administrator and handle daily decisions. **Assistant administrators** direct activities in clinical areas, such as nursing, surgery, and therapy, and in nonclinical areas, such as information technology and health information management.

In smaller facilities, top administrators handle more of the details of daily operations. For example, many nursing home administrators manage personnel, finances, facility operations, and admissions while also providing resident care.

Clinical managers have training or experience in a specific clinical area and, accordingly, have more specific responsibilities than do generalists. For example, directors of physical therapy are experienced physical therapists, and most health information administrators have a bachelor's degree in health information management. Clinical managers establish and implement **policies**, objectives, and procedures for their departments; evaluate personnel and work quality; develop reports and **budgets**; and **coordinate** activities with other managers.

In group medical practices, managers work closely with physicians. Whereas an office manager might handle business affairs in small medical groups, leaving policy decisions to the physicians themselves, larger groups usually employ a full-time administrator to help formulate business strategies and coordinate day-to-day business.

A small group of 10 to 15 physicians might employ one administrator to oversee personnel matters, billing and collection, budgeting, planning, equipment outlays, and patient flow. A large practice of 40 to 50 physicians might have a chief administrator and several assistants, each responsible for a different area of expertise.

Medical and health services managers in managed care settings perform functions like those of their counterparts in large group practices, except that they may have larger staffs to manage. In addition, they might do more community outreach and preventive care than do managers of a group practice.

Some medical and health services managers oversee the activities of a number of hospitals in health systems. Such systems might contain both inpatient and outpatient facilities and offer a wide range of patient services.

Managers in all settings will be needed to improve the quality and efficiency of health care while controlling costs, as insurance companies and Medicare demand higher levels of accountability. Managers also will be needed to oversee the creation, use, and storage of electronic patient records and ensure their security as required by law. Additional demand for managers will stem from the need to recruit workers and increase employee retention, to comply with changing regulations, to implement new technology, and to help improve the health of their communities by emphasizing preventive care.

Another aspect of professional management is the need to address the extensive oversight and scrutiny to which health facilities are subject. Both past performance and future plans are subject to review by a variety of groups and organizations, including consumer groups, government agencies, professional oversight bodies, insurance companies and other third-party payers, business coalitions, and even the courts. Preparing for inspection visits by observers from regulatory and accrediting bodies and submitting appropriate records and documentation can be time-consuming as well as technically demanding.

HEALTH SERVICES MANAGERS
Work Description

Health services manager is an inclusive term for individuals in many different positions who plan, organize, and coordinate the delivery of health care. Hospitals provide more than half of all jobs in this field. Other employers of health services managers include medical group practices; outpatient clinics; health maintenance organizations (HMOs); nursing homes; hospices; home health agencies; rehabilitation, community mental health, emergency care, and diagnostic imaging centers; and offices of doctors, dentists, and other health practitioners.

Three functional levels of administration are found in hospitals and other large facilities—executive, internal management, and specialized staff. The **chief executive officer (CEO)** provides overall management direction but also is concerned with community outreach, planning, policy making, response to government agencies and regulations, and **negotiation**. The CEO often speaks before civic groups, promotes public participation in health **programs**, and coordinates the activities of the hospital or facility with those of government or community agencies. Institutional planning is an increasingly important responsibility of chief administrators, who continually must assess the need for services, personnel, facilities, and equipment and periodically recommend changes such as shutting down a maternity ward or opening an outpatient clinic.

Chief administrators need leadership ability as well as technical skills to respond effectively to community requirements for health care while at the same time satisfying demand for **financial viability**, cost containment, and public and professional accountability. Within a single institution, such as a community hospital, the healthcare administrator is directly accountable to a board of trustees made up of community leaders who are voted onto the board to determine broad policies and objectives for the hospital. Day-to-day management, particularly in large facilities, may be the responsibility of one or more associate or assistant administrators, who work with service unit managers and staff specialists.

Depending on the size of the facility, assistant or **associate administrators** may be responsible for budget and finance; human resources, including personnel administration, education, and in-service training; information management; and direction of the medical, nursing, ancillary services, housekeeping, physical plant, and other operating departments. As the healthcare system becomes more specialized, skills in financial management, **marketing**, **strategic planning**, systems analysis, and labor relations will be needed as well.

Hospital and nursing home administration differ in important respects. Hospitals are complex organizations, housing as many as 30 highly specialized departments, including admissions, surgery, clinical laboratory, therapy, emergency medicine, nursing, physical plant, health information services, accounting, and so on. The hospital administrator works with the governing board in establishing general policies and operating **philosophy** and provides direction to the department heads and the assistant administrators (or vice presidents), who implement those policies. The hospital administrator coordinates the activities of the assistant administrators and department heads to ensure that the hospital runs efficiently, provides high-quality medical care, and recovers adequate revenue to remain solvent or profitable. Administrators represent the hospital to the community and the state. Nationally, they participate in professional associations such as the American Hospital Association, the American Public Health Association, and the Association of Mental Health Administrators.

Nursing home administrators need many of the same management skills as hospital administrators. Administrative staffs in nursing homes, however, are typically much smaller than those in hospitals. Nursing home administrators often have only one or two assistant administrators and sometimes none. As a result, nursing home administrators are involved in day-to-day management decisions much more often than hospital administrators in all but the smallest hospitals. Nursing home administrators wear various hats—personnel director, director of finance, director of facilities, and admissions director, for example. They analyze data and then make daily management decisions in all of these areas. In addition, because many nursing home residents stay for months or even years, administrators must try to create an environment that nourishes residents' psychological, social, and spiritual well-being as well as tends to their healthcare needs.

In the growing field of group practice management, administrators and managers need to be able to work effectively with the physicians who own the practice. An example of a health services manager meeting with a physician is seen in **FIGURE 25.1**. Specific job duties vary according to the size of the practice. While an office manager handles the business side in very small medical groups, leaving policy decisions to the physicians themselves, larger groups generally employ a full-time administrator to provide advice on business strategies and coordinate the day-to-day management of the practice.

A group of 10 or 15 physicians might employ a single administrator to oversee personnel matters, billing and collection, budgeting, planning, equipment outlays, advertising, and patient flow, whereas a practice of 40 or 50 physicians would require a chief administrator and several assistants, each responsible for a different area of management. In addition to providing overall management direction, the chief administrator of a group practice is responsible for ensuring that the practice maintains or strengthens its competitive position. This is no small task, given the rapidly changing nature of the healthcare environment. Ensuring competitiveness might entail market research to analyze the services the practice currently offers and those it might offer, negotiating contracts with hospitals or other healthcare providers to gain access to specialized facilities and equipment, or entering into joint ventures for the purchase of an expensive piece of medical equipment, such as a magnetic resonance imager.

Managers in HMOs perform all the functions of administrators and managers in large medical group practices plus one additional function—administering what amounts to an insurance company. HMO subscribers pay an annual fee that covers almost all of their care. HMO managers must establish a comprehensive medical benefits package with enrollment fees low enough to attract adequate enrollments but high enough to operate successfully. In addition, they may work more in the areas of community outreach and preventive care than do managers of a group practice. The size of the administrative staff in HMOs varies according to the size and type of HMO. Some health services managers

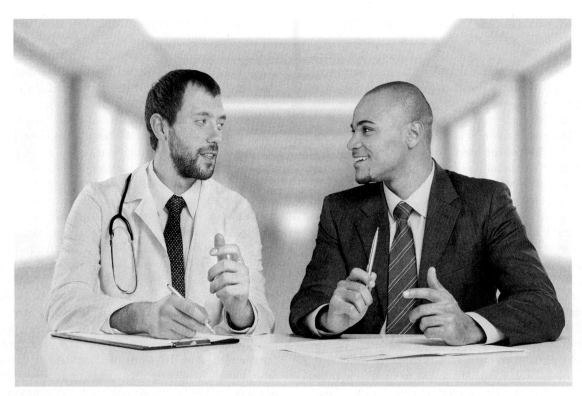

FIGURE 25.1 Meeting of health services manager and physician.
© BillionPhotos/Shutterstock.

oversee the activities of health systems that may encompass a number of inpatient and outpatient facilities and offer a wide range of patient services.

Work Environment

Health services managers often work long hours. Facilities such as nursing homes and hospitals operate around the clock, and administrators and managers may be called at all hours to deal with emergencies. The job also may include travel to attend meetings or to inspect healthcare facilities.

Employment Opportunities

Medical and health services managers held about 422,300 jobs in 2019. About 33% worked in hospitals, and another 22% worked in offices of physicians or in nursing and residential care facilities. Most of the remainder worked in home healthcare services, federal government healthcare facilities, outpatient care centers, insurance companies, and community care facilities for the elderly.

Educational and Legal Requirements

Health services managers must be familiar with management principles and practices. A master's degree in health services administration, long-term care administration, health sciences, public health, public administration, or business

administration is the standard credential for most generalist positions in this field. A bachelor's degree, however, is adequate for some entry-level positions in smaller facilities and for some entry-level positions at the departmental level within healthcare organizations. In addition, physicians' offices and some other facilities may accept on-the-job experience as a substitute for formal education.

Education and Training

For clinical department heads, a degree and work experience in the appropriate field may be sufficient for entry, but a master's degree in health services administration or a related field may be required to advance. For example, nursing services administrators are usually chosen from among supervisory registered nurses who have administrative abilities and a graduate degree in nursing or health services administration.

Bachelor's, master's, and doctoral degree programs in health administration are offered by colleges, universities, and schools of public health, medicine, allied health, public administration, and business administration. In 2021, 124 schools had accredited programs leading to a master's degree in health services administration, according to the Commission on Accreditation of Healthcare Management Executives (CAHME).[1]

Some graduate programs seek out students with undergraduate degrees in business or health administration; others prefer students with a liberal arts or health profession background. Candidates with previous work experience in health care may also have an advantage. Competition for entry into these graduate programs is keen, and applicants need above-average grades to gain admission.

Graduate degree programs usually last between two and three years. They may include as much as one year of supervised administrative experience and coursework in hospital organization and management, marketing, accounting and budgeting, human resource administration, strategic planning, law and ethics, biostatistics or epidemiology, health economics, and health information systems. Some programs allow students to specialize in one type of facility—hospitals, nursing homes, mental health facilities, or medical groups. Other programs encourage a generalist approach to health administration education. The types of concepts a health services manager must know are seen in the word cloud featured in **FIGURE 25.2**.

Recent graduates with master's degrees in health services administration may start as department managers or in staff positions. The level of the starting position varies with the experience of the applicant and the size of the organization. Hospitals and other health facilities offer postgraduate residencies and fellowships, which are usually staff positions. Graduates from master's degree programs also take jobs in HMOs, large group medical practices, clinics, mental health facilities, multi-facility nursing home corporations, and consulting firms.

Graduates with bachelor's degrees in health administration usually begin as administrative assistants or assistant department heads in larger hospitals or as department heads or assistant administrators in small hospitals or nursing homes.

Licensing and Certification

All states and the District of Columbia require nursing home administrators to have a bachelor's degree, pass a licensing examination, complete a state-approved training program, and pursue continuing education. Some states also require licenses for administrators in assisted-living facilities. A license is not required in other areas of medical and health services management.

Certification is another option for health services managers. The American College of Medical Practice Executives (ACMPE) offers the credentials of a Certified Medical Practice Executive and a Fellow.[2] The Professional Association of Healthcare Office Management (PAHCOM) offers two certification options: one in health information technology called the HIT Certified Manager (HITCM-PP)[3] and one in medical office management called the Certified Medical Manager (CMM).[4] The American College of Healthcare Administrators (ACHA) offers the Certified Nursing Home Administrator (CNHA) and the Certified Assisted Living Administrator (CALA) credentials.[5]

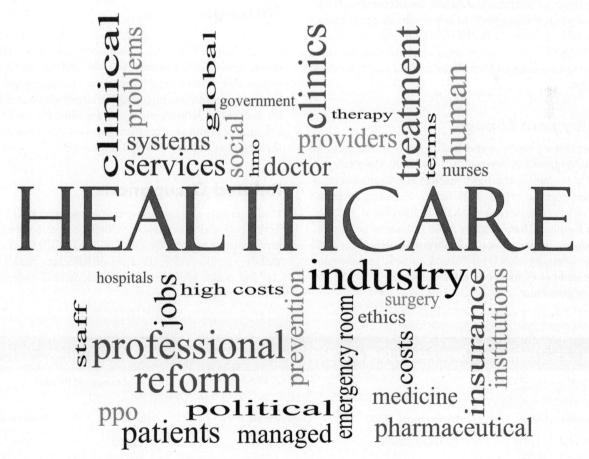

FIGURE 25.2 The types of concepts a health services manager must know can be very varied.
© Keith Bell/Shutterstock.

Other Qualifications

Health services managers often are responsible for millions of dollars in facilities and equipment and hundreds of employees. In order to make effective decisions, they need to be open to different opinions and be good at analyzing contradictory information. They must understand finance and information systems and be able to interpret data. They must be able to follow advances in laws, regulations, and healthcare technology. These managers need problem-solving skills so that they can reach creative solutions to complex problems. Motivating others to implement their decisions requires strong leadership abilities. Tact, diplomacy, flexibility, and communication skills are essential because health services managers spend most of their time interacting with others.

Advancement

Health services managers advance by moving into higher-paying positions with more responsibility, such as assistant or associate administrator, or by moving to larger facilities. Some experienced managers also may become consultants or professors of healthcare management.

Employment Trends

Employment of medical and health services managers is expected to grow faster than the average for all occupations. A demand for increase in health services overall will be seen as the large Baby Boom population ages and requires care, generating a need for additional medical and health services managers.

Employment Change

Employment of medical and health services managers is expected to grow 32% between 2019 and 2029. Hospitals will continue to employ the most medical and health services managers over the 2019 to 2029 decade. However, the number of new jobs created is expected to increase at a slower rate in hospitals than in many other industries because of the growing use of clinics and other outpatient care sites. Despite relatively slow employment growth in hospitals, a large number of new jobs will be created because of the industry's large size.

Employment will grow fast in offices of health practitioners. Many services previously provided in hospitals will continue to shift to these settings, especially as medical technologies improve. Demand in medical group practice management will grow as medical group practices become larger and more complex. As the population ages, there will be an increased demand for nursing home administrators. Managers with knowledge of health information management, health information technology, and informatics will be in demand to organize, manage, and integrate patient health records across the many areas of the healthcare industry.

Medical and health services managers also will be employed by healthcare management companies that provide management services to hospitals and other organizations and to specific departments such as emergency, information management systems, managed care contract negotiations, and physician recruiting. As insurance companies and Medicare demand higher levels of accountability, medical and health services managers will be needed in all healthcare settings to improve the quality and efficiency of health care while controlling costs, and hospitals will continue to be the largest employers of medical and health services managers over the 2019 to 2029 decade. **TABLE 25.1** shows some projection data provided by the U.S. Department of Labor.

Earnings

According to May 2020 data, median annual earnings of medical and health services managers were $104,280. The lowest 10% earned less than $59,980, and the highest 10% earned more than $195,630 per year. Median annual earnings in the industries employing the largest number of medical and health services managers are shown in **TABLE 25.2**. Earnings of health services managers vary by type and size of the facility as well as by level of responsibility.

Related Occupations

Health services managers have training or experience in both health care and management. Other occupations requiring knowledge of both fields are public health directors, social welfare administrators, directors of voluntary health agencies and health professional associations, and underwriters in health insurance companies.

TABLE 25.1 Projections Data for Medical and Health Services Managers, 2019–2029

Occupational Title	Employment, 2019	Projected Employment, 2029	Change, 2019–2029	
			Number	Percentage
Medical and health services managers	422,300	555,500	133,200	32%

Data from Bureau of Labor Statistics, U.S. Department of Labor. Occupational Outlook Handbook. U.S. Department of Labor; 2020. https://www.bls.gov/ooh/management/medical-and-health-services-managers.htm#tab-6

TABLE 25.2 Median Annual Earnings in the Industries Employing the Largest Number of Medical and Health Service Managers, 2020

Government	$116,380
Hospitals; state, local, and private	$112,870
Outpatient care centers	$100,690
Offices of physicians	$94,240
Nursing care facilities	$89,880

Data from Bureau of Labor Statistics, U.S. Department of Labor. Occupational Outlook Handbook. U.S. Department of Labor; 2020. https://www.bls.gov/ooh/management/medical-and-health-services-managers.htm#tab-5

Additional Information

General information about health administration is available from:

- American College of Healthcare Executives, One North Franklin St., Suite 1700, Chicago, IL 60606. https://www.ache.org

Information about undergraduate and graduate academic programs in this field is available from:

- Association of University Programs in Health Administration, 2000 14th St. North, Suite 780, Arlington, VA 22201. https://www.aupha.org

For a list of accredited graduate programs in health services administration, contact:

- Commission on Accreditation of Health Care Management Educators, 2111 Wilson Blvd., Suite 700, Arlington, VA 22201. https://www.cahme.org

For information about career opportunities in long-term care administration, contact:

- American College of Health Care Administrators, 1321 Duke St., Suite 400, Alexandria, VA 22314. https://achca.org

For information about career opportunities in medical group practices and ambulatory care management, contact:

- Medical Group Management Association, 104 Inverness Terrace East, Englewood, CO 80112. https://www.mgma.com
- American College of Medical Practice Executives, 104 Inverness Terrace East, Englewood, CO 80112. https://www.acmpe.com

For information about healthcare office managers, contact:

- Professional Association of Health Care Office Managers, 1576 Bella Cruz Dr., Suite 360, Lady Lake, FL 32159. http://www.pahcom.com

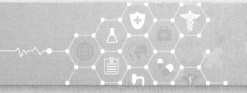

LEARNING PORTFOLIO

Issues for Discussion

1. Graduates of medical and health service management programs have been exposed to numerous specialized areas, including finance, government relations, human resources, information systems, marketing and public affairs, materials management (purchasing of equipment and supplies), medical staff relations, nursing administration, patient care services, and planning and development. Choose which of those areas you believe might be the most challenging to learn about and which area might be easiest to learn about. Discuss your reasoning with your instructor and classmates.

2. What attribute do you think is most important to possess when working as a health services manager? Why?

Enrichment Activities

1. View the following videos explaining careers in health services management: https://www.youtube.com/watch?v=XpMJL-f4pF8, https://www.youtube.com/watch?v=d6_0MxDMPBw, and https://www.youtube.com/watch?v=B3GMyZ87gMY. Discuss the roles performed by health services managers with your instructor and classmates.

2. Many students have questions about salaries for a chosen career. Review the following video that discusses healthcare administrator salaries: https://www.healthcarefinancenews.com/news/study-sheds-light-executive-pay-healthcare-industry Note how salaries vary according to the role played, and identify how a bonus can affect compensation.

CASE STUDY: AN ADMINISTRATOR'S WORK LIFE

Jillian is the assistant administrator at a small rehabilitation clinic in Johnstown, Pennsylvania. She is responsible for scheduling not only the staff but the patients as well. Jillian typically works during the daylight hours to assist with daily operations of the facility. She has also been assigned to handle personnel and financial responsibilities for the establishment.

Based on the information you have read about administrators, please answer the following questions.

1. True or false? As an assistant administrator, Jillian should not be responsible for handling the financial operations of the facility.

2. True or false? Jillian would most likely also be responsible for establishing and implementing policies and procedures in her clinical area.

3. True or false? Jillian has an obligation to handle more of the daily operations because this is a small facility.

4. True or false? Jillian most likely has a bachelor's degree in health information management.

5. True or false? Jillian should be expected to provide rehabilitation services to the patients.

References

1. Commission on Accreditation of Healthcare Management Education. CAHME Accredited Programs Database. https://cahme.org/healthcare-management-education-accreditation/about-cahme/ Accessed August 30, 2021.

2. American College of Medical Practice Executives, Board Certification Through ACMPE. https://www.mgma.com/certification/board-certification Accessed August 30, 2021.

3. Professional Association of Healthcare Office Management. HIT Certified Manager. https://my.pahcom.com/hit Accessed August 30, 2021.

4. Professional Association of Healthcare Office Management. Certified Medical Manager. https://my.pahcom.com/cmm Accessed August 30, 2021.

5. American College of Healthcare Administrators. Eligibility Requirements. https://www.achca.org/certification Accessed August 30, 2021.

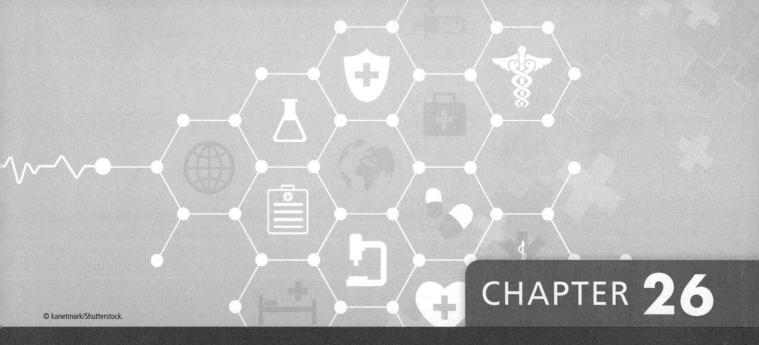

© kanetmark/Shutterstock.

CHAPTER **26**

Emergency Medical Technicians and Paramedics*

KEY TERMS

Advanced airway devices
Advanced emergency medical
  technician
Electrocardiograms (ECGs)
Emergency equipment
Emergency medical responder

Emergency medical services
  (EMS)
Emergency medical technician
  (EMT)
Emergency skills
Endotracheal intubations

First responder
National Registry of Emergency
  Medical Technicians (NREMT)
Paramedic
Trauma centers
Volunteer EMTs

* All information in this chapter, unless otherwise indicated, was obtained from Bureau of Labor Statistics. *Occupational Outlook Handbook 2020–2021 Edition*. Washington, DC: U.S. Department of Labor; 2021.

HIGH DRAMA IN HEALTH CARE

Paramedics, or **emergency medical technicians (EMTs)**, have a career that is often very dramatic, calling for immediate, calm application of the EMT's skills amid sometimes dangerous conditions. The September 11, 2001, attack on the World Trade Center was the most dramatic and deadly situation that paramedics, along with teams of firefighters and police, had ever faced, and they lived up to their potential and training with great heroism. If you watched the terrible events unfolding at that scene at the time or later in a video feed, you saw many of them in action as their ambulances drove through dangerous smoke, fire, and rubble to help rescue and transport the critically injured to hospitals. Their bravery in the face of peril speaks well of the crucial role played by paramedics in times of crisis as well as in everyday life.

Although not every call received by a paramedic team is a life-or-death situation, the potential for drama always exists. The remainder of this chapter details the dramatic as well as the mundane aspects of this healthcare profession.

EMT-PARAMEDICS
Significant Points

- Employment is projected to grow faster than the average for all occupations.
- Emergency medical technicians and paramedics need formal training and certification or licensure, but requirements vary by state.
- Emergency services function 24 hours a day, so EMTs and paramedics have irregular working hours.
- Opportunities will be best for those who have earned advanced certifications.

Work Description

People's lives often depend on the quick reaction and competent care of EMTs and paramedics. Incidents as varied as automobile accidents, heart attacks, slip and falls, childbirth, and gunshot wounds all require immediate medical attention. EMTs and paramedics provide this vital service as they care for and transport the sick or injured to a medical facility.

In an emergency, EMTs and paramedics are typically dispatched by a 911 operator to the scene, where they often work with police and firefighters. Collectively, EMTs, paramedics, police officers, and firefighters are often referred to as **first responders**. Once they arrive, EMTs and paramedics assess the nature of the patient's condition while trying to determine whether the patient has any preexisting medical conditions. Following medical protocols and guidelines, they provide appropriate emergency care and, when necessary, transport the patient. Some paramedics are trained to treat patients with minor injuries at the scene of an accident, or they may treat them at their home, without transporting them to a medical facility. Emergency treatment is carried out under the medical direction of physicians.

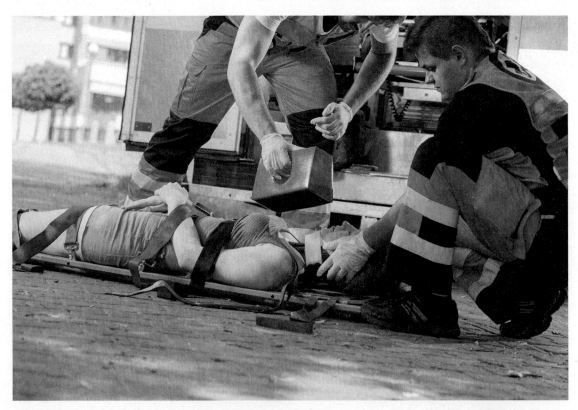

FIGURE 26.1 Paramedics placing patient on a backboard.
© Photographee.eu/Shutterstock.

EMTs and paramedics may use special equipment, such as backboards, to immobilize patients before placing them on stretchers and securing them in the ambulance for transport to a medical facility. An example of a patient placed on a backboard is seen in **FIGURE 26.1**. These healthcare workers generally go out in teams. During the transport of a patient, one EMT or paramedic drives while the other monitors the patient's vital signs and gives additional care as needed. Some paramedics work as part of a helicopter's flight crew to transport critically ill or injured patients to hospital **trauma centers**.

At the medical facility, EMTs and paramedics help transfer patients to the emergency department, report their observations and actions to emergency department staff, and may provide additional emergency treatment. They document the care they provided to the patient. After each run, EMTs and paramedics replace used supplies and check equipment. If a transported patient had a contagious disease, EMTs and paramedics decontaminate the interior of the ambulance and report cases to the proper authorities.

EMTs and paramedics also provide transportation for patients from one medical facility to another, particularly if they work for private ambulance services. Patients often need to be transferred to a hospital that specializes in their injury or illness or to a nursing home.

Beyond these general duties, the specific responsibilities of EMTs and paramedics depend on their level of qualification and training. The **National Registry of Emergency Medical Technicians (NREMT)** certifies emergency medical service providers at four levels: Emergency Medical Responder, Emergency Medical Technician, Advanced Emergency Medical Technician, and Paramedic.[1] Some states, however, have their own certification programs and use distinct names and titles.

The **emergency medical responder** represents the first component of the EMT system. An EMT trained at this level is prepared to care for patients at the scene of an accident and while transporting patients by ambulance to the hospital under medical direction. The emergency medical responder has the **emergency skills** to assess a patient's condition and manage respiratory, cardiac, and trauma emergencies.

The **EMT** represents the second component of the EMT system and has more advanced training. EMTs perform interventions with the basic equipment typically found on an ambulance. However, the specific tasks that those certified at this level are allowed to perform vary greatly from one state to another. **Advanced emergency medical technicians** represent the third component of the EMT system. They have the skills of an EMT plus the knowledge and skills necessary to operate both the basic and advanced equipment found on a typical ambulance. An example of EMTs with a patient in an ambulance is seen in **FIGURE 26.2**.

Paramedics represent the fourth component of the EMT system and provide the most extensive prehospital

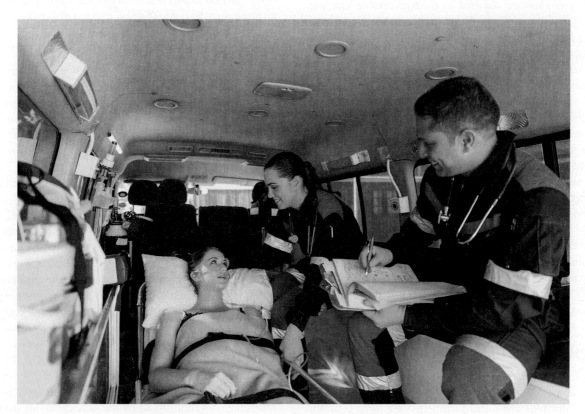

FIGURE 26.2 EMTs with a patient in an ambulance.
© michaeljung/Shutterstock.

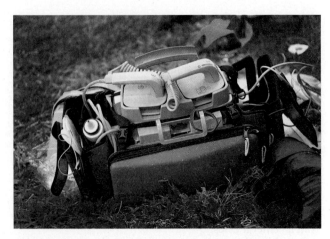

FIGURE 26.3 Portable defibrillator for cardiac emergencies.
© Kijja Pruchyathamkorn/Shutterstock.

care. In addition to carrying out the procedures of the other levels, paramedics may administer drugs orally and intravenously, interpret **electrocardiograms (ECGs),** perform **endotracheal intubations**, and use monitors and other complex equipment. An example of complex equipment is a heart defibrillator, seen in **FIGURE 26.3**. As with an advanced EMT, however, what paramedics are permitted to do varies by state.

Work Environment

EMTs and paramedics work both indoors and out in all types of weather. They are required to do considerable kneeling, bending, and heavy lifting. These workers risk noise-induced hearing loss from sirens and back injuries from lifting patients. In addition, EMTs and paramedics may be exposed to diseases such as hepatitis B and AIDS as well as violence from mentally unstable patients. The work not only is physically strenuous but can also be stressful, sometimes involving life-or-death situations and suffering patients. Nonetheless, many people find the work exciting and challenging and enjoy the opportunity to help others.

EMTs and paramedics employed by fire departments work about 50 hours a week. Those employed by hospitals frequently work between 45 and 60 hours a week, and those in private ambulance services work between 45 and 50 hours. Some of these workers, especially those in police and fire departments, are on call for extended periods. Some shifts are 12 hours in length, while other shifts are 24 hours in length. Because emergency services function 24 hours a day, EMTs and paramedics have irregular working hours.

Employment Opportunities

EMTs and paramedics held about 265,200 jobs in 2019. Most career EMTs and paramedics work in metropolitan areas. **Volunteer EMTs** and paramedics are more common in small cities, towns, and rural areas. These individuals volunteer for fire departments, **emergency medical services (EMS)**, or hospitals and may respond to only a few calls per month.

Paid EMTs and paramedics were employed in a number of industries. About 46% worked as employees of private ambulance services. About 28% worked in local governments. Another 19% worked in hospitals. The type of work or responsibility within each employment service is as follows:

1. Private ambulance services are usually contracted by private or public organizations for emergency situations.

2. Local governments are usually required to provide ambulance emergency medical services associated with the fire and police departments.

3. Hospitals obviously are required to provide the same services for patients in emergency situations.

Educational and Legal Requirements

Generally, a high school diploma and a cardiopulmonary resuscitation (CPR) certificate are required to enter a training program to become an EMT or paramedic. Workers must complete a formal training and certification process. Most of these training programs are postsecondary non-degree award programs that can be completed in less than one year; others last up to two years. Paramedics, however, may need an associate's degree.

Education and Training

A high school diploma and a cardiopulmonary resuscitation certificate are usually required to enroll in a formal EMT training program. A list of accredited programs for EMTs and paramedics, by state, is maintained by the Commission on Accreditation of Allied Health Education Programs.[2] Training is offered at progressive levels: Emergency Medical Responder, Emergency Medical Technician, Advanced Emergency Medical Technician, and Paramedic.

At the emergency medical responder and EMT levels, coursework emphasizes emergency skills, such as managing respiratory, trauma, and cardiac emergencies, and patient assessment. Formal courses are often combined with time in an emergency room or ambulance. The program provides instruction and practice in dealing with bleeding, fractures, airway obstruction, cardiac arrest, and emergency childbirth. Students learn how to use and maintain common **emergency equipment**, such as backboards, suction devices, splints, oxygen delivery systems, and stretchers. Graduates of approved emergency medical responder or EMT training programs must pass a written and practical examination administered by the state certifying agency or the NREMT.

At the Advance Emergency Medical Technician level, training requirements vary by state. The nationally defined level typically requires 300 to 350 hours of training based on the scope of practice. Students learn advanced skills, such as the use of **advanced airway devices**, intravenous fluids, and some medications. Advanced EMTs must pass a written and practical examination administered by the state certifying agency or the NREMT.

The most advanced level of training for this occupation is Paramedic. At this level, the caregiver receives training in anatomy and physiology as well as advanced medical skills. Most commonly, the training is conducted in community colleges and technical schools over one to two years and may result in an associate's degree. Such education prepares the graduate to take the NREMT examination and become certified as a paramedic. Extensive related coursework and clinical and field experience is required. Refresher courses and continuing education are available for EMTs and paramedics at all levels.

High school students interested in becoming an EMT or paramedic should take courses in health, biology, anatomy, and physiology. Courses that improve problem-solving skills will assist the future EMT or paramedic.

Licensure

All 50 states require certification for each of the EMT levels. In most states and the District of Columbia, registration with the NREMT is required at some or all levels of certification. Other states administer their own certification examination or provide the option of taking either the NREMT or state examination. To maintain certification, EMTs and paramedics must recertify, usually every two years. Generally, they must be working as an EMT or paramedic and meet a continuing education requirement.

Other Qualifications

EMTs and paramedics should be emotionally stable; have good dexterity, agility, and physical coordination; and be able to lift and carry heavy loads. They also need good eyesight—corrective lenses may be used—with accurate color vision. Strong listening and speaking skills are necessary so that the EMT or paramedic can determine the extent of a patient's illness or injury and give orders and direction for immediate care. Because most situations involve an emergency, EMTs and paramedics must be compassionate, especially with those patients who are in life-threatening situations or experiencing severe emotional or mental distress.

Advancement

Paramedics can become supervisors, operations managers, administrative directors, or executive directors of emergency services. Some EMTs and paramedics become instructors, dispatchers, or physician assistants; others move into sales or marketing of emergency medical equipment. A number of people become EMTs and paramedics to test their interest in health care before training as registered nurses, physicians, or other health workers.

Employment Trends

Employment for EMTs and paramedics is expected to grow faster than the average for all occupations through 2029. Job prospects should be good, particularly in cities and with private ambulance services.

Employment Change

Employment of EMTs and paramedics is expected to grow by 6% between 2019 and 2029, which is faster than the average for all occupations. Full-time, paid EMTs and paramedics will be needed to replace unpaid volunteers. It is becoming increasingly difficult for emergency medical services to recruit and retain unpaid volunteers because of the amount of training and the large time commitment these positions require. As a result, more paid EMTs and paramedics are needed. Furthermore, as a large segment of the population—aging members of the Baby Boom generation—becomes more likely to have medical emergencies, demand will increase for EMTs and paramedics. Demand for part-time, volunteer EMTs and paramedics will continue in rural areas and smaller metropolitan areas.

Job Prospects

Job prospects should be favorable. Many job openings will arise from growth and from the need to replace workers who leave the occupation because of the limited potential for advancement as well as the modest pay and benefits in private-sector jobs.

Job opportunities should be best in private ambulance services. Competition will be greater for jobs in local governments, including fire, police, and independent third-service rescue squad departments, which tend to have better salaries and benefits. As clients and patients expect and demand higher levels of care before arriving at the hospital, EMTs and paramedics who have advanced education and certifications, such as paramedic-level certification, should enjoy the most favorable job prospects. **TABLE 26.1** shows some projections data provided by the U.S. Department of Labor.

Earnings

Earnings of EMTs and paramedics depend on the employment setting and geographic location of their jobs, as well as their training and experience.

Median hourly wages of EMTs and paramedics were $17.62 in May 2020. The middle 50% earned between $14.03 and $22.99. The lowest 10% earned less than $11.85, and the highest 10% earned more than $29.88. Median hourly wages in the industries employing the largest numbers of EMTs and paramedics in May 2020 were $17.86 in

			Change, 2019–2029	
TABLE 26.1 Projections Data for Emergency Medical Technicians and Paramedics, 2019–2029				
Occupational Title	**Employment, 2019**	**Projected Employment, 2029**	**Number**	**Percentage**
Emergency medical technicians and paramedics	265,200	282,200	17,000	6%

Data from Bureau of Labor Statistics, U.S. Department of Labor. Occupational Outlook Handbook. U.S. Department of Labor; 2020. https://www.bls.gov/ooh/healthcare/emts-and-paramedics.htm#tab-6

other ambulatory healthcare services and $21.47 in local government.

Many EMTs participate in unions.

Related Occupations

Other workers in occupations that require quick and level-headed reactions to life-or-death situations are emergency management directors, firefighters, physician assistants, police officers and detectives, and registered nurses.

Additional Information

General information about EMTs and paramedics is available from:

- National Association of Emergency Medical Technicians, P.O. Box 1400, Clinton, MS 39060-1400. https ://www.naemt.org
- National Association of State EMS Officials, 201 Park Washington Court, Falls Church, VA 22046-4527. https://www.nasemso.org
- National Highway Traffic Safety Administration, Office of Emergency Medical Services, 1200 New Jersey Ave. SE, NTI-140, Washington, DC 20590. https://www .ems.gov
- National Registry of Emergency Medical Technicians, Rocco V. Morando Bldg., 6610 Busch Blvd., P.O. Box 29233, Columbus, OH 43229. https:// www .nremt.org

LEARNING PORTFOLIO

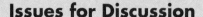

Issues for Discussion

1. All EMTs and paramedics are obligated to treat patients with dignity and respect. At the same time, they sometimes deal with patients in extreme emotional or mental distress. Discuss in class what difficulties, if any, EMTs or paramedics would experience treating such patients with dignity and respect in these situations.

2. When deciding on a career path as an EMT or paramedic, what are some of the more important aspects of the job you should consider? What aspects of your own personality make you well suited or not to pursue a career in this health field?

Enrichment Activities

1. Watch the career video Paramedic Careers—Life of an EMT from CareersOutThere.com: https://www.youtube.com/watch?v=1uB8kN_jeE8. Discuss the role of an EMT and how one copes with the difficulties involved in the job.

2. Use the internet to research your state's requirements for the EMT and paramedic professions discussed in this chapter. List these requirements if they exist. Compare and contrast licensing, certification, and registration for this career with any other career you have examined in this course.

CASE STUDY: AN EMT'S ETHICAL DILEMMA

Rosario is an EMT employed by an ambulance service in his community. He routinely attends to people in distress, evaluating each situation as part of his triage responsibility. One day Rosario's ambulance reported to the site of a vehicle accident. In evaluating the medical condition of one of the drivers involved in the vehicle accident, Rosario determined that the driver was injured and needed medical care beyond what could be provided by himself and his fellow crew member. Rosario informed the injured driver that he would transport the injured driver to a hospital for further care via the ambulance. The injured driver disagreed with Rosario, indicating the driver saw no need to go to the hospital or for any form of further medical care. The injured driver would prefer to go home and care for any injuries alone. How should Rosario respond?

References

1. National Registry of Emergency Medical Technicians. Become Involved as an EMS Professional. https://www.nremt.org Accessed August 30, 2021.

2. Commission on Accreditation of Health Education Programs. https://www.caahep.org/ Accessed August 30, 2021.

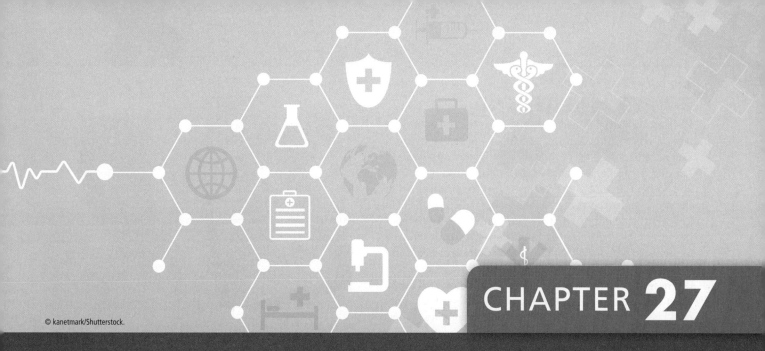

CHAPTER **27**

Radiation Technology*

KEY TERMS

Beam modification devices
Computed tomography (CT)
CT technologists
Dosimetrists
Fluoroscopy
Ionizing radiation

Magnetic resonance imaging
  (MRI)
Mammography
MRI technologist
Radiation oncologist
Radiation physicist

Radiation therapy
Radiographers
Radiologic technicians
Radiologic technologists
Radiologist

* All information in this chapter, unless otherwise indicated, was obtained from Bureau of Labor Statistics. *Occupational Outlook Handbook 2020–2021 Edition*. Washington, DC: U.S. Department of Labor; 2021.

X-RAYS AND BEYOND

Perhaps the most familiar use of the X-ray is the diagnosis of broken bones. Although this remains a major use, medical uses of radiation go far beyond that. Today, radiation is used not only to produce images of the interior of the body but also to treat disease and prevent its further progress. With the application of computer technology to radiology, the field has been revolutionized. Computer-enhanced equipment produces amazingly clear and sharp images. Thanks in part to the speed with which computerized scanners can read and organize the millions of messages involved in a single test, it is now possible to view soft tissues and organs such as the heart and brain, parts of the body that until quite recently could be examined only through invasive techniques such as exploratory surgery.

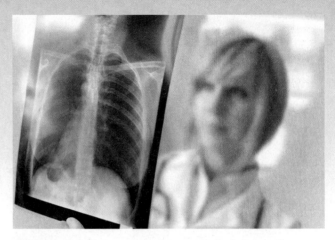

FIGURE 27.1 X-ray produced by radiographer.
© creo77/Shutterstock.

RADIOLOGIC TECHNOLOGISTS AND TECHNICIANS
Significant Points

- Employment is projected to grow faster than average; those with knowledge of more than one diagnostic imaging procedure will have the best employment opportunities.
- Formal training programs in radiography are offered in hospitals or colleges and universities and lead to a certificate, an associate's degree, or a bachelor's degree.
- Most states require licensure, and requirements vary.
- Although hospitals will remain the primary employers, a number of new jobs will be found in physicians' offices and diagnostic imaging centers.

Work Description

Radiologic technologists and technicians perform diagnostic imaging examinations. Radiologic technicians perform imaging examinations like X-rays, while technologists use other imaging modalities such as **computed tomography (CT)**, **magnetic resonance imaging (MRI)**, and mammography.

Radiologic technicians, sometimes referred to as **radiographers**, produce X-ray images (radiographs) of parts of the human body for use in diagnosing medical problems. They prepare patients for radiologic examinations by explaining the procedure, removing jewelry and other articles through which X-rays cannot pass, and positioning patients so that the parts of the body can be appropriately radiographed. To prevent unnecessary exposure to radiation, these workers surround the exposed area with radiation protection devices, such as lead shields, or limit the size of the X-ray beam. Radiographers position radiographic equipment at the correct angle and height over the appropriate area of a patient's body. Using instruments similar to a measuring tape, they may measure the thickness of the section

to be radiographed and set controls on the X-ray machine to produce radiographs of the appropriate density, detail, and contrast. An example of an X-ray produced through this effort is seen in **FIGURE 27.1**.

Radiologic technologists and technicians must follow physicians' orders precisely and conform to regulations concerning the use of radiation to protect themselves, their patients, and their coworkers from unnecessary exposure.

In addition to preparing patients and operating equipment, radiologic technologists and technicians keep patient records and adjust and maintain equipment. They also may prepare work schedules, evaluate purchases of equipment, or manage a radiology department.

Radiologic technologists perform more complex imaging procedures. When performing **fluoroscopy**, for example, radiologic technologists prepare a solution for the patient to drink, allowing the **radiologist** (a physician who interprets radiographs) to see soft tissues in the body.

Some radiologic technologists specialize in CT as **CT technologists**. CT scans produce a substantial number of cross-sectional X-rays of an area of the body. From those cross-sectional X-rays, a three-dimensional image is made. The CT uses **ionizing radiation**; therefore, it requires the same precautionary measures that are used with X-rays.

Radiologic technologists also can specialize in magnetic resonance imaging (MRI) as **MRI technologists**. MRI, like CT, produces multiple cross-sectional images to create a three-dimensional image. Unlike CT and X-rays, MRI uses nonionizing radio frequencies to generate image contrast. An example of an MRI machine is seen in **FIGURE 27.2**.

Radiologic technologists might also specialize in **mammography**. Mammographers use low-dose X-ray systems to produce images of the breast.

In addition to radiologic technologists, others who conduct diagnostic imaging procedures include cardiovascular technologists and technicians, diagnostic medical sonographers, and nuclear medicine technologists.

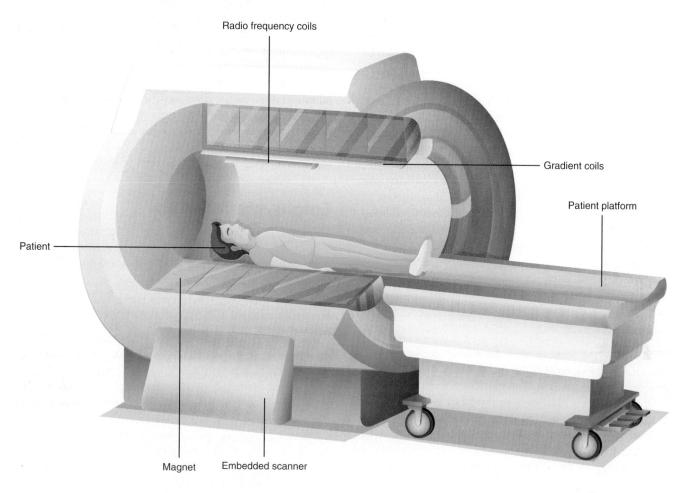

Radio frequency coils

Gradient coils

Patient platform

Patient

Magnet   Embedded scanner

FIGURE 27.2 Magnetic resonance imaging machine.
© BlueRingMedia/Shutterstock.

Work Environment

Physical stamina is important in this occupation because technologists and technicians are on their feet for long periods and may be required to lift or turn disabled patients. Technologists and technicians work at diagnostic machines but also may perform some procedures at patients' bedsides. Some travel to patients in large vans equipped with sophisticated diagnostic equipment.

Although radiation hazards exist in this occupation, they are minimized by the use of lead aprons, gloves, and other shielding devices and by instruments monitoring exposure to radiation. Technologists and technicians wear badges measuring radiation levels in the radiation area, and detailed records are kept on their cumulative lifetime dose.

Most full-time radiologic technologists and technicians work about 40 hours a week. They may, however, have evening, weekend, or on-call hours. Some radiologic technologists and technicians work part time for more than one employer; for those, travel to and from facilities must be considered.

Employment Opportunities

Radiologic technologists held about 212,000 jobs in 2019. About 60% of all jobs were in hospitals. Most other jobs were in offices of physicians; medical and diagnostic laboratories, including diagnostic imaging centers; and outpatient care centers.

Educational and Legal Requirements

There are multiple paths to entry into this profession offered in hospitals or colleges and universities. Most states require licensure, and requirements vary.

Education and Training

Formal training programs in radiography lead to a certificate, an associate's degree, or a bachelor's degree. An associate's degree is the most prevalent level of educational attainment among radiologic technologists and technicians.

Some may receive a certificate. Certificate programs typically last around 21 to 24 months.

The Joint Review Committee on Education in Radiologic Technology (JRCERT) accredits formal training programs in radiography. As of 2021, the committee accredited 725 radiography, radiation therapy, magnetic resonance, and medical dosimetry programs in the United States, the District of Columbia, and the Commonwealth of Puerto Rico. Only one state, Alaska, does not have a JRCERT-accredited program. Educational programs are sponsored by a variety of groups, including colleges and universities, for-profit institutions, private institutions, medical facilities, and the military. The programs provide both classroom and clinical instruction in anatomy and physiology, patient care procedures, radiation physics, radiation protection, principles of imaging, medical terminology, positioning of patients, medical ethics, radiobiology, and pathology.

Students interested in radiologic technology should take high school courses in mathematics, physics, chemistry, anatomy, physiology, and biology.

Licensure

Federal legislation protects the public from the hazards of unnecessary exposure to medical and dental radiation by ensuring that operators of radiologic equipment are properly trained. It is up to each state, however, to require the licensure of radiologic technologists. Most states require licensure for practicing radiologic technologists. Licensing requirements vary by state—for specific requirements, contact your state's health board.

Certification

The American Registry of Radiologic Technologists (ARRT) offers voluntary certification for radiologic technologists. In addition, a number of states use ARRT-administered exams for state licensing purposes. To be eligible for certification, technologists must graduate from an ARRT-approved accredited program and pass an examination.[1] Many employers prefer to hire certified radiologic technologists. In order to maintain an ARRT certification, 24 hours of continuing education must be completed every two years.

Other Qualifications

Radiologic technologists and technicians should be sensitive to patients' physical and psychological needs. They must pay attention to detail, follow instructions, and work as part of a team. In addition, operating complicated equipment requires mechanical ability and manual dexterity.

Advancement

With experience and additional training, staff technologists may become specialists, performing CT scanning, MRI, mammography, or bone densitometry. Technologists also may advance, with additional education and certification, to become a radiologist assistant. The ARRT offers specialty certification in many radiologic specialties, as well as a credentialing for radiologist assistants.

Experienced technologists also may be promoted to supervisor, chief radiologic technologist, and, ultimately, department administrator or director. Depending on the institution, courses or a master's degree in business or health administration may be necessary for the director's position.

Some technologists progress by specializing in the occupation to become instructors or directors in radiologic technology educational programs; others take jobs as sales representatives or instructors with equipment manufacturers.

Employment Trends

Employment is projected to grow faster than average. Those with knowledge of more than one diagnostic imaging procedure—such as CT, MRI, and mammography—will have the best employment opportunities.

Employment Change

Employment of radiologic technologists is expected to increase by about 7% from 2019 to 2029, faster than the average for all occupations. As the population grows and ages, there will be an increasing demand for diagnostic imaging. With age comes an increased incidence of illness and injury, which often requires diagnostic imaging for diagnosis. In addition to diagnosis, diagnostic imaging is used to monitor the progress of disease treatment. With the increasing success of medical technologies in treating disease, diagnostic imaging will increasingly be needed to monitor the progress of treatment.

The extent to which diagnostic imaging procedures are performed largely depends on cost and reimbursement considerations. Because accurate, early disease detection allows for lower cost of treatment in the long run, many third-party payers find use of diagnostic imaging procedures favorable.

Although hospitals will remain the principal employer of radiologic technologists, a number of new jobs will be found in offices of physicians and diagnostic imaging centers. As technology advances, many imaging modalities are becoming less expensive and more feasible to have in physicians' offices.

Job Prospects

In addition to job growth, job openings also will arise from the need to replace technologists who leave the occupation. Those with knowledge of more than one diagnostic imaging procedure—such as CT, MRI, and mammography—will have the best employment opportunities as employers seek to control costs by using multi-credentialed employees.

Demand for radiologic technologists and technicians can tend to be regional, with some areas having great demand while other areas are saturated. Technologists and technicians willing to relocate may have better job prospects.

CT is continuing to become a frontline diagnosis tool. Instead of taking X-rays to decide whether a CT is needed, as was the practice before, it is often the first choice for

TABLE 27.1 Projections Data for Radiologic Technologists and Technicians, 2019–2029

Occupational Title	Employment, 2019	Projected Employment, 2029	Change, 2019–2029	
			Number	Percentage
Radiologic technologists and technicians	212,000	226,100	14,100	7%

Data from Bureau of Labor Statistics, U.S. Department of Labor. Occupational Outlook Handbook. U.S. Department of Labor; 2020. https://www.bls.gov/ooh/healthcare/radiologic-technologists.htm#tab-6

TABLE 27.2 Median Annual Earnings in the Industries Employing the Largest Number of Radiologic Technologists, May 2020

Medical and diagnostic laboratories	$61,410
Federal government	$69,960
Hospitals: state, local, and private	$62,850
Outpatient care centers	$66,780
Offices of physicians	$56,340

Data from Bureau of Labor Statistics, U.S. Department of Labor. Occupational Outlook Handbook. U.S. Department of Labor; 2020. https://www.bls.gov/ooh/healthcare/radiologic-technologists.htm#tab-5

imaging because of its accuracy. MRI also is increasingly used. Technologists with credentialing in either of these specialties will be very marketable to employers. **TABLE 27.1** shows some projection data provided by the U.S. Department of Labor.

Earnings

The median annual wage of radiologic technologists was $61,900 in May 2020. The lowest 10% earned less than $42,180, and the highest 10% earned more than $92,660. Median annual wages in the industries employing the largest numbers of radiologic technologists in 2020 are shown in **TABLE 27.2**.

Related Occupations

Radiologic technologists operate sophisticated equipment to help physicians, dentists, and other health practitioners diagnose and treat patients. Workers in related healthcare occupations include cardiovascular technologists and technicians, diagnostic medical sonographers, nuclear medicine technologists, and radiation therapists.

Additional Information

For information on careers in radiologic technology, contact:

- American Society of Radiologic Technologists, 15000 Central Ave. SE, Albuquerque, NM 87123. https://www.asrt.org

For the current list of accredited education programs in radiography, contact:

- Joint Review Committee on Education in Radiologic Technology, 20 N. Wacker Dr., Suite 2850, Chicago, IL 60606-3182. https://www.jrcert.org

For certification information, contact:

- American Registry of Radiologic Technologists, 1255 Northland Dr., St. Paul, MN 55120-1155. http://www.arrt.org

RADIATION THERAPISTS
Significant Points

- A bachelor's degree, associate's degree, or certificate in radiation therapy is generally required.
- Employment is projected to grow much faster than the average for all occupations.
- Good job opportunities are expected.
- Earnings are relatively high.

Work Description

Radiation therapy is used to treat cancer in the human body. As part of a medical radiation oncology team, radiation therapists use machines called linear accelerators to administer radiation treatment to patients. Linear accelerators are most commonly used in a procedure called external beam therapy, which projects high-energy X-rays at targeted cancer cells. As the X-rays collide with human tissue, they produce highly energized ions that can shrink and eliminate cancerous tumors. Radiation therapy is sometimes used as the sole treatment for cancer, but it is usually used in conjunction with chemotherapy or surgery.

Before treatment can begin, the oncology team must develop a treatment plan. To create this plan, the radiation therapist must first use an X-ray imaging machine or CT scan to pinpoint the location of the tumor. Then a **radiation oncologist** (a physician who specializes in therapeutic radiology) and a **radiation physicist** (a worker who calibrates the linear accelerator simulator and checks that radiation output is accurate) determine the best way to administer treatment. The therapist completes the plan by positioning the patient, adjusting the linear accelerator simulator to the specifications

Professional Profiles

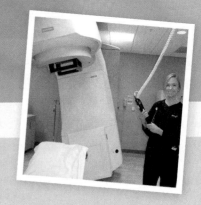

Name: Nicole, RT(T)
Title: Radiation Therapist RT(T)
Education: BS in Radiation Therapy

Q: Tell us about your job and the organization in which you work.

A: I am a radiation therapist at an outpatient cancer treatment center, located on the campus of a major county hospital. I have worked at this facility for a little over four years, and this career is beyond rewarding to me. I deliver radiation treatments to cancer patients daily, using treatment machines called linear accelerators. These machines electrically produce photon and electron radiation, which is then delivered to the patient through a shaped beam, according to tumor location.

I also work with patients needing HDR (high-dose radiation) and LDR (low-dose radiation) treatments, in which a live radioactive source is placed inside the patient in the necessary treatment area. Some of these cases may be performed in a procedure room; other cases may require an operating room.

In addition to their direct treatment, I am also involved in the patient's simulation. During the simulation, I will find the best possible position for the patient to be in for treatment. This includes creating necessary immobilization devices and placing any appropriate positioning marks on the patient. The patient is then imaged in this position for the radiation oncologist and dosimetrists (treatment planners) to derive a treatment plan.

Q: Describe a typical workday.

A: I treat from 20 to 30 patients on a daily basis. I position the patient on the treatment table, using appropriate immobilization devices, positioning marks, and any other special instructions from the radiation oncologist or dosimetrists. Next, I perform any imaging required to verify patient position and ensure only the targeted area will receive radiation. This can be done with films, fluoroscopy, CT imaging, or a number of other image-guidance technologies. After verifying patient position and making any necessary adjustments, the patient is then treated.

Q: Why did you choose this profession?

A: I started out majoring in a different healthcare field. Sometimes it's hard to know exactly what you want to do until you figure out what you don't want to do. I knew I wanted a career in health care, so I explored until I found a career that fit my passions and interests.

Q: What do you like most about this profession?

A: I love the technical side but also the compassionate side of this profession. I like problem-solving and

being challenged, working with different machines and gadgets. But most of all I care for people, and that's why I do what I do.

Q: What kind of training is involved in this field, and how long does it take?

A: Radiation therapy is a bachelor's degree, most commonly beginning with an associate's degree in radiology. After completing the program, the ARRT (American Registry of Radiologic Technologists) requires you take and pass the radiation therapy registry exam to become a certified and registered radiation therapist. Coursework includes radiobiology, radiophysics, radiation safety, treatment planning and delivery, clinical concepts, and patient care. Along with the didactic coursework, students are required to complete at least nine months of clinical work where they will complete different competency tests within the scope of practice.

Q: Name and explain the academic training that most prepared you for this profession.

A: The scientific coursework is absolutely necessary, but the clinical work is what prepares you most for your career as a therapist. Not only are you able to apply classroom knowledge, but you also learn the flow of a radiation therapy department; how to work as a team alongside radiation oncologists, dosimetrists, nurses, and fellow therapists; and how to effectively communicate with patients. All of this is vital in the job of an RT.

Q: What do you wish you had known in high school/college about pursuing this career?

A: I wish I had known this field existed in high school! I feel that a lot of students don't realize all of the options and opportunities available within health care, and I was no different. Talk to an academic counselor and do some digging. Most important: job shadow, job shadow, job shadow!

Q: What skills are essential for being effective in this career?

A: Really take advantage of your clinical time. Don't be afraid to ask questions! Stay professional. It's easy to get comfortable and mesh into the team at your clinic, but every day is a job interview, and your behavior and attitude will be remembered first before anything else.

developed by the team, and then recording the details so that those conditions can be replicated during treatment. The therapist later explains the treatment plan to the patient and answers any questions that the patient may have. An example of a linear accelerator simulator is seen in **FIGURE 27.3**.

The next step in the process is treatment. To begin each treatment session, the radiation therapist uses the guidelines developed during the planning phase to position the patient and adjust the linear accelerator. Then, from a separate room that is protected from the X-ray radiation, the therapist operates the linear accelerator and monitors the patient's condition through a TV monitor and an intercom system. Treatment can take anywhere from 10 to 30 minutes.

During the treatment phase, the radiation therapist monitors the patient's physical condition to determine whether the patient is having any adverse reactions to the treatment. The therapist must also be aware of the patient's emotional well-being. Because many patients are under stress and are emotionally fragile, it is important for the therapist to maintain a positive attitude and provide emotional support.

Radiation therapists keep detailed records of their patients' treatments. These records include information such as the dose of radiation used for each treatment, the total amount of radiation used to date, the area treated, and the patient's reactions. Radiation oncologists and **dosimetrists** (technicians who calculate the dose of radiation that will be used for treatment) review these records to ensure that the treatment plan is working, to monitor the amount of radiation exposure that the patient has received, and to keep side effects to a minimum. Therapists also may assist dosimetrists with routine aspects of dosimetry, the process used to calculate radiation dosages.

Work Environment

Radiation therapists work in hospitals, physician offices, outpatient centers, or cancer treatment centers. These places are clean, well lit, and well ventilated. Therapists do a considerable amount of lifting and must be able to help disabled patients get on and off treatment tables. They spend most of their time on their feet.

Radiation therapists generally work 40 hours a week, and unlike workers in some other healthcare occupations, they normally work only during the day because most procedures are scheduled in advance. Because radiation therapy emergencies do occur, some therapists are required to be on call and may have to work outside their normal hours.

Working with cancer patients can be stressful, but many radiation therapists also find it rewarding. Because they work around radioactive materials, radiation therapists take great care to ensure that they are not exposed to dangerous levels of radiation. By following standard safety procedures, radiation therapists can prevent overexposure.

Employment Opportunities

Radiation therapists held about 18,500 jobs in 2019. About 63% worked in hospitals, and about 24% worked in the offices of physicians. A small proportion worked in outpatient care centers and medical and diagnostic laboratories.

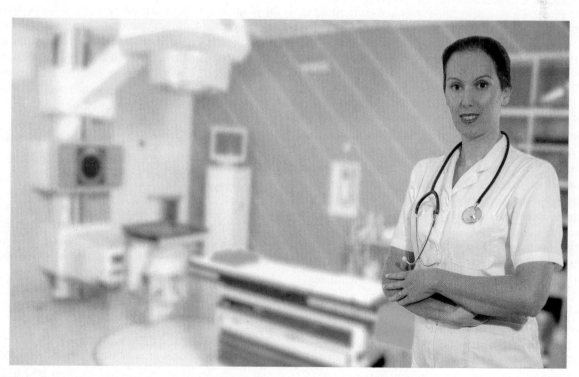

FIGURE 27.3 Radiation therapist with linear accelerator simulator.

Educational and Legal Requirements

A bachelor's degree, associate's degree, or certificate in radiation therapy generally is required. Many states require radiation therapists to be licensed, and most employers require certification. With experience, therapists can advance to managerial positions.

Education and Training

Employers usually require applicants to complete an associate's or a bachelor's degree program in radiation therapy. Individuals also may become qualified by completing an associate's or a bachelor's degree program in radiography, which is the study of radiological imaging, and then by completing a 12-month certificate program in radiation therapy. Radiation therapy programs include core courses on radiation therapy procedures and the scientific theories behind them. In addition, such programs often include courses on human anatomy and physiology, physics, algebra, precalculus, writing, public speaking, computer science, and research methodology. In 2021, there were 89 radiation therapy programs in the United States and 20 abroad that were accredited by the American Registry of Radiologic Technologists (ARRT).[2]

Licensure

More than 75% of states required radiation therapists to be licensed by a state accrediting board in 2021.[3] Licensing requirements vary by state, but many states require applicants to pass the ARRT certification examination. Further information is available from individual state licensing offices.

Certification

Some states, as well as many employers, require radiation therapists to be certified by the ARRT. To become ARRT certified, an applicant must complete an accredited radiation therapy program, adhere to ARRT ethical standards, and pass the ARRT certification examination. The examination covers radiation protection and quality assurance, clinical concepts in radiation oncology, treatment planning, treatment delivery, and patient care and education. Candidates also must demonstrate competency in several clinical practices including patient care activities; simulation procedures; dosimetry calculations; fabrication of **beam modification devices**; low-volume, high-risk procedures; and the application of radiation.

ARRT certification is valid for one year, after which therapists must renew their certification. Requirements for renewal include abiding by the ARRT ethical standards, paying annual dues, and satisfying continuing education requirements. Continuing education requirements must be met every two years and include either the completion of 24 course credits related to radiation therapy or the attainment of ARRT certification in a discipline other than radiation therapy. States or employers that require initial certification may not require certification renewal.

Other Qualifications

All radiation therapists need good communication skills because their work involves a great deal of interaction with patients. Individuals interested in becoming radiation therapists should be psychologically capable of working with cancer patients. They should be caring and empathetic because they work with patients who are ill and under stress. They should be able to keep accurate, detailed records. They also should be physically fit because they work on their feet for long periods and lift and move disabled patients. They also need technical skills so that they can operate properly with computers and technological equipment.

Advancement

Experienced radiation therapists may advance to manage radiation therapy programs in treatment centers or other healthcare facilities. Managers generally continue to treat patients while taking on management responsibilities. Other advancement opportunities include teaching, technical sales, and research. With additional training and certification, therapists also can become dosimetrists, who use complex mathematical formulas to calculate proper radiation doses.

Employment Trends

Employment is expected to increase much faster than average, and job prospects should be good.

Employment Change

Employment of radiation therapists is projected to grow by 7% between 2019 and 2029, which is much faster than the average for all occupations. The growing older adult population is expected to cause an increase in the number of people needing treatment. In addition, as radiation technology becomes safer and more effective and sophisticated treatment techniques are employed, it will be prescribed more often, leading to an increased demand for radiation therapists. Growth is likely to be rapid across all practice settings, including hospitals, physicians' offices, and outpatient centers.

Job Prospects

Job prospects are expected to be good. Job openings will result from employment growth and from the need to replace workers who retire or leave the occupation for other reasons. Applicants with a bachelor's degree and related work experience may have the best opportunities. TABLE 27.3 shows some projections data from the U.S. Department of Labor.

Earnings

Median annual wages of radiation therapists were $86,850 in May 2020. The lowest 10% earned less than $60,080, and the highest 10% earned more than $132,950. Some employers also

TABLE 27.3 Projections Data for Radiation Therapists, 2019–2029

| Occupational Title | Employment, 2019 | Projected Employment, 2029 | Change, 2019–2029 | |
			Number	Percentage
Radiation therapists	18,500	19,900	1,300	7%

Data from Bureau of Labor Statistics, U.S. Department of Labor. Occupational Outlook Handbook. U.S. Department of Labor; 2020. https://www.bls.gov/ooh/healthcare/radiation-therapists.htm?view_full#tab-6

TABLE 27.4 Median Annual Earnings in the Industries Employing the Largest Number of Radiation Therapists, 2019–2029

Outpatient care centers	$112,280
Offices of physicians	$89,060
Hospitals: state, local, and private	$84,630

reimburse their employees for the cost of continuing education. Median annual wages in the industries employing the largest number of radiation therapists in 2020 are shown in **TABLE 27.4**.

Related Occupations

Other occupations that administer medical treatment to patients include cardiovascular technologists and technicians, dental hygienists, diagnostic medical sonographers, nuclear medicine technologists, nursing and psychiatric aides, physical therapist assistants and aides, radiologic technologists and technicians, and registered nurses.

Additional Information

Information on certification by the American Registry of Radiologic Technologists and on accredited radiation therapy programs may be obtained from:

- American Registry of Radiologic Technologists, 1255 Northland Dr., St. Paul, MN 55120. https://www.arrt.org

Information on careers in radiation therapy may be obtained from:

- American Society of Radiologic Technologists, 15000 Central Ave. SE, Albuquerque, NM 87123. https://www.asrt.org

LEARNING PORTFOLIO

Issues for Discussion

1. Review the requirements for becoming a radiologic technician and a radiation therapist. Compare the requirements for preparing for these two careers in terms of length of training, cost of training, job opportunities, and lifetime income. Which of these careers best matches your career goals?

2. Several leading agencies, such as the Environmental Protection Agency and the International Agency for Research on Cancer, classify X-rays as cancer-causing agents. By following standard safety procedures, radiation therapists can prevent overexposure to these agents. Discuss whether the risks associated with this exposure would influence your choice of career as a radiation therapist.

Enrichment Activities

1. The history of X-rays goes back to the late nineteenth century. Create a timeline (either as a narrative piece, a poster, or an infographic) tracing the progression of this science and include the names of key theorists and advancements in the field.

2. Many individuals who will receive radiation therapy are concerned about the side effects of treatment. Download the pamphlet titled "Radiation Therapy and You" from the National Cancer Institute, a division of the National Institutes for Health (https://www.cancer.gov/Publications/patient-education/radiation-therapy-and-you). Review the ways by which an individual can manage the side effects of radiation therapy, including how to monitor foods and liquids that play a role in these side effects.

CASE STUDY: AN X-RAY TECHNICIAN'S WORK

Shane is working in the radiology department at Cooper Medical Center. He is a radiologic technician and has been working there for the past 6 months. Today, Shane is caring for a patient who came in to have an X-ray of his right arm. Shane begins to prepare the patient for his test by explaining the procedure. During the testing, Shane will help prevent any unnecessary exposure to radiation for the patient as well as himself. After he has completed the procedure, Shane is responsible for documenting in the patient's medical record.

Based on the information you have read about radiation technology, answer the following questions.

1. True or false? As a radiologic technician, Shane is working within his scope of practice by completing this X-ray film.

2. True or false? While preparing the patient, Shane must insist that the patient remove all jewelry and any articles that would not allow X-rays to pass through.

3. True or false? Shane should position the patient so that the patient's entire body is accessible for the X-ray equipment.

4. True or false? Shane should apply a plastic shield to the patient and to himself to reduce the risk of any unnecessary exposure to radiation.

5. True or false? In order to achieve the best image of the patient's arm, Shane should position the equipment at the correct angle and height directly over the patient's right arm.

References

1. American Association of Radiologic Technicians. Initial AART Certification and Registration. https://www.arrt.org/Certification Accessed August 30, 2021.

2. American Registry of Radiologic Technologists. Radiation Therapy Schools. https://www.arrt.org/Education/Educational-Programs Accessed August 30, 2021.

3. American Registry of Radiologic Technologists. State Licensing. https://www.arrt.org/pages/resources/state-licensing Accessed August 30, 2021.

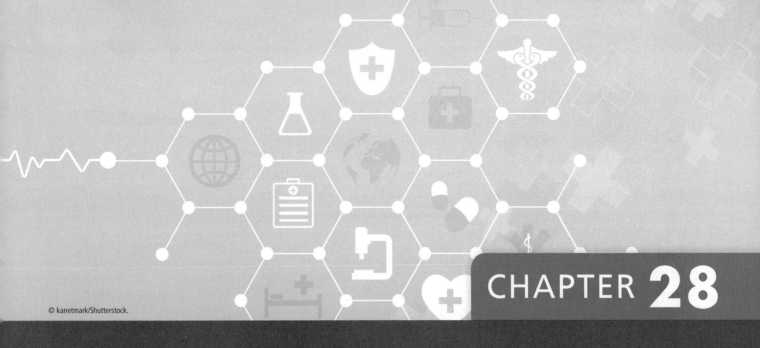
© kanetmark/Shutterstock.

CHAPTER 28

Diagnostics and Related Technology*

KEY TERMS

Abdominal sonographer
Breast sonographer
Cardiographic technician
Cardiopulmonary technologists
Cardiovascular invasive
　specialist
Cardiovascular technician
Cardiovascular technologist
Diagnostic imaging
Diagnostic medical sonography
Echocardiographer
Electrocardiogram (ECG)
Electrocardiograph technician

Gamma scintillation camera
High-frequency transducers
Holter monitoring
Invasive cardiology
Magnetic resonance scanners
Neurosonographer
Noninvasive procedure
Nuclear cardiology (NCT)
　technologists
Nuclear medicine
Nuclear medicine computer
　tomography (CT)
　technologists

Obstetric and gynecologic
　sonographer
Positron emission scanners
Positron emission tomography
　(PET) technologists
Radionuclides
Radiopharmaceuticals
Sonographers
Stress testing
Surgical technologist
Transesophageal echocardiography
Ultrasound machines
Vascular technologist

* All information in this chapter, unless otherwise indicated, was obtained from Bureau of Labor Statistics. *Occupational Outlook Handbook 2020–2021 Edition*. Washington, DC: U.S. Department of Labor; 2021.

Introduction

The rapidly growing use of imaging techniques that do not involve X-rays has transformed the healthcare field. Computer-enhanced equipment produces amazingly clear and sharp images. Thanks in part to the speed with which computerized scanners can read and organize the millions of messages involved in a single test, it is now possible to view soft tissues and organs such as the heart and brain—parts of the body that until quite recently could be examined only through invasive techniques such as exploratory surgery. The impact of these imaging techniques has resulted in the creation of new terminology and a number of new roles in health care.

DIAGNOSTIC MEDICAL SONOGRAPHERS
Significant Points

- Job opportunities should be favorable.
- Employment will grow as sonography becomes an increasingly attractive alternative to radiological procedures.
- Hospitals employ about 61% of all sonographers.
- Sonographers may receive education and training in hospitals, vocational-technical institutions, colleges and universities, or the armed forces.

Work Description

Remarkable strides have occurred in the development of imaging equipment that does not involve the use of radiation, thereby reducing the risk of adverse side effects. Examples include **ultrasound machines**, which use sound waves; **magnetic resonance scanners**, which use radio waves; and **positron emission scanners.** Although discovered many years ago, some of these imaging techniques became clinically practical only during the 1990s, as a result of improvements in electronic circuitry that enable computers to handle the vast amount of data involved.

Future generations of imaging equipment are certain to be even more sophisticated than machines in use today. Physicians seeking to confirm a diagnosis or monitor a patient's condition will obtain better information, and patients will be subjected to less risk or discomfort. There is ample reason to believe that technological advances in this field will continue to occur very rapidly and that the clinical benefits will spur even more extensive use of diagnostic imaging procedures.

Diagnostic imaging embraces several procedures that aid in diagnosing ailments. The most familiar procedures are the X-ray and magnetic resonance imaging (MRI); however, not all imaging technologies use ionizing radiation or radio waves. Sonography, or ultrasonography, uses sound waves to generate an image for the assessment and diagnosis of various medical conditions. Sonography commonly is associated with obstetrics and the use of ultrasound imaging during pregnancy, but this technology has many other applications in the diagnosis and treatment of medical conditions throughout the body. Concepts associated with sonography are seen in **FIGURE 28.1**.

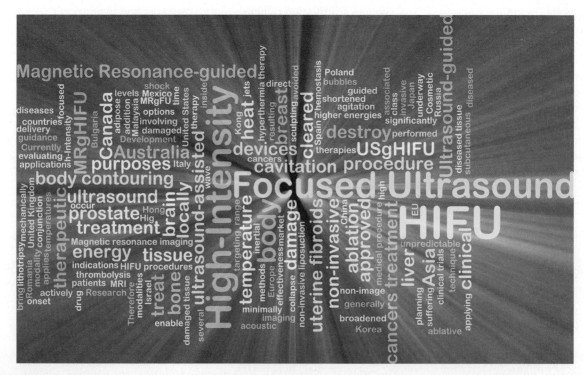

FIGURE 28.1 Concepts associated with sonography.
© Kheng Guan Toh/Shutterstock.

Diagnostic medical **sonographers** use special equipment to direct nonionizing, high-frequency sound waves into areas of the patient's body. Sonographers operate the equipment, which collects reflected echoes and forms an image that may be videotaped, transmitted, or photographed for interpretation and diagnosis by a physician.

Sonographers begin by explaining the procedure to the patient and recording any medical history that may be relevant to the condition being viewed. They then select appropriate equipment settings and direct the patient to move into positions that will provide the best view. To perform the exam, sonographers use a transducer, which transmits sound waves in a cone- or rectangle-shaped beam. Although techniques vary with the area being examined, sonographers usually spread a special gel on the skin to aid the transmission of sound waves.

Viewing the screen during the scan, sonographers look for subtle visual cues that contrast healthy areas with unhealthy ones. They decide whether the images are satisfactory for diagnostic purposes and select which ones to store and show to the physician. Sonographers take measurements, calculate values, and analyze the results in preliminary findings for the physicians.

In addition to working directly with patients, diagnostic medical sonographers keep patient records and adjust and maintain equipment. They also may prepare work schedules, evaluate equipment purchases, or manage a sonography or diagnostic imaging department.

Diagnostic medical sonographers may specialize in obstetric and gynecologic sonography (the female reproductive system), abdominal sonography (the liver, kidneys, gallbladder, spleen, and pancreas), neurosonography (the brain), or breast sonography. In addition, sonographers may specialize in vascular sonography musculoskeletal sonography, pediatric sonography, or cardiac sonography.

Obstetric and gynecologic sonographers specialize in the imaging of the female reproductive system. Included in the discipline is one of the better-known uses of sonography: examining the fetus of a pregnant woman to track the baby's growth and health. These sonographers work closely with physicians in detecting congenital birth defects. An example of a patient undergoing an obstetrical ultrasound is seen in **FIGURE 28.2**.

Abdominal sonographers inspect a patient's abdominal cavity to help diagnose and treat conditions primarily involving the gallbladder, bile ducts, kidneys, liver, pancreas, spleen, and male reproductive system. Using ultrasound, abdominal sonographers may assist with biopsies or other examinations. Abdominal sonographers also are able to scan parts of the chest, although echocardiographers usually perform studies of the heart using sonography. An example of abdominal sonography is seen in **FIGURE 28.3**.

Neurosonographers focus on the nervous system, including the brain. In neonatal care, neurosonographers study and diagnose neurological and nervous system disorders in premature infants. They also may scan blood vessels to check for abnormalities indicating a stroke in children diagnosed with sickle-cell anemia. Like other sonographers, neurosonographers operate transducers to perform the sonogram, but they use frequencies and beam shapes different from those used by obstetric and abdominal sonographers.

Breast sonographers use sonography to study diseases of the breast. Sonography aids mammography in the detection of breast cancer and can confirm the presence of a cyst or tumor detected by the patient or doctor. Breast sonography can also track tumors and blood supply conditions and assist in the accurate biopsy of breast tissue. Breast sonographers use **high-frequency transducers**, made exclusively to study breast tissue.

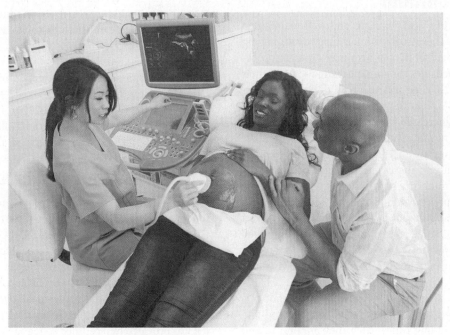

FIGURE 28.2 Pregnant woman undergoing ultrasound.
© monkeybusinessimages/iStockPhoto.

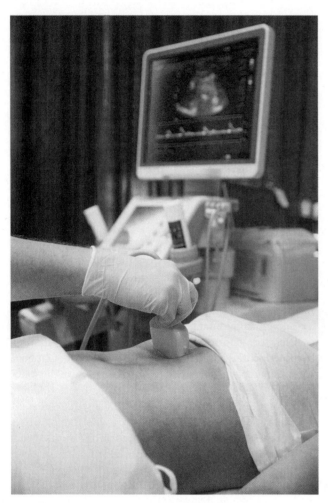

FIGURE 28.3 Patient undergoing abdominal ultrasound.
© zlikovec/Shutterstock.

Work Environment

Sonographers typically work in clean and well-maintained healthcare facilities. They usually work at diagnostic imaging machines in darkened rooms but also may perform procedures at patients' bedsides. Sonographers may be on their feet for long periods of time and may have to lift or turn disabled patients. In addition, the nature of their work can put sonographers at an increased risk for musculoskeletal disorders such as carpal tunnel syndrome or neck, back, and eye strain. The increasing use of ergonomically correct equipment, combined with an increasing awareness of potential problems, will help minimize such risks.

Some sonographers work as contract employees and may travel to several different healthcare facilities within a given area. Similarly, some sonographers travel with mobile imaging service providers and bring mobile diagnostic imaging services to patients in areas who otherwise lack access to them.

Most full-time sonographers work about 40 hours a week. Hospital-based sonographers may have evening and weekend hours, including times when they are on call and must be ready to report to work on short notice.

Employment Opportunities

Diagnostic medical sonographers held about 74,300 jobs in 2019. About 61% of all sonographer jobs were in public and private hospitals. The remainder worked typically in physicians' offices, medical and diagnostic laboratories, and outpatient care centers.

Educational and Legal Requirements

Employers hiring in **diagnostic medical sonography** recognize and accept several levels of education and methods of acquiring it. Although no one level of education is preferred, employers do prefer registered sonographers who trained in accredited programs.

Education and Training

Several avenues exist for entry into the field of diagnostic medical sonography. Sonographers may train in hospitals, vocational-technical institutions, colleges and universities, or the armed forces. Some training programs prefer applicants with a background in science or experience in other healthcare professions. Some training programs also may consider high school graduates with courses in mathematics and science as well as applicants with liberal arts backgrounds, but this practice is infrequent.

Colleges and universities offer formal training in both two- and four-year programs, culminating in an associate's or a bachelor's degree. Two-year programs are most prevalent. Coursework includes classes in anatomy, physiology, instrumentation, basic physics, patient care, and medical ethics. A limited number of master's degree programs are available.

Employers also accept a few one-year programs, some of which result in a certificate, as appropriate education. These programs typically are satisfactory education and training for workers already in health care who seek to increase their marketability by training in sonography. These programs are often not accredited.

The Commission on Accreditation of Allied Health Education Programs (CAAHEP) accredited 394 diagnostic medical sonography training programs in 2020.[1] These programs typically are the formal training programs offered by colleges and universities. Some hospital programs are accredited as well.

Certification and Other Qualifications

Although no state requires licensure in diagnostic medical sonography, organizations such as the American Registry for Diagnostic Medical Sonographers (ARDMS) certify the skills and knowledge of sonographers through credentialing, including registration. Registration provides an independent, objective measure of an individual's professional standing, and many employers prefer to hire registered sonographers. Some insurance providers will only pay for a patient's ultrasound services if it was provided by a certified sonographer. Sonographers registered by the ARDMS are referred to as registered diagnostic medical sonographers (RDMS). Registration with the ARDMS requires passing a general physical principles and instrumentation examination, in addition to passing an exam in a specialty such as obstetric and gynecologic sonography, abdominal sonography, or neurosonography. Sonographers must complete a required number of continuing education hours to maintain registration with the ARDMS and to stay abreast of technological advancements related to the occupation.[2]

Sonographers need good communication and interpersonal skills because they must be able to explain technical procedures and results to their patients, some of whom may be nervous about the exam or the problems it may reveal. Good hand-eye coordination is particularly important to obtain quality images. Sonographers should also enjoy learning because continuing education is the key to them staying abreast of the ever-changing field of diagnostic medicine. A background in mathematics and science is helpful for sonographers as well.

Advancement

Sonographers specializing in one particular discipline often seek competency in other specialties. For example, obstetric sonographers might seek training in abdominal sonography to broaden their opportunities and increase their marketability. Sonographers may also have advancement opportunities in education, administration, research, sales, or technical advising.

Employment Trends

Faster-than-average employment growth is expected. Job opportunities should be favorable.

Employment Change

As the U.S. population ages, demand for diagnostic imaging and therapeutic technology will increase. Employment of diagnostic medical sonographers is expected to increase by about 17% through 2029—faster than the average for all occupations.

Additional job growth also is expected as patients seek safer treatment methods and sonography becomes an increasingly attractive alternative to radiologic procedures. Unlike most diagnostic imaging methods, sonography does not involve radiation, so harmful side effects and complications from repeated use are less likely for both the patient and the sonographer. Sonographic technology is expected to evolve rapidly and to spawn many new sonography procedures, such as 3D and 4D sonography, for use in obstetric and ophthalmologic diagnosis. High costs and necessary

approval by the federal government, however, may limit the rate at which some promising new technologies are adopted.

Hospitals will remain the principal employer of diagnostic medical sonographers. Employment is expected to grow more rapidly in physicians' offices and in medical and diagnostic laboratories, including diagnostic imaging centers. Healthcare facilities such as these are expected to increase very rapidly because of the strong shift toward outpatient care, encouraged by third-party payers and made possible by technological advances that permit more procedures to be performed outside the hospital.

With members of the large Baby Boom generation remaining more active later in life, the need to diagnose medical conditions associated with aging (e.g., blood clots and tumors) will likely increase. The expansion of health insurance as a result of the Affordable Care Act has allowed more patients to have access to health insurance, likely increasing the use of imaging technology in making a diagnosis. Diagnostic medical sonographers will be needed to use and maintain the equipment employed for diagnosis and treatment.

Job Prospects

Job opportunities should be favorable. In addition to job openings from growth, some openings will arise from the need to replace sonographers who retire or leave the occupation permanently for some other reason. Pain caused by musculoskeletal disorders has made it difficult for some sonographers to perform well. Some are forced to leave the occupation early because of such disorders. TABLE 28.1 shows some projection data provided by the U.S. Department of Labor.

Earnings

Median annual earnings of diagnostic medical sonographers were $75,920 in May 2020. The lowest 10% earned less than $53,790, and the highest 10% earned more than 105,340. Median annual wages of diagnostic medical sonographers in May 2020 were $96,780 for those employed in outpatient care centers, $75,270 for those employed in offices of physicians, and $76,060 for those working in general medical and surgical hospitals.

Related Occupations

Diagnostic medical sonographers operate sophisticated equipment to help physicians and other health practitioners diagnose and treat patients. Workers in related occupations

TABLE 28.1 Projections Data for Diagnostic Medical Sonographers, 2019–2029			Change, 2019–2029	
Occupational Title	Employment, 2019	Projected Employment, 2029	Number	Percentage
Diagnostic medical sonographers	74,300	86,800	12,500	17%

Data from Bureau of Labor Statistics, U.S. Department of Labor. Occupational Outlook Handbook. U.S. Department of Labor; 2020. https://www.bls.gov/ooh/healthcare/diagnostic-medical-sonographers.htm#tab-6

include cardiovascular technologists and technicians, clinical laboratory technologists and technicians, nuclear medicine technologists, and respiratory therapists.

Additional Information

For information on a career as a diagnostic medical sonographer, contact:

- Society of Diagnostic Medical Sonography, 2745 Dallas Pkwy., Suite 350, Plano, TX 75093-8730. https://www.sdms.org

For information on becoming a registered diagnostic medical sonographer, contact:

- American Registry for Diagnostic Medical Sonography, 1401 Rockville Pike, Suite 600, Rockville, MD 20852-1402. https://www.ardms.org

For certification information, contact:

- American Registry of Radiologic Technologists, 1255 Northland Dr., St. Paul, MN 55120-1155. https://www.arrt.org

For more information on ultrasound in medicine, contact:

- American Institute of Ultrasound in Medicine, 14750 Sweitzer Ln., Suite 100, Laurel, MD 20707-5906. https://www.aium.org

For a current list of accredited education programs in diagnostic medical sonography, contact:

- Joint Review Committee on Education in Diagnostic Medical Sonography, 6021 University Boulevard, Suite 500, Ellicott City, MD 21043. https://www.jrcdms.org
- Commission on Accreditation for Allied Health Education Programs, 1361 Park St., Clearwater, FL 33756. https://www.caahep.org

CARDIOVASCULAR TECHNOLOGISTS AND TECHNICIANS
Significant Points

- Employment is expected to grow much faster than average.
- Technologists and technicians with multiple professional credentials, trained to perform a wide range of procedures, will have the best prospects.
- About 79% of jobs are in hospitals.
- Workers typically need a two-year associate's degree at a junior or community college; most employers also require a professional credential.

Work Descriptions

Cardiovascular technologists and technicians assist physicians in diagnosing and treating cardiac (heart) and peripheral vascular (blood vessel) ailments. Cardiovascular technologists and technicians schedule appointments, perform ultrasound or cardiovascular procedures, review doctors' interpretations and patient files, and monitor patients' heart rates. They also operate and maintain testing equipment, explain test procedures, and compare test results to a standard to identify problems. Other day-to-day activities vary significantly between specialties. A **cardiovascular technologist** assists physicians by performing complex medical tests involving the heart and pulmonary system whereas a **cardiovascular technician** generally performs less complex tests. Cardiovascular technologists and technicians may specialize in any of four areas of practice: **invasive cardiology**, echocardiography, vascular technology, or cardiopulmonary technology.

Invasive Cardiology

Cardiovascular technologists specializing in invasive procedures are called **cardiovascular invasive specialists**. They assist physicians with cardiac catheterization procedures in which a small tube, or catheter, is threaded through a patient's artery from a spot on the patient's groin to the heart. The procedure can determine whether a blockage exists in the blood vessels that supply the heart muscle. The procedure also can help diagnose other problems. Part of the procedure may involve balloon angioplasty, which can be used to treat blockages of blood vessels or heart valves without the need for heart surgery. Cardiology technologists assist physicians as they insert a catheter with a balloon on the end to the point of the obstruction. Another procedure using the catheter is the electrophysiology test, which helps locate the specific areas of heart tissue that give rise to the abnormal electrical impulses that cause arrhythmias.

Technologists prepare patients for cardiac catheterization by first positioning them on an examining table and then shaving, cleaning, and administering anesthesia to the top of their leg near the groin. During the catheterization procedures, they monitor patients' blood pressure and heart rate with electrocardiogram (ECG) equipment and notify the physician if something appears to be wrong. Technologists also may prepare and monitor patients during open-heart surgery and during the insertion of pacemakers and stents that open blockages in arteries to the heart and major blood vessels.

Noninvasive Technology

Technologists who specialize in vascular technology or echocardiography perform noninvasive tests. Tests are called noninvasive if they do not require the insertion of probes or other instruments into the patient's body. For example, procedures such as Doppler ultrasound transmit high-frequency sound waves into areas of the patient's body and then process reflected echoes of the sound waves to form an image. Technologists view the ultrasound image on a screen and may record the image on videotape or photograph it for interpretation and diagnosis by a physician. As the technologist uses the instrument to perform scans and record images, technologists check the image on the screen for subtle differences between healthy and diseased areas, decide which images to include in the report to the physician, and judge whether the images are satisfactory for diagnostic purposes. They also explain the procedure to patients, record any additional medical history the patient relates, select appropriate equipment settings, and change the patient's position as necessary.

Vascular Technology

Technologists who assist physicians in the diagnosis of disorders affecting the circulation are known as **vascular technologists** or vascular sonographers. Vascular technologists complete patients' medical history, evaluate pulses and assess blood flow in arteries and veins by listening to vascular flow sounds for abnormalities, and confirm that the appropriate vascular test has been ordered. Once confirmed, they perform a **noninvasive procedure** using ultrasound instruments to record vascular information such as vascular blood flow, blood pressure, oxygen saturation, cerebral circulation, peripheral circulation, abdominal circulation, and the presence of blood clots in the body. Many of these tests are performed during or immediately after surgery. Vascular technologists then provide a summary of findings to the physician to aid in patient diagnosis and management.

Cardiopulmonary Technology

For those cardiovascular professionals who are also interested in treating the lungs, they can become **cardiopulmonary technologists**. Using specialized equipment, they work with physicians to help diagnose and treat diseases and illnesses related to both the heart and lungs. They prepare patients for tests and explain procedures to them. Cardiopulmonary technologists monitor the patient's well-being throughout these tests, watching for abnormalities that might require an emergency response.

Electrocardiography and Echocardiography

This area of practice includes taking **electrocardiograms (ECGs)** and sonograms of the heart. Cardiovascular technicians who specialize in ECGs and **stress testing** and perform Holter monitor procedures are known as **cardiographic** or **electrocardiograph technicians**.

A basic ECG, which traces electrical impulses transmitted by the heart, requires technicians to attach electrodes to the patient's chest, arms, and legs and then manipulate switches on an ECG machine to obtain a reading. An ECG is printed out for interpretation by the physician. This test is done before most kinds of surgery or as part of a routine physical examination, especially on persons who have reached middle age or who have a history of cardiovascular problems.

Electrocardiograph technicians with advanced training perform Holter monitor and stress testing. For **Holter monitoring**, technicians place electrodes on the patient's chest and attach a portable ECG monitor to the patient's belt. Following 24 or more hours of normal activity by the patient, the technician removes a tape from the monitor and places it in a scanner. After checking the quality of the recorded impulses on an electronic screen, the technician usually prints the information from the tape for analysis by a physician. Physicians use the output from the scanner to diagnose heart ailments, such as heart rhythm abnormalities or problems with pacemakers. An example of a Holter monitor is seen in **FIGURE 28.4**.

For a treadmill stress test, ECG technicians document the patient's medical history, explain the procedure, connect the patient to an ECG monitor, and obtain a baseline reading and resting blood pressure. Next, they monitor the heart's performance while the patient is walking on a treadmill, gradually increasing the treadmill's speed to observe the effect of increased exertion. Like vascular technologists and cardiac sonographers, cardiographic technicians who perform ECG, Holter monitor, and stress tests are known as "noninvasive" technicians.

Technologists who use ultrasound to examine the heart chambers, valves, and vessels are referred to as cardiac sonographers, or **echocardiographers**. They use ultrasound instrumentation to create images called echocardiograms. An echocardiogram may be performed while the patient is either resting or physically active. Technologists may administer medication to physically active patients to assess their heart function. Cardiac sonographers also may assist physicians who perform **transesophageal echocardiography**, which involves placing a tube in the patient's esophagus to obtain ultrasound images.

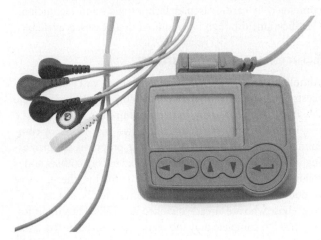

FIGURE 28.4 Holter monitor.
© Brittny/Shutterstock.

Work Environment

Cardiovascular technologists and technicians spend a lot of time walking and standing. Heavy lifting may be involved to move equipment or transfer patients. These workers wear heavy protective aprons while conducting some procedures. Those who work in catheterization laboratories may face stressful working conditions because they are in close contact with patients with serious heart ailments. For example, some patients may encounter complications that have life-or-death implications.

Some cardiovascular technologists and technicians may have the potential for radiation exposure, which is kept to a minimum by strict adherence to radiation safety guidelines. In addition, those who use sonography can be at an increased risk for musculoskeletal disorders such as carpel tunnel syndrome, neck and back strain, and eyestrain. The greater use of ergonomically correct equipment and an increased awareness of hazards will continue to minimize such risks.

Technologists and technicians generally work a five-day, 40-hour week that may include weekends. Those in catheterization laboratories tend to work longer hours and may work evenings. They also may be on call during the night and on weekends.

Employment Opportunities

Cardiovascular technologists and technicians held about 57,400 jobs in 2019. About 79% of jobs were in public and private hospitals, primarily in cardiology departments. The remaining jobs were mostly in offices of physicians, including cardiologists, or in medical and diagnostic laboratories, including diagnostic imaging centers.

Educational and Legal Requirements

An associate's degree is the most common level of education completed by cardiovascular technologists and technicians. Certification, although not required in all cases, is available.

Education and Training

Although a few cardiovascular technologists, vascular technologists, and cardiac sonographers are currently trained on the job, most receive training in two- to four-year programs. The majority of technologists complete a two-year junior or community college program, but four-year programs are increasingly available. The first year is dedicated to core courses and is followed by a year of specialized instruction in either invasive or noninvasive cardiovascular or noninvasive vascular technology. Those who are already qualified in an allied health profession need to complete only the year of specialized instruction.

The Joint Review Committee on Education in Cardiovascular Technology reviews education programs seeking accreditation. The Commission on Accreditation of Allied Health Education Programs (CAAHEP) accredits these education programs; as of September 2020, there were 97 accredited programs in cardiovascular technology in the United States.[3] Similarly, students who want to study echocardiography or vascular sonography may also attend CAAHEP-accredited programs in diagnostic medical sonography. In 2020, there were 394 diagnostic medical sonography programs accredited by CAAHEP. Those who attend these accredited programs are eligible to obtain professional certification.

Unlike most other cardiovascular technologists and technicians, most ECG technicians are trained on the job by an ECG supervisor or a cardiologist. On-the-job training usually lasts about four to six weeks. Most employers prefer to train people already in the healthcare field—nursing aides, for example. Some ECG technicians are students enrolled in two-year programs to become technologists, working part time to gain experience and make contact with employers. For technicians who perform Holter monitoring, on-the-job training may last around 18 to 24 months.

Licensure and Certification

Some states require workers in this occupation to be licensed. For information on a particular state, contact that state's medical board. Certification is available from two organizations: Cardiovascular Credentialing International (CCI) and the American Registry for Diagnostic Medical Sonographers (ARDMS). The CCI offers nine certifications—Certified Cardiographic Technician (CCT), Registered Cardiac Sonographer (RCS), Registered Vascular Specialist (RVS), Registered Cardiovascular Invasive Specialist (RCIS), Registered Cardiac Electrophysiology Specialist (RCES), Registered Congenital Cardiac Sonographer (RCCS), Advanced Cardiac Sonographer (ACS), Certified Rhythm Analysis Technician (CRAT), and Registered Phlebology Sonographer (RPhS).[4] The ARDMS offers Registered Diagnostic Cardiac Sonographer (RDCS) and Registered Vascular Technologist (RVT) credentials.[5] Some states require certification as part of licensure. In other states, certification is not required, but many employers prefer it.

Other Qualifications

Cardiovascular technologists and technicians must be reliable, have mechanical aptitude, and be able to follow detailed instructions. A pleasant, relaxed manner for putting patients at ease is an asset. Cardiovascular technologists and technicians must be articulate and well spoken, as they must communicate in technical detail with physicians and also explain procedures in a simple manner to patients.

Advancement

Technologists and technicians can advance to higher levels of the profession as many institutions structure the occupation in multiple levels, each having an increasing amount of responsibility. Technologists and technicians also can advance into supervisory or management positions. Other common possibilities include working in an educational setting or conducting laboratory work.

Employment Trends

Employment is expected to grow faster than average; technologists and technicians with multiple professional credentials, trained to perform a wide range of procedures, will have the best prospects.

Employment Change

Employment of cardiovascular technologists and technicians is expected to increase by 5% through the year 2029, faster than the average for all occupations. Growth will occur as the population ages because older people have a higher incidence of heart disease and other complications of the heart and vascular system. Noninvasive procedures, such as ultrasound, are being performed more often as an alternative to more expensive and invasive procedures. Due to advances in medicine and greater public awareness, signs of vascular disease can be detected earlier, creating demand for cardiovascular technologists and technicians to perform various procedures.

Employment of vascular technologists and echocardiographers will grow as advances in vascular technology and sonography reduce the need for more costly and invasive procedures. Electrophysiology is also becoming a rapidly growing specialty. Fewer ECG technicians will be needed, however, as hospitals train nursing aides and others to perform basic ECG procedures. Individuals trained in Holter monitoring and stress testing are expected to have more favorable job prospects than those who can perform only a basic ECG.

Medicaid has relaxed some of the rules governing reimbursement for vascular exams, which is resulting in vascular studies becoming a more routine practice. As a result of the increased use of these procedures, individuals with training in vascular studies should have more favorable employment opportunities.

Job Prospects

Some additional job openings for cardiovascular technologists and technicians will arise from replacement needs as individuals transfer to other jobs or leave the labor force. Job prospects will be best for those with multiple professional credentials, trained to perform a wide range of procedures. Those willing to relocate or work irregular hours also will have better job opportunities.

It is not uncommon for cardiovascular technologists and technicians to move between the specialties within the occupation by obtaining certification in more than one specialty. TABLE 28.2 shows some projection data provided by the U.S. Department of Labor.

Median annual earnings of cardiovascular technologists and technicians were $59,100 in May 2020. The lowest 10% earned less than $30,140, and the highest 10% earned more than $96,790. Median annual earnings of cardiovascular technologists and technicians in 2020 were $75,430 in outpatient care centers, $63,250 in offices of physicians, and $57,850 in general medical and surgical hospitals.

Related Occupations

Cardiovascular technologists and technicians operate sophisticated equipment that helps physicians and other health practitioners to diagnose and treat patients. Other occupations include diagnostic medical sonographers, nuclear medicine technologists, radiation therapists, radiologic technologists and technicians, and respiratory therapists.

Additional Information

For general information about a career in cardiovascular technology, contact:

- Alliance of Cardiovascular Professionals, P.O. Box 2007, Midlothian, VA 23113. https://www.acp-online.org

For a list of accredited programs in cardiovascular technology, contact:

- Committee on Accreditation for Allied Health Education Programs, 1361 Park St., Clearwater, FL 33756. https://www.caahep.org
- Society for Vascular Ultrasound, 4601 Presidents Dr., Suite 260, Lanham, MD 20706-4381. https://www.svunet.org

TABLE 28.2 Projections Data for Cardiovascular Technologists and Technicians, 2019–2029				
			Change, 2019–2029	
Occupational Title	Employment, 2019	Projected Employment, 2029	Number	Percentage
Cardiovascular technologists and technicians	57,400	60,500	3,100	5%

Data from Bureau of Labor Statistics, U.S. Department of Labor. Occupational Outlook Handbook. U.S. Department of Labor; 2020. https://www.bls.gov/ooh/healthcare/diagnostic-medical-sonographers.htm#tab-6

For information regarding registration and certification, contact:

- Cardiovascular Credentialing International, 1500 Sunday Dr., Suite 102, Raleigh, NC 27607. https://www.cci-online.org
- American Registry of Diagnostic Medical Sonographers, 51 Monroe St., Plaza East One, Rockville, MD 20850-2400. http://www.ardms.org

NUCLEAR MEDICINE TECHNOLOGISTS
Significant Points

- Job opportunities should be favorable.
- Technologists with training in multiple diagnostic methods or in nuclear cardiology should have the best prospects.
- Nuclear medicine technology programs range in length from one to four years and lead to a certificate, an associate's degree, or a bachelor's degree.
- About 73% of nuclear medicine technologists work in hospitals.

Work Description

Diagnostic imaging embraces several procedures that aid in diagnosing ailments, the most familiar being the X-ray. In **nuclear medicine**, **radionuclides**—unstable atoms that emit radiation spontaneously—are used to diagnose and treat disease. Radionuclides are purified and compounded to form **radiopharmaceuticals**. Nuclear medicine technologists administer radiopharmaceuticals to patients and then monitor the characteristics and functions of tissues or organs in which the drugs localize. Abnormal areas show higher-than-expected or lower-than-expected concentrations of radioactivity. An example of a radiopharmaceutical used for imaging plaques associated with Alzheimer's disease is seen in **FIGURE 28.5**. Nuclear medicine differs from other diagnostic imaging technologies because it determines the presence of disease on the basis of metabolic changes rather than changes in organ structure.

Nuclear medicine technologists operate cameras that detect and map the radioactive drug in a patient's body to create diagnostic images. After explaining test procedures to patients, technologists prepare a dose of the radiopharmaceutical and administer it by mouth, injection, inhalation, or other means. They position patients and start a **gamma scintillation camera**, or "scanner," which creates images of

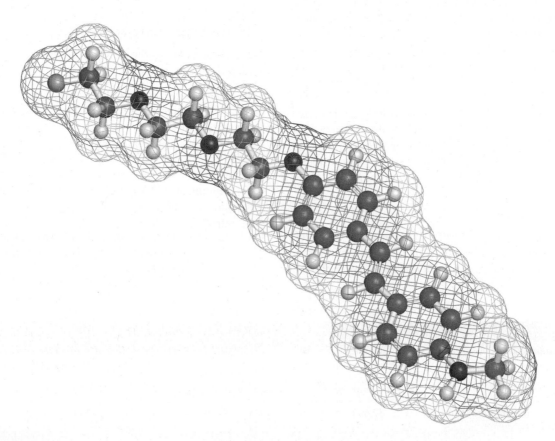

FIGURE 28.5 Radiopharmaceutical associated with diagnosing Alzheimer's disease.
© molekuul_be/Shutterstock.

the distribution of a radiopharmaceutical as it localizes in, and emits signals from, the patient's body. The images are produced on a computer screen or on film for a physician to interpret. Additionally, they may treat medical conditions by delivering prescribed doses to specific areas, such as tumors, as an alternative to surgery.

When preparing radiopharmaceuticals, technologists adhere to safety standards that keep the radiation exposure as low as possible to workers and patients. Technologists maintain patient records and document the amount and type of radionuclides that they receive, use, and discard. They comply with established protocols for the disposal of the radionuclides.

In the event of an emergency involving radiation or a nuclear disaster, technologists may serve as emergency responders. Their knowledge of detecting radiation and monitoring its presence is useful in such an event.

Work Environment

Physical stamina is important because nuclear medicine technologists are on their feet much of the day and may have to lift or turn disabled patients. In addition, technologists must operate complicated equipment that requires mechanical ability and manual dexterity.

Although the potential for radiation exposure exists in this field, it is minimized by the use of shielded syringes, gloves, and other protective devices and by adherence to strict radiation safety guidelines. The amount of radiation in a nuclear medicine procedure is comparable to that received during a diagnostic X-ray procedure. Technologists also wear badges that measure radiation levels. Because of safety programs, badge measurements rarely exceed established safety levels. Detailed measurements are kept over a lifetime to determine how much radiation technologists receive.

Nuclear medicine technologists generally work a 40-hour week, perhaps including evening or weekend hours, in departments that operate on an extended schedule. Opportunities for part-time and shift work also are available. In addition, technologists in hospitals may have on-call duty on a rotational basis, and those employed by mobile imaging services may be required to travel to several locations.

There are three areas of specialty for nuclear medicine technologists—**nuclear cardiology (NCT)**, **positron emission tomography (PET)**, and **nuclear medicine computer tomography (CT) technologists**. Nuclear cardiology typically involves myocardial perfusion imaging, which, like most nuclear medicine, uses radiopharmaceuticals and cameras to image the body. Myocardial perfusion imaging, however, requires that patients perform exercise so the technologist can image the heart and blood flow. Technologists specializing in PET operate a special medical imaging device that produces a 3D image of the body. CT technologists combine the use of radioisotopes with X-rays to create two-dimensional or three-dimensional images inside the human body.

Employment Opportunities

Nuclear medicine technologists held about 18,500 jobs in 2019. About 73% of all nuclear medicine technologist jobs were in hospitals—private and public. Most of the rest were in offices of physicians or in medical and diagnostic laboratories, including diagnostic imaging centers.

Educational and Legal Requirements

Nuclear medicine technology programs range in length from one to four years and lead to a certificate, an associate's degree, or a bachelor's degree. Many employers and an increasing number of states require certification or licensure. Aspiring nuclear medicine technologists should check the requirements of the state in which they plan to work.

Education and Training

Completion of a nuclear medicine technology program takes one to four years and leads to a certificate, an associate's degree, or a bachelor's degree. Generally, certificate programs are offered in hospitals, associate's degree programs in community colleges, and bachelor's degree programs in four-year colleges and universities. Courses cover the physical sciences, the biological effects of radiation exposure, radiation protection and procedures, the use of radiopharmaceuticals, imaging techniques, and computer applications.

One-year certificate programs are for health professionals who already possess an associate's degree—especially radiologic technologists and diagnostic medical sonographers—but who wish to specialize in nuclear medicine. The programs also attract medical technologists, registered nurses, and others who wish to change fields or specialize.

The Joint Review Committee on Education Programs in Nuclear Medicine Technology accredits most formal training programs in nuclear medicine technology. In 2021, there were more than 70 accredited programs available.[6]

Licensure and Certification

Educational requirements for nuclear medicine technologists vary from state to state, so it is important that aspiring technologists check the requirements of the state in which they plan to work. In 2021, all 50 states, the District of Columbia, and Puerto Rico licensed nuclear medicine technologists. In addition, many third-party payers require nuclear medicine technologists to be certified in order for the healthcare facility to receive reimbursement for imaging procedures. Certification is available from the American Registry of Radiologic Technologists (ARRT) and from the Nuclear Medicine Technology Certification Board (NMTCB). Although not required, some workers receive certification from both agencies. Nuclear medicine technologists must meet the minimum federal standards on the administration of radioactive drugs and the operation of radiation detection equipment.

The most common way to become eligible for certification by ARRT or NMTCB is to complete a training program recognized by those organizations. Other ways to become eligible are completing a bachelor's or associate's degree in biological science or a related health field, such as registered nursing, or acquiring, under supervision, a certain number of hours of experience in nuclear medicine technology. ARRT and NMTCB have different requirements, but in all cases, one must pass a comprehensive exam to become certified.

In addition to the general certification requirements, certified technicians also must complete a certain number of continuing education hours. Continuing education is required primarily because of the frequent technological and innovative changes in the field of nuclear medicine. Typically, technologists must register annually with both the ARRT and the NMTCB.

Other Qualifications

Nuclear medicine technologists should have excellent communication skills, be detail oriented, and have a desire to continue learning. Technologists must effectively interact with patients and their families and should be sensitive to patients' physical and psychological needs. Nuclear medicine technologists must be able to work independently as they usually have little direct supervision. Technologists also must be detailed oriented and meticulous when performing procedures to ensure that all regulations are being followed. Technologists require physical stamina when lifting and moving patients who need their help and in standing for long periods of time.

Advancement

Technologists may advance to supervisor, then to chief technologist, and to department administrator or director. Some technologists specialize in a clinical area, such as nuclear cardiology or computer analysis, or leave patient care to take positions in research laboratories. Some become instructors in or directors of nuclear medicine technology programs, a step that usually requires a bachelor's or master's degree in the subject. Others leave the occupation to work as sales or training representatives for medical equipment and radiopharmaceutical manufacturing firms or as radiation safety officers in regulatory agencies or hospitals.

Employment Trends

Faster-than-average job growth will arise from an increase in the number of middle-aged and elderly persons, who are the primary users of diagnostic and treatment procedures. The number of job openings each year will increase because of technological advancements in the profession.

Employment Change

Employment of nuclear medicine technologists is expected to increase by 5% from 2019 to 2029, faster than the average for all occupations. Growth will arise from technological advancement, the development of new nuclear medicine treatments, and an increase in the number of middle-aged and older persons, who are the primary users of diagnostic procedures, including nuclear medicine tests.

Technological innovations may increase the diagnostic uses of nuclear medicine. New nuclear medical imaging technologies, including positron emission tomography (PET) and single photon emission computed tomography (SPECT), are expected to be used increasingly and to contribute further to employment growth. The wider use of nuclear medical imaging to observe metabolic and biochemical changes during neurology, cardiology, and oncology procedures also will spur demand for nuclear medicine technologists.

Nonetheless, cost considerations will affect the speed with which new applications of nuclear medicine grow. Some promising nuclear medicine procedures, such as positron emission tomography, are extremely costly, and hospitals contemplating these procedures will have to consider equipment costs, reimbursement policies, and the number of potential users.

Job Prospects

In spite of fast growth in nuclear medicine, the number of openings in the occupation each year remain steady because new workers will replace those who retire or transfer to different occupations. Technologists who have additional training in other diagnostic methods, such as radiologic technology or diagnostic medical sonography, will enjoy the best prospects. TABLE 28.3 shows some projection data provided by the U.S. Department of Labor.

Earnings

Median annual earnings of nuclear medicine technologists were $79,590 in May 2020. The lowest 10% earned less than $57,830, and the highest 10% earned more than $109,070. Median annual earnings of nuclear medicine technologists in 2020 were $116,800 in outpatient care centers, $79,210 in physician offices, and $79,750 in general medical and surgical hospitals.

TABLE 28.3 Projections for Nuclear Medicine Technologists, 2019–2029

Occupational Title	Employment, 2019	Projected Employment, 2029	Change, 2019–2029 Number	Percentage
Nuclear medicine technologists	18,500	19,500	1000	5%

Data from Bureau of Labor Statistics, U.S. Department of Labor. Occupational Outlook Handbook. U.S. Department of Labor; 2020. https://www.bls.gov/ooh/healthcare/nuclear-medicine-technologists.htm#tab-6

Related Occupations

Nuclear medicine technologists operate sophisticated equipment to help physicians and other health practitioners diagnose and treat patients. Cardiovascular technologists and technicians, clinical laboratory technologists and technicians, diagnostic medical sonographers, radiation therapists, radiologic technologists and technicians, and respiratory therapists perform similar functions.

Additional Information

Additional information on a career as a nuclear medicine technologist is available from:

- Society of Nuclear Medicine and Molecular Imaging, 1850 Samuel Morse Dr., Reston, VA 20190. https://www.snmmi.org

For a list of accredited programs in nuclear medicine technology, contact:

- Joint Review Committee on Educational Programs in Nuclear Medicine Technology, 2000 W. Danforth Rd., Suite 130 #203, Edmond, OK 73003. https://www.jrcnmt.org

Information on certification is available from:

- Nuclear Medicine Technology Certification Board, 3558 Habersham at Northlake, Building 1, Tucker, GA 30084. https://www.nmtcb.org
- American Registry of Radiologic Technologists, 1255 Northland Dr., St. Paul, MN 55120-1155. https://www.arrt.org

SURGICAL TECHNOLOGISTS
Significant Points

- Employment is expected to grow faster than average.
- Job opportunities will be best for technologists who are certified and for those who are willing to relocate.
- Training programs last 9 to 24 months and lead to a certificate, diploma, or associate's degree.
- Hospitals will continue to be the primary employers, although much faster employment growth is expected in other healthcare industries.

Work Descriptions

Surgical technologists, also called scrubs and surgical or operating room technicians, assist in surgical operations under the supervision of surgeons, registered nurses, or other surgical personnel. Surgical technologists are members of operating room teams, which most commonly include surgeons, anesthesiologists, and circulating nurses.

Before an operation, surgical technologists help prepare the operating room by setting up surgical instruments and equipment, sterile drapes, and sterile solutions. They assemble both sterile and nonsterile equipment as well as check and adjust it to ensure that it is working properly. Technologists also get patients ready for surgery by washing, shaving, and disinfecting incision sites. They transport patients to the operating room, help position them on the operating table, and cover them with sterile surgical drapes. Technologists also observe patients' vital signs, check charts, and help the surgical team put on sterile gowns and gloves.

During surgery, technologists pass instruments and other sterile supplies to surgeons and surgeon assistants. They may hold retractors, cut sutures, and help count sponges, needles, supplies, and instruments. Surgical technologists help prepare, care for, and dispose of specimens taken for laboratory analysis and help apply dressings. Some operate sterilizers, lights, or suction machines and help operate diagnostic equipment.

After an operation, surgical technologists may help transfer patients to the recovery room and clean and restock the operating room. Certified surgical technologists with additional specialized education or training also may act as the surgical first assistant or circulator. The surgical first assistant, as defined by the American College of Surgeons (ACS), plays a hands-on role, providing aid in exposure, hemostasis (controlling blood flow and stopping or preventing hemorrhage), and other technical functions under the surgeon's direction to assist the surgeon in carrying out a safe operation. A circulating technologist is the "unsterile" member of the surgical team. The circulator interviews and prepares the patient prior to surgery, assists with anesthesia, obtains and opens packages from which the "sterile" team members remove sterile contents during the procedure, keeps a written account of the surgical procedure, and answers the surgeon's questions about the patient during the surgery.

Work Environment

Surgical technologists work in clean, well-lit, cool environments. They must stand for long periods and remain alert during operations. At times, they may be exposed to communicable diseases and unpleasant sights, odors, and materials. They must wear special sterile clothing called scrubs while they are in the operating room. Most surgical technologists work a regular 40-hour week, although they may be on call or work nights, weekends, and holidays on a rotating basis.

Employment Opportunities

Surgical technologists held about 111,300 jobs in 2019. About 73% of jobs for surgical technologists were in hospitals, mainly in operating and delivery rooms. Other jobs were in offices of physicians or dentists who perform outpatient surgery and in outpatient care centers, including ambulatory surgical centers. A few technologists, known as private scrubs, are employed directly by surgeons who maintain specialized surgical teams, such as those for liver transplants.

Educational and Legal Requirements

Training programs last 9 to 24 months and lead to a certificate, diploma, or associate's degree. Professional certification can help in getting jobs and promotions.

Education and Training

Surgical technologists receive their training in formal programs offered by community and junior colleges, vocational schools, universities, hospitals, and the military. In 2011, the Commission on Accreditation of Allied Health Education Programs (CAAHEP) recognized about 500 accredited training programs.[7] Programs last from 9 to 24 months and lead to a certificate, diploma, or associate's degree. High school graduation normally is required for admission. Recommended high school courses include health, biology, chemistry, and mathematics.

Surgical technologist training programs provide classroom education and supervised clinical experience. Students take courses in anatomy, physiology, microbiology, pharmacology, professional ethics, and medical terminology. Other topics covered include the care and safety of patients during surgery, sterile techniques, and surgical procedures. Students also learn to sterilize instruments, prevent and control infection, and handle special drugs, solutions, supplies, and equipment.

Certification and Other Qualifications

Most employers prefer to hire certified surgical technologists. Technologists may obtain voluntary professional certification from the National Board of Surgical Technology and Surgical Assisting by graduating from a CAAHEP-accredited program and passing a national certification examination.[8] They may then use the Certified Surgical Technologist (CST) designation. Continuing education or reexamination is required to maintain certification, which must be renewed every four years.

Certification also may be obtained from the National Center for Competency Testing (NCCT).[9] Candidates qualify for the exam by following one of three paths: (1) they complete an accredited training program, (2) undergo a two-year hospital on-the-job training program, or (3) acquire three years of experience working in the field. After passing the exam, individuals may use the designation Tech in Surgery-Certified (TS-C). This certification must be renewed every five years through either continuing education or reexamination.

Surgical first assistants can obtain certification from three organizations: the Certified First Surgical Assistant (CFSA) designation from the National Board of Surgical Technology and Surgical Assisting, the Surgical Assistant Certified (SA-C) designation from the American Board of Surgical Assistants, or the Certified Surgical Assistant (CSA) designation from the National Surgical Assistants Association.[10]

Surgical technologists need manual dexterity sufficient to handle instruments quickly. They also must be conscientious, orderly, and emotionally stable to handle the demands of the operating room environment. Technologists must respond quickly and be familiar enough with operating room procedures to have instruments on hand for surgeons as needed. They are expected to keep abreast of new developments in the field.

Advancement

Technologists advance by specializing in a particular area of surgery, such as neurosurgery or open-heart surgery. They also may work as circulating technologists. With additional training, some technologists advance to surgical first assistant. Some surgical technologists manage central supply departments in hospitals or take positions with insurance companies, sterile supply services, and operating equipment firms.

Employment Trends

Employment of surgical technologists is expected to grow faster than the average for all occupations. Job opportunities will be best for technologists who are certified and for those who are willing to relocate.

Employment Change

Employment of surgical technologists is expected to grow 7% between 2019 and 2029, faster than the average for all occupations, as the volume of surgeries increases. Surgeries are safer due to advances in medical technology, allowing for an increase in operations for a variety of injuries and illnesses. The number of surgical procedures is expected to rise as the population grows and ages. Older people, including the Baby Boom generation, who generally require more surgical procedures, will account for a larger portion of the general population. In addition, technological advances, such as fiber optics and laser technology, will permit an increasing number of new surgical procedures to be performed and also will allow surgical technologists to assist with a greater number of procedures.

Hospitals will continue to be the primary employer of surgical technologists, although much faster employment growth is expected in offices of physicians and in outpatient care centers, including ambulatory surgical centers.

Job Prospects

Job opportunities will be best for technologists who are certified. TABLE 28.4 shows some projection data provided by the U.S. Department of Labor.

Earnings

Median annual earnings of wage and salary surgical technologists were $49,710 in May 2020. The lowest 10% earned less than $34,120, and the highest 10% earned more than $73,110. Median annual earnings in the industries employing the largest numbers of surgical technologists are shown in TABLE 28.5.

TABLE 28.4 Projections Data for Surgical Technologists, 2019–2029

Occupational Title	Employment, 2019	Projected Employment, 2029	Change, 2019–2029	
			Number	Percentage
Surgical technologists	111,300	118,900	7,600	7%

Data from Bureau of Labor Statistics, U.S. Department of Labor. Occupational Outlook Handbook. U.S. Department of Labor; 2020. https://www.bls.gov/ooh/healthcare/surgical-technologists.htm#tab-6

TABLE 28.5 Median Annual Earnings in Industries Employing Surgical Technologists, May 2020

Outpatient care centers	$52,120
Hospitals: state, local and private	$49,500
Offices of physicians	$49,670
Offices of dentists	$46.940

Data from Bureau of Labor Statistics, U.S. Department of Labor. Occupational Outlook Handbook. U.S. Department of Labor; 2020. https://www.bls.gov/ooh/healthcare/surgical-technologists.htm?view_full#tab-5

Wages of surgical technologists vary with their experience and education, the responsibilities of the position, the working hours, and the economy of a given region of the country. Benefits provided by most employers include paid vacation and sick leave; health, medical, vision, dental, and life insurance; and retirement programs. A few employers also provide tuition reimbursement and child-care benefits.

Related Occupations

Other health occupations requiring approximately one year of training after high school include dental assistants, licensed practical and licensed vocational nurses, clinical laboratory technologists and technicians, and medical assistants.

Additional Information

For additional information on a career as a surgical technologist and a list of CAAHEP-accredited programs, contact:

- Association of Surgical Technologists, 6 West Dry Creek Cir., Suite 200, Littleton, CO 80120. https://www.ast.org

For information on becoming a certified surgical technologist, contact:

- National Board of Surgical Technologists and Surgical Assistants, 6 West Dry Creek Cir., Suite 100, Littleton, CO 80120. https://www.nbstsa.org

For information on becoming a Tech in Surgery-Certified, contact:

- National Center for Competency Testing, 7007 College Blvd., Suite 385, Overland Park, KS 66211. https://www.ncctinc.com

For information on becoming certified as a surgical assistant, contact:

- National Board of Surgical Technologists and Surgical Assistants, 6 West Dry Creek Cir., Suite 100, Littleton, CO 80120. https://www.nbstsa.org
- American Board of Surgical Assistants, 11414 West Park Place , Milwaukee, WI 53224. https://www.absa.net
- National Surgical Assistant Association, 1775 Eye Street NW, Washington DC 20006. https://www.nsaa.net

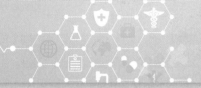

LEARNING PORTFOLIO

Issues for Discussion

1. Review the requirements for becoming a diagnostic medical sonographer, a cardiovascular technologist, a nuclear medicine technologist, and a surgical technologist. Compare the requirements for preparing for these four careers in terms of length of training, cost of training, job opportunities, and lifetime income. Which of these careers best matches your career goals?

2. Diagnostic medical sonographers and cardiovascular technologists each have opportunities to specialize in certain areas of their respective fields. Discuss these specializations and identify which one is of most interest to you.

Enrichment Activities

1. View the career video developed by the Society of Diagnostic Medical Sonography. (https://www.youtube.com/watch?v=4K6tf27z6wU). Discuss your impressions.

2. View the career video on about cardiovascular technologists and technicians. (https://www.youtube.com/watch?v=MRixkfg2jFM). Discuss your impressions.

CASE STUDY: NUCLEAR MEDICINE SAFETY & HEALTH

Breanna is studying to be a nuclear medicine technologist. She will complete her educational program in May and expects to obtain employment at the local community hospital. Today, Breanna is shadowing in the nuclear medicine department where she will see exactly how the technologists perform their job duties.

Based on the information you have read about nuclear medicine technologists, answer the following questions.

1. Breanna realized half way through her shift that _____ stamina is important because technologists spend most of the day on their feet, in addition to lifting or turning patients.
   A. mental
   B. physical
   C. emotional
   D. financial

2. In order to reduce the risk of radiation exposure, Breanna was required to wear _____ during her day in the department.
   A. gloves and shields
   B. hats and boots
   C. helmets and face masks
   D. a respirator and jumpsuit

3. Breanna had the opportunity to visit one of the specialty areas of nuclear medicine where myocardial perfusion imaging is performed. This area is most likely:
   A. nuclear neurology.
   B. nuclear psychology.
   C. nuclear gynecology.
   D. nuclear cardiology.

4. Breanna learned that technologists specializing in positron emission tomography operate a special imaging device that produces a(n) _____ image.
   A. black-and-white
   B. color
   C. 3D
   D. life-size

5. Breanna is completing her four-year bachelor's degree in May and will have covered courses such as:
   A. physical sciences.
   B. imaging techniques.
   C. computer applications.
   D. All of these are correct.

References

1. Commission on Accreditation of Allied Health Education Programs. Diagnostic Medical Sonography Accredited Programs. https://www.caahep.org/Students/Find-a-Program.aspx Accessed August 30, 2021.

2. American Registry of Diagnostic Medical Sonographers. Registered Diagnostic Medical Sonographer. https://www.ardms.org/get-certified/rdms/ Accessed August 30, 2021.

3. Commission on Accreditation of Allied Health Education Programs. Cardiovascular Technology Accredited Programs. https://www.caahep.org/Students/Find-a-Program.aspx Accessed August 30, 2021.

4. Cardiovascular Credentialing International. Certifications. https://cci-online.org/CCI/Credentials/CCI/Content/Credentials.aspx?hkey=8770022b-951e-4b38-aa50-c2920ea6a7d6 Accessed August 30, 2021.

LEARNING PORTFOLIO

5. American Registry of Diagnostic Medical Sonographers. Get Certified. https://www.ardms.org/ Accessed August 30, 2021.

6. Joint Review Committee on Education Programs in Nuclear Medicine Technology. Accredited Programs. https://jrcnmt .org/find-a-program/ Accessed August 30, 2021.

7. Commission on Accreditation of Allied Health Education Programs. Surgical Technology. https://www.caahep .org/Students/Find-a-Program.aspx Accessed August 30, 2021.

8. National Board of Surgical Technology and Surgical Assisting, CST Examinations. https://www.nbstsa.org/cst-certification Accessed August 30, 2021.

9. National Center for Competency Testing. Tech-In-Surgery. https://www.ncctinc.com/Certifications/tsc Accessed August 30, 2021.

10. National Board of Surgical Technology and Surgical Assisting. CSFA Examinations. https://www.nbstsa.org/csfa-certification Accessed August 30, 2021.

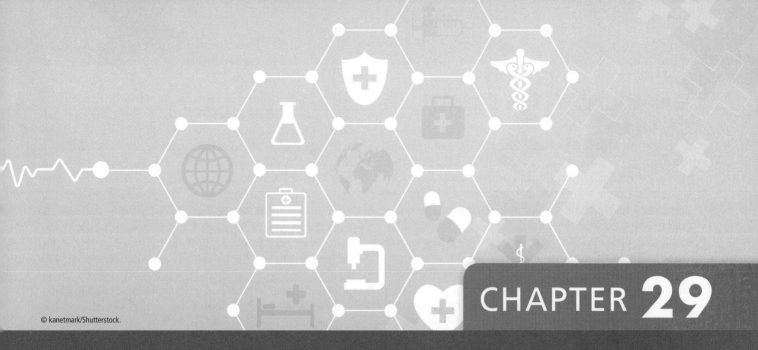

© kanetmark/Shutterstock.

CHAPTER **29**

Respiratory Care Practitioners*

KEY TERMS

Aerosol
Arterial blood sample
Blood pH
Cardiopulmonary disorders
Certified Respiratory
  Therapist (CRT)

Chest physiotherapy
Commission on Accreditation
  for Respiratory Care (Co-ARC)
Lung capacity
National Board for Respiratory
  Care (NBRC)

Oxygen or oxygen mixtures
Polysomnography
Registered Respiratory
  Therapist (RRT)
Respiratory therapy technicians
Ventilators

* All information in this chapter, unless otherwise indicated, was obtained from Bureau of Labor Statistics. *Occupational Outlook Handbook 2020–2021 Edition*. Washington, DC: U.S. Department of Labor; 2021.

MAINTAINING THE BREATH OF LIFE

A person can live without water for a few days and without food for a few weeks, but if someone stops breathing for more than a few minutes, serious brain damage occurs. If oxygen is cut off for more than nine minutes, death usually results. Respiratory therapists, also known as respiratory care practitioners, specialize in the evaluation, treatment, education, and care of patients with breathing disorders. Whenever the breath of life is at risk, the respiratory therapist is called upon to intervene. Respiratory therapists perform procedures that are crucial in maintaining the lives of seriously ill patients with breathing problems and assist in the treatment of patients with cardiopulmonary (heart and lung) diseases and disorders.

RESPIRATORY THERAPISTS
Significant Points

- Job opportunities should be very good.
- Hospitals will account for the vast majority of job openings, but a growing number of openings will arise in other settings.
- An associate's degree is the minimum educational requirement, but a bachelor's or master's degree may be important for advancement in management or education.
- All states except Alaska require respiratory therapists to be licensed.

Work Description

Respiratory therapists—also known as respiratory care practitioners—evaluate, treat, educate, and care for patients with breathing or other **cardiopulmonary disorders**. Practicing under the direction of a physician, respiratory therapists assume primary responsibility for all respiratory care therapeutic treatments and diagnostic procedures, including the supervision of respiratory therapy technicians. They consult with physicians and other healthcare staff to help develop and modify patient care plans. Therapists also provide complex therapy requiring considerable independent judgment, such as caring for patients on life support in intensive care units of hospitals.

Respiratory therapists evaluate and treat all types of patients, ranging from premature infants whose lungs are not fully developed to older adults whose lungs are diseased. They provide temporary relief to patients with chronic asthma or emphysema and give emergency care to patients who are victims of a heart attack, stroke, drowning, trauma, or shock. Cystic fibrosis—an inherited genetic disease of the lungs—requires ongoing respiratory therapy. The mucus secreted by the lungs is thick and sticky, which increases the risk for lung infections, requiring ongoing respiratory therapy to prevent and treat lung infections.

Respiratory therapists interview patients, perform limited physical examinations, and conduct diagnostic tests. For example, respiratory therapists test patients' breathing capacity and determine the concentration of oxygen and other gases in their blood. They also measure a **blood pH**, which indicates the acidity or alkalinity of the blood. To evaluate a patient's **lung capacity**, respiratory therapists have the patient breathe into an instrument—a spirometer—that measures the volume and flow of oxygen during inhalation and exhalation. An example of how a patient inhales and exhales is seen in **FIGURE 29.1**. By comparing the reading with the norm for the patient's age, height, weight, and sex, respiratory therapists can provide information that helps determine whether the patient has any lung deficiencies. To analyze oxygen, carbon dioxide, and blood pH levels, therapists draw an **arterial blood sample**, place it in a blood gas analyzer, and relay the results to a physician, who then makes treatment decisions.

To treat patients, respiratory therapists use **oxygen or oxygen mixtures**, **chest physiotherapy**, and **aerosol** medications—liquid medications suspended in a gas that forms a mist that is inhaled. They teach patients how to inhale the aerosol properly to ensure its effectiveness. When a patient has difficulty getting enough oxygen into his or her blood, therapists increase the patient's concentration of oxygen by placing an oxygen mask or nasal cannula on the patient and setting the oxygen flow at the level prescribed by a physician. Therapists also connect patients who cannot breathe on their own to **ventilators** that deliver pressurized oxygen into the lungs. The therapists insert a tube into the patient's trachea, or windpipe; connect the tube to the ventilator; and set the rate, volume, and oxygen concentration of the oxygen mixture entering the patient's lungs. A demonstration of a respiratory therapist inserting a tube into a patient mannequin is seen in **FIGURE 29.2**.

Therapists perform regular assessments of patients and equipment. If a patient appears to be having difficulty breathing or if the oxygen, carbon dioxide, or pH level of the blood is abnormal, therapists change the ventilator setting according to the doctor's orders or check the equipment for mechanical problems.

Respiratory therapists perform chest physiotherapy on patients to remove mucus from their lungs and make it easier for them to breathe. Therapists place patients in positions that help drain mucus—usually the patient lies down with the head facing down—and the therapist vibrates the patients' rib cages, often by tapping on the chest and telling the patients to cough. Chest physiotherapy may be needed after surgery, for example, because anesthesia depresses respiration. As a result, physiotherapy may be prescribed to help get the patient's lungs back to normal and to prevent congestion. Chest physiotherapy also helps patients suffering from lung diseases, such as cystic fibrosis.

Therapists who work in home care teach patients and their families to use ventilators and other life-support systems. In addition, these therapists visit patients in their homes to inspect and clean equipment, evaluate the home environment, and ensure that patients have sufficient knowledge of their diseases and the proper use of their medications

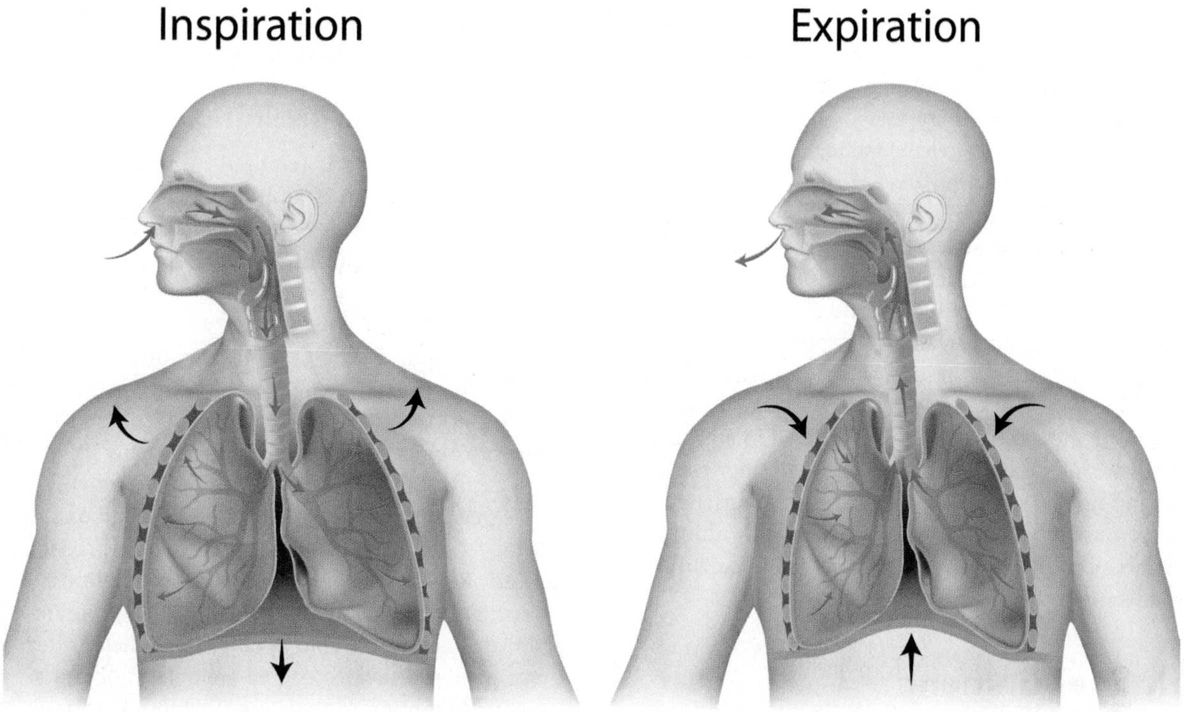

Inspiration   Expiration

FIGURE 29.1 Example of patient breathing.
© Alila Medical Media/Shutterstock.

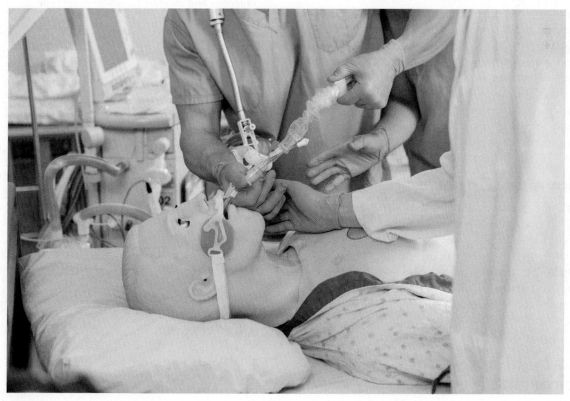

FIGURE 29.2 Insertion of breathing tube.
© Tyler Olson/Shutterstock.

and equipment. Therapists also make emergency visits if equipment problems arise.

In some hospitals, therapists perform tasks that fall outside their traditional role. Therapists are becoming involved in areas such as pulmonary rehabilitation, smoking-cessation counseling, disease prevention, case management, and **polysomnography**—the diagnosis of breathing disorders during sleep, such as sleep apnea. Respiratory therapists also increasingly treat critical-care patients in intensive care units in the hospital and as part of surface and air transport teams or as part of rapid-response teams in hospitals.

The respiratory therapist is often part of a team of health professionals who work in pulmonary rehabilitation—a program of education and exercise—offered to a group of individuals with lung disease (e.g., COPD) to improve lung function and muscle strength so that patients can participate in physical activity without shortness of breath. Additional team members on the rehab team are doctors, nurses, physical therapists, exercise specialists, and dietitians.[1]

Work Environment

Respiratory therapists generally work between 35 and 40 hours a week. The majority work in hospitals—81%—or nursing care facilities. Because these facilities operate around the clock, therapists can work evenings, nights, or weekends. Physical stamina is a necessary quality for therapists because they spend long periods standing and walking between patients' rooms and may also need to lift or turn disabled patients. In an emergency, therapists work under the stress of the situation. Respiratory therapists employed in home health care must travel frequently to patients' homes.

Respiratory therapists are trained to work with gases stored under pressure. Adherence to safety precautions and the regular maintenance and testing of equipment minimize the risk of injury. As in many other health occupations, respiratory therapists are exposed to infectious diseases, but by carefully following proper infection control procedures, they can minimize these risks.

Employment Opportunities

Respiratory therapists held about 135,800 jobs in 2019. About 82% of jobs were in hospitals, mainly in departments of respiratory care, anesthesiology, or pulmonary medicine. Most of the remaining jobs were in offices of physicians or other health practitioners, consumer-goods rental firms that supply respiratory equipment for home use, nursing care facilities, employment services, and home healthcare services.

Educational and Legal Requirements

An associate's degree is the minimum educational requirement, but a bachelor's or master's degree may be important for advancement. All states except Alaska require respiratory therapists to be licensed.

Education and Training

An associate's degree is required to become an entry-level respiratory therapist. Training is offered at the postsecondary level by colleges and universities, medical schools, vocational-technical institutes, and the armed forces. Most programs award associate's or bachelor's degrees and prepare graduates for jobs as entry-level respiratory therapists. According to the **Commission on Accreditation for Respiratory Care (Co-ARC)**, 438 respiratory care programs held Co-ARC accreditation status in 2020.[2] The majority offered associate degrees, although many offered bachelor's degrees and a few offered master's degrees. There are 17 Degree Advancement (DA) programs and one Advanced Practice (APRT) education program for practicing **Registered Respiratory Therapists (RRT)** holding Co-ARC accreditation. Students enrolled in a DA program with an associate's degree are able to obtain a bachelor's degree, and those with a bachelor's degree are able to obtain a master's degree.[2] According to the Commission on Accreditation of Allied Health Education Programs (CAAHEP), 16 perfusion programs and 41 polysomnographic technology programs were accredited in the United States in 2020.[3]

Among the areas of study in respiratory therapy programs are human anatomy and physiology, pathophysiology, chemistry, physics, microbiology, pharmacology, medical terminology, and mathematics. Other courses deal with therapeutic and diagnostic procedures and tests, equipment, patient assessment, cardiopulmonary resuscitation, the application of clinical practice guidelines, patient care outside of hospitals, cardiac and pulmonary rehabilitation, respiratory health promotion and disease prevention, and medical record keeping and reimbursement. An example of the medical terminology with which a respiratory therapist must be familiar when treating asthma patients is seen in **FIGURE 29.3**.

High school students interested in applying to respiratory therapy programs should take courses in health, biology, mathematics, chemistry, and physics. Respiratory care involves basic mathematical problem solving and an understanding of chemical and physical principles. For example, respiratory care workers must be able to compute dosages of medication and calculate gas concentrations.

Licensure and Certification

A license is required to practice as a respiratory therapist, except in Alaska. The majority of states require completion of continuing education hours for license renewal. Also, most employers require respiratory therapists to maintain a cardiopulmonary resuscitation (CPR) certification.

Licensure is usually based, in large part, on meeting the requirements for certification from the **National Board for Respiratory Care (NBRC)**.[4] The board offers the **Certified Respiratory Therapist (CRT)** credential to those who

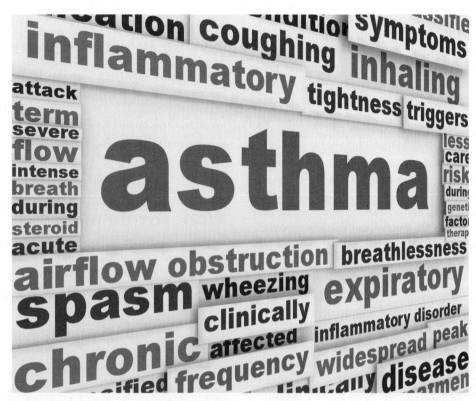

FIGURE 29.3 Medical terminology used by respiratory therapists.
© Andrii Kondiuk/Shutterstock.

graduate from entry-level or advanced programs accredited by the Commission on Accreditation for Respiratory Care (CoARC) and who also pass the CRT exam.

The board also awards the Registered Respiratory Therapist (RRT) credential to CRTs who have graduated from advanced programs and pass two separate examinations. Supervisory positions and intensive-care specialties usually require the RRT. Six states now require the RRT credential for licensure. Specialty certification is available through the National Board for Respiratory Care (NBRC). NBRC credentialed practitioners become eligible to apply for specialty credential examinations after earning the RRT or CRT credential. Work experience is also required to apply for some specialty areas. The four specialty areas are[4]:

- Adult critical care
- Neonatal/pediatric respiratory care
- Sleep disorders testing and therapeutic intervention
- Pulmonary function technology

Specialty credentialing can improve job opportunities and salaries.

Other Qualifications

Therapists should be sensitive to patients' physical and psychological needs. Respiratory care practitioners must pay attention to detail, follow instructions, and work as part of a team. In addition, operating advanced equipment requires proficiency with computers.

Advancement

Respiratory therapists advance in clinical practice by moving from general care to the care of critically ill patients who have significant problems in other organ systems, such as the heart or kidneys. Respiratory therapists, especially those with a bachelor's or master's degree, also may advance to supervisory or managerial positions in a respiratory therapy department. Respiratory therapists in home health care and equipment rental firms may become branch managers. Some respiratory therapists advance by moving into teaching positions. Others use the knowledge gained as a respiratory therapist to work in another industry, such as developing, marketing, or selling pharmaceuticals and medical devices.

Employment Trends

Much faster than average growth is projected for respiratory therapists. The 2020–2021 COVID-19 pandemic increased the demand for respiratory therapists to provide ventilator support for patients in intensive care units.

Employment Change

Employment of respiratory therapists is expected to grow by 19% from 2019 to 2029, much faster than the average for all occupations. The increasing demand will come from substantial growth in the middle-aged and older adult populations—a development that will heighten the incidence of chronic obstructive pulmonary disease (COPD), which can permanently damage the lungs or restrict lung function. Growth in demand also will result from the expanding role of respiratory therapists in case management, disease prevention, emergency care, and research.

Older Americans suffer most from respiratory ailments and cardiopulmonary diseases, such as pneumonia, chronic bronchitis, emphysema, and heart disease. As the number of older persons increases, the need for respiratory therapists is expected to increase as well. In addition, advances in inhalable medications and in the treatment of lung transplant patients, heart attack and accident victims, and premature infants—many of whom depend on a ventilator during part of their treatment—will increase the demand for the services of respiratory care practitioners. Other conditions affecting the general population, such as respiratory problems due to smoking and air pollution, along with respiratory emergencies, will continue to create demand for respiratory therapists.

Job Prospects

Job opportunities are expected to be very good, especially for those with a bachelor's degree and certification and those with cardiopulmonary care skills or experience working with infants. The vast majority of job openings will continue to be in hospitals. However, a growing number of openings are expected to be outside hospitals, especially in home healthcare services, offices of physicians or other health practitioners, consumer-goods rental firms, or the employment services industry as temporary workers in various settings. TABLE 29.1 provides projections data from the National Employment Matrix.

Earnings

Median annual wages of respiratory therapists were $62,810 in May 2020. The lowest 10% earned less than $45,940, and the highest 10% earned more than $89,170.

RESPIRATORY THERAPY TECHNICIANS
Significant Points

- Job opportunities will be in decline because of changes in credentialing in the field of respiratory therapy.
- Completion of a one-year certification program is the minimum educational requirement.

Work Description

Respiratory therapy technicians follow specific, well-defined respiratory care procedures under the direction of respiratory therapists and physicians. They help evaluate, treat, and care for patients with breathing or other cardiopulmonary disorders. They administer oxygen and breathing treatments to ensure their patients are breathing properly. They prepare and test equipment before procedures begin, analyze samples, and maintain patient records.

Work Environment

Respiratory therapy technicians typically work between 35 and 40 hours per week. Some healthcare facilities require patient care continuously, requiring technicians to work evenings and weekends. Direct patient care involves exposure to disease and technicians can minimize their risk of attracting a disease by following proper hygiene protocols. They may be required to stand and walk for long periods of time.

Educational and Legal Requirements

A one-year certification program is the requirement to work as a respiratory therapy technician. However, students who have completed the first year of an associate's degree program in respiratory therapy are sometimes designated as a respiratory therapy technician.

Employment Trends
Employment Change

Employment decline is projected for respiratory therapy technicians. The NBRC eliminated the Certified Respiratory Therapy Technician designation in 1999 and transitioned to Certified Respiratory Therapist (CRT). Also, the Bureau of Labor Statistics eliminated respiratory therapy technician from the *Occupational Outlook Handbook* index after 2018.[5] Most work in respiratory care is being done by respiratory therapists, resulting in limited demand for respiratory therapy technicians. In 2018 there were 9,300 respiratory therapy technicians.

			Change, 2019–2029	
Occupational Title	Employment, 2019	Projected Employment, 2029	Number	Percentage
Respiratory therapists	135,800	162,000	26,300	19%

TABLE 29.1 Projections Data for Respiratory Therapists, 2019–2029

Data from Bureau of Labor Statistics, U.S. Department of Labor. Occupational Outlook Handbook. U.S. Department of Labor; 2020. https://www.bls.gov/ooh/healthcare/respiratory-therapists.htm#tab-6

Job Prospects

Respiratory therapy technicians can expect keen competition. Very few openings for respiratory therapy technicians are expected, as the work is increasingly performed by respiratory therapists. Accredited entry level respiratory therapy programs now require an associate's degree for the credential, Certified Respiratory Therapist (CRT).

Earnings

Median annual wages for respiratory therapy technicians were $51,210 in May 2018.

Related Occupations

Workers in related healthcare occupations include physicians, surgeons, and respiratory therapists.

Additional Information

Information concerning a career in respiratory care is available from:

- American Association for Respiratory Care, 9425 N. MacArthur Blvd., Suite 100, Irving, TX 75063-4706. http://www.aarc.org

For a list of accredited educational programs for respiratory care practitioners, contact either of the following organizations:

- Commission on Accreditation for Allied Health Education Programs, 9355 - 113th St. N, #7709, Seminole, FL 33775. http://www.caahep.org
- Commission on Accreditation for Respiratory Care, Precision Blvd, 264 Telford, TN 37690. https://coarc .com/students/find-an-accredited-program/

Information on gaining credentials in respiratory care can be obtained from:

- National Board for Respiratory Care, Inc., 18000 W. 105th St., Olathe, KS 66061. http://www.nbrc.org

A list of state licensing agencies can be obtained from:

- American Association for Respiratory Care, 9425 N MacArthur Blvd, Suite 100, Irving, TX 75063. https ://www.aarc.org/advocacy/

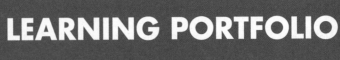

LEARNING PORTFOLIO

Issues for Discussion

1. Because respiratory therapists deal with a fundamental aspect of living, namely breathing, they often encounter patients with both significant breathing difficulties and anxiety about their health. Identify and discuss what traits are most important to a respiratory therapist to be successful in dealing with this patient population.

2. Go to the American Association for Respiratory Care website to learn more about preparing for a career as a respiratory therapist. https://c.aarc.org/career/be_an_rt/more_information.cfm

3. Some problems respiratory therapists treat are created by patients themselves, such as the side effects from smoking regular or vapor cigarettes. Discuss in class the effects smoking may have on patients, those who surround them, and those who treat them. Review "Quit Smoking" on the Centers for Disease Control and Prevention website and view the video "Tips from Former Smokers." List at least two suggestions for quitting based on the information on this site. Centers for Disease Control and Prevention. "Tips from Former Smokers." https://www.cdc.gov/tobacco/campaign/tips/stories/tonya.html

Enrichment Activities

1. View the 25-minute video "Life and Breath" to learn about the roles and responsibilities of respiratory therapists. http://d3vbuoemguibb4.cloudfront.net/life_and_breath_complete.mp4
   - Describe three different work settings for respiratory therapists shown in the video.
   - Explain three conditions treated by pediatric respiratory therapists.

2. Respiratory therapists often work with patients who suffer from chronic obstructive pulmonary disease (COPD). Use Chronic Obstructive Pulmonary Disease Prevalence Maps from the CDC to learn more about pulmonary problems in the United States, including the state in which you live. Which states have the highest rates of COPD, and which states have the lowest rates of COPD? https://www.cdc.gov/copd/data.html

3. Assume you have a friend who is interested in becoming a respiratory therapist. Summarize the advice you would give that person in a one- or two-page paper.

CASE STUDY: RESPIRATORY CARE PRACTITIONERS

Annie completed her degree at the local university and was hired on at S.L. Medical Center as a respiratory therapist last fall. She works with a team of healthcare professionals to treat patients who are critically ill and having breathing problems. Most recently Annie was called to assist with a patient who was in distress and needed ventilatory support. Annie performed an arterial blood gas analyzer, and after conferring with the attending physician, Annie inserted a breathing tube into the patient's trachea and connected the tube to a ventilator for breathing support.

Based on the information you have read about respiratory therapists, answer the following questions.

1. It is most likely that Annie has completed at least a(n) _____ degree, the minimally accepted degree that is required to become a respiratory therapist.

2. Because Annie is not working in Alaska, it is highly likely that she has obtained her _____ to practice as a respiratory therapist.

3. As a respiratory therapist, Annie typically uses oxygen, chest physiotherapy, and _____ medications to treat her patients.

4. As a more noninvasive approach to increase a patients' concentration of oxygen, Annie can apply an oxygen _____ or nasal cannula.

5. After inserting a breathing tube into the patient's trachea, Annie must then attach the _____ to the tube that will deliver the pressurized oxygen into the lungs.

LEARNING PORTFOLIO

References

1. American Lung Association. *The Basics of Pulmonary Rehabilitation*. https://www.lung.org/lung-health-diseases/lung-procedures-and-tests/pulmonary-rehab Accessed July 1, 2020.

2. Commission on Accreditation for Respiratory Care (CoARC). *Find an Accredited Program*. https://coarc.com/students/find-an-accredited-program/ Accessed July 2, 2020.

3. Commission on Accreditation of Allied Health Education Programs. *Find a Program*. https://www.caahep.org/Students/Find-a-program.aspx Accessed August 28, 2021.

4. National Board for Respiratory Care. *Examinations*. https://www.nbrc.org/Pages/examinations.aspx Accessed July 2, 2020.

5. Willden H. *Job Outlook is Good for Respiratory Therapists*. May 2, 2019. American Association for Respiratory Therapy. https://www.aarc.org/nn19-job-outlook-good-for-respiratory-therapists/ Accessed August 27, 2021.

PART FOUR

Healthcare Support Personnel

This section addresses professionals who have limited decision-making responsibilities or have little or no direct contact with patients. Instead, support personnel deliver care under the recommendation and supervision of another health professional. For example, a nursing assistant may be supervised by a registered nurse. Categories of health professionals without direct patient contact are Medical Laboratory Personnel and Health Information Personnel.

OBJECTIVES

The following objectives are for all chapters in Part IV. After studying these chapters, the student should be able to:

- Describe the responsibilities and work of each profession.
- Classify the specialties in each profession.
- Discuss the environment in which the work takes place.
- Identify any healthcare personnel who assist the professionals with their work.
- Compare and contrast the following factors among the professions: educational requirements, employment trends, opportunities for advancement, salary potential, and career ladders.
- Identify other professionals who do similar tasks or have similar responsibilities.
- Discuss the advantages of the national organizations to which professionals belong.
- Explain the concept and process of interprofessional education (IPE) and interprofessional practice (IPP) in healthcare.

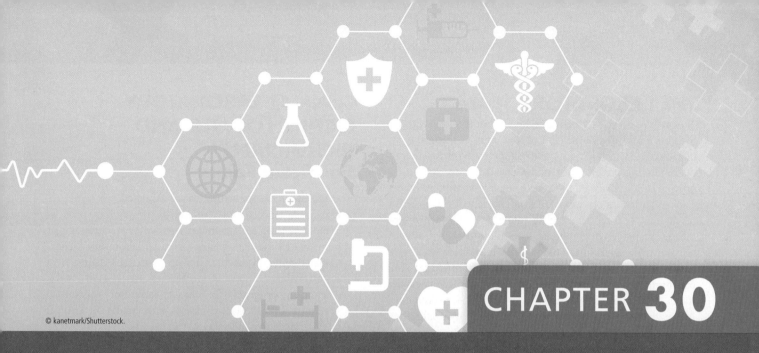
© kanetmark/Shutterstock.

CHAPTER 30

Clinical Laboratory Personnel*

KEY TERMS

American Association of
  Bioanalysts (AAB)
American Medical Technologists
  (AMT)
American Society for Clinical
  Pathology (ASCP)
Automated analyzer
Blood bank technologist
Board of Certification (BOC)
Cell counters
Clinical chemistry specialist

Clinical Laboratory Improvement
  Amendment (CLIA)
Clinical laboratory scientists
Clinical laboratory technicians
Clinical laboratory technologists
Cytotechnologist
Hematology specialists and
  technologists
Histotechnicians and
  histotechnologists

Immunology scientists and
  technologists
Microbiology specialist
National Accrediting Agency for
  Clinical Laboratory Sciences
  (NAACLS)
Phlebotomist
Prescribed drug regimen
Skin puncture
Venipuncture

* All information in this chapter, unless otherwise indicated, was obtained from Bureau of Labor Statistics. *Occupational Outlook Handbook 2020–2021 Edition*. Washington, DC: U.S. Department of Labor; 2021.

THE LABORATORY TEAM

The practice of modern medicine would be impossible without the tests performed in the clinical laboratory. A medical team of pathologists, technologists, and technicians work together to determine the presence, extent, or absence of disease and to provide data to evaluate the effectiveness of treatment. Physicians order laboratory work for a wide variety of reasons: Test results may be used to establish values against which future measurements can be compared; to monitor treatment, as with tests for drug levels in the blood that can indicate whether a patient is adhering to a **prescribed drug regimen**; to reassure patients that a disease is absent or under control; or to assess the status of a patient's health, as with cholesterol measurements. Although physicians depend heavily on laboratory results, they do not ordinarily perform the tests themselves. This job falls to clinical laboratory personnel. Clinical laboratory testing plays a crucial role in the detection, diagnosis, and treatment of disease. Medical and clinical laboratory technologists and technicians perform most of these tests.

The Occupational Outlook Handbook developed by the Bureau of Labor Statistics within the U.S. Department of Labor describes bachelor's degree level–trained laboratory personnel as **clinical laboratory technologists** and associate's degree level–trained personnel as **clinical laboratory technicians**. The American Society for Clinical Pathology—the professional organization that offers certification for laboratory personnel—designates graduates of a bachelor's program as **clinical laboratory scientists**. Academic training programs also designate graduates of a bachelor's program as clinical laboratory scientists. Both *scientist* and *technologist* are terms used to describe professionals in the clinical laboratory who have completed a bachelor's training program in clinical laboratory science.

This chapter will describe clinical laboratory technologists, technicians, and phlebotomists in detail and introduce other lab personnel with specialized training.

CLINICAL LABORATORY TECHNOLOGISTS AND TECHNICIANS
Significant Points

- Excellent job opportunities are expected.
- Clinical laboratory technologists usually have a bachelor's degree with a major in medical technology or in one of the life sciences; clinical laboratory technicians generally need either an associate's degree or a certificate.
- Training programs for clinical laboratory personnel require both didactic classes and hands-on clinical experience in a laboratory.
- Most jobs will continue to be in hospitals, but employment will grow rapidly in other settings as well.

Work Description

Clinical laboratory testing plays a crucial role in the detection, diagnosis, and treatment of disease. Medical and clinical laboratory technologists, also referred to as medical and clinical laboratory scientists, and medical and clinical laboratory technicians perform most of these tests. Clinical laboratory personnel examine and analyze body fluids and cells. They look for bacteria, parasites, and other microorganisms; analyze the chemical content of fluids; match blood types for transfusions; and test for drug levels in the blood that show how a patient is responding to treatment. Scientists also prepare specimens for examination, count cells, and look for abnormal blood cells and other abnormalities in body fluids. They use microscopes, **cell counters**, and other sophisticated laboratory equipment (**FIGURE 30.1**).

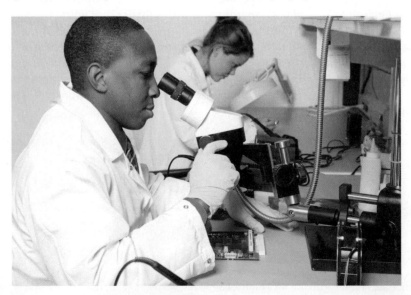

FIGURE 30.1 Laboratory technologists use a microscope to identify abnormal cells or the presence of bacteria or viruses.
© Stephen Coburn/Shutterstock.

They also use automated equipment and computerized instruments capable of performing a number of tests simultaneously. After testing and examining a specimen, they analyze the results and relay them to physicians; the results may also be automatically transmitted to the patient's electronic health record. With increasing automation and the use of computer technology, the work of technologists and technicians has become less hands-on and more analytical. The complexity of tests performed, the level of judgment needed, and the amount of responsibility workers assume depend largely on the amount of education and experience they have. Clinical laboratory technologists usually do more complex tasks than clinical laboratory technicians. Clinical laboratory technologists perform complex chemical, biological, hematological, immunologic, microscopic, and bacteriological tests. Technologists and technicians examine blood and other body fluids with a microscope. They make cultures of body fluid and tissue samples to determine the presence of bacteria, fungi, parasites, or other microorganisms (**FIGURE 30.2**).

Technologists and technicians analyze samples for chemical content or a chemical reaction and determine concentrations of compounds such as blood glucose and cholesterol levels. They also type and cross-match blood samples for transfusions and type tissue samples for kidney or other organ transplants. Clinical laboratory scientists evaluate test results, develop and modify procedures, and establish and monitor programs to ensure the accuracy of tests. Some technologists supervise other clinical laboratory technologists and technicians.

Technologists in small laboratories perform many types of tests, whereas those in large laboratories generally specialize in clinical chemistry, microbiology, immunology, cytology, or blood banking. **Clinical chemistry specialists**, for example, prepare specimens and analyze the chemical and hormonal content of body fluids. **Microbiology specialists** examine and identify bacteria and other microorganisms. **Blood bank technologists**, or **hematology specialists**

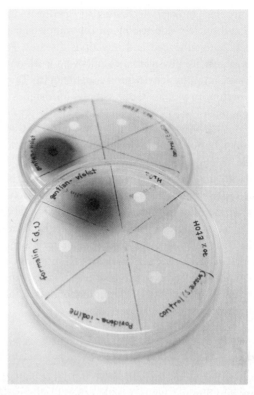

FIGURE 30.2 Microbiologists grow cultures of body fluids to determine the presence of bacteria.
© Tinydevil/Shutterstock.

and technologists, collect, type, and prepare blood and its components for transfusions. **Immunology scientists and technologists** examine elements of the human immune system—antigens and antibodies, for example—and response to foreign bodies, most commonly viruses and bacteria. **Cytotechnologists** prepare slides of body cells and examine these cells with a microscope for abnormalities that may signal the beginning of a cancerous growth (**FIGURE 30.3**).

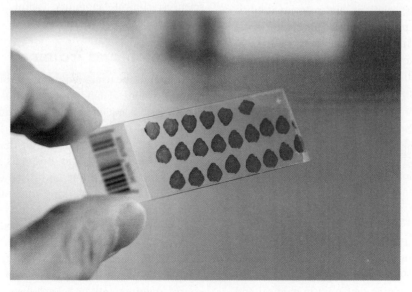

FIGURE 30.3 Cytotechnologists prepare slides of cells and examine for abnormalities.
© science photo/Shutterstock.

Molecular biology technologists perform complex protein and nucleic acid testing on cell samples for genetic testing of both inherited and infectious diseases. Pathologists' assistants are physician assistants who work under the supervision of a physician who is a pathologist. They work in a laboratory to prepare tissue samples for diagnostic tests and for autopsy.[1]

Medical laboratory technicians perform less complex tests and laboratory procedures than medical laboratory scientists. Technicians may prepare specimens and operate **automated analyzers**, for example, or they may perform manual tests in accordance with detailed instructions. They usually work under the supervision of a medical laboratory technologist or laboratory manager, pathologist, or research scientist. Like technologists, clinical laboratory technicians may work in several areas of the clinical laboratory or specialize in just one. For example, histotechnicians prepare tissue specimens for microscopic examination by pathologists, and **phlebotomists** collect blood samples.

Work Environment

Laboratory personnel generally have no direct contact with patients and limited contact with other health personnel except for physicians who depend on lab results to make a diagnosis and monitor treatment. Pathologists depend on **histotechnicians and histotechnologists** to prepare slides to use in making a diagnosis. Clinical laboratory personnel are trained to work with specimens that may contain viruses or bacteria with a potential for causing a serious infectious disease such as the flu or pneumonia. When proper methods of infection control and sterilization are followed, few hazards exist. Protective masks, gloves, and goggles often are necessary to ensure the safety of laboratory personnel (**FIGURE 30.4**).

Working conditions vary with the size and type of employment setting. Laboratories usually are well lit and clean; however, specimens, solutions, and reagents used in the laboratory sometimes produce fumes. Laboratory workers may spend a great deal of time on their feet.

The hours that clinical laboratory technologists and technicians work vary with the size and type of employment setting. Laboratories within large hospitals and large independent laboratories often operate continuously. Therefore, personnel may work a day, evening, or night shift as well as weekends and holidays. Laboratory personnel in small facilities may work on rotating shifts rather than on a regular shift. In some facilities, laboratory personnel are on call several nights a week or on weekends in case of an emergency.

Employment Opportunities

Clinical laboratory technologists and technicians held about 337,800 jobs in 2019. Nearly half of the jobs were in hospitals. Most of the remaining jobs were in medical and diagnostic laboratories. A small proportion was in offices

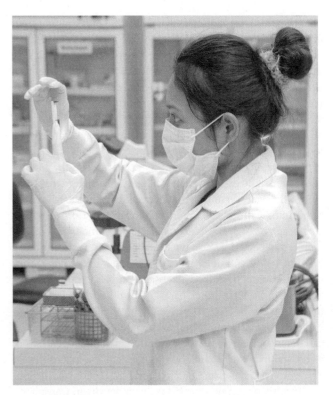

FIGURE 30.4 Lab personnel wearing protective gloves and a mask to prevent contact with infectious organisms from human body fluids.
© Milkovasa/Shutterstock.

of physicians, educational services, and other ambulatory healthcare services.

Educational and Legal Requirements

Clinical laboratory technologists generally require a bachelor's degree in medical technology or in one of the life sciences; clinical laboratory technicians usually need an associate's degree or a certificate.

Education and Training

Even though the usual requirement for an entry-level position as a clinical laboratory technologist is a bachelor's degree with a major in medical technology or one of the life sciences, it is possible to qualify for some jobs with a combination of education and on-the-job and specialized training. Universities and hospitals offer medical technology programs. Online and distance programs provide access to training for working students and those living in rural areas. All programs require a combination of didactic classes and a clinical laboratory practicum where students receive one-on-one training and supervision from a laboratory staff, usually in a hospital setting. Some programs can be completed in two years after completing didactic course requirements or a bachelor's degree in biology or chemistry. There is strong competition among students to obtain clinical rotations in hospitals and inadequate staff to mentor and supervise students because of vacancies in laboratory departments, especially in the Northeastern United States.[2]

Bachelor's degree programs in medical technology include courses in chemistry, biological sciences, microbiology, mathematics, and statistics, as well as specialized courses devoted to knowledge and skills used in the clinical laboratory. Many programs also offer or require courses in management, business, and computer applications. The **Clinical Laboratory Improvement Amendment (CLIA)** requires personnel who perform highly complex tests to have at least an associate's degree.[3]

Medical and clinical laboratory technicians generally have either an associate's degree from a community or junior college or a certificate from a hospital, a vocational or technical school, or the armed forces. A few technicians learn their skills on the job. The **National Accrediting Agency for Clinical Laboratory Sciences (NAACLS)** accredits 236 associate degree programs for medical laboratory technicians and 241 bachelor's programs for medical laboratory scientists/technologists. NAACLS also approves 58 programs in phlebotomy and six programs in clinical assisting.[4] Other nationally recognized agencies that accredit specific areas for clinical laboratory workers include the Commission on Accreditation of Allied Health Education Programs (CAAHEP) and the Accrediting Bureau of Health Education Schools (ABHES).

Licensure

As of 2020, 11 states and Puerto Rico required licensure for laboratory personnel.[5] Information on licensure is available from state departments of health or boards of occupational licensing.

Certification and Other Qualifications

Many employers prefer applicants who are certified by a recognized professional association. Those associations offering certification include the Board of Registry of the **American Society for Clinical Pathology (ASCP)**, the **American Medical Technologists (AMT)**, and the Board of Registry of the **American Association of Bioanalysts (AAB)**. These associations have different requirements for certification and different organizational sponsors. Graduates of a bachelor's program in medical technology are eligible to take the national exam administered by the **Board of Certification (BOC)** within the American Society for Clinical Pathology (ASCP). Medical laboratory technologists who become certified under ASCP can use the initials MLS behind their name[6] and the initials MT if certified under the American Association of Bioanalysts (AAB).[7] Those who meet the requirements for technicians are designated as MLT by both the AAB and ASCP.[6,7] For technologists, there are various paths to certification including meeting educational requirements plus experience in a NAACLS-accredited laboratory.

Educational requirements are either a bachelor's degree in medical laboratory science plus one year of work experience in a laboratory or a master's degree plus six months work experience in a laboratory. For technicians, the AAB awards Medical Laboratory Technician certification for those who have met postsecondary training requirements and successfully passed the MLT (AAB) generalist examination.[6] Both ASCP and AAB recognize military training and experience in clinical laboratory science for certification of technicians.[6,7]

In addition to certification, employers seek clinical laboratory personnel with good analytical judgment and the ability to work under pressure. Technologists in particular are expected to be good at problem solving. Close attention to detail is also essential for laboratory personnel because small differences or changes in test substances or numerical readouts can be crucial to a diagnosis. Manual dexterity and normal color vision are highly desirable, and with the widespread use of automated laboratory equipment, computer skills are necessary. The ability to use complex and specialized laboratory equipment is also necessary for most personnel. A personal characteristic valued by employers is the ability to work independently and as part of the laboratory team. Laboratory personnel usually have no direct contact with patients except in smaller laboratories, where staff may draw blood from patients in addition to conducting laboratory tests. However, they often communicate results to physicians.

Advancement

Technicians can advance and become technologists through additional education and experience. Technologists can advance to supervisory positions in laboratory work or become chief medical or clinical laboratory scientists or laboratory managers in hospitals. Technologists can also assume the role of quality improvement for a laboratory. Manufacturers of home diagnostic testing kits and laboratory equipment and supplies also seek experienced technologists to work in product development, marketing, and sales. Professional certification and a graduate degree in medical technology, one of the biological sciences, chemistry, management, or education usually speed advancement. A doctorate usually is needed to become a laboratory director. Many laboratory directors are pathologist physicians or other physicians with training and experience in a laboratory. Federal regulation requires directors of moderately complex laboratories to have either a master's degree or a bachelor's degree, combined with the appropriate amount of training and experience. Specialization is another path to advancement. The NAACLS website lists programs for specialty training including pathologists' assistant, cytogenic technologist, diagnostic molecular scientist, histotechnician, and histotechnologist. Programs that require a master's degree are pathologists' assistant and molecular biologist.[4]

TABLE 30.1 Projections Data for Clinical and Medical Laboratory Technologists and Technicians, 2019–2029

Occupational Title	Employment, 2019	Projected Employment, 2029	Change, 2019–2029	
			Number	Percent
Clinical laboratory technologists and technicians	337,800	362,500	24,700	7%

Data from Bureau of Labor Statistics, U.S. Department of Labor. Occupational Outlook Handbook. U.S. Department of Labor; 2020. https://www.bls.gov/ooh/healthcare/clinical-laboratory-technologists-and-technicians.htm#tab-6

TABLE 30.2 Facilities Employing the Largest Numbers of Clinical Laboratory Technologists and Technicians, 2019

	Percent
Hospitals	47%
Medical and diagnostic laboratories	20%
Offices of physicians	9%
Colleges, universities, and professional schools	6%
Outpatient care centers	3%

Data from Bureau of Labor Statistics, U.S. Department of Labor. Occupational Outlook Handbook. U.S. Department of Labor; 2020. https://www.bls.gov/ooh/healthcare/clinical-laboratory-technologists-and-technicians.htm#tab-3

Employment Trends

Rapid job growth and excellent job opportunities are expected. Most jobs will continue to be in hospitals, but employment will grow rapidly in other settings as well.

Employment Change

Employment of medical laboratory technologists and technicians is expected to grow by 7% from 2019 to 2029, faster than the average for all occupations. The volume of laboratory tests continues to increase with both population growth and the development of new types of tests.

Technological advances will continue to have opposing effects on employment. On the one hand, new, increasingly powerful diagnostic tests and advances in genomics—the study of the genetic information of a cell or organism—will encourage additional testing and spur employment. On the other hand, research and development efforts targeted at simplifying and automating routine testing procedures may enhance the ability of non laboratory personnel—physicians, nurses, and patients in particular—to perform tests now conducted in laboratories. TABLE 30.1 provides some projections data from the National Employment Matrix.

Although hospitals are expected to continue to be the major employer of clinical laboratory workers, employment is expected also to grow rapidly in medical and diagnostic laboratories, offices of physicians, and all other ambulatory healthcare services. TABLE 30.2 lists major employers of clinical laboratory workers in 2019.

Job Prospects

Job opportunities are expected to be excellent because the number of job openings is expected to continue to exceed the number of job seekers. An increase in the aging population will lead to a greater need to diagnose medical conditions, such as cancer or type 2 diabetes, through laboratory procedures. Prenatal testing for various types of genetic conditions also is increasingly common. Medical laboratory technologists and technicians will be in demand to use and maintain the equipment needed for diagnosis and treatment.

Earnings

Clinical laboratory technologists and technicians had a median annual salary of $54,180 in May 2020 and a median hourly wage of $26.05 in May 2020. Based on a salary survey conducted in 2017, the average hourly wage was $22.38 for technicians and $30.49 for technologists/scientists; the average yearly salary of technologists/scientists was about $15,000 higher than the salary for technicians.[8] Median annual salaries are listed for clinical laboratory technologists and technicians by industry in 2020 (TABLE 30.3).

Average hourly wages are higher for laboratory workers with more education, training, and certification in subspecialties (TABLE 30.4). Supervisors and lead staff also earn higher salaries.

Related Occupations

Clinical laboratory technologists and technicians analyze body fluids, tissue, and other substances using a variety of tests. Chemists and materials scientists, science technicians, and veterinary technologists and technicians perform similar or related procedures.

PHLEBOTOMISTS
Significant Points

- Employment of phlebotomists is expected to grow faster than average and faster than other health professions.
- Phlebotomists require postsecondary training including both classroom and clinical experience to qualify for the certification exam.

TABLE 30.3 Median Annual Wages for Clinical Laboratory Technologists and Technicians by Industry, May 2020

Industry	Salary
Outpatient care centers	$57,640
Hospitals	$56,630
Colleges, universities, and professional schools	$52,260
Medical and diagnostic laboratories	$52,250
Offices of physicians	$48,260

TABLE 30.4 Hourly Wages of Certified Clinical Laboratory Scientists and Technicians by Various Specialties, 2019

Specialty	Hourly Wage
Cytogenetic technologist (CG)	$34.01
Cytotechnologist (CT)	$36.82
Histotechnician (HT)	$28.83
Histotechnologist (HTL)	$29.30
Medical laboratory technician (MLT)	$23.66
Medical laboratory technologist/scientist (MT/MLS)	$31.41
Pathologists' assistant (PA)	$45.97
Phlebotomy technician (PBT)	$17.15
Specialist in blood banking (SBB)	$35.49

Data from Garcia E, Kundu I, Fong K. The American Society for Clinical Pathology's 2019 wage survey of medical laboratories in the United States. *Am J Clin Pathol.* 2021; *155*(5): 649–673. https://doi.org /10.1093/ajcp/aqaa197

- Most jobs for phlebotomists are in hospitals, diagnostic laboratories, and outpatient clinics. Some phlebotomists travel to different sites to draw blood (e.g., hospitals, clinics, assisted-living facilities, and nursing homes).
- Phlebotomists may specialize in population groups that require greater skill in drawing blood—for example, newborns or the elderly.
- Competition from other health professionals who become certified as phlebotomists may reduce employment opportunities for phlebotomists.

Work Description

Phlebotomists draw blood for tests, research, or blood donations. Some phlebotomists draw blood for other purposes, such as at blood drives where people donate blood. Some of them explain their work to patients and provide assistance if patients have adverse reactions after their blood is drawn. Phlebotomists primarily draw blood, which is then used for different kinds of medical laboratory testing. In medical and diagnostic laboratories, patient interaction is often only with the phlebotomist. Some phlebotomists in blood donor centers may do simple lab procedures such as using a centrifuge to spin a blood sample to separate red blood cells from plasma to determine hematocrit—that is, to determine if a donor has a normal amount of red blood cells—before donating blood. Phlebotomists use both **venipuncture** and **skin puncture** to collect blood. Venipuncture is the insertion of a needle into a vein, usually inside the elbow; the needle is attached to a blood-collecting tube. A skin puncture is another method of taking a small sample of blood for glucose monitoring or blood typing (**FIGURE 30.5**).

Because of the high volume of blood samples taken by a phlebotomist, they often become very skilled in obtaining samples quickly without causing the patient pain. A skilled phlebotomist who can put a tense patient at ease during the blood draw is valued by the healthcare team.

Work Environment

Phlebotomists work in hospitals, diagnostic laboratories, blood donor centers, and large outpatient clinics or travel to assisted-living facilities or nursing homes to collect blood samples. Phlebotomists may specialize in age groups for whom it is difficult to obtain blood samples because of small or collapsed veins—for example, in infants, children, or the elderly. Because all blood samples look the same, phlebotomists must identify the patient before drawing blood, label collecting tubes, and enter patient information into a database. In order to avoid causing infection or other complications, phlebotomists must keep their work area and instruments clean and sanitary. Phlebotomists often spend a lot of time standing. Walking is required by phlebotomists who travel to patients' rooms or to assisted-living facilities or nursing homes.

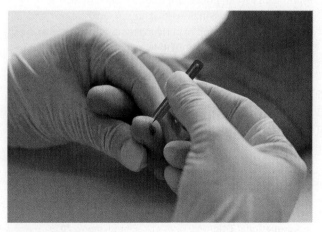

FIGURE 30.5 Phlebotomists doing a skin puncture to draw blood to determine hematocrit at a blood donor center.
© pittawut/Shutterstock.

Employment Opportunities

Blood analysis remains an essential function in medical laboratories and hospitals. Demand for phlebotomists will remain high as doctors and other healthcare professionals require blood work for analysis and diagnoses. As hospitals and medical laboratories evaluate their staffing needs, phlebotomists may be replaced by other, more skilled healthcare workers. For example, nurses often become certified as phlebotomists in small hospitals or clinics.

Educational and Legal Requirements

Phlebotomists typically enter the occupation with a postsecondary non-degree award from a phlebotomy program.

Educational and Training

Programs for phlebotomy are available from community colleges, vocational schools, or technical schools. These programs usually take less than one year to complete and lead to a certificate or diploma. Programs have classroom and laboratory portions and include instruction in anatomy, physiology, and medical terminology. Some phlebotomists may enter the occupation with a high school diploma and are trained to be a phlebotomist on the job. Beginning January 1, 2021, those applying to a training program will be required to submit official high school transcripts to verify high school graduation to be eligible for the training program.[9]

Licensure

Individual states determine licensure requirements. States do not require phlebotomists to be licensed except for the state of California. Information on licensure is available from state departments of health or boards of occupational licensing.

Certification and Other Qualifications

Many employers prefer applicants who are certified by a recognized professional association. Certification typically includes education and experience requirements and successful completion of an examination, which may include demonstration of the ability to carry out the tasks of a phlebotomist, both venipuncture and skin puncture. Laboratory experience must be in a CLIA-regulated laboratory. Those associations offering certification include the Board of Registry of the American Society for Clinical Pathology (ASCP), the National Center for Competency Testing (NCCT), and the American Medical Technologists (AMT). These associations have different requirements for education and experience. Other qualifications are excellent eyesight including color vision, good hand–eye coordination, accuracy, basic computer skills, and the ability to work in stressful situations and to put nervous patients at ease.

Advancement

Phlebotomists may specialize in working with an age group that presents a challenge to obtaining a blood sample. For example, newborns may require that blood be drawn from a capillary in the heel, or an elderly patient may require an experienced phlebotomist to locate a vein for drawing blood in a location other than the inner arm. Some phlebotomists take additional training to become a medical laboratory technician or a medical assistant or complete another professional degree program in the healthcare field. For students who are unsure of enrolling in a health career program, working as a phlebotomist provides exposure to the healthcare environment before investing the time and money in a career that requires longer training.

Employment Trends

Blood analysis remains an essential function in medical laboratories and hospitals. Demand for phlebotomists will remain high as doctors and other healthcare professionals require blood work for analysis and diagnoses. As hospitals and medical laboratories evaluate their staffing needs, phlebotomists may be replaced by other more skilled healthcare workers. For example, there may be competition from licensed practical nurses and registered nurses who are eligible to take the exam to become certified as a phlebotomist.

Employment Change

Employment of phlebotomists is projected to grow 17% from 2019 to 2029, much faster than average for all occupations. Hospitals, diagnostic laboratories, blood donor centers, and other locations will need phlebotomists to perform blood draws. **TABLE 30.5** provides some projections data from the National Employment Matrix.

Job Prospects

Job prospects are best for phlebotomists who receive certification from one of several reputable organizations.

TABLE 30.5 Projections Data for Phlebotomists, 2019–2029

Occupational Title	Employment, 2019	Projected Employment, 2029	Change, 2019–2029 Number	Percent
Phlebotomists	132,600	155,500	22,800	17%

Data from Bureau of Labor Statistics, U.S. Department of Labor. Occupational Outlook Handbook. U.S. Department of Labor; 2020. https://www.bls.gov/ooh/healthcare/phlebotomists.htm#tab-6

Earnings

The median hourly wage for phlebotomists in May 2020 was $17.46 per hour, and the median annual salary for phlebotomists was $36,320.

Related Occupations

Dental assistants, medical assistants, medical and clinical laboratory technicians and technologists, medical records and health information technologists, medical transcriptionists, veterinary technologists and technicians, veterinary assistants, lab animal caretakers, and physician assistants perform similar or related procedures.

Additional Information

Contact one of the following accredited and approved educational programs for clinical laboratory personnel:

- Accrediting Bureau of Health Education Schools, 7777 Leesburg Pike, Suite 314 N., Falls Church, VA 22043. http://www.abhes.org
- Commission on Accreditation of Allied Health Education Programs, 9355-113th St. N, #7709 Seminole, FL 33775 https://www.caahep.org
- National Accrediting Agency for Clinical Laboratory Sciences, 5600 N. River Rd., Suite 720, Rosemont, IL 60018-5119. https://www.naacls.org/Students.aspx

Information on certification is available from:

- American Association of Bioanalysts, Board of Registry, 906 Olive St., Suite 1200, St. Louis, MO 63101. https://www.aab.org/
- American Medical Technologists, 10700 W. Higgins Rd., Suite 150, Rosemont, IL 60018. https://www.americanmedtech.org/
- American Society for Clinical Pathology, 33 West Monroe St., Suite 1600, Chicago, IL 60603. https://www.ascp.org/content/about-ascp

Additional career information is available from:

- American Association of Blood Banks, 4550 Montgomery Ave., Suite 700, North Tower, Bethesda, MD 20814. https://www.aabb.org
- American Society for Clinical Laboratory Science, 1861 International Dr., Suite 200, McLean, VA 22102. https://ascls.org

- American Society for Cytopathology, 100 West 10th St., Suite 605, Wilmington, DE 19801. http://cytologyedlab.org/
- Clinical Laboratory Management Association, 330 N. Wabash Ave., Suite 2000, Chicago, IL 60611. https://www.clma.org
- ExploreHealthCareers. *Medical Laboratory Scientist/ Technician.* https://explorehealthcareers.org/career/allied-health-professions/clinical-laboratory-scientist-technician/
- National Society for Histotechnology, 3545 Ellicott Mills Dr., Ellicott City, MD 20143. https://www.nsh.org/home

Information regarding licensure of medical laboratory personnel is available from:

- The American Society for Clinical laboratory Science, 1861 International Dr., Suite 200, McLean, VA 22102. https://www.ascls.org/advocacy-issues/licensure

General information on phlebotomists can be found at:

- ExploreHealthCareers.org. *Phlebotomist.* https://explorehealthcareers.org/career/allied-health-professions/phlebotomist/ U.S. Department of Labor. CareerOne Stop. *Phlebotomists.* https://www.careeronestop.org/Videos/CareerVideos/career-videos.aspx

Information on training programs is available from these organizations:

- Center for Phlebotomy Education, 520 N. Main St., Suite 208, Cheboygan, MI 49721 https://www.phlebotomy.com
- National Accrediting Agency for Clinical Laboratory Sciences, 5600 N. River Rd., Suite 720, Rosemont, IL 60018. https://www.naacls.org

Information on becoming certified as a phlebotomist is available from these organizations:

- American Medical Technologists, 10700 W. Higgins Rd., Suite 150, Rosemont, IL 60018. https://www.americanmedtech.org
- American Society for Clinical Pathology, Board of Certification, 33 W. Monroe, #1600, Chicago, IL 60603. https://www.ascp.org/content
- National Center for Competency Testing, 7007 College Blvd., Suite 385, Overland Park, KS 66211. https://www.ncctinc.com
- National Healthcareer Association, 11161 Overbrook Rd., Leawood, KS 66211. https://www.nhanow.com

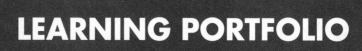

LEARNING PORTFOLIO

Issues for Discussion

1. Go to the American Society for Clinical Pathology (ASCP) website to learn more about different careers as a lab professional. Review careers requiring two years or less of education and careers requiring four years or more of education. Review the bios of laboratory personnel. List two careers for each and describe what they do in their job. American Society for Clinical Pathology. *What's My Next.* https://www .whatsmynext.org/#1562853518541-99e2cb15-7698

2. Go to the Laboratory Science Careers website and link to *Meet a Professional.* Review the bios of a medical laboratory technician, a medical laboratory scientist, and a director of laboratory services. Review the bio of Abou, who describes his responsibilities as a clinical laboratory scientist as well as a phlebotomist in a rural area of Montana. Discuss during class. Which of these professionals or settings appeals to you? https://www.laboratorysciencecareers.com/meet-a -laboratory-science-professional-860335.html

3. Use the online resource *U.S. Procedures for Examination & Certification*, January 2021, from the American Society of Clinical Pathology (ASCP) Board of Certification (BOC). Choose one laboratory professional, review the different pathways to become certified, and report what you found during class. Is this information helpful in making a decision about becoming a laboratory professional? https://www.ascp.org/ content/docs/default-source/boc-pdfs/exam-content -outlines/ascp-boc-us-procedures-book-web.pdf

4. Discuss the pros and cons of obtaining certification as a specialist in an area of medical laboratory technology: blood banking, chemistry, microbiology, hematology, or cytotechnology.

5. Discuss the advantages and disadvantages of automation in a laboratory. How will automation impact employment opportunities for medical laboratory personnel?

6. Review the one-minute video that explains the job responsibilities of a phlebotomist. Compare the responsibilities of a phlebotomist with a medical laboratory technician. U.S. Department of Labor. CareerOneStop. *Phlebotomists.* https://www .careeronestop.org/videos/careeronestop-videos .aspx?videocode=31909700

Enrichment Activities

1. Review the four-minute video "Clinical Laboratory Technician, Technologist & Scientist." Describe the options for becoming a clinical laboratory technologist for students who already have a bachelor's degree in biology or chemistry. https://www.youtube.com /watch?v=wdQEjRDyzIk

2. Review the 5 ½-minute video from the National Society for Histotechnology titled "Preparing for a Histotechnology Career in the US." Describe tools used by a histology technician or technologist. What personal characteristics are important for a career as a histotechnician or histotechnologist? https://www .youtube.com/watch? v=sBfA30Ouc8w

3. Review the ASCP Certification options to become a certified phlebotomist. There are two certifications, Phlebotomy Technician (PBT) and Donor Phlebotomy Technician (DPT). https://nationalphlebotomysolutions .com/cpt-certification/

CASE STUDY: LABORATORY PERSONNEL

Cortez is completing a bachelor's degree in biology and was planning to apply for medical school but discovered that he enjoys laboratory work, which is more suitable to his inquisitive mind. Cortez has been working part-time in a cancer research lab and has been offered a full-time job upon graduation and plans to accept the job. However, he would like to explore other career options.
The following questions relate to this case study.

1. True or false? Cortez is eligible to apply for certification as a technologist in blood banking from the American Society of Clinical Pathology (ASCP).

2. If Cortez meets all of the requirements for certification as a technologist in blood banking through the American Society of Clinical Pathology, which designation would he be able to use after his name?
   A. MLS
   B. CT
   C. PBT
   D. BB

3. Graduates of a bachelor's degree program in Medical Laboratory Science are eligible to apply for certification

LEARNING PORTFOLIO

and to use which of the following designations after their name?

A. MLT

B. MT

C. HT

D. HTL

4. Medical laboratory technicians can obtain the necessary education and laboratory clinical training through:

A. an associate's degree in medical laboratory science.

B. training and laboratory experience in the armed services.

C. training leading to a certificate from a vocational school.

D. all of the above.

5. True or false? Phlebotomists have very little contact with patients. Instead, they spend most of their time labeling and transporting vials of blood.

References

1. *Definition and History.* Duke Pathology. Duke University School of Medicine. Pathologists' Assistant Program. https://pathology.duke.edu/education/pathologists-assistant-program/definition-history Accessed October 4, 2021.

2. Position Paper of the American Society for Clinical Laboratory Science (ASCLS). *Addressing the Clinical Laboratory Workforce Shortage.* The American Society for Clinical Laboratory Science, August 2018. http://www.ccclw.org/uploads/6/3/4/9/63493369/clinical_laboratory_workforce_final_20180824.pdf Accessed September 3, 2020.

3. Electronic Code of Federal Regulation. Title 42: Public Health; (5) 493. Laboratory Requirements. 1489. Standard: Testing personnel qualifications. https://www.ecfr.gov/cgi-bin/text-idx?SID=60935fc838c3686717826687221cd863&mc=true&node=pt42.5.493&rgn=div5 Updated September 2, 2020. Accessed September 4, 2020.

4. National Accrediting Agency for Clinical Laboratory Sciences. (NAACL). *Find a Program.* https://www.naacls.org/Find-a-Program.aspx Accessed August 30, 2021.

5. The American Society for Clinical laboratory Science. *Personnel Licensure.* https://ascls.org/licensure/ Accessed August 25, 2020.

6. ASCP Board of Certification. *U.S. Certification.* https://www.ascp.org/content/board-of-certification/get-credentialed Accessed August 25, 2020.

7. American Association of Bioanalysts (AAB). *Types of Certification.* https://www.aab.org/aab/Types_of_Certification.asp Accessed August 30, 2021.

8. Garcia E, Kundu I, Fong K. The American Society for Clinical Pathology's 2019 wage survey of medical laboratories in the United States. *Am J Clin Pathol.* 2021; *155* (5): 649–673. https://doi.org/10.1093/ajcp/aqaa197

9. ASCP Board of Certification. *Examination Eligibility Assistant.* https://apps.ascp.org/BOCROUTEFINDER Accessed October 4, 2021.

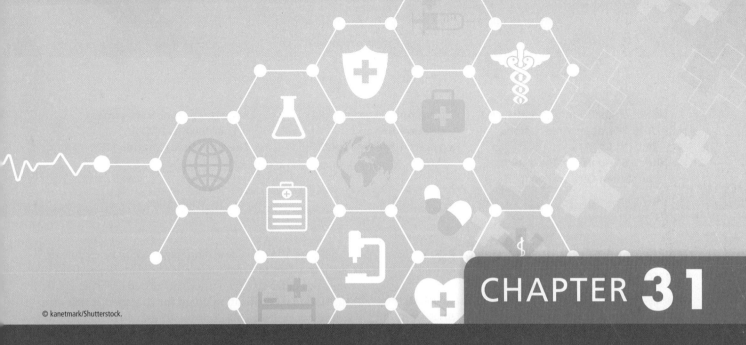

© kanetmark/Shutterstock.

CHAPTER **31**

Alternative Therapy: Massage, Recreation, Art, Dance, and Music Therapists*

KEY TERMS

American Art Therapy
Association (AATA)
American Dance Therapy
Association (ADTA)
American Music Therapy
Association (AMTA)
American Therapeutic
Recreation Association (ATRA)
Art Therapist (AT)
Arts Therapy Credentials Board
(ATCB)
Art Therapist Registered-Board
Certified (ATR-BC)

Board Certified-Dance/
Movement Therapist (BC-DMT)
Cardiopulmonary resuscitation
(CPR)
Certified Therapeutic Recreation
Specialist (CTRS)
Commission on Accreditation
of Allied Health Education
Programs (CAAEP)
Complementary and alternative
medicine
Dance Movement Therapist
(DMT)

Federation of State Massage
Therapy Boards (FSMTB)
Manual dexterity
Massage and Bodywork
Licensing Examination
(MBLEx)
Massage therapy
Music Therapist (MT)
Music Therapist-Board Certified
(MT-BC)
National Certification Board
for Therapeutic Massage &
Bodywork (NCBTMB)

* All information in this chapter, unless otherwise indicated, was obtained from Bureau of Labor Statistics. *Occupational Outlook Handbook 2020–2021 Edition*. Washington, DC: U.S. Department of Labor; 2021.

405

National Coalition of Creative
Arts Therapies Associations,
Inc. (NCCATA)
National Council for Therapeutic
Recreation Certification (NCTRC)

Recreational Therapist (RT)
Recreation therapy
Registered Art Therapist
(ATR)

Registered Dance/Movement
Therapist (R-DMT)
Therapeutic Recreation (TR)

ALTERNATIVE AND OTHER THERAPIES

Massage has been part of traditional Chinese medicine for 4,000 years but has been slow to be recognized as a health profession in the United States. Swedish massage was introduced to the United States in 1850 and was practiced by some physicians. However, only since the 1970s, as part of the **complementary and alternative medicine** movement, has massage therapy become popular.[1] The expected demand for massage therapists is currently at an all-time high with a projected growth of 21% between 2019 and 2029 according to the U.S. Department of Labor (**FIGURE 31.1**).

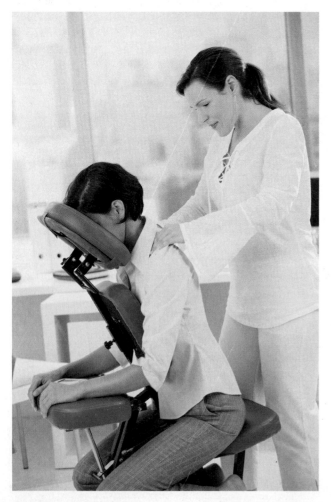

FIGURE 31.1 The demand for massage therapists is expected to increase by 21% between 2019 and 2029.
© StockLite/Shutterstock.

Before 1988 very few states regulated massage therapy. The movement to license massage therapists began in 1992 when two different organizations developed licensing exams. The **National Certification Board for Therapeutic Massage & Bodywork (NCBTMB)** was founded in 1992 and administered the first licensing exam the same year. Also, in 1992, the **Federation of State Massage Therapy Boards (FSMTB)** created the licensure exam **Massage and Bodywork Licensing Examination (MBLEx)** to allow reciprocity between states. In 2014, the NCBTMB and FSMTB agreed that only FSMTB would administer the licensure exam MBLEx for all new graduates and that NCBTMB would be responsible for board certification of licensed massage therapists.[2]

In contrast, **recreation therapy** originated as "Special Services" in the U.S. Army during World War II in the 1940s and in 1945 became known as "recreation," a section under the Rehabilitation Medicine Service Office of the Veterans Administration (VA).[3] By 1953, the National Association of Recreational Therapy was organized,[4] and credentialing of recreational therapists began in 1956 through the Commission for the Advancement of Hospital Recreation.[5] Since 1981, the **National Council for Therapeutic Recreation Certification (NCTRC)** has certified recreational therapists.[5] Currently, the VA's therapeutic recreation program offers social activities, games and sports, outdoor recreation, and arts and crafts. The program also includes music therapy, dance therapy, and psychodrama.[3]

Even though recreational therapists may include art, music, or dance as part of their treatment plan, each of these artistic fields offers a career that combines artistic skills with the skills as a therapist. All of these health careers developed in response to a need to serve armed services personnel affected by the trauma of war. Music therapy began after World War I,[6] while recreation therapy, art therapy, and dance therapy began after World War II.

The **National Coalition of Creative Arts Therapies Associations, Inc. (NCCATA)** is an alliance of professional associations that promotes the arts as a therapeutic modality for treating disabilities and illness. The coalition includes art therapy, dance/movement therapy, and music therapy as well as poetry therapy and psychodrama.[7] Dance and art techniques are used as nonverbal means of communication and expression and, along with music, are often useful in helping patients improve physical, emotional, cognitive, and social functioning. Art therapy emerged in the mental health field in the 1940s as an approach to explore feelings and conflicts and manage behavior and addictions. The **American Music**

Therapy Association (AMTA) was founded in the 1950s to gain professional status for music therapists who used vocal and instrumental music with individuals and groups to promote social, emotional, and cognitive function. Dance therapy integrates body, mind, and spirit through movement.[8]

Education, training, and licensure requirements for therapies described in this chapter vary from a postsecondary certificate to a master's degree. A postsecondary certificate is required for massage therapy, while a bachelor's degree is required for recreational therapy and music therapy. Art and dance therapy require a master's degree.

This chapter will discuss massage therapy and recreation therapy in detail with only a brief overview of art, music, and dance therapies since these are not included in the *Occupational Outlook Handbook*.

MASSAGE THERAPISTS
Significant Points

- Massage therapy is a rapidly growing healthcare profession.
- One to two years of postsecondary education training combining classroom study and clinical experience are required to become eligible for certification or registration.
- The majority of new massage therapists already have a career in either body movement or health care.
- Most massage therapists are self-employed and work an average of 27 hours a week.

Work Description

Massage therapists use touch to manipulate the soft tissues, muscles, tendons, and connective tissue. Stimulation from massage often improves joint mobility and range of motion; however, direct work on the skeleton is considered outside the scope of practice. Massage promotes circulation, relaxes muscle tightness, and relieves the stress of pain. There is scientific evidence that **massage therapy** may alleviate back pain and improve the quality of life for individuals with depression, cancer, and HIV/AIDS.[9]

For an initial visit, a massage therapist will obtain a medical history, including symptoms or areas of pain from a client. During therapy, the therapist is able to identify tense and painful areas of the body and manipulate muscles to release muscle tightness. Therapists talk with clients about what they hope to achieve through massage. Usually, the type of massage depends on the client's needs and physical condition. For example, therapists may use a special technique for elderly clients that they would not use for athletes. Some forms of massage are given solely to one type of client; for example, prenatal massage is given to pregnant women.

Massage therapists knead muscles and soft tissues with their hands, fingers, forearms, and elbows while their clients lie on a massage table. For massage of the neck, face, shoulders, hands, or arms, the client may be placed on a massage chair. Therapists often use lotions and oils during massage to facilitate the process. The massage can be gentle or forceful depending on the modality, or type of massage. Therapists often specialize in many different types of massage—for example, Swedish massage, deep-tissue massage, or sports massage. Different modalities require different techniques. A massage session can be as short as 5 to 10 minutes or could last more than an hour; however, most last at least 30 minutes.

Once the therapist identifies the source of muscle tightness, injury, or stress for a client, the therapist may give instructions on techniques for the client to practice at home such as stretching, body positioning to improve posture, or strengthening exercises to prevent injury. Instructions may also include relaxation techniques to reduce stress. The therapist documents each treatment session and recommends follow-up therapy visits.

Work Environment

Therapeutic massage is employed throughout the healthcare system for patients ranging from premature infants to the elderly. Massage therapists work in a variety of healthcare settings, such as hospitals, offices of other health professionals, sports medicine clinics, substance use disorder treatment centers, and pain clinics as well as assisted-living and skilled nursing facilities. Other locations include hotels, spas, airports, cruise ships, and fitness centers. Many have a home-based private practice or travel to clients' homes; those who are self-employed provide their own equipment such as a massage table, sheets, pillows, candles, and body lotions or oils.

A massage therapist's working conditions depend on the location and whether the client has an injury or is seeking therapy to reduce psychological stress and muscle tightness. For example, a massage meant to help rehabilitate a client with an injury may be conducted in a sports clinic or chiropractor's office. When the purpose of massage is to help clients relax, therapists usually work in a dimly lit room; use candles, incense, and body oils; and play calm, soothing music.

Massage therapists must feel comfortable using touch to treat clients. Most massage therapists are sole practitioners, and many work part time either because massage therapy is a second career or because the work is physically demanding. Therapy requires **manual dexterity** and strength to exert pressure during deep-muscle massage; therapists can injure themselves if they do not use the proper techniques. Repetitive-motion injuries are common, and therapists often experience fatigue from standing for prolonged periods. Injuries can be prevented with the use of good body mechanics, maintaining physical fitness, limiting the number of clients seen per day, and receiving regular massage themselves.

Good listening skills are important to identify sources of the client's pain and response to massage therapy. Since most therapists are self-employed they often do business-related tasks such as marketing and maintaining financial records. In addition, massage therapists may work closely with other members of the healthcare team, including physicians, physical therapists, chiropractors, athletic trainers, and acupuncturists.

TABLE 31.1 Facilities with the Largest Numbers of Massage Therapists, 2019

Self-employed	35%
Personal care services	33%
Offices of other health practitioners	31%
Offices of chiropractors	8%
Travelers accommodation (hotels)	6%

Data from Bureau of Labor Statistics, U.S. Department of Labor. Occupational Outlook Handbook. U.S. Department of Labor; 2020. https://www.bls.gov/ooh/healthcare/massage-therapists.htm#tab-3

Employment Opportunities

There were 166,700 individuals employed as massage therapists in May 2019. According to an American Massage Therapy Association survey of members conducted in 2020, most massage therapists enter the profession as a second career from a first career that may include other forms of bodywork or work as a healthcare professional.[10] About one-third each were self-employed or worked in personal care services for massage therapy franchises, and nearly 20% worked in the offices of other health professionals (**TABLE 31.1**).

Educational and Legal Requirements

Educational standards and requirements for massage therapists vary by state or locality. Most states regulate massage therapy and require massage therapists to be licensed.

Education and Training

Massage therapists typically complete a postsecondary education program of 500 to 1,000 hours of study and clinical experience, although standards and requirements vary by state. Educational programs usually require a high school diploma for admission and are typically found in private or public postsecondary vocational institutions or community colleges. Programs offer either a certificate or an associate's degree upon graduation and therefore vary in length from one to two years. The section *Additional Information* at the end of this chapter lists accredited educational programs under the Commission on Massage Therapy Accreditation (CMTA)[11] and the National Certification Board for Therapeutic Massage and Bodywork (NCBTMB) which lists approved schools (designated as assigned schools).[12] Programs generally include both classroom study and hands-on practice of massage techniques and include courses in anatomy, physiology, kinesiology, pathology (a study of diseases), business management, and ethics. The length of the program will vary with the program and educational and work background of the applicant. For example, students already working in a healthcare field will be able to finish the program more quickly because prerequisite courses such as physiology, anatomy, and medical

terminology will not be required. Programs may concentrate on certain modalities, or specialties, of massage. Several programs also offer job placement and continuing education. Both full-time and part-time programs are available.

Licensure

The FSMTB governs and administers the MBLEx, the national entry-level licensure examination for massage therapists. As of 2021, MBLEx was required for licensure of massage therapists in 49 states, Puerto Rico, and the Virgin Islands. Regulations may also exist by city or county.[13] Most states have continuing education requirements for license renewal.

The FSMTB administers the MBLEx for all states that require it for licensure for massage therapists. As of 2021, Wyoming was the only state that did not require licensure for massage therapists.[13] However, since successful completion of the MBLEx exam is required for licensure, new graduates will often take the exam upon graduation.

Certification and Other Qualifications

Board certification is awarded by the NCBTMB and is considered a more advanced level of practice. The requirements for becoming board certified are as follows: (1) graduate from a NCBTMB Assigned School, (2) have state licensure as a massage therapist, (3) successfully pass the Board Certification Exam for Therapeutic Massage & Bodywork (BCTMB), (4) pass a national criminal background check, and (5) agree to practice the NCBTMB's Standards of Practice and Code of Ethics. Board certification must be renewed every two years; renewal requires a national criminal background check and continuing education.[14] The NCBTMB also offers specialty certification, which requires additional course work and successful completion of a specialty examination. Specialty certification enhances skills for a particular population or condition, for example oncology massage care, pain and palliative care, sports massage, and reflexology.[14] Personal qualifications needed to be successful as a massage therapist are excellent communication skills to identify the client's goals of therapy and to explain the process of therapy and expected outcome of therapy—reducing muscle tightness and pain, for example. Empathy and the ability to build trust is necessary for repeated visits and referrals from other health professionals. Decision-making skills are also necessary to evaluate the client's needs and provide treatment to meet the needs of each individual client. Massage therapists use their hands, arms, and elbows to carry out their work and must have a level of physical fitness and stamina to carry out their work.

Those wishing to practice massage therapy should look into legal and other requirements for the state and other locality in which they intend to practice. However, certification in **cardiopulmonary resuscitation (CPR)** and liability insurance are usually required regardless of work location.

Advancement

Board certification is required by some hospitals and high-end spas. Massage therapists with board certification and specialty certification can expect to be more competitive in obtaining jobs with higher salaries. Other advancement opportunities are becoming an instructor or supervisor for training new massage therapists and initiating or participating in research to demonstrate the health benefits of massage.

Employment Trends

The use of massage therapy is expected to increase with greater recognition through licensure requirements. Licensure is also the pathway for massage therapy to be reimbursed by health insurance. Research demonstrating the medical benefits of massage therapy will also increase third-party reimbursement. Reimbursement will make therapy more affordable for clients and generate more business for therapists.

Massage also offers specific benefits to particular groups of people whose continued demand for massage services will lead to overall growth for the occupation. For example, some sports teams hire massage therapists to help give their athletes relief from pain and to rehabilitate clients with injuries. Massage therapy is being recognized as an alternative to medication for the treatment of pain, regardless of the cause of pain. Seniors in nursing homes or assisted-living facilities also are learning the benefits of massage, such as increased energy levels and reduced health problems. Demand for massage therapy should grow among older age groups because many are enjoying longer, more active lives.

In addition, the number of massage clinic franchises has increased in recent years, allowing massage to be more affordable for a wider variety of clients. As with many services paid by the consumer, demand for massage services may be limited by the overall state of the economy. During tough economic times, both the number of people who seek massage therapy and the frequency of their massages may decline.

Employment Change

Employment of massage therapists is projected to grow 21% from 2019 to 2029, much faster than the average for all occupations. Continued growth in the demand for massage services will lead to new openings for massage therapists.

Job Prospects

Opportunities should be available to those who complete formal programs and become board certified. New massage therapists should expect to work as an employee until they can build their own client base. Even though the total number of massage therapists is high (**TABLE 31.2**), the majority work an average of 27 hours a week, and 72% work as an independent practitioner instead of as an employee.[10]

Because referrals are an important source of work for massage therapists, marketing and networking will increase the number of job opportunities. According to a 2020 survey, referrals to massage therapists are from chiropractors, physical therapists, mental health professionals, and physicians.[10] It may also be helpful for massage therapists who are seeking to attract new clients to obtain specialty certification in sports massage, pain and palliative care, or other specialties. Those with specialty certification are more likely to find positions in a hospital or a clinic or work as a solo practitioner in a salon or in the client's home.[15] Other massage therapists may specialize in massage during pregnancy to relieve back pain or swelling of the feet and legs or oncology massage care after breast surgery for cancer to stimulate lymphatic drainage.

Earnings

The median hourly wage was $20.97 and the median annual salary for massage therapists was $43,620 in May 2020. Hourly fees for massage therapy vary widely depending upon geographic location and work setting. Fees are typically higher in high-end spas and hospitals. A 2019 survey reported that massage therapists charged an average of $75 for one hour of massage.[16] Most therapists earn a combination of wages and tips. Because therapists work by appointment, in most cases, their schedules and the number of hours worked each week can vary considerably, as can weekly income. Often, health professionals become licensed massage therapists to complement their work as a nurse or physical therapist or work as a massage therapist first and then complete course work to become a registered nurse or physical therapist.

Related Occupations

Similar occupations are athletic trainers and exercise physiologists, physical therapists, physical therapy assistants, and aides.

RECREATIONAL THERAPISTS
Significant Points

- Applicants for recreational therapist jobs will experience competition.
- A bachelor's degree in therapeutic recreation is the usual educational requirement.
- Only a few states require licensure, but certification is generally required for employment.
- Most recreational therapists are employed by hospitals, clinics, or nursing care facilities.

TABLE 31.2 Projections Data for Massage Therapists, 2019–2029				
Occupational Title	Employment, 2019	Projected Employment, 2029	Change, 2019–2029 Number	Percentage
Massage therapist	166,700	201,100	34,400	21%

Data from Bureau of Labor Statistics, U.S. Department of Labor. Occupational Outlook Handbook. U.S. Department of Labor; 2020. https://www.bls.gov/ooh/healthcare/massage-therapists.htm#tab-6

Work Descriptions

The **American Therapeutic Recreation Association (ATRA)** defines recreational therapy as "a treatment service designed to restore, remediate and rehabilitate a person's level of functioning and independence in life activities, to promote health and wellness as well as reduce or eliminate the activity limitations and restrictions to participation in life situations caused by an illness or disabling condition."[17] **Recreational Therapists (RTs)** are employed in **Therapeutic Recreation (TR)** services, and they plan, direct, and coordinate recreation-based treatment programs for people with disabilities, injuries, or illnesses.

RTs use a variety of activities to maintain or improve the emotional, physical, and social functioning of their clients. These could include, arts and crafts, sports, and games as well as community reintegration field trips where clients with limited mobility can participate in aquatic therapy or learn to use public transportation. RTs sometimes use the arts such as dance or music to encourage movement and recover basic motor functioning.

Therapists plan activities for clients to reduce depression, stress, and anxiety and to build confidence and reduce the impact of the illness or disability on physical and mental functioning. For example, a therapist may introduce a therapy dog to patients who need help managing their depression or anxiety (**FIGURE 31.2**).

RTs assess clients by gathering information from observations of the patient in different settings, review of medical records, conducting standardized assessments, and discussions with the patient and their families as well as other members of the healthcare team. Based on this information, they develop and carry out therapeutic interventions consistent with the clients' needs and interests. For example, they may encourage clients who are isolated or who have limited social skills to play games with others. RTs modify activities for those with physical limitations—for example, using chair yoga for those who have difficulty moving from the floor to a standing position or using a large ball for tossing from person to person in a group of patients sitting in a circle. RTs observe and document a patient's participation, reactions, and progress.

Work Environment

In *acute healthcare settings*, RTs may work at the bedside when doing an assessment, especially for someone newly hospitalized after experiencing trauma or undergoing surgery. In *mental health settings*, RTs treat individuals with specific mental health conditions such as substance use disorder/addiction, serious mental illness, or post-traumatic stress disorder. In *physical rehabilitation settings*, RTs provide recreational therapy for those with severe physical injuries requiring extensive rehabilitation—for example, spinal cord or traumatic brain injuries. In *hospice and palliative care settings*, RTs may focus on activities that promote relaxation to relieve stress and pain—for example, listening to music or participating in musical activities.

In *long-term and residential care facilities*, RTs use leisure activities, especially structured group programs, to improve and maintain physical and mental health. They also may provide interventions to prevent the client from suffering further medical problems and complications—for example, stretching and limbering exercises, proper body mechanics for participation in recreational activities, and pacing and energy conservation techniques. Another example is an RT initiating a structured walking group in the park for those adjusting to a new prosthesis after amputation of a lower leg.

Community-based RTs may work in parks and recreation departments; special education programs for school districts; or assisted-living, adult day care, and substance use disorder rehabilitation centers. In these programs, therapists use interventions to develop specific skills while providing opportunities for exercise, mental stimulation, creativity, and fun. Those who work in schools help counselors, teachers, and parents address the special needs of students, including easing disabled students' transition into adult life.

Therapists usually work in collaboration with physicians, nurses, psychologists, social workers, and physical and occupational therapists. RTs provide services in special activity rooms in assisted-living and skilled nursing facilities but also use offices to plan their activities and prepare documentation. Working with clients in community integration programs involves traveling to parks, swimming pools, theaters, sports stadiums, or other places of interest to the client. Therapists need physical strength since they often lift and carry equipment used to support activities. RTs generally work a 40-hour week but also some evenings, weekends, and holidays to accommodate the schedules of the clients and their families.

Employment Opportunities

Recreational therapists held about 19,900 jobs in 2019. The majority of RTs work in hospitals. Other RTs work in state and local government agencies, skilled nursing facilities, and ambulatory care services (**TABLE 31.3**).

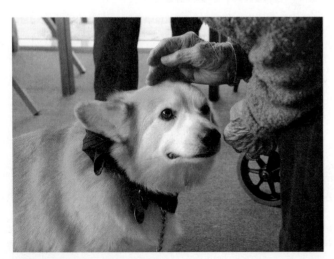

FIGURE 31.2 Recreational therapists use therapy dogs to treat anxiety and depression.
© Sue McDonald/Shutterstock.

TABLE 31.3 Facilities Employing the Largest Numbers of Recreational Therapists, 2019	
Hospitals	38%
Government	17%
Nursing care facilities	13%
Ambulatory healthcare services	9%

Data from Bureau of Labor Statistics, U.S. Department of Labor. Occupational Outlook Handbook. U.S. Department of Labor; 2020. https://www.bls.gov/ooh/healthcare/recreational-therapists.htm#tab-3

Many RTs in the United States work for the VA system in hospitals, community-based outpatient clinics, and tele-rehabilitation.[18] Only a small number of therapists are self-employed, generally contracting with long-term care facilities or community agencies to develop and oversee programs.

Educational and Legal Requirements

A bachelor's degree with a major or concentration in therapeutic recreation is the usual requirement for entry-level positions. Some states regulate RTs, but requirements vary.

Education and Training

Most entry-level RTs need a bachelor's degree in therapeutic recreation or in recreation with a concentration in therapeutic recreation. Bachelor level programs are listed on the Commission on Accreditation of Allied Health Education Programs webpage and on the American Therapeutic Recreation Association webpage. Some programs offer master's or doctoral degrees.[19,20]

The necessary background courses include human anatomy, physiology, abnormal psychology, medical and psychiatric terminology, characteristics of illnesses and disabilities, and professional ethics. Courses specific to therapeutic recreation include assessment, treatment, and program planning; intervention of individual clients; and the use of assistive devices and technology. Students also learn how to design and evaluate recreational therapy programs.

Licensure

States regulate RTs through licensure, registration, or the regulation of titles. Requirements vary by state. In 2021, five states—New Hampshire, New Jersey, North Carolina, Oklahoma, Utah—and the District of Columbia required licensure to practice as a recreational therapist, while California and Washington had other regulations that apply to RT professionals.[21]

Certification and Other Qualifications

Most employers, particularly those in hospitals and other clinical settings, prefer to hire certified RTs. The NCTRC offers the **Certified Therapeutic Recreation Specialist (CTRS)** credential. Certification requires a bachelor's degree with a concentration in therapeutic recreation, completion of a supervised internship (normally completed as part of the degree program) of at least 560 hours, and passing an exam. An alternative path to certification is a bachelor's degree in another field plus courses in anatomy and physiology, abnormal psychology, human growth and development, and therapeutic recreation. An additional requirement is work experience using the therapeutic recreation process.[22] Therapists must also take continuing education classes to maintain certification.

NCTRC also offers specialty certification in seven areas of practice: behavioral health, community inclusion services, developmental disabilities, geriatrics, pediatrics, adaptive sports and recreation, and physical medicine/rehabilitation.[23] Therapists may also earn certificates from other organizations to show proficiency in specific therapy techniques such as aquatic therapy (**FIGURE 31.3**).

Recreational therapists need to be comfortable working with people who are ill or disabled and be patient, tactful, and persuasive when working with people who have a variety of special needs. A sense of humor and imagination are needed to adapt activities to individual needs, and good physical coordination is necessary to demonstrate or participate in recreational activities. Other important qualities are speaking skills needed to give clear instructions and leadership skills to plan, develop, and evaluate interventions for individuals and groups.

Advancement

Therapists may advance to supervisory or administrative positions or obtain specialty certification. Some teach, conduct research, or consult for health or social service agencies.

Employment Trends

Overall employment of RTs is expected to grow about as fast as average for all occupations. Competition for jobs is expected.

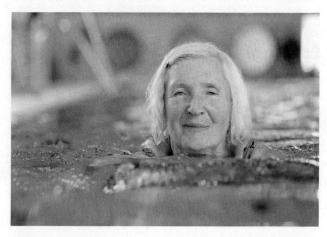

FIGURE 31.3 Recreational therapists may specialize in aquatic therapy.
© CroMary/Shutterstock.

Employment Change

Employment of RTs is expected to increase 8% from 2019 to 2029, about as fast as average for all occupations. As the large Baby Boom generation ages, its members will need RTs to help treat age-related injuries and illnesses. Older persons are more likely to suffer from stroke, Alzheimer's disease, and mobility-related injuries that require recreational therapy. Continued growth is expected in nursing care facilities, adult day care programs, senior centers, and assisted-living facilities that care for geriatric patients. RTs employed by VA hospitals and clinics help veterans manage service-related conditions such as post-traumatic stress disorder, brain injuries, or the loss of a limb. RTs help veterans reintegrate into their homes and communities and adjust to physical, social, or cognitive limitations.

In addition, the number of people with chronic conditions such as diabetes and obesity is growing. Recreational therapists will be needed to help patients maintain mobility and to teach patients to adapt to changes in mobility. Therapists will also be needed to plan and lead programs designed to maintain overall wellness through participation in activities such as camps, day trips, and sports. Healthcare facilities will support a growing number of jobs in settings offering short-term mental health and substance use disorder treatment services. Rehabilitation, home health care, and transitional programs will provide additional jobs. Because of the Americans with Disabilities Act of 1990, public spaces are more accessible to students and adults with physical and intellectual disabilities, resulting in more employment opportunities for RTs who are needed to teach clients how to access these spaces.[24]

Job Prospects

Job prospects will be best for RTs with both a bachelor's degree and certification. Therapists who specialize in working with the elderly or who earn certification in geriatric therapy may have the best job prospects. Opportunities also should be good for therapists who hold specialized certifications. Since many RTs are employed by the VA system, jobs will be more plentiful in states with VA hospitals and rehabilitation centers. **TABLE 31.4** shows some projection data provided by the U.S. Department of Labor.

Earnings

Median annual earnings of RTs were $47,710 in May 2020, and median hourly wages were $22.94 per hour in May 2020.

TABLE 31.5 Median Annual Earnings in the Industries Employing the Largest Numbers of Recreational Therapists, 2020

Government	$64,100
Hospitals: state, local, private	$52,130
Ambulatory healthcare services	$49,260
Nursing care facilities	$43,480
Social assistance	$37,900

Data from Bureau of Labor Statistics, U.S. Department of Labor. Occupational Outlook Handbook. U.S. Department of Labor; 2020. https://www.bls.gov/ooh/healthcare/recreational-therapists .htm#tab-5

Median annual earnings in the industries employing the largest numbers of RTs in May 2020 are included in **TABLE 31.5**.

Related Occupations

Recreational therapists primarily design activities to help people with disabilities lead more fulfilling and independent lives. Other workers who have similar jobs are athletic trainers, exercise physiologists, occupational therapists, physical therapists, rehabilitation counselors, social workers, speech-language pathologists, special education teachers, and school and career counselors.

ART THERAPISTS

Art therapy emerged as a mental health profession in the 1940s in veterans' hospitals as part of the treatment for soldiers returning from war.

Work Descriptions

The most practical application of art therapy has been with those suffering from mental disorders, developmental disorders, or other problems of social and psychological development, but innovative work has also been done on a variety of other problems. For example, art therapy is helpful to distract the focus on pain to creative activities in those with chronic pain, and in those with Alzheimer's, art therapy is used to trigger short- and long-term memory and reduce agitation. Participation in

TABLE 31.4 Projections Data for Recreational Therapists, 2019–2029

Occupational Title	Employment, 2019	Projected Employment, 2029	Change, 2019–2029	
			Number	Percentage
Recreational therapists	19,900	21,600	1,700	8%

Data from Bureau of Labor Statistics, U.S. Department of Labor. Occupational Outlook Handbook. U.S. Department of Labor; 2020. https://www.bls.gov/ooh/healthcare/recreational-therapists.htm#tab-6

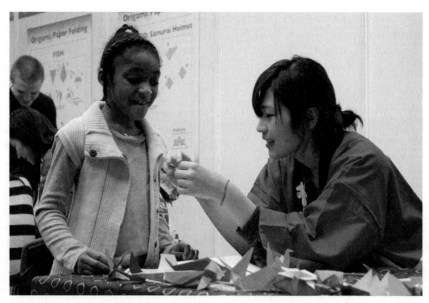

FIGURE 31.4 Art therapists work with people of all ages with physical and mental disabilities.
© Nando Machado/Shutterstock.

art therapy facilitates cognitive retraining in those with head injuries. Art therapy is also beneficial for those who have experienced trauma through combat, abuse, or natural disasters.[25]

Art Therapists (ATs) apply theories and techniques of human development, psychology, and counseling together with their knowledge and skills in the creative process of visual art forms such as drawing, painting, and sculpture to treat clients. Art therapy is based on the use of art as a tool for nonverbal expression and communication. The goal of art therapy is to resolve emotional conflicts, manage behavior and addictions, reduce anxiety and depression, and encourage personal growth and self-understanding.[26]

Work Environment

ATs work with people of all ages who have various degrees of mental or physical impairment. They practice with individuals, groups, or families in clinical, educational, or rehabilitative settings. These include private psychiatric hospitals and clinics, home health agencies, hospice, community health centers, substance use disorder clinics, nursing homes, halfway houses, prisons, public and private schools, and institutions for the emotionally disturbed, intellectually or physically disabled, brain injured, and hearing and visually impaired. Many ATs who work in clinics also teach art therapy in colleges or universities and may do research on some aspect of therapy. However, the primary involvement of most ATs is with clients in some type of clinical setting[27] (**FIGURE 31.4**).

ATs consult with members of the medical health team to diagnose patients' problems. Combining art, education, and insight, ATs assess their patients' problems, strengths, and weaknesses and determine a course of treatment best suited to accomplish specific treatment goals. ATs plan art activities, provide art instruction, and observe and record the various interactions that occur during therapy sessions. Emphasis is placed not on the quality of the product but rather on the well-being of the patient. ATs often work as members of

teams of other professionals and coordinate their activities with those of other therapists.

ATs normally work a 40-hour week, although the hours and degree of responsibility vary with the setting. The facilities in which they work are usually fully equipped with art materials, tables, chairs, art desks, and storage areas; general working conditions are good.

Educational and Legal Requirements

Educational requirements for an entry-level AT is the completion of a master's degree in art therapy. Master's degree programs also require that applicants submit an art portfolio to demonstrate proficiency in different forms of art media.[28]

Education and Training

There are several paths to becoming an AT. Although they are not required to do so, undergraduates often obtain a degree in art, psychology, or both. Recommended art courses are studio art in a variety of media to allow expression with different materials—for example, drawing, painting, and working in clay. Although there are undergraduate degrees in art therapy, educational requirements for the entry-level AT are the completion of a master's degree in art therapy.

Master's level programs include courses in human growth and development, psychopathology, psychological assessment, counseling theories, history and theory of art therapy, materials and techniques of practice in art therapy, and application of art therapy in different treatment settings. A thesis or project is required as well as 100 hours of supervised practicum and 600 hours of a supervised art therapy clinical internship.[28]

The **Commission on Accreditation of Allied Health Education Programs (CAAEP)** accredits master's level programs in art therapy,[19] and the **American Art Therapy Association (AATA)** approves art therapy programs at the undergraduate, master's, and doctoral level.[28]

Licensure

As of 2021, a total of 18 states and Washington DC regulate licensure for art therapists, allow licensure under another professional license (e.g., for psychotherapists), or have title protection. An additional 12 states are in the process of seeking licensure.[29]

Certification and Other Qualifications

To become a **Registered Art Therapist (ATR)**, a candidate must complete a supervised clinical experience after completing a CAAEP- or AATA-approved master's degree program. ATRs can become board certified as an **Art Therapist Registered-Board Certified (ATR-BC)** with successful completion of an exam administered by the **Arts Therapy Credentials Board (ATCB)**.[30]

DANCE THERAPISTS

Dance therapy got its start in the United States in the 1940s as a way to treat psychosis, anxiety, and depression in traumatized World War II veterans before the availability of psychiatric medications.

Work Description

Today, **dance/movement therapy** is used to treat those with both mental and physical disabilities associated with trauma and aging. Dance/movement therapy has recently had an upswing in popularity as a career among college students.[31] The **American Dance Therapy Association (ADTA)** defines dance/movement therapy as the "psychotherapeutic use of movement to further the emotional, cognitive, physical, and social integration of the individual."[32] **Dance/Movement Therapists (DMTs)** work with individuals, couples, families, and groups for those with developmental, social, physical, and psychological impairment (**FIGURE 31.5**).

DMTs use movement as the primary medium for observation, assessment, and therapeutic interaction/interventions for individual clients. They assess emotional and social behavior, movement capabilities, and general posture. Dance therapy helps clients develop communication skills and relationships and gain insight into their patterns of behavior as well as creating a broader range of options for coping with problems. Some benefits of dance therapy are a connection between mind and body, improved body image and social relationships, and relief from physical and emotional blocks.[30]

Dance movement therapy provides an avenue to communicate through movement for those with cognitive or neurological disorders unable to communicate verbally. For example, individuals who have had a traumatic brain injury or those with Parkinson's disease are able to communicate with others through movement and thus reduce feelings of isolation. Dance movement therapy improves physical mobility by enhancing coordination and gait and improves cognitive function by reconfiguring neural pathways in the brain.[33] For the treatment of mental or emotional disorders, dance therapists use body posture and movement to evaluate patients who have experienced physical or psychological

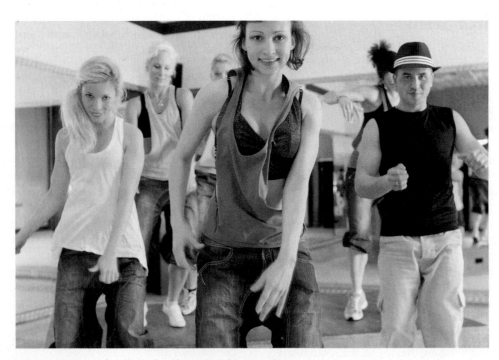

FIGURE 31.5 Dance therapy is a tool for physical and emotional integration.
© Kzenon/Shutterstock.

trauma. Anxiety and depression associated with trauma are reduced through the expansion of movement vocabulary.[31] DMTs develop treatment plans and goals, document their work in clinical records, and collaborate with professionals from other disciplines.

Work Environment

DMTs practice in a variety of settings with individuals of all ages and abilities in mental health centers, psychiatric hospitals, developmental centers, day care centers, correctional facilities, and nursing homes as well as health promotion programs and in private practice.[32]

DMTs participate in case conferences, staff meetings, community meetings, verbal therapy sessions, and other activities, depending on the setting in which they work. Some engage in research on movement behavior, teach or train others in educational or employment settings, or act as consultants to various agencies or organizations.

Hours and other working conditions vary. Most aspects of dance therapy involve close physical contact with different types of patient groups as well as a good deal of physical activity. In all instances, strength, flexibility, stamina, and a strong desire to relate to and help others are necessary.

Educational and Legal Requirements

Education and Training

Entry-level positions require a master's degree, including an internship. The American Dance Therapy Association approves master's level programs in dance therapy. As of 2021 there were seven approved programs in dance therapy.[34] Although each program has different requirements, a bachelor's level degree in either dance or psychology is encouraged. In addition, applicants are required to have dance experience with a proficiency in at least one dance form plus a background in dance education, choreography, or improvisation as well as other body/mind practices such as meditation or yoga. Some programs require a dance audition or a video for faculty to evaluate how prospective students express themselves and communicate through movement.

A dance therapy curriculum includes core courses in human development, neuroscience, neuropsychology, psychopathology, and group psychology. Courses specific to dance therapy are the history, theory, and practice of dance therapy; principles of dance and movement therapy; body/mind integration; multidisciplinary psychodiagnostics; and movement observation, assessment, and analysis. Programs also include at least 700 hours of supervised clinical training through fieldwork and internship experiences.[34]

Licensure

As of 2021 only two states (Wisconsin and New York) required DMTs to be licensed.[35]

Certification and Other Qualifications

After successful completion of the master's degree and internship, students are eligible to become a **Registered Dance/Movement Therapist (R-DMT)**.[36] Certification as a **Board-Certified Dance/Movement Therapist (BC-DMT)** is required to be able to supervise and train others and to work independently in private practice. Requirements for applying for the BC-DMT certification are having registration status, R-DMT, for at least one year; two years of employment; and completion of clinical supervision by a BC-DMT. For detailed requirements, refer to the handbook.[37]

In addition to having a regular dance practice, other qualifications needed to be an effective DMT are an interest and experience in working with people. Since DMTs develop a therapeutic relationship with their clients, most enter therapy as part of their training process. Helpful experience would include working or volunteering with people of different ages in various settings such as summer camps, after school programs, the YMCA, schools, hospitals, assisted living facilities, senior centers, and nursing homes. Physical strength, flexibility, stamina, and a strong desire to relate to and help others are necessary.

MUSIC THERAPISTS

Music therapy began as a profession after World War I and World War II when musicians volunteered to perform at VA hospitals for veterans suffering from service-related physical and emotional trauma. The positive response of the veterans to music led to hospitals hiring musicians and by the 1940s a formal training for music therapy emerged.[38]

Music therapists (MTs) combine knowledge and skills in both music and therapy to assess client needs and develop an intervention using music as the medium. Similar to art and dance/movement therapy, music therapy provides an avenue for expression for those who find it difficult to express themselves in words because of cognitive, emotional, or physical limitations. Unlike most music programs, the focus of music therapy is on the well-being of the client rather than a perfected musical product.

Work Description

Music therapy is used to facilitate motor skills, cognitive abilities, communication, and positive social outcomes for individuals of all ages. The MT is trained to select music most appropriate to the physical and cognitive abilities of the client. Individual or group therapy is chosen based on the clients' abilities, interests, and needs. Voice and traditional and nontraditional instruments and music are used. In addition, instrumental and vocal music are often combined with body movements as a part of therapy.

The MT often works as a member of an interdisciplinary team that may include other therapists, primary care physicians, psychiatrists, neurologists, psychologists, nurses, social workers, special educators, physical and occupational therapists, speech-language pathologists and audiologists as well as the patient and caregivers.[39] MTs participate in interdisciplinary treatment planning and determine how a client might be helped through a music program. They determine what goals and objectives can be met and plan musical activities and experiences that are likely to meet them, on both an individual and a group basis.[39]

Music therapy can achieve changes in the behavior of a person with mental illness that give them a new understanding of themselves and of the world around them. This new understanding can serve as a basis for improved mental health and a more effective adjustment to normal living. MTs treat patients of all ages, ranging from disturbed small children and adolescents to adults who suffer from mental illnesses of many types and various degrees of severity. The developmentally disabled, those with cerebral palsy, individuals with physical impairments, and the blind make up a group that is second only to the mentally ill in the number receiving music therapy.

Work Environment

MTs find employment in a variety of settings including hospitals, clinics, community mental health centers, physical rehabilitation centers, geriatric care programs, residential facilities, day treatment programs, correctional facilities, home health and hospice programs, public and private schools, special education programs, and prevention and wellness programs, Some music therapists maintain private practices or serve as consultants.[40]

At the most basic level, an individual may listen to the therapist play the guitar and sing in a hospice setting or for someone with Alzheimer's disease. In a group setting, the client might participate with others who are singing and playing instruments, clapping, or moving to the music. Therapy is beneficial for those undergoing physical rehabilitation; therapy provides emotional support for clients and their families after experiencing trauma or surgery. Music therapy can also ease the pain of childbirth as well as chronic pain associated with an injury or rheumatoid arthritis.

Standard work hours are common in most settings; however, those who work in a hospital or hospice program or in private practice may have weekend and evening hours. Music therapists work in close cooperation with professionals in other disciplines and often share physical facilities to plan and schedule activities.

Education and Legal Requirements

There are different options to becoming a certified music therapist; however, the minimum requirement is a bachelor's degree in music therapy. There are also master's degree programs in music therapy. The bachelor's degree in music therapy includes 1,200 hours of clinical training including a supervised internship. Students who complete

degree requirements are eligible to become board certified by successfully completing the national board certification exam and to use the title **Music Therapist-Board Certified (MT-BC)**.[41]

Education and Training

Application to a music therapy program requires an audition to evaluate music competency.[41] There are 36 undergraduate and master's programs in music therapy in the United States approved by the American Music Therapy Association (AMTA). The AMTA website lists each program with details about admission and course requirements.[42]

Course requirements for an undergraduate program in music therapy include biology, physiology, and psychology in addition to courses in music including music theory, conducting, and improvisation. Students may have a primary instrument when applying for a program but are usually required to take additional classes in piano, guitar, and percussion to broaden the number of instruments that can be used with individuals and groups during therapy. A practicum in music therapy introduces the student to music therapy through the observation of a music therapist in practice, and an internship is also required.[43]

Licensure

As of 2021, licensure was required for music therapists in 15 states.[44] Requirements for licensure can be found for each state.

Certification and Other Qualifications

Students who have completed academic and clinical training requirements are eligible to sit for the national board certification exam. Successful candidates are able to use the title MT-BC. Certification is often required by states that require licensure, certification, or a registry.[45]

Music therapists work very closely with their clients and must be able to relate to them and their problems in a warm, professional manner. The therapist's efforts to change behavior can precipitate resistance and negative attitudes in the client. Creativity, resourcefulness, and flexibility are qualities needed to be successful as a music therapist. Having a broad range of experience and skills as a musician with different instruments and styles of music is also important for someone interested in becoming a music therapist.

Additional Information

For information and materials on careers and academic programs in massage therapy, contact:

- Accrediting Commission of Career Schools and Colleges, 2101 Wilson Blvd., Suite 302, Arlington, VA 22201. http://www.accsc.org/Directory/index.aspx
- Associated Bodywork & Massage Professionals. 25188 Genesee Trail Rd., Suite 200, Golden, CO 60401. https://www.abmp.com/home

- American Massage Therapy Association, 600 Davis St., Suite 900, Evanston, IL 60201. https://www.amtamassage.org/index.html
- Commission on Massage Therapy Accreditation, 900 Commonwealth Place, Suite 200-331, Virginia Beach, VA 23464. https://comta.org/contact

For more information on national testing and national certification for massage therapists, visit:

- Federation of State Massage Therapy Boards, 7300 College Blvd., Suite 650, Overland Park, KS 66210. https://www.fsmtb.org/
- National Certification Board for Therapeutic Massage & Bodywork, 1333 Burr Ridge Parkway, Suite 200, Burr Ridge, IL 60527. http://www.ncbtmb.org/

For information on license requirements by state, visit:

- Federation of State Massage Therapy Boards. *States That Regulate Massage.* https://www.fsmtb.org/consumer-information/regulated-states/

For information and materials on careers and academic programs in recreational therapy, contact:

- American Therapeutic Recreation Association, 25 Century Blvd., Suite 505 | Nashville, TN 37214. https://www.atra-online.com
- Commission on Accreditation of Allied Health Education Programs, 9355 - 113th St. N, Suite 7709 Seminole, FL 33775. www.caahep.org

- National Therapeutic Recreation Society, 22377 Belmont Ridge Rd., Ashburn, VA 20148-4501. https://www.nrpa.org

Information on certification of RTs may be obtained from:

- National Council for Therapeutic Recreation Certification, 16 Squadron Blvd., Suite 101 New City, NY 10956. https://www.nctrc.org

For information on licensure requirements, contact the appropriate recreational therapy regulatory agency for your state.

For career information on art, dance, and music therapy, visit:

- American Art Therapy Association (AATA), 4875 Eisenhower Ave., Suite 240, Alexandria, VA 22304. https://www.arttherapy.org
- American Dance Therapy Association, 230 Washington Ave. Extension, Suite 101, Albany, NY 12203-3539. https://www.adta.org
- American Music Therapy Association, Inc., 8455 Colesville Rd., Suite 1000, Silver Spring, MD 20910. https://www.musictherapy.org
- Art Therapy Credentials Board (ATCB), 7 Terrace Way, Greensboro, NC. https://www.atcb.org/
- National Coalition of Creative Arts Therapy Associations, c/o AMTA, 8455 Colesville Rd., Suite 1000, Silver Spring, MD 20910. https://www.nccata.org/
- Certification Board for Music Therapists. 506 E. Lancaster Ave., Suite 102, Downington, PA 19335. https://www.cbmt.org

LEARNING PORTFOLIO

Issues for Discussion

1. Discuss the differences between licensure and certification for massage therapists. What are the advantages for a massage therapist to become certified?

2. Review the 13-minute YouTube video "Therapeutic Recreation: Who We Are, What We Do," produced by the Therapeutic Recreation Association of Atlantic Canada. Using examples from the video, describe different work settings for RTs and differences between recreation and therapeutic recreation. https://www.youtube.com/watch?v=yRmHnFEzoV0

3. Discuss the similarities and differences between recreation therapy, art therapy, dance therapy, and music therapy in terms of the typical patient or client. What do academic programs in art, dance, and music therapy require that is not required for a degree in recreation therapy?

4. Go to the American Art Therapy Association (AATA) and view one video clip from *Art Therapy in Action* (for example, children in hospitals, memory care, eating disorders, or military service members and veterans). https://arttherapy.org/art-therapy-action/

5. Learn more about music therapy and settings in which music therapy is used as part of a treatment program by viewing the 9-minute YouTube video "The Healing Power of Music." What are some of the ages and health conditions of those receiving music therapy? https://www.youtube.com/watch?v=Ketz-mJ-x-Q

Enrichment Activities

1. Learn more about being a massage therapist by viewing a video from the U.S. Department of Labor. *CareerOneStop. Career Videos: Massage Therapy.* https://www.careeronestop.org/videos/careeronestop-videos.aspx?videocode=31901100

2. Learn more about the work settings of a recreational therapist by viewing a video from the U.S. Department of Labor. *CareerOneStop. Career Videos: Recreation Therapy.* https://www.careeronestop.org/videos/careeronestop-videos.aspx?videocode=29112500

3. Learn how recreation therapy and art therapy were used in the rehabilitation of a young woman after a spinal cord injury. *Spinal Cord Injury: Michele Lee's Story.* Rehabilitation Institute of Chicago (RIC). https://spinalcordinjuryzone.com/news/9450/michele-lees-spinal-cord-injury-patient-story

4. Read profiles of dance/movement therapists to learn how movement and psychotherapy are combined in a career. American Dance Therapy Association. *Profiles of Dance/Movement Therapists.* https://www.adta.org/profiles-of-dmts

CASE STUDY: MASSAGE THERAPY

Linda Rae works full-time as a massage therapist. Her first client for the day is Annie Dullen. Annie is pregnant with her first child and is anxious to receive her massage. She works long hours on her feet, and as a result, she has been experiencing lower back pain. This is the first time Annie has scheduled a massage with Linda.

Based on the information you have read about massage therapists, answer the following questions.

1. During Annie's initial massage visit, Linda will:
   A. present her with a gift card for a return appointment.
   B. obtain a medical history.
   C. insist that she pay in advance for services.
   D. provide her with a tour of the facilities.

2. Annie should acknowledge which of the following?
   A. Tense and painful areas on her body
   B. Goals she would like to achieve through massage
   C. Sensitivity to certain oils and lotions
   D. All of these are correct.

3. Because of Annie's pregnancy, Linda must:
   A. cancel the appointment.
   B. limit the massage to 10 minutes.
   C. use a different technique.
   D. eliminate all use of oils and lotions.

4. After Linda completes Annie's massage, she should:
   A. insist that Annie sleep for the next hour.
   B. document the treatment session.
   C. recommend that Annie no longer receive therapy.
   D. offer Annie a light lunch and beverage.

5. In order to limit the risk of injury to herself, Linda knows that she must:
   A. use proper technique.
   B. space sessions properly.
   C. exercise regularly.
   D. receive massage herself.
   E. All of these are correct.

LEARNING PORTFOLIO

References

1. Kish KS. Massage, the Oldest Form of Medicine. *Blog.* December 23, 2015. https://www.kristeenkish.com/2015/12/23/massage-the-oldest-form-of-medicine/ Accessed September 16, 2020.

2. National Certification board for Therapeutic Massage & Bodywork (NCBTMB). *About NCBTMB.* https://www.ncbtmb.org/about-ncbtmb Accessed July 2, 2020.

3. U.S. Department of Veteran Affairs. *A History of Recreation Therapy in the VA.* https://www.rehab.va.gov/PROSTHETICS/rectherapy/history.asp Accessed July 2, 2020.

4. Mansfield JA. *Recreation Therapy History by Categories.* http://www.recreationtherapy.com/history/rthistory4.htm Accessed September 17, 2020.

5. National Council for Therapeutic Recreation Certification (NCTRC). *About NCTRC.* http://www.nctrc.org/about-ncrtc/ Accessed September 17, 2020.

6. American Music Therapy Association. *History of Music Therapy.* https://www.musictherapy.org/about/history/ Accessed September 17, 2020.

7. National Coalition of Creative Arts Therapies Associations, Inc. (NCCATA). *About NCCATA.* https://www.nccata.org/aboutnccata Accessed July 2, 2020.

8. National Coalition of Creative Arts Therapies Associations, Inc. (NCCATA). *Membership: Membership Associations.* https://www.nccata.org/membership Accessed September 3, 2021.

9. National Center for Complementary and Integrative Health. *Massage Therapy for Health Professionals: What You Need to Know.* https://www.nccih.nih.gov/health/massage-therapy-what-you-need-to-know Accessed July 2, 2020.

10. American Massage Therapy Association. *State of the Massage Therapy Profession. 2020 Fact Sheet.* https://www.amtamassage.org/globalassets/documents/publications-and-research/amta-2020-student-fact-sheet.pdf Accessed September 3, 2021.

11. Commission on Massage Therapy Accreditation. *Massage Therapy Training.* https://comta.org/massage-therapy-training/ Accessed September 18, 2020.

12. National Certification Board for Therapeutic Massage & Bodywork. *Assigned Schools FAQs.* https://www.ncbtmb.org/faqs/assigned-schools-faqs/ Accessed September 18, 2020.

13. Federation of State Massage Therapy Boards (FSMTB). *States that Regulate Massage.* https://www.fsmtb.org/consumer-information/regulated-states/ Accessed August 30, 2021.

14. National Certification Board for Therapeutic Massage & Bodywork. *About Specialty Certificates.* https://exam.ncbtmb.org/about/ Accessed September 2, 2021.

15. National Certification Board for Therapeutic Massage & Bodywork. *About Specialty Certificates.* https://exam.ncbtmb.org/about/ Accessed September 3, 2021.

16. American Massage Therapy Association. *Massage Therapy Industry Fact Sheet.* https://www.amtamassage.org/publications/massage-industry-fact-sheet/ Accessed September 3, 2021.

17. American Therapeutic Recreation Association. *About Recreational Therapy.* https://www.atra-online.com/page/AboutRecTherapy Accessed October 4, 2021.

18. U.S. Department of Veteran's Affairs. Rehabilitation and Prosthetics Services. *Recreation Therapy Service Fact Sheet.* February 2019. https://www.rehab.va.gov/PROSTHETICS/factsheet/RecTherapy-FactSheet.pdf Accessed September 3, 2021.

19. Commission on Accreditation of Allied Health Education Programs. *Find a Program.* https://www.caahep.org/Students/Find-a-program.aspx Accessed September 18, 2020.

20. American Therapeutic Recreation Association. *Become a Recreational Therapist.* https://www.atra-online.com/page/BecomeAnRT Accessed September 18, 2020.

21. American Therapeutic Recreation Association. *Certification and Licensure.* https://www.atra-online.com/page/CertandLicense Accessed July 2, 2020.

22. American Therapeutic Recreation Association. *Paths to Certification.* https://www.nctrc.org/new-applicants/paths-to-certification/ Accessed September 18, 2020.

23. American Therapeutic Recreation Association. *Specialization Area Designation.* https://www.nctrc.org/about-certification/specialty-certification/ Accessed September 18, 2020.

24. United States Department of Justice. Civil Rights Division. *Information and Technical Assistance on the Americans with Disabilities Act.* https://www.ada.gov/ Accessed September 18, 2020.

25. National Coalition of Creative Arts Therapies Associations, Inc. *Research on the Efficacy of the Arts Therapies.* https://www.nccata.org/research Accessed September 18, 2020.

26. American Art Therapy Association. *Definition.* https://www.arttherapy.org/upload/2017_DefinitionofProfession.pdf Updated June 2017. Accessed October 4, 2016.

27. National Coalition of Creative Arts Therapies Associations, Inc. *About NCCATA.* https://www.nccata.org/aboutnccata Accessed September 18, 2020.

28. American Art Therapy Association. *Becoming an Art Therapist.* https://arttherapy.org/becoming-art-therapist/ Accessed September 18, 2020.

29. American Art Therapy Association. *State Advocacy.* https://arttherapy.org/state-advocacy/ Accessed September 3, 2021.

30. Art Therapy Credentials Board (ATCB). *Board Certified Registered Art Therapist (ATR-BC)*. https://www.atcb.org/board-certified-registered-art-therapist-atr-bc/ Accessed October 4, 2021.

31. Molzahn L. Dance heals: Newly popular therapy makes big strides with movement. *Chicago Tribune*. June 6, 2015: 1, 6. https://www.chicagotribune.com/entertainment/theater/ct-dance-movement-therapy-20150604-column.html Accessed September 3, 2021.

32. *American Dance Therapy Association. Frequently Asked Questions*. https://www.adta.org/faq Accessed October 4, 2021.

33. Luc KA. Deerfield Woman Mixes Dance, Psychology, in Unique Session. *Chicago Tribune*. April 2, 2015. https://www.chicagotribune.com/suburbs/buffalo-grove/ct-dfr-north-shore-dance-therapy-tl-0409-20150402-story.html Accessed October 4, 2021.

34. American Dance Therapy Association. *Approved Masters Programs*. https://adta.memberclicks.net/approved-masters-programs Accessed September 18, 2020.

35. American Dance Therapy Association. *Advisory for Those Seeking State Licensure*. https://adta.wildapricot.org/StateLicensingTools Accessed September 18, 2020.

36. American Dancer Therapy Association. *R-DMT*. https://www.adta.org/r-dmt Accessed September 20, 2020.

37. Dance Movement Therapy Board. *Dance/Movement Therapy Board, Inc.* https://www.adta.org/assets/docs/BCDMT-HANDBOOK-Final-Copy-3.pdf Accessed September 18, 2020.

38. American Music Therapy Association. *History of Music Therapy.* http://www.musictherapy.org/about/history/ Accessed July 2, 2020.

39. American Music Therapy Association/Certification Board for Music Therapists. *Scope of Music Therapy Practice*, January 11, 2018. https://www.cbmt.org/wp-content/uploads/2019/10/CBMT-AMTA-Scope-of-Music-Therapy-Practice.pdf Accessed September 3, 2021.

40. Certification Board for Music Therapists. *About Us.* https://www.cbmt.org/about/ Accessed October 4, 2021.

41. American Music Therapy Association. *Professional Requirements for Music Therapists*. https://www.musictherapy.org/about/requirements/ Accessed October 4, 2021.

42. American Music Therapy Association. *Organization Directory Search*. https://netforumpro.com/eweb/DynamicPage.aspx?Site=AMTA2&WebCode=OrgSearch& Accessed September 18, 2020.

43. Major in Music (B.M.), *Music Therapy Concentration*. https://catalog.colostate.edu/general-catalog/colleges/liberal-arts/music-theatre-dance/music-bm-therapy-concentration/ Accessed September 18, 2020.

44. Certification Board for Music Therapists. *State Licensure*. https://www.cbmt.org/state-requirements/ Accessed September 18, 2020.

45. Certification Board for Music Therapists. *Board Certification*. https://www.cbmt.org/candidates/certification/ Accessed October 4, 2021.

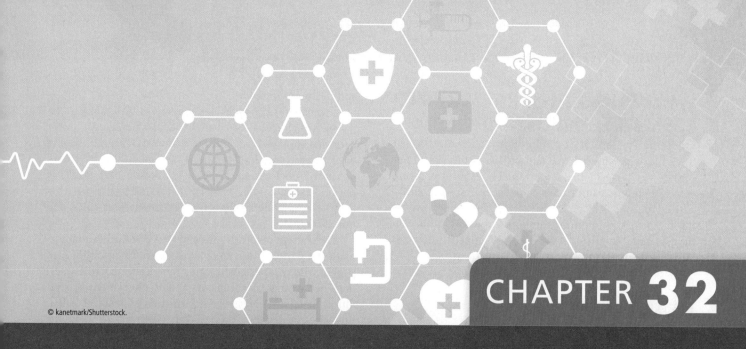
© kanetmark/Shutterstock.

CHAPTER **32**

Health Information Personnel*

KEY TERMS

Assessment
Cancer registrar
Clinical documentation
  improvement (CDI) specialist
Coder
Diagnosis and treatment plan
Diagnosis-related groups (DRG)
DRG validator
Documentation
Electronic health records (EHR)

Electronic health record support
  specialist
Health data analyst
Health informatics
Health information
  administrator
Health information
  management (HIM)
Health information personnel
Health information technician

Health record
Insurance claims
Medical or health science
  librarian
Medical transcriptionists
Medicare reimbursement
Privacy officer
Quality improvement analyst
Statistics
Symptoms and response

* All information in this chapter, unless otherwise indicated, was obtained from Bureau of Labor Statistics. *Occupational Outlook
Handbook 2020–2021 Edition*. Washington, DC: U.S. Department of Labor; 2021.

PROVIDING AND PRESERVING ESSENTIAL INFORMATION

Providing and preserving information of ethical, scientific, and legal value to the appropriate professional personnel are some of the most valuable aspects of health care. Managing an information system that meets medical, administrative, ethical, and legal requirements involves the teamwork of administrators, technicians, transcriptionists, and medical librarians, collectively known as **health information personnel**.

HEALTH INFORMATION MANAGEMENT
Significant Points

- Employment is expected to grow much faster than average.
- Job prospects should be very good, particularly for technicians with strong computer software skills.
- Entrants usually have an associate's degree for a technician role and a bachelor's degree for an administrator role.
- This is one of the few health-related occupations in which there is no direct hands-on patient care.

Health information management (HIM) professionals work to acquire, analyze, and protect digital and traditional health information that is considered vital to the delivery of quality patient care.[1] HIM is at the heart of health care because health records and health information systems serve as the backbone of healthcare systems, hospitals, clinics,

and healthcare provider offices. Just as schools and colleges keep transcripts of grades and employers maintain personnel records, doctors and hospitals set up a permanent file for every patient they treat. This file is known by multiple names but is most commonly known as the patient's health record or chart. It includes the patient's medical history, results of physical examinations, results of X-ray and laboratory tests, diagnoses, treatment plans, doctors' orders and notes, and nurses' notes.[2]

The **health record** is the centerpiece of the health information system because it contains the entire history of each patient who receives health care. This health record—a permanent document of the history and progress of one person's illness or injury—preserves information of medical, scientific, legal, and planning value. The health record shows the **diagnosis and treatment plan** and the patient's **symptoms and response** to treatment. It is compiled from observations and findings recorded by the patient's physician and other professional members of the medical team. An example of healthcare professionals viewing a traditional (paper) health record is seen in **FIGURE 32.1**. The entries and reports noted in it originate from various points in the hospital, clinic, nursing home, health center, or other healthcare facility. Through a network of communications systems, they are entered in the individual patient's health record. This vital medical profile constitutes each patient's unique medical history.

Although accurate and orderly records are essential for clinical purposes, health records have other important uses as well. They provide background and **documentation** for **insurance claims** and **Medicare reimbursement**, legal actions, professional review of treatment and medications prescribed, and training of health professions personnel. Health records are used for research and planning purposes.

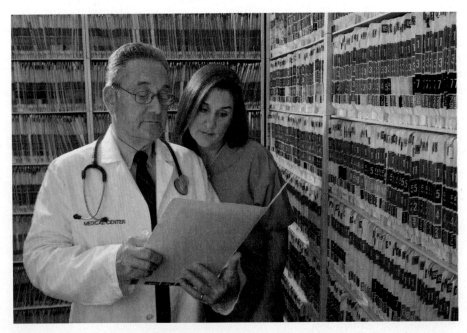

FIGURE 32.1 Healthcare professionals viewing a traditional paper record.
© Kent Weakley/Shutterstock.

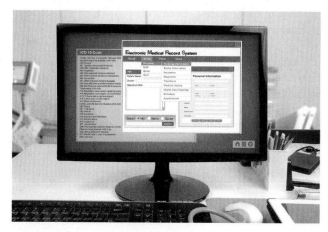

FIGURE 32.2 Electronic health record.
© pandpstock001/Shutterstock.

They provide data for clinical studies, evaluations of the benefits and costs of various medical and surgical procedures, and **assessments** of community health needs.

The increasing use of **electronic health records (EHRs)** continues to broaden and alter the job responsibilities of health information management professionals. For example, HIM professionals must be familiar with EHR computer software, maintaining EHR security, and analyzing electronic data to improve healthcare information. HIM professionals use EHR software to maintain data on patient safety, patterns of disease, and disease treatment and outcomes and to conduct clinical research. HIM professionals also may assist with improving EHR software usability and may contribute to the development and maintenance of health information networks. An example of an electronic health record is seen in **FIGURE 32.2**.

HEALTH INFORMATION ADMINISTRATORS
Work Description

Traditionally, **health information administrators** directed and controlled the activities of the health information department. While some continue to do so today, many others often work in a variety of different settings, possessing an array of different job titles. They possess skills in health data management, information policy, information systems, and administrative and clinical workflow. They train and supervise the health information staff and develop systems for documenting, storing, and retrieving health information. They manage the workflow for capturing data in a variety of healthcare settings, from large hospital systems to small physician practices. They organize, maintain, and disclose content considered part of the patient's health record in accordance with healthcare requirements, professional practice standards, and numerous state and federal regulations. Health information administrators compile **statistics** required by federal and state agencies, assist the medical staff in evaluations of patient care or research studies, and

sometimes testify in court about patient health records and procedures of record keeping.

Health information administrators are focused on operations management, specifically working to ensure an accurate and complete health record and cost-effective information processing. The deployment of health information technology and EHRs by the majority of healthcare providers has influenced the skills needed by a health information administrator. As a result, health information managers must possess skills and training regarding evolving information technology and specialized software technology, analysis of electronic data, disclosure of electronic health information, current and proposed laws about health information systems, and trends in managing large amounts of complex data. In addition, because patient data is central to quality management and medical research, health information managers ensure that databases are complete, accurate, and available only to authorized personnel.

Health information managers are responsible for the maintenance and security of all patient records. Recent regulations enacted by the federal government require that all healthcare providers maintain secure electronic patient records. Health information administrators ensure confidentiality and security of patient information and protect patients' health information from unauthorized access and use. Health information administrators work with a team to employ security measures, such as authentication and permission protocols, encryption, and damage prevention techniques. They address breaches of protected health information, whether those breaches occur because of identity theft, unauthorized access to data, or theft or loss of laptop computers and mobile devices. They ensure that notification to patients of breaches of protected health information is completed according to standards and regulations. An example of the many terms a health information administrator must understand regarding a data breach is seen in **FIGURE 32.3**.

Health information administrators are viewed as key members of the management team, and they work closely

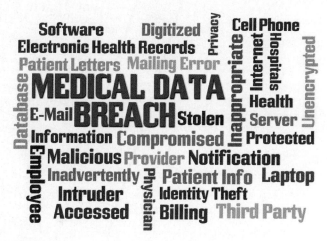

FIGURE 32.3 Word cloud illustrating the concepts involved in a data breach.
© Rob Wilson/Shutterstock.

with the finance department to monitor revenue cycle and hospital spending patterns. As part of the management team, health administrators establish and implement policies, objectives, and procedures for the protection and security of health information; evaluate personnel and work performance; develop reports and budgets; and coordinate activities with other managers.

This teamwork approach extends to the interaction between the health information administrator and clinical staff. Some health information administrators work as **clinical documentation improvement (CDI) specialists**; they are responsible for review of the patient's electronic health record and serve as the liaison to the clinical treatment team in documenting clinical care. The CDI specialist works to obtain appropriate clinical documentation to ensure that the level of service rendered to the patient and the clinical complexity of the patient's condition are completely and accurately documented. The CDI specialist identifies gaps in clinical documentation and ensures that the severity of the patient's illness, the intensity of services, and the risk of mortality are appropriately reflected in the health record.

Some health information administrators specialize in protecting the confidentiality of health information, serving as privacy officers. A **privacy officer** develops and implements requisite privacy policies and procedures, receives complaints, and disseminates information about an entity's privacy practices. A privacy officer must have knowledge of numerous federal laws and regulations and industry and institutional standards governing the protection of patient health information. Privacy officers provide extensive compliance training to physicians, associates, and board members and investigate reported privacy concerns.

Other health information administrators specialize as **health data analysts**. They work to acquire, manage, analyze, interpret, and transform data into accurate, consistent, and timely information. They focus on a variety of data points, calculate numerous rates, trend public health data, and measure costs. They balance the big picture strategic vision with day-to-day details of patient care.

Other health information administrators pursue the path of health informatics. **Health informatics** refers to the science of how health information is technically captured, transmitted, and utilized. Often the focus of education at the graduate level, health informatics addresses information systems, informatics principles, and information technology as applied to the continuum of healthcare delivery. Health informatics professionals work to develop more efficient, effective, and intuitive ways of controlling stored health information, managing clinical workflow tasks, and improving the general security of health information. For example, they work to create an EHR system that contains health history information according to a standardized fashion, whether from a traditional paper form or through direct data entry. An example of a traditional health history form is seen in **FIGURE 32.4**. By focusing on health information technology, these professionals strive to improve healthcare quality and efficiency, thereby resulting in lower costs and greater accessibility.

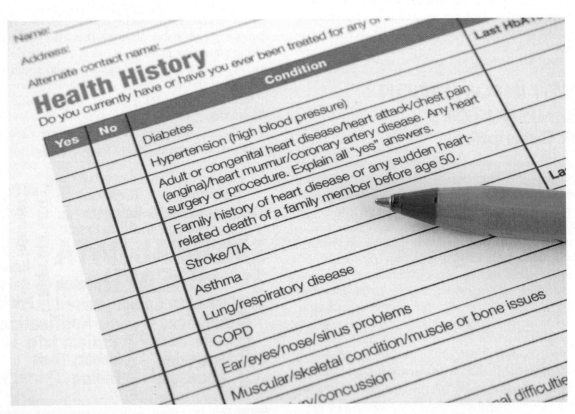

FIGURE 32.4 Traditional health history form.
© Ekaterina_Minaeva/Shutterstock.

Professional Profiles

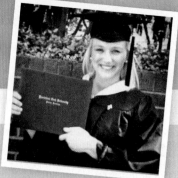

Name: Amanda, MHI, RHIA
Title: ICD-10 Implementation Team Leader
Education: BS in Health Informatics and Information Management;
MS in Health Informatics (MHI)

Q: Tell us about your job and the type of organization you work in.

A: I am currently working at a large nonprofit medical center with a cardiology department ranking in the top 50 in the United States. It is an urban facility located in the middle of a large city. I am on the ICD-10 implementation team working with the order validation team to ensure the standards for the ICD-10 codes received are correct. I also provide training and guidance for the order validation team. I also have been working with DRG Denial Review Appeal letters. I write appeal letters and send them to insurance companies and provide appropriate documents to support our coding and findings.

Q: Describe a typical workday.

A: My typical work week is split between two different locations that my facility operates. I work in their electronic health record on a daily basis to look at orders and to pull information for denial letters. I do not have any patient interaction in this position.

Q: Why did you choose this profession?

A: I chose this profession because I believe in it. I chose this profession because what health information management (HIM) professionals do is a vital step in patient care. The data that is collected and used in the HIM Department can be used in so many ways to enhance patient quality of care. Health informatics and information management is cutting edge, and it combines health care, technology, and clinical care all in one profession.

Q: What do you like most about this profession, and what challenges you?

A: I love how HIM is always changing. You are constantly learning something new. A new puzzle presents itself every day, and you have the knowledge to solve it. I love to learn, and this profession allows me to learn every day.

Q: Is there room for advancement in this field?

A: The room for advancement is never ending! With a degree in HIM you can find your niche in so many different venues of health care. It opens so many doors. It is overwhelming the amount of opportunity that comes with this profession. Since health care is moving into the realm of technology, there are even more positions available. Technology just opened a new door of health informatics and data-driven decision making now that facilities have that capability.

Q: What kind of academic training is required in this field, and how long does it take?

A: At my alma mater, we did a lot of academic training. I learned ICD-10 coding and took three database technology classes. These classes were geared toward using database query tools to gather information to enhance patient care. We also covered healthcare law, research, and statistics. We also learned EHR infrastructure and used a real EHR to follow a patient through admission to discharge. The coursework that I went through was extensive, but it prepared me for every aspect of the HIM department in a large hospital facility.

Q: Name and explain what part of your academic training most prepared you for this profession.

A: What most prepared me for my experiences in my job were the relationships and the things I learned from my professors. I learned a lot in all of our courses, but the lessons that they taught me on a day-to-day basis are invaluable in my career today.

Q: Did you face obstacles in pursuing your goals? If so, describe them and how you overcame them.

A: I think every new graduate will face obstacles in getting their foot in the door, but it is all about networking. I had the once-in-a-lifetime opportunity to work with the AHIMA (American Health Information Management Association) Board of Directors and staff. I ensured that I soaked up everything I heard from them at every meeting and convention I went to. Learning from the subject matter experts in a field that means so much to you is a great way to get over the obstacles you face as a new graduate. It also gives you the opportunity to network with the best in the business and always gives you an opportunity to learn. So getting involved at your state level and of course volunteering at the national level is a great way to get started and to learn.

Q: What do you wish you had known in high school/college about pursuing this career?

A: I wish I would have known more about it! I feel like HIM is the best-kept secret. It really can open so many doors in health care and can take your career in so many different directions. I wish that this profession was given more recognition.

Q: What advice would you give someone who is considering this career?

A: Do your research. If you know you want to work in health care but you aren't sure which avenue to go into, really consider an undergraduate degree in HIM. Having an undergraduate degree in HIM can lead you to many different opportunities to continue your education at the master's level and the doctoral level. Since I found my love in data and data-driven decision making, I got my master's degree in informatics.

Work Environment

Most health information administrators work in pleasant and comfortable offices or on hospital patient floors, but they may work long hours if they are called in to help solve unexpected problems. Some aspects of the job can be stressful. The utmost accuracy is essential, which demands concentration and close attention to detail. The emphasis on accuracy can cause fatigue and mental strain. Those who work at computers for prolonged periods may experience muscle pain and eyestrain.

Employment Opportunities

Employment of medical and health services managers is expected to grow 32% from 2019 to 2029, much faster than the average for all occupations. The healthcare industry as a whole is expected to see an increase in demand because of the aging population and the fact that people stay more active in life longer. Managers will be needed to manage and organize health information, oversee the digitization of patient records, and ensure their security as required by law. Additional demand for managers will stem from the need to recruit workers and increase employee retention, to comply with changing regulations, and to implement new technology. Hospitals will continue to employ the majority of medical and health services managers; however, the number of new jobs created in hospitals is expected to increase at a slower rate than in many other industries because of the growing use of clinics and other outpatient care sites. Employment will grow fastest in practitioners' offices, ambulatory care centers, home healthcare agencies, and consulting firms.

Educational and Legal Requirements

The minimum educational program for a registered health information administrator is a bachelor's degree in health information administration. In 2021, there were 73 accredited bachelor's degree programs, 19 master's degree programs in informatics, and 10 master's degree programs in health information management, according to the Commission on Accreditation for Health Informatics and Information Management Education (CAHIIM).[3] The pre-professional curriculum includes studies in the humanities and behavioral, biological, and physical sciences. The professional curriculum covers leadership, regulatory compliance, data content, structures and standards, informatics, analytics, data use, information protection, revenue management, medical terminology, medical care organizations, disease classification systems, organization, supervision, healthcare statistics, and principles of law.

Certification and Other Qualifications

Health information managers who hold a bachelor's degree or post-baccalaureate degree from an approved program and who pass an exam can earn certification as a Registered Health Information Administrator (RHIA) from the American Health Information Management Association (AHIMA).[4] AHIMA offers additional credentials to those health information administrators who specialize, including the Certified Document Improvement Practitioner (CDIP) credential, the Certified Health Data Analyst credential (CHDA), the Certified in Healthcare Privacy and Security (CHPS) credential.[5]

Health information administrators need good interpersonal skills so that they can communicate effectively when discussing patient information, discrepancies, and data requirements with the healthcare team. They need strong analytical skills, must be detail oriented, and must be able to adapt to new laws and regulations governing health care. Because they work to protect confidential patient information, health information administrators must possess integrity.

Earnings

Earnings of health information administrators vary by type and size of the facility as well as by the level of education and responsibility. Salaries also vary according to geographic region. According to the latest statistics available in 2019 from AHIMA, mean annual earnings for health information administrators for those with a single credential were $75,540 and for those with four or more credentials were $113,950.

Related Occupations

Health information administrators receive training and experience in both health sciences and management. Other occupations and services requiring knowledge of both fields include hospital and nursing home administrators, public health directors, health agency directors, clinical laboratory workers, nursing services, physical therapists, rehabilitation services, radiology, respiratory therapists, and outpatient services administrators.

Additional Information

Information on careers in health information management may be obtained from

- American Health Information Management Association, 233 N. Michigan Ave., 21st Floor, Chicago, IL 60601-5800. https://www.ahima.org

HEALTH INFORMATION TECHNICIANS
Work Description

Every time a patient receives health care, a record is maintained of the observations, medical or surgical interventions, and treatment outcomes. This record includes information that the patient provides concerning his or her symptoms and medical history, the results of examinations, results of X-rays and laboratory tests, diagnoses, and treatment plans. **Health information technicians** organize and evaluate these records and the data contained within them for timeliness, completeness, accuracy, appropriateness, and compliance. They organize and manage health information and data using various applications and databases and track patient outcomes for quality assessment. They ensure health record and data quality, accuracy, accessibility, and security in both paper and electronic systems. They organize, maintain, and disclose content considered part of the patient's electronic health record in accordance with healthcare requirements, professional practice standards, and numerous state and federal regulations. They ensure confidentiality and security of patient information and protect patients' health information from unauthorized access and use. They regularly interact with physicians and other healthcare professionals to maintain complete and accurate health information and records.[6]

Technicians regularly use software tools to electronically record data for collection, storage, analysis, retrieval, and reporting. They organize, maintain, and report data for clinical databases and registries. These efforts serve to improve patient care, contain costs, and provide documentation for use in legal actions or research studies.

Some health information technicians use various classification systems to code, categorize, and report patient information for insurance reimbursement purposes, for databases and registries, and to maintain patients' medical and treatment histories. These technicians are often referred to as **coders**. Coders use classification software to assign clinical codes to each diagnosis and procedure, relying on their knowledge of disease processes and multiple classification systems, such as the Current Procedural Terminology (CPT) and the International Statistical Classification of Diseases and Related Health Problems, 10th edition, or ICD-10 for short. In turn, coders use classification systems software to assign the patient to one of several hundred **diagnosis-related groups (DRGs)**. The DRG determines the amount for which Medicare or other insurance programs using the DRG system will reimburse the healthcare provider if the patient is covered. In addition to the DRG system, coders use other coding systems, such as those required for ambulatory settings, physician offices, or long-term care. Some coders advance to the position of **DRG validator**, where they perform quality review of records and data coded by the coding staff. The DRG validators effectively use abstracting databases, internal and external audit results, Quality Improvement Organization reports, and revenue cycle edit/denial information to perform their jobs.

Some health information technicians specialize as **quality improvement analysts**. In that role, they analyze, review, forecast, trend, and present information directed at improving the quality of patient care. They use analytical and statistical methodologies and techniques to measure trends, progress, or change in the delivery of patient care. They focus on patient safety, patient outcomes, patient satisfaction, utilization management, and cost and functional outcomes.

Some technicians specialize as **cancer registrars**. These individuals maintain a hospital-based registry of cancer patients. They review patient records and abstract data from inpatient and outpatient records, death certificates, pathology reports, and autopsy reports. They assist the hospital with its cancer program and compliance with regulatory requirements.

Another specialization for health information technicians is to work as an **electronic health record support specialist**. These specialists provide ongoing end-user support, maintenance, training, and customization of the EHR. They develop and maintain EHR documentation and system-related workflow processes. They may create templates and train physicians and members of the healthcare team on how to use EHR systems. They may configure software to meet the needs of clinicians.

Health information technicians' duties vary according to the size and needs of the facility. In large to medium facilities, technicians may specialize in one aspect of health information, supervise health information clerks and transcribers, or work with revenue cycle managers or information technology staff. In small facilities, a registered health information technician sometimes manages the department.

Work Environment

Health information personnel generally work a standard 40-hour week. Some overtime may be required. In hospitals where health information management departments are open 18 to 24 hours a day, seven days a week, health information management personnel work on day, evening, and night shifts. Both part-time and remote work is generally available.

This is one of the few health occupations in which there is little or no physical contact with patients. The work environment is usually pleasant and comfortable, but some aspects of the job can be stressful. The utmost accuracy is essential, which demands concentration and close attention to detail. The emphasis on accuracy can cause fatigue and mental strain. Health information technicians whose use computer monitors for prolonged periods may experience eyestrain and musculoskeletal pain.

Employment Opportunities

Health information technicians held about 341,600 jobs in 2019. About one out of three jobs were in hospitals. The rest were mostly in offices of physicians; professional, scientific, and technical services; nursing care facilities; outpatient care centers; and home healthcare services.

Insurance firms that deal in health matters employ health information technicians to tabulate and analyze health information. Public health departments also employ technicians to supervise data collection from healthcare institutions and to assist in research.

Educational and Legal Requirements

Health information technicians entering the field usually have a two-year associate's degree from a community or junior college. Associate's degree course work includes classes in medical terminology and diseases, anatomy and physiology, legal aspects of health information management, coding and classification systems, statistics, health data standards and requirements, databases, quality assurance methods, healthcare reimbursement methods, and information technology systems, as well as general education. High school students can improve their chances of acceptance into a health information education program by taking courses in biology, chemistry, health, and especially computer training.

Experienced health information technicians usually advance in one of two ways—by specializing or by managing. Many senior health information technicians specialize in cancer registry, EHR support positions, database management, revenue cycle management, quality improvement analyst positions, or coding, particularly Medicare coding, and may obtain voluntary certification.

Certification and Other Qualifications

Many employers favor technicians who have become Registered Health Information Technicians (RHIT). RHITs must pass a written examination offered by AHIMA.[7] To take the examination, a person must graduate from a two-year associate's degree program accredited by CAHIIM. Technicians trained in non-CAHIIM-accredited programs or trained on the job are not eligible to take the examination. In 2021, there were about 250 CAHIIM-accredited programs in Health Information Management at the associate's degree level.[8]

Health information technicians who specialize as coders may become certified through several organizations. AHIMA offers the Certified Coding Associate (CCA) credential for new coders who have graduated from a training program or spent at least six months coding and pass a comprehensive examination. AHIMA offers the Certified Coding Specialist (CCS) credential for those who graduated from a more comprehensive training program, possess two years' experience in the field, or possess the CCA credential and have one year of professional coding experience and pass a comprehensive examination.[9] The American Association of Professional Coders (AAPC) offers the Certified Coding Professional credential.[10] This credential is available to persons with two years' experience in the field who pass a certification examination. AAPC recommends but does not require candidates

to graduate from an associate's degree program in medical cording or health information management.

Some health information technicians who specialize in cancer registry can become a Certified Tumor Registrar (CTR). The certification is offered by the National Cancer Registrars Association and requires completion of an examination with a passing score and maintenance of continuing education credits.[11]

Health information technicians need good interpersonal skills so that they can communicate well when discussing patient information, discrepancies, and data requirements with the healthcare team. They need strong analytical skills and must be detail oriented. Because they work to protect confidential patient information, health information technicians must possess integrity.

Employment Trends

Employment of health information technicians is expected to increase by 8%, faster than the average for all occupations through 2029. Employment growth will result from the increase in the number of medical tests, treatments, and procedures that will be performed. As the population continues to age, the occurrence of health-related problems will increase. Cancer registrars should experience job growth as the incidence of cancer increases from an aging population. In addition, with the prevalence of electronic health records, more technicians will be needed to meet the responsibilities associated with electronic data management.

Job Prospects

New jobs are expected in offices of physicians because of increasing use of electronic health records and demand for detailed data to support reimbursement. New jobs also are expected in home healthcare services, outpatient care centers, and nursing and residential care facilities. Although employment growth in hospitals will not keep pace with growth in other healthcare industries, many new jobs will, nevertheless, be created. Cancer registrars should experience job growth, along with the need for registrars for other special purposes or diseases. As the population continues to age, the incidence of cancer may increase because many illnesses are detected and treated later in life. **TABLE 32.1** shows some projection data provided by the U.S. Department of Labor.

Earnings

According to information from 2019, median annual earnings of health information technicians were $44,090. The lowest 10% earned less than $28,800, and the highest 10% earned more than $73,370 per year. Median annual earnings in the industries employing the largest number of health information technicians are shown in **TABLE 32.2**. According to the latest statistics available in 2019 from AHIMA, mean annual earnings for health information technicians were $70,300.

TABLE 32.1 Projections Data for Health Information Technicians, 2019–2029

Occupational Title	Employment, 2019	Projected Employment, 2029	Change, 2019–2029	
			Number	Percentage
Health information technician	341,600	370,600	29,000	8%

Data from Bureau of Labor Statistics, U.S. Department of Labor. Occupational Outlook Handbook. U.S. Department of Labor; 2020. https://www.bls.gov/ooh/healthcare/medical-records-and-health-information-technicians.htm#tab-6

TABLE 32.2 Median Annual Earnings in the Industries Employing the Largest Number of Health Information Technicians, May 2020

General medical and surgical hospitals	$46,880
Administrative and support services	$43,840
Professional, scientific, and technical services	$43,460
Management companies and enterprises	$50,010
Offices of physicians	$39,190

Data from Bureau of Labor Statistics, U.S. Department of Labor. Occupational Outlook Handbook. U.S. Department of Labor; 2020. https://www.bls.gov/ooh/healthcare/medical-records-and-health-information-technicians.htm#tab-5

Related Occupations

Health information technicians need strong clinical background knowledge to analyze the contents of health records. Other occupations that require knowledge of medical terminology, anatomy, and physiology but do not interact directly with patients are medical secretaries, transcriptionists, writers, and illustrators.

Additional Information

Information on careers in health information management and technology, including a list of accredited programs and certifications, is available from:

- American Health Information Management Association, 233 N. Michigan Ave., 21st Floor, Chicago, IL 60601-5800. https://www.ahima.org

For information about the medical coding profession and certifications, visit:

- American Health Information Management Association, 233 N. Michigan Ave., 21st Floor, Chicago, IL 60601-5800. https://www.ahima.org
- American Association of Professional Coders, 2233 S. Presidents Dr., Salt Lake City, UT 84120. https://www.aapc.com

For information about the cancer registrar profession and certification, visit:

- National Cancer Registrars Association, 12030 Sunrise Valley Dr., Suite 400, Reston, VA 20191. https://ncra.org

MEDICAL TRANSCRIPTIONISTS
Significant Points

- Jobs are expected to decline by 2%.
- Training requirements involve postsecondary education.
- Most transcriptionists work full time.

Work Description

Medical transcriptionists translate and edit voice recordings made by physicians and other healthcare providers regarding patient assessment and treatment. They use headsets and transcribing machines to listen to voice recordings made by physicians and other healthcare professionals. They use word-processing software, specialized computer software such as speech recognition technology, and medical reference materials to accomplish their work. These workers transcribe and edit a variety of medical reports, including those about emergency room visits, diagnostic imaging studies, operations, chart reviews, and final summaries.

To understand and accurately transcribe dictated reports into a format that is clear and comprehensible for the reader, the medical transcriptionist must understand the language of medicine, anatomy and physiology, diagnostic procedures, and treatment. They also must be able to translate medical jargon and abbreviations into their expanded forms. After reviewing and editing for grammar and clarity, the medical transcriptionist transcribes the dictated reports and returns them in either printed or electronic form to the dictating physician or care provider for review and signature or correction. The medical transcriptionist identifies any inaccuracies in the transcripts initially prepared by speech recognition technology and makes corrections as appropriate. For inaccuracies that cannot be resolved by the transcriptionist, the inaccuracies are identified and conveyed to the dictating physician or care provider so that the patient will receive effective treatment. The medical transcriptionist may be responsible for filing these reports in the patient's electronic health record, while other transcriptionists may share this responsibility for filing these reports with others in the healthcare field. These reports eventually become a part of the patient's permanent file. An example of a medical transcriptionist listening to voice recordings, editing, and transcribing a report is seen in **FIGURE 32.5**.

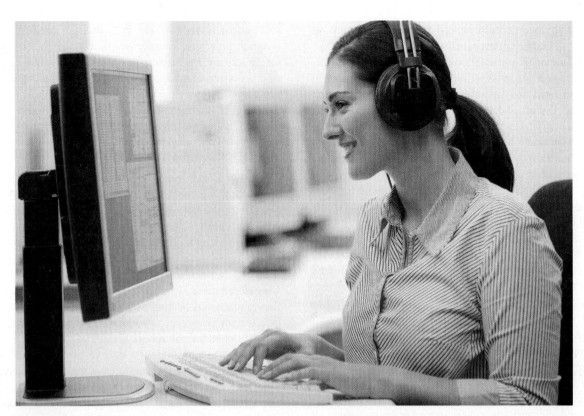

FIGURE 32.5 Woman transcribing dictation.
© Monkey Business Images/Shutterstock.

Accuracy and confidentiality are important aspects of a medical transcriptionist's role. The need for accuracy is vital because accurate information is important for improving patient safety and reducing the chance that a patient may receive an ineffective or even harmful treatment. Medical transcriptionists engage in quality assurance activities related to medical documentation and the security of that documentation. Medical transcriptionists must observe strict confidentiality requirements and only discuss confidential patient information with those medical personnel who are involved in treating the patient.

Medical transcriptionists must be familiar with electronic health record systems. They may need to enter reports, create templates, help develop documentation policies, and train physicians on how to use EHR systems. They may work with clinicians to improve documentation created by clinicians using features of EHR systems such as speech recognition software, drop-down menus, and templates.

Work Environment

The majority of medical transcriptionists are employed in comfortable settings. They usually work in hospitals, doctors' offices, or medical transcription services. An increasing number of medical transcriptionists work from home-based offices as subcontractors for hospitals and transcription services. In these settings, the medical transcriptionist receives voice recordings electronically, transcribes documents, and returns them quickly to their client for approval.

The work presents few hazards. Sitting in the same position for long periods can be tiring, however, and workers can suffer wrist, back, neck, or eye problems due to strain and risk incurring repetitive motion injuries such as carpal tunnel syndrome. The pressure to be both accurate and fast also can prove stressful.

Most medical transcriptionists work a standard 40-hour week, although about one out of three works part time. A substantial number of medical transcriptionists are self-employed, which may allow for irregular working hours.

Employment Opportunities

Medical transcriptionists held about 58,500 jobs in 2019. Employment of medical transcriptionists is projected to decline by 2% from 2019 to 2029. An aging population may spur demand for medical transcription services because older age groups receive proportionately greater numbers of medical tests, treatments, and procedures requiring documentation. The continuing need for electronic documentation that can be shared easily among providers, third-party payers, regulators, consumers, and health information systems will sustain a level of demand for transcription services. Medical transcriptionists will be needed to amend patients' records, edit documents produced by speech recognition systems, and identify discrepancies in medical reports.

Outsourcing of transcription work overseas and advancements in speech recognition technology are not expected to reduce the need for well-trained medical transcriptionists within the United States. Outsourcing transcription work abroad—to countries such as India, Pakistan, Philippines, and the Caribbean—has grown more popular as transmitting confidential health information over the internet has become more secure; however, the demand for overseas transcription services is expected only to supplement the demand for well-trained domestic medical transcriptionists. In addition, reports transcribed by overseas medical transcription services usually require editing for accuracy by domestic medical transcriptionists before they meet U.S. quality standards. Concerns over patient confidentiality and data security suggest a continued need for transcriptionists within the United States. Speech recognition technology allows physicians and other health professionals to dictate medical reports into a computerized program that converts speech to text. In spite of advancements in this technology, speech recognition software has been slow to grasp and analyze the human voice, the English language, and the medical vernacular with all its diversity. As a result, there will continue to be a need for skilled medical transcriptionists to identify and appropriately edit the inevitable errors created by speech recognition systems and to create a final document.

Job opportunities should be best for those who earn an associate's degree or certification from the Association for Healthcare Documentation Integrity (AHDI).

Education and Legal Requirements

Employers prefer to hire transcriptionists who have completed postsecondary training in medical transcription offered by many vocational schools, community colleges, and distance-learning programs.

Completion of a two-year associate's degree or one-year certificate program—including course work in anatomy, medical terminology, legal issues relating to healthcare documentation, risk management, and English grammar and punctuation—is highly recommended but not always required. Many of these programs include supervised on-the-job experience. Some transcriptionists, especially those already familiar with medical terminology from previous experience as a nurse or medical secretary, become proficient through refresher courses and training.

Formal accreditation is not required for medical transcription programs. However, the Credentialing Commission for Healthcare Documentation (CCHD)—established by the AHDI—offers voluntary accreditation for medical transcription programs.[12] Although voluntary, completion of an American Academy of Professional Coders (AAPC)-approved program may be required for transcriptionists seeking certification.

Certification and Other Qualifications

The AHDI awards two voluntary designations, the Registered Healthcare Documentation Specialist (RHDS) and the Certified Healthcare Documentation Specialist (CHDS).[13] Medical transcriptionists who are recent graduates of medical transcription educational programs or have fewer than two years' experience in acute care may become a RHDS. The RHDS credential is awarded upon successfully passing the AHDI level 1 registered medical transcription exam. The CHDS designation requires certification as an RHDS and at least two years of acute care experience working in multiple specialty areas using different format, report, and dictation types. Candidates also must earn a passing score on a certification examination. Because medicine is constantly evolving, medical transcriptionists are encouraged to update their skills regularly. RHDSs and CHDSs must earn continuing education credits every three years to be recertified. As in many other fields, certification is recognized as a sign of competence.

For those seeking work as medical transcriptionists, understanding medical terminology is essential. Good English grammar and punctuation skills are required, as is familiarity with personal computers and word-processing software. Good listening skills are also necessary because some doctors and healthcare professionals speak English as a second language. Time management skills are helpful because transcriptionists often work under short, tight deadlines.

Job Prospects

Those medical transcriptionists with formal education and experience working with electronic health records should encounter good job prospects. Opportunities for new transcriptionists will arise from the retirement of existing transcriptionists who retire over the next decade. **TABLE 32.3** shows projection data provided by the U.S. Department of Labor.

Earnings

Medical transcriptionists had median wages of $35,270 in May 2020. The lowest 10% earned less than $21,790, and

TABLE 32.3 Projections Data for Medical Transcriptionists, 2019-2029

Occupational Title	Employment, 2019	Projected Employment, 2029	Change, 2019–2029	
			Number	Percentage
Medical transcriptionists	58,500	57,200	−1,300	−2%

Data from Bureau of Labor Statistics, U.S. Department of Labor. Occupational Outlook Handbook. U.S. Department of Labor; 2020. https://www.bls.gov/ooh/healthcare/medical-transcriptionists.htm#tab-6

TABLE 32.4 Median Annual Wages in the Industries Employing the Largest Numbers of Medical Transcriptionists, May 2020

Medical and diagnostic laboratories	$42,070
Hospitals; state, local, and private	$40,810
Offices of physicians	$36,860
Administrative and support services	$29,730

Data from Bureau of Labor Statistics, U.S. Department of Labor. Occupational Outlook Handbook. U.S. Department of Labor; 2020. https://www.bls.gov/ooh/healthcare/medical-transcriptionists.htm#tab-5

the highest 10% earned more than $55,220. Median annual wages in the industries employing the largest numbers of medical transcriptionists are detailed in **TABLE 32.4**.

Compensation methods for medical transcriptionists vary. Some are paid based on the number of hours worked or on the number of lines transcribed. Others receive a base pay per hour with incentives for extra production. Large hospitals and healthcare organizations usually prefer to pay for the time an employee works. Independent contractors and employees of transcription services usually receive production-based pay.

Related Occupations

A number of other workers type, record information, and process paperwork. Among these are administrative assistants, bookkeepers, receptionists, secretaries, information clerks, and human resource clerks. Medical secretaries may also transcribe as part of their job. Other workers who provide medical support include medical assistants and health information technicians.

Additional Information

For information on a career as a medical transcriptionist, contact:

- Association for Healthcare Documentation Integrity, 4230 Kierman Ave., Suite 130, Modesto, CA 95356. https://www.ahdionline.org

MEDICAL LIBRARIANS
Significant Points

- Job prospects are expected to grow 5%, faster than the national average.
- Medical librarians require knowledge of both library science and health science.
- Salaries vary depending on individual qualifications and the type, size, and location of the library.

Work Description

Medical or health science librarians provide essential services to professional staff and personnel in medicine, dentistry, nursing, pharmacy, the allied health professions, and other related technologies. Because health and other related fields are growing rapidly, professional staff need quick and efficient access to large volumes of information and materials to keep abreast of developments, new procedures and techniques, and other relevant data. Relevant information and materials are used in education and training programs, in exchange-of-information activities among different health professions, and in biomedical research. Health science librarians may provide information about new clinical trials and medical treatments and procedures, teach medical students how to locate medical information, or answer consumers' health questions. They make this information available to those who need it, utilizing knowledge of both library science and health science in their work.

Depending on the size of the facility where they work, health science librarians may take charge of an entire library or be assigned to specific functions. They select and order books, journals, and other materials and classify and catalog acquisitions to allow their easy retrieval. Other duties include preparing guides to reference materials, compiling bibliographies, and selecting and acquiring films and other audiovisual materials.

Readers and researchers frequently call on the specialized skills of the librarian to track down information on a particular subject. The material may be bound in obscure documents or scattered in many places, requiring detective work to locate it. If the document is in another language, the librarian may be called on to obtain a translation. Frequently, the librarian is asked to compile a bibliography or to provide a comprehensive review or summary on a particular subject.

Aside from assisting patrons in person, the medical librarian also responds to mail, e-mail, and phone inquiries. Success in handling these inquiries depends largely on the librarian's skill. Librarians may have only very general knowledge of medicine, but they must know how and where to locate all types of information on short notice.

In hospitals, services offered by the medical library may depend on whether the hospital conducts research and training or on the categories of illness treated there. Some hospitals have separate medical, nursing, and patient libraries. Increasingly, however, these collections are grouped together under the direction of one chief librarian, with assistants in charge of the separate services.

The medical librarian also plays an important role in the hospital's rehabilitation services. In addition, librarians serving patients provide book cart services, develop programs of interest for ambulatory patients, and visit new patients to learn about their reading interests.

Work Environment

In addition to hospitals, medical librarians work in schools of medicine, nursing, dentistry, and pharmacy; research institutes; pharmaceutical and related industries; health departments; professional societies; and voluntary health agencies. Medical libraries are found in numerous locations throughout the country but tend to be concentrated in or near population centers. Individual size and working conditions vary greatly from library to library. For instance, hospital libraries may range from a staff size of 1 to slightly fewer than 100. Some librarians have private offices, while others share space. In ill-equipped offices, librarians may risk eyestrain, backache, and carpal tunnel syndrome. Nevertheless, surroundings are usually pleasant and free of hazards or unusual environmental working conditions.

Employment Opportunities

Employment of librarians is expected to grow by 5% between 2019 and 2029, which is faster than the average for all occupations. Growth in the number of librarians will be driven in part by the availability and growth of electronic information and media materials, resulting in requests for help sorting through the large amount of digital information and collection materials available. Many libraries are equipped for users to access library resources directly from their homes or offices through library websites, allowing users to conduct research on their own. Librarians will still be needed, however, to manage staff, help users define their research needs and develop database search techniques, address complicated reference requests, and choose appropriate materials.

Over the next decade, jobs for medical librarians outside traditional settings will grow fastest. These settings include private industry, nonprofit organizations, and consulting firms. Examples of jobs in industry for medical librarians include the biotechnology, insurance, pharmaceutical, publishing, and medical equipment industries.

Many companies are turning to librarians because of their research and organizational skills and their knowledge of computer databases and library automation systems. Librarians also are hired by organizations to organize information on the internet. Librarians working in these settings may be classified as systems analysts, database specialists and trainers, webmasters or web developers, or local area network (LAN) coordinators.

Most recently, medical and other librarians held about 146,500 jobs. Most were in school and academic libraries; others were in public and special libraries. A small number of librarians worked for hospitals and religious organizations. Others worked for government agencies. Entrepreneurial librarians sometimes start their own consulting practices, acting as freelance librarians or information brokers and providing services to other libraries, business, or government agencies. Replacement needs will account for more job openings over the next decade, as more than two out of three librarians are age 45 or older, which will result in many job openings as these librarians retire. Faster than average employment growth, coupled with an increasing number of graduates with master's degrees in library

science (MLS), will result in more applicants competing for the projected 13,800 openings per year. Applicants for librarian jobs in large cities or suburban areas will face competition, while those willing to work in rural areas should have better job prospects.

Educational and Legal Requirements

A master of library science (MLS) degree is necessary for librarian positions in most public, academic, and special libraries and in some school libraries. The federal government requires an MLS or the equivalent in education and experience. Many colleges and universities offer MLS programs, but employers often prefer graduates of the approximately 63 schools accredited by the American Library Association.[14] Most MLS programs require a bachelor's degree; a major in liberal arts is appropriate preparation for such graduate work.

Most MLS programs take one year to complete, but some take two years. A typical graduate program includes courses in the foundations of library and information science, including the history of books and printing, intellectual freedom and censorship, and the role of libraries and information in society. Other basic courses cover learning different research methods and strategies, online reference systems, internet search techniques, material selection and processing, the organization of information, automated circulation systems, and user services. Computer-related course work is an increasingly important component of an MLS degree.

An MLS degree provides general preparation for library work, but some individuals specialize in one particular area. The minimum qualifications for librarians specializing in medicine are as follows:

- A master's degree in library and information science from an American Library Association–accredited school
- Strong oral and written communication skills
- Strong interpersonal skills
- Strong computer skills
- Strong organizational skills
- Strong problem-solving skills

Librarians participate in continuing training once they are on the job to keep abreast of new information systems brought about by changing technology. Most MLS schools offer courses in Health Sciences Information, which is recommended for those interested in becoming a medical librarian.

Certification and Other Qualifications

Certification as a medical librarian is offered through membership in the Academy of Health Information

Professionals (AHIP), a subsidiary of the Medical Library Association.[15] Certification is based on three levels of achievement: academic preparation, professional work experience, and individual professional accomplishments. Depending on the level of work experience a medical librarian has, membership levels differ: Provisional for those with five years or less experience; Member or Senior for those with five or more years of experience; and Distinguished for those with 10 years or more experience. A point system addressing professional accomplishments corresponds with each level.

Because medical librarians interact with and must convey information to a wide variety of users, they must possess strong communication skills. Computer skills are a necessity, as new information, technology, and resources change what a medical librarian can do. Problem-solving skills are needed to conduct research, along with excellent reading skills.

Earnings

Salaries of librarians vary according to the individual's qualifications and the type, size, and location of the library. Librarians with primarily administrative duties often have greater earnings. Median annual wages of librarians in May 2020 were $60,820. The lowest 10% earned less than $34,810, and the highest 10% earned more than $97,460. The Medical Library Association reports that the average starting salary was $49,060 in 2012. The overall average salary for medical librarians in 2012 was $66,622. Library directors can earn from a low average of $52,293 up to a high average of $116,200 per year.[16]

Related Occupations

Librarians play an important role in the transfer of knowledge and ideas by providing people with access to the information they need and want. Jobs requiring similar analytical, organizational, and communication skills include physicians, nurses, health educators, community health workers, allied healthcare professionals, administrators, and information technology programmers and specialists.

Additional Information

Information on librarianship, including information on scholarships or loans, is available from the American Library Association. Consult its website for a listing of accredited library education programs.

- American Library Association, Office for Human Resource Development and Recruitment, 50 East Huron St., Chicago, IL 60611. http://www.ala.org

For information on employment opportunities as a health science librarian, scholarship information, credentialing information, and a list of MLA-accredited schools offering programs in health sciences librarianship, contact:

- Medical Library Association, 65 East Wacker Pl., Suite 1900, Chicago, IL 60601-7246. https://www.mlanet.org

For information about medical librarians in academic settings, contact:

- Association of Academic Health Sciences Libraries (AAHSL), 2150 North 107th St., Suite 205, Seattle, WA 98133-9009. https://aahsl.org

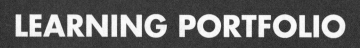

LEARNING PORTFOLIO

Issues for Discussion

1. Imagine you are a patient who has entrusted your healthcare provider with your personal health information. Brainstorm with your classmates and instructor what problems may arise if that personal health information is not kept confidential as the law requires and you expect.

2. Unfortunately, data breaches have been in the news over recent years, ranging from those occurring at banks and department stores to government agencies. Discuss with your classmates whether any of you have been the victim or know a victim of a data breach. If so, describe what kind of breach was involved (e.g., bank data, credit cards, health information, etc.), what type of notice was received about the breach, and what remedies were offered as part of the notification.

Enrichment Activities

1. Visit the website https://www.ahima.org/careers /healthinfo to hear health information management students and professionals speak about their career choice.

2. Visit the career map for health information management careers found at https://myahima.org/careermap. Navigate the map to understand current and emerging careers, promotional paths, job descriptions, and salary information in this discipline.

3. Learn more about personal health records by visiting the websites https://webmd.com/phr and http ://phrplus.com and learn how you can create your own personal health record. Choose one of the free offerings and create a personal health record for yourself or a loved one.

4. Learn about the career of a medical coder by viewing the videos at https://www.careerstep.com/career -profile-medical-coding-billing-video?uid=pub 140514 and https://www.youtube.com/watch?v=_0tbR Ax2Xgc

5. Learn more about medical transcription as a career by viewing the video at https://youtube.com/watch ?v=hMwitgRW63A

6. Visit the "HackLibrarySchool" blog at https://hackli braryschool.com/2014/10/27/medical-librarianship / and read interviews with four medical librarians and their take on specializing in library school.

CASE STUDY: HEALTH INFORMATION ADMINISTRATOR CAREER

Theresa is a health information administrator at a large city hospital. Many of her work duties require her to possess skills in health data management as well as customer service. She is responsible for the administrative and clinical workflow of the health information department and collaborates with administrators by providing updated statistics and informational data that will help in the research department.

Based on the information you have read about health information administrators, answer the following questions.

1. True or false? Compiling statistics and providing informational data may be required of health information administrators by federal or state agencies.

2. True or false? As a health information administrator, Theresa should possess skills in health data management, information policy, and information systems.

3. True or false? Theresa should not be held responsible for the administrative and clinical workflow of the health information department.

4. True or false? Theresa may be called to testify in court about patient health records and procedures of record keeping because of her job title.

5. True or false? Theresa not only should be skilled at her job, but she should also display good interpersonal skills and communication skills in her role as the health information administrator.

LEARNING PORTFOLIO

References

1. American Health Information Management Association. *What Is Health Information.* https://www.ahima.org/careers/healthinfo Accessed August 30, 2021.

2. Much of the information included in this section of the text comes from the American Health Information Management Association. https://www.ahima.org Accessed August 30, 2021.

3. Commission on Accreditation for Health Informatics and Information Management Education. *Program Directory.* https://www.cahiim.org/programs/program-directory. Accessed August 30, 2021.

4. American Health Information Management Association. *Registered Health Information Administrator.* https://www.ahima.org/certification/RHIA Accessed August 30, 2021.

5. American Health Information Management Association. *Specialty Certifications.* https://www.ahima.org/certification-careers/certification-exams/ Accessed August 30, 2021.

6. Much of the information included in this section of the text comes from the American Health Information Management Association. https://www.ahima.org Accessed August 30, 2021.

7. American Health Information Management Association. *Registered Health Information Technician.* https://www.ahima.org/certification/RHIT Accessed August 30, 2021.

8. Commission on Accreditation for Health Informatics and Information Management Education. *Program Directory.* https://www.cahiim.org/programs/program-directory Accessed August 30, 2021.

9. Coding credentials issued by the American Health Information Management Association. Coding Certifications. https://www.ahima.org/certification-careers/certifications-overview/ Accessed August 30, 2021.

10. American Association of Professional Coders. *Medical Coding Certification.* https://www.aapc.com/certification/ Accessed August 30, 2021.

11. National Cancer Registrars Association. *Certification.* https://www.ncra-usa.org/About/Paths-to-the-Profession Accessed August 30, 2021.

12. Association for Healthcare Documentation Integrity. *Find an Approved Program.* https://www.ahdionline.org/page/find_approved_prgm Accessed August 30, 2021.

13. Association for Healthcare Documentation Integrity. *Types of Credentials.* https://www.ahdionline.org/page/typescredentials Accessed August 30, 2021.

14. American Library Association. *Directory of Institutions Offering ALA-Accredited Master's Programs in Library and Information Sciences* http://www.ala.org/educationcareers/accreditedprograms/directory Accessed August 30, 2021.

15. Academy of Health Information Professionals. *AHIP Credentialing.* https://www.mlanet.org/academy Accessed August 30, 2021.

16. Medical Library Association. *Explore a Career in Health Science Information.* https://www.mlanet.org/page/explore-this-career Accessed August 30, 2021.

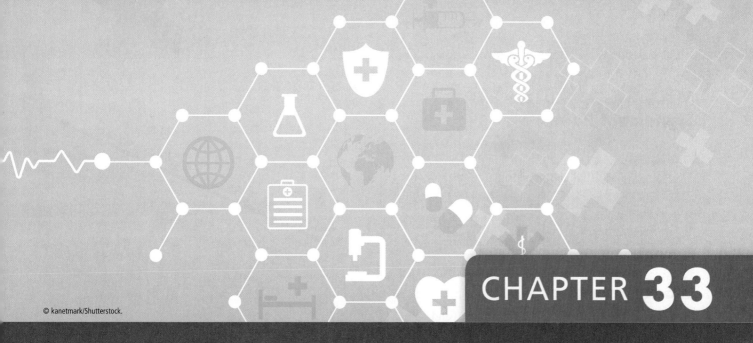
© kanetmark/Shutterstock.

CHAPTER **33**

Medical and Nursing Assistants*

KEY TERMS

Administrative medical
 assistants
Clinical medical assistants

Medical assistants
Nursing assistants
Ophthalmic medical assistants

Optometric medical assistants
Orderlies
Podiatric medical assistants

* All information in this chapter, unless otherwise indicated, was obtained from Bureau of Labor Statistics. *Occupational Outlook Handbook 2020–2021 Edition*. Washington, DC: U.S. Department of Labor; 2021.

MEDICAL ASSISTANTS
Significant Points

- Employment is projected to grow much faster than average.
- Job prospects should be excellent.
- More than half of all medical assistants work in offices of physicians.
- Some medical assistants are trained on the job, but many complete one- or two-year programs.

Work Descriptions

Medical assistants perform administrative and clinical tasks to keep the offices of physicians, podiatrists, chiropractors, and other health practitioners running smoothly. They should not be confused with physician assistants, who examine, diagnose, and treat patients under the direct supervision of a physician. Physician assistants are discussed in a separate chapter.

The duties of medical assistants vary from office to office, depending on the location and size of the practice and the practitioner's specialty. In small practices, medical assistants usually perform many different kinds of tasks, handling both administrative and clinical duties and reporting directly to an office manager, physician, or other health practitioner. Those in large practices tend to specialize in a particular area, under the supervision of department administrators. Many physician offices have adopted electronic health records (EHRs), requiring medical assistants to understand the computer software their EHR uses. Medical assistants who handle patient records must observe strict confidentiality requirements and only discuss patient confidential information with those medical personnel who are involved in treating the patient.

Administrative medical assistants perform many duties. They update and file patients' health records, fill out insurance forms, and arrange for hospital admissions and laboratory services. They also perform tasks less specific to medical settings, such as answering telephones, greeting patients, scheduling appointments, and handling correspondence, billing, and bookkeeping.

For **clinical medical assistants**, duties vary according to what is allowed by state law. Some common tasks include taking medical histories and recording vital signs, explaining treatment procedures to patients, preparing patients for examinations, and assisting physicians during examinations. An example of a medical history is seen in **FIGURE 33.1**. Medical assistants collect and prepare laboratory specimens and sometimes perform basic laboratory tests on the premises, dispose of contaminated supplies, and sterilize medical instruments. An example of a blood draw that would be used for laboratory testing is seen in **FIGURE 33.2**. They might instruct patients about medications and special diets, prepare and administer medications as directed by a physician, authorize drug refills as directed, telephone prescriptions to a

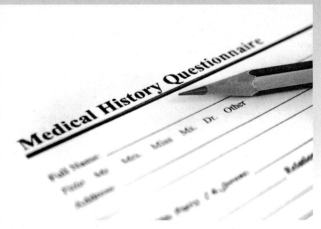

FIGURE 33.1 A medical history questionnaire.
© alexskopje/Shutterstock.

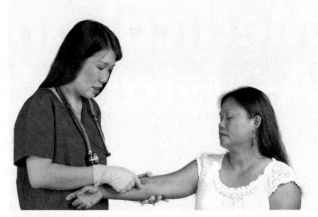

FIGURE 33.2 A medical assistant drawing blood from a patient.
© Orchidflower/Shutterstock.

pharmacy, draw blood, prepare patients for X-rays, take electrocardiograms, remove sutures, and change dressings. Medical assistants also may arrange examining room instruments and equipment, purchase and maintain supplies and equipment, and keep waiting and examining rooms neat and clean.

Ophthalmic medical assistants, optometric assistants, and podiatric medical assistants are examples of specialized medical assistants who have additional duties. **Ophthalmic medical assistants** help ophthalmologists provide eye care. They conduct diagnostic tests, measure and record vision, and test eye muscle function. They also show patients how to insert, remove, and care for contact lenses, and they apply eye dressings. Under the direction of the physician, ophthalmic medical assistants may administer eye medications. They also maintain optical and surgical instruments and may assist the ophthalmologist in surgery. **Optometric assistants** also help provide eye care, working with optometrists. They provide chair side assistance, instruct patients about contact lens use and care, conduct preliminary tests on patients, and otherwise provide assistance while working directly with an optometrist. **Podiatric medical assistants** make castings of feet, expose and develop X-rays, and assist podiatrists in surgery.

Professional Profiles

Name: Marin, COA, CPO
Job Title: Certified Ophthalmic Assistant (COA) and Certified Paraoptometric (CPO)

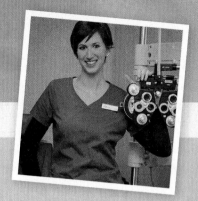

Q: Tell us about your job and the type of organization you work in.

A: I work in a private ophthalmology practice with four doctors, two specializing in "front of the eye" (cornea, cataracts, etc.) and two specializing in "back of the eye" (retina, diabetes, macular degeneration, and other eye diseases). There are 10 exam rooms for patients. On an average day we see about 50 patients.

Q: Describe a typical workday.

A: On a typical day, I am working up patients (histories, chief complaints, refractions, and general exams) and getting them ready for the doctor. Between workups, I do special testing, such as retinal photography, optical coherence tomography (OCT), visual fields, or specular microscopy. Some patients wear contact lenses, so I am also the person to fit them in their lenses. In our office, we have a minor surgery suite where minor procedures and surgeries are performed. As a certified assistant, I can assist in those procedures as needed.

Q: Why did you choose this profession?

A: After "falling into" a job at an optometrist's office and later becoming certified as a paraoptometric, I chose to advance my career into ophthalmology.

Q: What do you like most about this profession?

A: What I like most about my job is the relationship I build with the patients. So many treat me like family. Working in a smaller private practice, I am able to get to know the patients and really focus on their individual needs. I love knowing that I am helping people every day and being surrounded by staff that is just as happy to be there doing the same type of work. One other thing to note is no two patients are the same. Every day brings a learning experience, and my knowledge of eye care is continually expanding.

Q: Is there room for advancement in this field?

A: There is definitely room for advancement, continuing education, and further certification. I am currently studying for my COT (Certified Ophthalmic Technician), which will show that I have learned more skills that can be used to help the doctors.

Q: Name and explain what part of your academic training most prepared you for this profession.

A: The best training I had for my job was hands-on training in the workplace. Learning from doctors and senior technicians prepared me for the test to be certified. It also taught me how to interact with patients and how to be good at special tests.

Q: What do you wish you had known in high school/college about pursuing this career?

A: First of all, I wish I had known this career existed! When I started going to college, I had a different major every semester, it seemed. If I had known that I was going to find a job like the one I have, I would have stuck with my schooling and finished getting my degree. A bachelor's degree would give me many more opportunities to grow and advance in this field, and I could make more money.

Q: What advice would you give someone who is considering this career?

A: I would suggest to someone considering this career to call their local ophthalmologist or optometrist and ask about setting up a day to shadow as a student. I would definitely urge them to continue their education and finish their degree.

Work Environment

Medical assistants work in well-lit, clean environments. They constantly interact with other people and may have to handle several responsibilities at once. Most full-time medical assistants work a regular 40-hour week. Many medical assistants, however, work part time, evenings, or weekends to cover shifts in medical facilities that are always open.

Employment Opportunities

Medical assistants held about 725,200 jobs in 2019. More than half worked in offices of physicians; 15% worked in public and private hospitals, including inpatient and outpatient facilities; and 12% worked in outpatient care centers and offices of other health practitioners, such as chiropractors, optometrists, and podiatrists. Most of the remainder worked in other healthcare industries such as nursing and residential care facilities and employment services.

Educational and Legal Requirements

Some medical assistants are trained on the job, but many complete one- or two-year programs.

Education and Training

Postsecondary medical assisting programs are offered in vocational-technical high schools, postsecondary vocational schools, and community and junior colleges. Programs usually last either one year and result in a certificate or diploma or two years and result in an associate's degree. Courses cover anatomy, physiology, and medical terminology as well as typing, transcription, record keeping, accounting, and insurance processing. Students learn laboratory techniques, clinical and diagnostic procedures, pharmaceutical principles, the administration of medications, and first aid. They study office practices, patient relations, medical law, and ethics. Medical assistants also learn how to code both paper and EHRs and how to record patient information. There are various organizations that accredit medical assisting programs. Accredited programs often include an internship that provides practical experience in physicians' offices, hospitals, or other healthcare facilities.

Formal training in medical assisting, while generally preferred, is not always required. Some medical assistants are trained on the job, although this practice is less common than in the past. Applicants usually need a high school diploma or the equivalent. Recommended high school courses include mathematics, health, biology, typing, bookkeeping, computers, and office skills. Volunteer experience in the healthcare field also is helpful. Medical assistants who are trained on the job usually spend their first few months attending training sessions and working closely with more experienced workers. Some states allow medical assistants to perform more advanced procedures, such as giving injections, after passing a test or taking a course.

Certification and Other Qualifications

Employers prefer to hire experienced or certified workers. Although not required, certification indicates that a medical assistant meets certain standards of competence. The certification process varies. There are various associations—some listed among the sources of information that follow—that award certification credentials to medical assistants. One credential is the Certified Medical Assistant (CMA). This credential allows the CMA to take medical histories, draw blood, perform basic laboratory tests, and remove sutures, among other duties.[1] Another credential is the Certified Clinical Medical Assistant (CCMA). This credential allows the CCMA to interview and educate patients, assist the physician with medical exams, measure and record vital signs, and administer injections. A medical assistant may choose to become certified in a specialty, such as podiatry, optometry, chiropractic, or ophthalmology.[2]

Medical assistants deal with the public; therefore, they must be neat and well groomed, have a courteous, pleasant manner, and be able to put patients at ease and explain physicians' instructions. They must respect the confidential nature of medical information. They must be able to understand and follow health records and diagnoses and may be required to code a patient's medical record for billing purposes. Clinical duties require a reasonable level of manual dexterity and visual acuity in order to use basic clinical instruments.

Advancement

Medical assistants may advance to other occupations through experience or additional training. For example, some may go on to teach medical assisting, and others pursue additional education to become nurses or other healthcare workers. Administrative medical assistants may advance to office manager or qualify for a variety of administrative support occupations.

Employment Trends

Employment is projected to grow much faster than average. Job opportunities should be excellent, particularly for those with formal training or experience and certification.

Employment Change

Employment of medical assistants is expected to grow 19% from 2019 to 2029, much faster than the average for all occupations. As the healthcare industry expands because of technological advances in medicine and the growth and aging of the population, an increased need for all healthcare workers will be felt. The increasing use of medical assistants in the rapidly growing healthcare industry will further stimulate job growth.

Helping to drive job growth is the increasing number of group practices, clinics, and other healthcare facilities that need a high proportion of support personnel, particularly medical assistants who can handle both administrative and clinical duties. As more and more physicians' practices switch to an EHR, medical assistants' job responsibilities will continue to change. Assistants will need to become familiar with EHR computer software, including maintaining EHR security and analyzing electronic data, to improve healthcare information. In addition, medical assistants work primarily in outpatient settings, a rapidly growing sector of the healthcare industry.

Job Prospects

Job seekers who want to work as medical assistants should encounter excellent job prospects. Medical assistants are projected to account for a very large number of new jobs, and many other opportunities will come from the need to replace workers leaving the occupation. Those with formal training or experience—particularly those with certification—should have the best job opportunities. **TABLE 33.1** shows some projection data provided by the U.S. Department of Labor.

Earnings

The earnings of medical assistants vary, depending on experience, skill level, and location. Median annual earnings of wage and salary medical assistants were $35,850 in May 2020. The lowest 10% earned less than $26,930, and the highest 10% earned more than $50,580. Median annual earnings in the industries employing the largest numbers of medical assistants in May 2020 are shown in **TABLE 33.2**.

Related Occupations

Medical assistants perform work similar to the tasks completed by other workers in medical support occupations. Administrative medical assistants do work similar to that of medical secretaries, medical transcriptionists, and medical records and health information technicians. Clinical medical assistants perform duties similar to those of dental assistants; dental hygienists; occupational therapist assistants and aides; pharmacy aides; licensed practical and licensed vocational nurses; surgical technologists; physical therapist assistants and aides; and nursing, psychiatric, and home health aides.

Additional Information

Information about career opportunities and certification for medical assistants is available from:

TABLE 33.2 Median Annual Earnings in the Industries Employing the Largest Numbers of Medical Assistants, May 2020

Hospitals: state, local, and private	$37,050
Offices of physicians	$35,870
Outpatient care centers	$38,860
Offices of chiropractors	$31,470

Data from Bureau of Labor Statistics, U.S. Department of Labor. Occupational Outlook Handbook. U.S. Department of Labor; 2020. https://www.bls.gov/ooh/healthcare/medical-assistants.htm#tab-5

- American Association of Medical Assistants, 20 North Wacker Dr., Suite 1575, Chicago, IL 60606. https://www.aama-ntl.org
- American Medical Technologists, 10700 West Higgins Rd., Suite 150, Rosemont, IL 60018. https://www.americanmedtech.org
- National Healthcareer Association, 11161 Overbrook Rd., Leawood, KS 66211. https://www.nhanow.com

For lists of accredited educational programs in medical assisting, contact:

- Accrediting Bureau of Health Education Schools, 7777 Leesburg Pike, Suite 314 N, Falls Church, VA 22043. https://www.abhes.org
- Commission on Accreditation of Allied Health Education Programs, 9355 113th St. N, #7709, Seminole, FL 33775. https://www.caahep.org

Information about career opportunities, training programs, and certification for ophthalmic medical personnel is available from:

- Joint Commission on Allied Health Personnel in Ophthalmology, 2025 Woodlane Dr., St. Paul, MN 55125. https://www.jcahpo.org

Information about career opportunities, training programs, and certification for optometric assistants is available from:

- American Optometric Association, 243 N. Lindbergh Blvd., St. Louis, MO 63141. https://www.aoa.org

Information about certification for podiatric assistants is available from:

- American Society of Podiatric Medical Assistants, 109 First St., Itasca, IL 60143-2114 . https://www.aspma.org

TABLE 33.1 Projections Data for Medical Assistants, 2019–2029

Occupational Title	Employment, 2019	Projected Employment, 2029	Change, 2019–2029	
			Number	Percentage
Medical assistants	725,200	864,400	139,200	19%

Data from Bureau of Labor Statistics, U.S. Department of Labor. Occupational Outlook Handbook. U.S. Department of Labor; 2020. https://www.bls.gov/ooh/healthcare/medical-assistants.htm#tab-6

Information about certification for chiropractic assistants is available from:

- Federation of Chiropractic Licensing Boards, 5401 W. 10th St., Suite 101, Greeley, CO 80634. https://www.fclb.org/Services/ChiroAssistants.aspx

NURSING ASSISTANTS AND ORDERLIES
Significant Points

- Numerous job openings and excellent job opportunities are expected.
- Most jobs are in nursing and residential care facilities and in hospitals.
- A high school diploma is required for many jobs; specific qualifications vary by occupation, state laws, and work setting.
- This occupation is characterized by modest entry requirements, low pay, high physical and emotional demands, and limited advancement opportunities.

Work Description

Nursing assistants and orderlies help care for physically or mentally ill, injured, disabled, or infirm individuals in hospitals, nursing care facilities, and mental health settings. Nursing assistants and orderlies are among the occupations commonly referred to as direct care workers due to their role in working with patients who need long-term care. The specific care they give depends on their specialty. Nursing assistants and orderlies work under the supervision of licensed practical nurses or registered nurses.

Nursing assistants, also known as nurse aides, certified nursing assistants, or geriatric aides, are trained professionals who support the nursing staff in hospitals, long-term care facilities, rehabilitation clinics, and doctor offices. Nursing assistants provide hands-on care and perform routine tasks under the supervision of nursing and medical staff. Specific tasks vary, with assistants handling many aspects of a patient's care. They often help patients eat, dress, and bathe. They also answer calls for help, deliver messages, serve meals, make beds, and tidy up rooms. Assistants sometimes are responsible for taking a patient's temperature, pulse rate, respiration rate, or blood pressure. They also may help provide care to patients by helping them get out of bed and walk, escorting them to operating and examining rooms, or providing skin care. Some assistants help other medical staff by setting up equipment, storing and moving supplies, and assisting with some procedures. Assistants also observe patients' physical, mental, and emotional conditions and report any change to the nursing or medical staff. An example of a nursing assistant pushing a patient in a wheelchair is seen in **FIGURE 33.3**.

Nursing assistants employed in nursing care facilities often are the principal caregivers and have more contact with

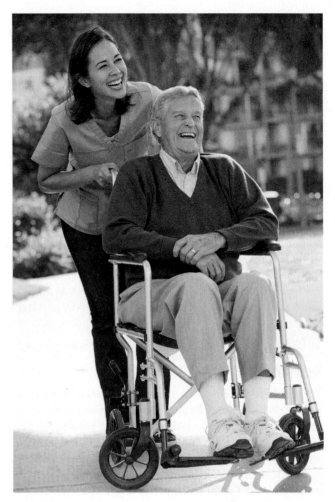

FIGURE 33.3 A nursing assistant pushing a patient in a wheelchair.
© Monkey Business Images/Shutterstock.

residents than do other members of the staff. Because some residents may stay in a nursing care facility for months or even years, many assistants develop positive, caring relationships with their patients.

Orderlies, also known as hospital attendants or unlicensed assistive personnel, work in a hospital and are responsible for the nonmedical care of patients and the maintenance of order and cleanliness. Orderlies sometimes transport patients to wards, may assist housekeepers with changing bed linen, provide patients with meals, and clean equipment and wards. When they do assist patients, their duties often include helping patients with bathing and dressing or assisting patients out of bed. Often, they are assigned daily responsibilities based on the operational needs of the hospital, which means their duties may differ from day to day.

Work Environment

Work as an assistant or orderly can be physically demanding. Assistants and orderlies spend many hours standing and walking, and they often face heavy workloads. Nursing assistants and orderlies must guard against back injury because they may have to move patients into and out of bed or help them stand or walk. It is important for nursing assistants and orderlies to be trained in and to follow the proper procedures for lifting and moving patients. Nursing assistants also may face hazards from minor infections and major diseases, such as hepatitis, but can avoid infections by following proper procedures. Nursing aides, orderlies, and attendants had some of the highest nonfatal injuries and illness rates for all occupations in 2021.

Nursing assistants and orderlies also perform tasks that some may consider unpleasant, such as emptying bedpans and changing soiled bed linens. The patients they care for may be disoriented, irritable, or uncooperative. Although their work can be emotionally demanding, many aides gain satisfaction from assisting those in need.

Most full-time nursing assistants and orderlies work about 40 hours per week, but because patients need care 24 hours a day, some work evenings, nights, weekends, and holidays. Most nursing assistants and orderlies work full time.

Employment Opportunities

Nursing assistants held about 1.5 million jobs in 2019. Orderlies held about 50,600 jobs in 2019. About 37% of nursing assistants and attendants worked in nursing care facilities, and another 27% worked in hospitals. About 78% of orderlies worked in hospitals. Others were employed in residential care facilities, government agencies, outpatient care centers, and individual and family services.

Educational and Legal Requirements

In many cases, a high school diploma or equivalent is necessary for a job as an orderly, and a high school diploma plus specific training is necessary for a job as a nursing assistant. Specific qualifications vary by occupation, state laws, and work setting. Advancement opportunities are limited.

Education and Training

Nursing assistants must complete a state-approved education program and must pass their state's competency exam to become certified. Orderlies generally have at least a high school diploma and receive on-the-job training. Nursing assistant training is offered in high schools, vocational-technical centers, some nursing care facilities, and some community colleges. Basic nursing skills are taught, and clinical work is supervised. Courses cover body mechanics, nutrition, anatomy and physiology, infection control, communication skills, and resident rights. Personal care skills, such as how to help patients bathe, eat, and groom themselves, also are taught. Hospitals may require previous experience as a nursing aide or home health aide.

Some employers provide classroom instruction for newly hired aides, while others rely exclusively on informal on-the-job instruction by a licensed nurse or an experienced aide. Such training may last from several days to a few months. Aides also may attend lectures, workshops, and in-service training.

Licensure and Certification

Federal government requirements exist for nursing assistants who work in nursing care facilities.[3] These assistants must complete a minimum of 75 hours of state-approved training and pass a competency evaluation. Aides who complete the program are known as Certified Nurse Assistants (CNAs) and are placed on the state registry of nurse assistants. Nursing assistants must be on the state registry in order to work in nursing homes. Additional requirements may exist, such as for continuing education and a criminal background check, but they vary by state. Therefore, individuals should contact their state board directly for applicable information.

Some state-approved training programs allow nursing assistants to earn additional credentials. One such credential is the Certified Medication Assistant (CMA). This credential allows the CMA to give patients medications. Some states permit nursing assistants to become certified in specialized areas, such as geriatrics.

Orderlies do not require a license. Nonetheless, many jobs require a Basic Life Support certification, which shows evidence of training in CPR.

Other Qualifications

Assistants must be in good health. Physical stamina is needed because assistants and orderlies spend much of their work time on their feet. A physical examination, including state-regulated disease tests, may be required. A criminal background check also is usually required for employment. Applicants should be tactful, patient, understanding, emotionally stable, and dependable and should have a desire to help people. They also should be able to work as part of a team, have good communication skills, and be willing to perform repetitive, routine tasks.

Advancement

Opportunities for advancement within these occupations are limited. Assistants and orderlies generally need additional formal training or education to enter other health occupations. The most common healthcare occupations for former assistants are licensed practical nurse, registered nurse, and medical assistant.

For some individuals, these occupations serve as entry-level jobs. For example, some high school and college students gain experience working in these occupations while attending school. Also, experience as an assistant can help individuals decide whether to pursue a career in health care.

Employment Trends

Employment is projected to grow faster than the average. Excellent job opportunities are expected.

TABLE 33.3 Projection Data for Employment Trends for Nursing Assistants and Orderlies, 2019–2029				
			Change, 2019–2029	
Occupational Title	Employment, 2019	Projected Employment, 2029	Number	Percentage
Nursing assistants and orderlies	1,579,100	1,698,600	119,500	8%
Nursing assistants	1,528,500	1,645,500	116,900	8%
Orderlies	50,600	53,100	2,500	5%

Data from Bureau of Labor Statistics, U.S. Department of Labor. Occupational Outlook Handbook. U.S. Department of Labor; 2020. https://www.bls.gov/ooh/healthcare/nursing-assistants.htm#tab-6

Employment Change

Overall employment of nursing assistants is projected to grow 8% between 2019 and 2029, faster than the average for all occupations. Growth will vary for individual occupations however. Employment for orderlies and attendants will grow 5% for the same time period, predominantly in response to the long-term care needs of an increasing older adult population. Financial pressures on hospitals to discharge patients as soon as possible should boost admissions to nursing care facilities. As a result, new jobs will be more numerous in nursing and residential care facilities than in hospitals, and growth will be especially strong in community care facilities for the elderly. Modern medical technology will also drive demand for nursing assistants because as the technology saves and extends more lives, it increases the need for long-term care provided by aides. Employment growth is not expected to be as fast as for other healthcare support occupations, largely because nursing aides are concentrated in the relatively slower-growing nursing and residential care facilities industry sector. In addition, growth will be hindered by nursing facilities' reliance on government funding, which does not increase as fast as the cost of patient care. Government funding limits the number of nursing assistants nursing facilities can afford to have on staff.

Job Prospects

High replacement needs for nursing assistants reflect modest entry requirements, low pay, high physical and emotional demands, and limited opportunities for advancement within the occupation. For these same reasons, the number of people looking to enter the occupation will be limited. Many assistants leave the occupation to attend training programs for other healthcare occupations. Therefore, people who are interested in and suited for this work should have good job opportunities. **TABLE 33.3** shows some projection data provided by the U.S. Department of Labor.

Earnings

Median annual wages of nursing assistants were $30,850 in May 2020. The lowest 10% earned less than $22,750, and

TABLE 33.4 Median Annual Wages in the Industries Employing the Largest Numbers of Nursing Assistants, 2020	
Government	$37,240
Hospitals: state, local, and private	$32,160
Nursing care facilities (skilled nursing facilities)	$30,120
Continuing care retirement communities and assisted-living facilities for the elderly	$30,020
Home healthcare services	$29,210

Data from Bureau of Labor Statistics, U.S. Department of Labor. Occupational Outlook Handbook. U.S. Department of Labor; 2020. https://www.bls.gov/ooh/healthcare/nursing-assistants.htm#tab-5

wages in the industries employing the largest numbers of nursing assistants in May 2020 is shown in **TABLE 33.4**.

Median annual wages of orderlies were $30,030 in May 2020. The lowest 10% earned less than $22,260, and the highest 10% earned more than $44,550. Median hourly wages in the industries employing the largest numbers of orderlies in May 2020 is shown in **TABLE 33.5**.

Related Occupations

Other occupations that help people who need routine care or treatment include child care workers, home health aides and personal and home care aides, licensed practical and licensed vocational nurses, medical assistants, occupational therapist assistants and aides, registered nurses, and social and human service assistants.

Additional Information

Information about employment opportunities may be obtained from local hospitals, nursing care facilities, home healthcare agencies, psychiatric facilities, state boards of nursing, and local offices of the state employment service.

Information on licensing requirements for nursing assistants and lists of state-approved nursing assistant programs are available from state departments of public health, departments of occupational licensing, and boards of nursing.

TABLE 33.5 Median Annual Wages in the Industries Employing the Largest Numbers of Orderlies	
Government	$33,920
Hospitals: state, local, and private	$30,070
Ambulatory healthcare services	$32,450

Data from Bureau of Labor Statistics, U.S. Department of Labor. Occupational Outlook Handbook. U.S. Department of Labor; 2020. https://www.bls.gov/ooh/healthcare/nursing-assistants.htm#tab-5

For more information on nursing assistants, orderlies, and attendants, contact:

- National Association of Health Care Assistants, 501 East 15th St., Joplin, MO 64804. https://www.nahcacna.org

- National Network of Career Nursing Assistants, 3577 Easton Rd., Norton, OH 44203. https://www.cna-network.org
- National Association for Home Care and Hospice, 228 7th St. SE, Washington, DC 20003. https:www.nahc.org

For more information on the assisted-living, nursing facilities, developmentally disabled, and subacute care provider industry, contact:

- American Health Care Association, 1201 L St. NW, Washington, DC 20005. https://www.ahcancal.org/Pages/default.aspx

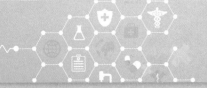

LEARNING PORTFOLIO

Issues for Discussion

1. Identify a non-healthcare-related profession in which the basic responsibilities are similar to those of a medical assistant or a nursing assistant. Discuss the job you chose and why you think it is similar.

2. Which of the jobs discussed in this chapter would you most likely recommend to a friend or acquaintance interested in working in the healthcare field? Explain your selection and rationale.

Enrichment Activities

1. View the following videos: "A Day-in-the-Life of a Medical Assistant" at https://www.youtube.com /watch?v=6jbS5bLzQoU and A Day-in-the-Life of an Ophthalmic Assistant at https://www.youtube.com /watch?v=PGw93dlFReU" and review the profiles found at Discover Eye Careers (https://www.discov-ereyecareers.org/Profiles/). Discuss the roles of a medical assistant and an ophthalmic assistant with your instructor and classmates.

2. Develop a chart to compare and contrast the following factors among the professions discussed in this chapter: educational requirements, employment trends, opportunities for advancement, salary potential, and possible career ladders.

3. Use the internet to research your state's requirements for any of the professions discussed in this chapter. List these requirements if they exist. Compare and contrast licensing, certification, and registration for this career with any other career you have examined in this course.

CASE STUDY: MEDICAL ASSISTANT OPPORTUNITIES

Victoria is graduating from community college with her medical assisting associate's degree in May. She is currently searching the job market for available opportunities in her field. Victoria realizes that she has gained many skills, both administrative and clinical, which will make her very versatile in an office setting. During her job search, Victoria identifies specialty areas where medical assistants are needed and has considered applying for open positions.

Based on the information you have read about medical assistants, answer the following questions:

1. Which higher education course would Victoria most likely have taken in her medical assisting program?
   A. Medical terminology
   B. Transcription
   C. Pharmaceutical principles
   D. First aid
   E. All of these are correct.

2. Which of the following would most likely explain why Victoria would be very versatile in an office setting?
   A. She will have access to medical records.
   B. She has excellent communication skills.

C. She received clinical and administrative training.
D. She understands medical insurance and billing.

3. During her training, Victoria learned administrative skills such as:
   A. answering telephones.
   B. handling correspondence.
   C. bookkeeping.
   D. All of these are correct.

4. One job opportunity that Victoria is considering is a specialty position where she would help ophthalmologists provide eye care. This position would be for:
   A. ophthalmic medical assistant.
   B. optometric medical assistant.
   C. podiatric medical assistant.
   D. All of these are correct.

LEARNING PORTFOLIO

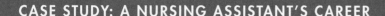

CASE STUDY: A NURSING ASSISTANT'S CAREER

After graduating high school, Eva knew that she wanted to start a career in health care. Eva registered for a nursing assistant course offered by the community college. She graduated from the program and was offered a full-time job on the medical-surgical unit at the local hospital.

Based on the information you have read about nursing assistants, answer the following questions:

1. When compared to orderlies, nursing assistants like Eva typically:
   A. receive only on-the-job training.
   B. attend training offered at technical schools and community colleges.
   C. do not need to complete state-approved education programs.
   D. do not provide hands-on care to patients.

2. During her training program, Eva most likely studied:
   A. nutrition.
   B. body mechanics.
   C. infection control.
   D. All of these are correct.

3. While working as a nursing assistant, Eva will be expected to perform:
   A. patient care.
   B. equipment setup.
   C. skin care.
   D. vitals assessment.
   E. All of these are correct.

4. While assisting with a procedure, Eva noted a drop in the patient's blood pressure. Her first response should be to:
   A. continue to monitor the patient.
   B. report the change to the medical staff.
   C. wait 10 minutes and reassess.
   D. do nothing. Eva is not required to do anything because she is not performing the procedure.

5. Eva was asked to assist a patient with grooming and ambulation. This task is most likely:
   A. beneath her abilities to perform.
   B. not within her scope of practice.
   C. within her trained duties.
   D. None of the above.

References

1. American Association of Medical Assistants. *What Is a Medical Assistant?* https://www.aama-ntl.org/medical-assisting/what-is-a-medical-assistant#.Vu4NdW2v_x8 Accessed September 2, 2021.

2. National Healthcareer Association. *Certified Clinical Medical Assistant.* https://www.nhanow.com/certifications/clinical-medical-assistant Accessed September 2, 2021.

3. Office of Inspector General, U.S. Department of Health & Human Services. *State Nurse Aide Training: Program Information and Data.* https://oig.hhs.gov/oei/reports/oei-05-01-00031.pdf Accessed September 2, 2021.

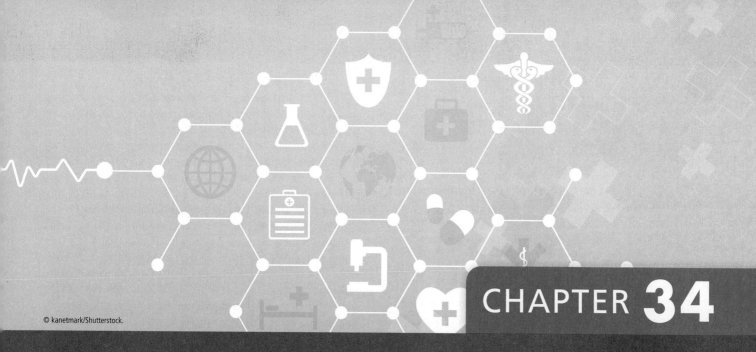

© kanetmark/Shutterstock.

CHAPTER 34

Home, Personal, and Psychiatric Aides*

KEY TERMS

Direct support professionals
Home health aides

Personal and home care aides
Psychiatric aides

Psychiatric technicians

* Information in this chapter, unless indicated otherwise, was obtained from Bureau of Labor Statistics, *Occupational Outlook Handbook 2020–2021 Edition*. Washington, DC: U.S. Department of Labor; 2021.

HOME HEALTH AND PERSONAL CARE AIDES
Significant Points

- Job opportunities are expected to be excellent because of rapid growth in home health care and high replacement needs.
- Training requirements vary from state to state, the type of home services agency, and the funding source covering the costs of services.
- Most personal care aides have high school diplomas and on-the-job training.
- Many of these workers work part time and weekends or evenings to suit the needs of their clients.

Work Description

Home health aides and personal and home care aides help people who are disabled, chronically ill, or cognitively impaired. They help older adults who may need assistance to live in their own homes or in residential facilities instead of in health facilities or institutions. They may assist people in hospices and day programs and help individuals with disabilities go to work and remain engaged in their communities. Most aides work with older adults or physically or mentally disabled clients who need more care than family or friends can provide. Others help discharged hospital patients who have relatively short-term needs.

Aides provide light housekeeping and homemaking tasks such as laundry, changing bed linens, shopping for food, and planning and preparing meals. Aides also may help clients get out of bed, bathe, dress, and groom. Some accompany clients to doctors' appointments or on other errands.

Home health aides provide instruction and psychological support to their clients. They may advise families and patients on nutrition, cleanliness, and household tasks.

Aides' daily routine may vary. They may go to the same home every day or week for months or even years, and they often visit four or five clients on the same day. Some aides, however, may work solely with one client who is in need of more care and attention. In some situations, this may involve working with other aides in shifts so that the client has an aide throughout the day and night. Aides also work with clients, particularly younger adults, at schools or at the client's work site. In general, home health aides and personal and home care aides have similar job duties. However, there are some small differences.

Home health aides typically work for certified home health or hospice agencies that receive government funding and therefore must comply with regulations to receive funding. This means that they must work under the direct supervision of a medical professional, usually a nurse. These aides keep records of services performed and of clients' condition and progress. They report changes in the client's condition to the supervisor or case manager. Aides also work with therapists and other medical staff.

Home health aides may provide some basic health-related services, such as checking patients' pulse rate, temperature, and respiration rate. An example of a home health aide taking a patient's blood pressure at home is seen in **FIGURE 34.1**. They also

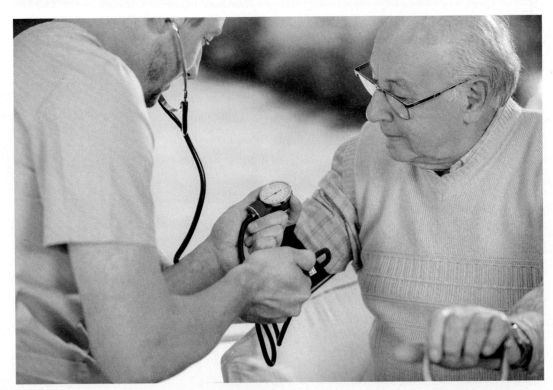

FIGURE 34.1 A home health aide taking a patient's blood pressure.
© Tyler Olson/Shutterstock.

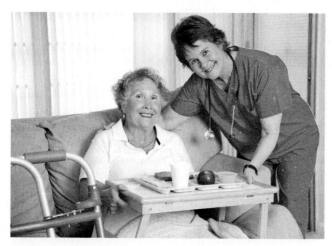

FIGURE 34.2 A personal care aide assisting an elderly patient with a meal.
© Lisa F. Young/Shutterstock.

may help with simple prescribed exercises and assist with medications administration. Occasionally, they change simple dressings, give massages, provide skin care, or assist with braces and artificial limbs. With special training, experienced home health aides also may assist with medical equipment such as ventilators, which help patients breathe.

Personal and home care aides—also called homemakers, caregivers, companions, and personal attendants—work for various public and private agencies that provide home care services. In these agencies, caregivers are likely supervised by a licensed nurse, social worker, or other nonmedical managers. Aides receive detailed instructions explaining when to visit clients and what services to perform for them. Personal and home care aides work independently, however, with only periodic visits by their supervisors. These caregivers may work with only one client each day or five or six clients once a day every week or every two weeks.

Personal and home care aides provide companionship to clients and help them with daily tasks. For example, they may fix meals and/or feed patients, as seen in **FIGURE 34.2**.

Some aides are hired directly by the patient or the patient's family. In these situations, personal and home care aides are supervised and assigned tasks directly by the patient or the patient's family. Personal and home care aides provide instruction and psychological support to their clients. They may advise families and patients on nutrition, cleanliness, and household tasks.

Aides may also work with individuals who are developmentally or intellectually disabled. These workers are often called **direct support professionals**, and they may assist in implementing a behavior plan, teaching self-care skills, and providing employment support as well as providing a range of other personal assistance services.

Work Environment

Work as an aide can be physically demanding. Aides must guard against back injury because they may have to move patients into and out of bed or help them stand or walk. Aides also may face hazards from minor infections and exposure to communicable diseases, such as hepatitis; they can avoid infections by following proper procedures. Because mechanical lifting devices available in institutional settings are not as frequently available in patients' homes, home health aides must take extra care to avoid injuries resulting from overexertion when they assist patients. These workers experience a larger-than-average number of work-related injuries or illnesses.

Aides also perform tasks that some may consider unpleasant, such as emptying bedpans and changing soiled bed linens. The patients they care for may be disoriented, irritable, or uncooperative. Although their work can be emotionally demanding, many aides gain satisfaction from assisting those in need.

Most aides work with a number of different patients, each job lasting a few hours, days, or weeks. They often visit multiple patients on the same day. Surroundings differ by case. Some homes are neat and pleasant, whereas others are untidy and depressing. Some clients are pleasant and cooperative; others are angry, abusive, depressed, or otherwise difficult.

Home health aides and personal and home care aides generally work alone, with periodic visits from their supervisor. They receive detailed instructions explaining when to visit patients and what services to perform. Aides are responsible for getting to patients' homes, and they may spend a good portion of the workday traveling from one patient to another. Many of these workers work part time and weekends or evenings to suit the needs of their clients.

Personal care aides may work in a client's home, in a group home setting, or in a large care community. Many are employed by organizations or agencies that provide in-home support services. These aides may assist individuals receiving hospice care or in day service programs. They may also help individuals with disabilities go to work and stay engaged in their communities.

Because of the physically demanding nature of the job, personal care aides suffer a higher rate of injuries and illnesses than the national average. They may become injured when assisting a patient out of beds or wheelchairs or when lifting patients. Some aides experience danger when working with patients who suffer from emotional and mental disorders or cognitive impairments and become violent or combative. Some aides working with patients who suffer from infections or communicable diseases (e.g., influenza) may contract these diseases.

Employment Opportunities

Home health aides and personal and home care aides held about 3,439,700 jobs in 2019. The majority of jobs were in home healthcare services, individual and family services, residential care facilities, and private households.

Educational and Legal Requirements

Home health aides must receive formal training and pass a competency test to work for certified home health or hospice agencies that receive reimbursement from Medicare or

Medicaid. Personal and home care aides are not required to meet formal educational requirements, but most have a high school diploma.

Education and Training

Home health aides are generally not required to have a high school diploma. They usually are trained on the job by registered nurses, licensed practical nurses, experienced aides, or their supervisor. Aides are instructed on how to cook for clients, including those on special diets. Furthermore, they may be trained in basic housekeeping tasks, such as making a bed and keeping the home sanitary and safe for the client. Generally, they are taught how to respond to an emergency, learning basic safety techniques. Employers also may train aides to conduct themselves in a professional and courteous manner while in a client's home. Some clients prefer that tasks are done a certain way and will teach the aide. A competency evaluation may be required to ensure that the aide can perform the required tasks.

The U.S. Department of Labor operates a Registered Apprentice Program for home health aides employed in long-term care facilities.[1] This program is designed to help employers recruit and retain skilled employees. For workers, these programs provide an opportunity to learn on the job and advance their careers. The apprentice progresses through a structured training and on-the-job learning program established by the employer that includes incremental wage increases associated with steps on a career ladder.

Many personal and home care aides are trained on the job by registered nurses or other personal care aides or directly by their employer. They may receive training in specific tasks, such as helping client's prepare meals or learning how to deal with a client who has a cognitive impairment.

States vary in their requirements for formal education or training programs. Some states may require aides to complete formal training or education programs offered by community colleges, vocational schools, elderly care programs, or home health agencies. Some states require personal and home care aides to undergo a criminal background check, and some require aides to undergo a competency evaluation to ensure the aide can perform the required tasks.

Employers may impose their own training requirements. For example, they may require aides to have training in first aid, cardiopulmonary resuscitation (CPR), or infection control.

The U.S. Department of Labor operates a Registered Apprentice Program for direct support professionals employed in long-term care facilities.[2] This program is designed to help employers recruit and retain skilled employees. For workers, these programs provide an opportunity to learn on the job and advance their careers. The apprentice progresses through a structured training and on-the-job learning program established by the employer that includes incremental wage increases associated with steps on a career ladder.

Licensure

Home health aides who work for agencies that receive reimbursement from Medicare or Medicaid must receive a minimum level of training. They must complete both a training program consisting of a minimum of 75 hours and a competency evaluation or state certification program. Training includes information regarding personal hygiene, safe transfer techniques, reading and recording vital signs, infection control, and basic nutrition. Aides may take a competency exam to become certified without taking any of the training. At a minimum, 16 hours of supervised practical training are required before an aide has direct contact with a resident. These certification requirements represent the minimum, as outlined by the federal government. Some states may require additional hours of training to become certified.

Other Qualifications

Aides should have a desire to help people. They should be responsible, compassionate, patient, emotionally stable, and cheerful. In addition, aides should be tactful, honest, and discreet because they work in private homes. They should possess good time-management skills so that they can follow agreed-upon schedules and arrive at a client's home on time. Aides also must be in good health. A physical examination, including state-mandated tests for tuberculosis and other diseases, may be required. A criminal background check and a good driving record also may be required for employment.

Personal and home care aides work with the public; therefore, they must be neat and well groomed and possess a courteous, pleasant manner. They must be sensitive to a patient's emotions and be able to place patients at ease. They need physical stamina and must be comfortable performing physical tasks. They should possess good time-management skills so that they can follow agreed-upon schedules and arrive at a client's home on time. Aides must follow strict rules and protocols when assisting patients, requiring them to be detail oriented. To succeed as a personal and home care aide, they must enjoy helping people.

Certification and Advancement

While offered for some time, certification for home care aides was discontinued by the National Association for Home Care and Hospice (NAHC). Home care associations at the state level offer some forms of certification.

Advancement for home health aides is limited. In some agencies, workers start out performing homemaker duties, such as cleaning. With experience and training, they may take on more personal care duties. Some aides choose to receive additional training to become nursing aides, licensed practical nurses, or registered nurses. Some may start their own home care agency or work as a self-employed aide. Self-employed aides have no agency affiliation or supervision and accept clients, set fees, and arrange work schedules on their own.

Personal and home care aides are not required to be certified in most states. For those aides who offer services paid for through a state's Medicaid plan, they often must meet certification requirements, such as a minimum number of hours of training with a state-approved curriculum and a competency evaluation.

Opportunities for advancement as a personal and home care aide are limited. To enter other healthcare occupations, aides need additional training and education. The most common occupations for former aides are licensed practical nurses, registered nurses, nurse's aides, and medical assistants.

These positions are considered entry-level positions. Some individuals work as aides while pursuing further schooling in the healthcare field. The experience as a personal and home care aide can help someone decide whether to pursue a career in health care.

Employment Trends

Excellent job opportunities are expected for this occupation because rapid employment growth and high replacement needs are projected to produce a large number of job openings. Pressures for additional aides will come from the increase in the older adult population predicted for the near future. Many of these older adults are predicted to develop health or mobility problems and require assistance with daily tasks.

Employment Change

Employment of home health and personal care aides is projected to grow by 34% between 2019 and 2029. The expected growth is due, in large part, to the projected rise in the number of older adults, an age group that often has mounting health problems and that needs some assistance with daily activities. Older adults and other clients, such as the mentally disabled, increasingly rely on home care.

This trend reflects several developments. Inpatient care in hospitals and nursing homes can be extremely expensive, so more patients return to their homes from these facilities as quickly as possible in order to contain costs. Patients, who need assistance with everyday tasks and household chores rather than medical care, can reduce medical expenses by returning to their homes. Furthermore, most patients—particularly the elderly—prefer care in their homes rather than in nursing homes or other inpatient facilities because it allows for a more personal experience. Patient families frequently choose personal and home

care aides to care for their loved ones if their loved ones do not require medical care or other services. Some studies have shown that treatment received in the home is more effective than treatment received in a hospital or nursing home. Receiving care in familiar surroundings contributes to the effectiveness of treatment.

Job Prospects

In addition to job openings created by the increased demand for these workers, replacement needs are expected to lead to many openings. The relatively low skill requirements, low pay, and high emotional demands of the work result in high replacement needs. For these same reasons, many people are reluctant to seek jobs in the occupation. Therefore, persons who are interested in and suited for this work—particularly those with experience or training as personal care, home health, or nursing aides—should have excellent job prospects.

Job prospects for personal and home care aides are excellent. High replacement needs reflect modest barriers to entry into the field. Some aides leave the occupation to attend additional training, while other aides leave due to low pay and high emotional demands. This means they will need to be replaced, creating further demand. **TABLE 34.1** shows projection data provided by the U.S. Department of Labor for jobs as home health and personal care aides.

Earnings

Median annual wages of home health and personal care aides were $27,080 in May 2020. The lowest 10% earned less than $20,130, and the highest 10% earned more than $36,990. Median hourly wages in the industries employing the largest numbers of home health and personal care aides in May 2020 are shown in **TABLE 34.2**.

Aides receive slight pay increases with experience and added responsibility. Usually they are paid only for the time worked in the home, not for travel time between jobs, and must pay for their travel costs from their earnings. Most employers hire only on-call hourly workers.

Related Occupations

Home health aides combine the duties of caregivers and social service workers. Workers in related occupations that involve personal contact to help others include childcare workers, licensed practical and licensed vocational nurses,

TABLE 34.1 Projections Data for Home Health and Personal Care Aides, 2019–2029

| Occupational Title | Employment, 2019 | Projected Employment, 2029 | Change, 2019–2029 | |
			Number	Percentage
Home health and personal care aides	3,439,700	4,599,200	1,159,500	34%

Data from Bureau of Labor Statistics, U.S. Department of Labor. Occupational Outlook Handbook. U.S. Department of Labor; 2020. https://www.bls.gov/ooh/healthcare/home-health-aides-and-personal-care-aides.htm#tab-6

TABLE 34.2 Median Annual Wages in the Industries Employing the Largest Numbers of Home Health and Personal Care Aides, May 2020

Continuing care retirement communities and assisted-living facilities for the elderly	$27,430
Residential intellectual and developmental disability facilities	$27,300
Home healthcare services	$26,220
Individual and family services	$27,360

Data from Bureau of Labor Statistics, U.S. Department of Labor. Occupational Outlook Handbook. U.S. Department of Labor; 2020. https://www.bls.gov/ooh/healthcare/home-health-aides-and-personal-care-aides.htm#tab-5

medical assistants, nursing and psychiatric aides, occupational therapist assistants and aides, physical therapist assistants and aides, radiation therapists, registered nurses, and social and human service assistants.

Additional Information

Information on licensing requirements for nursing and home health aides, as well as lists of state-approved nursing aide programs, are available from state departments of public health, departments of occupational licensing, boards of nursing, and home care associations.

For information about voluntary credentials for personal and home care aides, contact:

- National Association for Home Care and Hospice, 228 Seventh St. SE, Washington, DC 20003. https://www.nahc.org

For information about becoming a home health care aide, visit:

- Paraprofessional Healthcare Institute, 400 E. Fordham Rd, 11th Floor, Bronx, NY 10458. https://phinational.org/

PSYCHIATRIC TECHNICIANS AND AIDES
Significant Points

- Most psychiatric technicians and aides work in psychiatric hospitals and residential mental health facilities.
- Psychiatric technicians require post-secondary education and aides need at least a high school diploma.
- Demand for psychiatric technicians and aides is projected to grow 12%, about as fast as the national average.

Work Description

Psychiatric technicians, also known as mental health technicians, provide therapeutic care to patients who are mentally impaired, developmentally disabled, or emotionally disabled. They work with an interdisciplinary team that includes physicians, psychiatrists, psychologists, psychiatric nurses, social workers, counselors, and therapists. They lead patients in therapeutic and recreational activities, monitor patient's vital signs, give medication, observe and record patient behavior, and, when necessary, restrain patients who have become violent. Because of their closeness to patients, they often serve as the eyes and ears of the diagnosing professional, reporting unusual symptoms that need professional attention. Additionally, psychiatric technicians help with admitting and discharging patients and assist patients with activities involved in daily living, such as bathing and eating.

Psychiatric aides, also known as mental health assistants or psychiatric nursing assistants, also care for mentally impaired or emotionally disturbed individuals. They work under a team that may include psychiatrists, psychologists, psychiatric nurses, social workers, counselors, and therapists. In addition to helping patients to dress, bathe, groom themselves, and eat, psychiatric aides socialize with patients and lead them in educational and recreational activities. As a general rule, psychiatric aides do not engage in therapeutic activities with patients in the same way psychiatric technicians do. Psychiatric aides may play card games or other games with patients, watch television with them, or participate in group activities, such as playing sports or going on field trips. They observe patients and report any physical or behavioral signs that might be important for the professional staff to know. They accompany patients to and from therapy and treatment. Because they have such close contact with patients, psychiatric aides can have a great deal of influence on patients' outlook and treatment.

Both psychiatric technicians and aides work with patients having a variety of needs. Some patients may be receiving treatment for drug and alcohol addiction, while others are severely developmentally disabled and require intensive care. Regardless of patient need, psychiatric technicians and aides strive to provide a safe, clean environment for patients.

Work Environment

Psychiatric technicians and aides must be prepared to care for patients whose illnesses may cause violent behavior or cause them to become disoriented or uncooperative, making the work unpleasant at times. Although their work can be emotionally demanding, many aides gain satisfaction from assisting those in need. Much of their shifts involves standing on their feet for long periods of time and considerable time walking. Psychiatric technicians and aides are prone to injury due to the performance of physically demanding tasks, such as lifting patients.

Both psychiatric technicians and aides generally work a 40-hour week. Full- or part-time work is available for both technicians and aides and shifts may cover nights, weekends, and holidays when caring for patients.

Employment Opportunities

Psychiatric technicians held about 82,800 jobs in 2019. About 76% of psychiatric technicians worked in hospitals. The remaining psychiatric technicians worked in residential care facilities, outpatient care centers, and the offices of healthcare practitioners.

Psychiatric aides held about 59,500 jobs in 2019. Around 64% of psychiatric aides worked in hospitals. The remaining psychiatric aides worked in residential care facilities and individual, family, community, and vocational rehabilitation services.

Education and Legal Requirements

In most cases, graduation from a certificate program is necessary for a job as a psychiatric technician. In many cases, a high school diploma or equivalent is necessary for a job as a psychiatric aide.

Education and Training

Psychiatric technicians generally complete a postsecondary certificate or associate's degree program. These programs are commonly offered by community colleges and technical schools. Courses cover biology, psychology, and mental health counseling. Supervised structured work experience is typically included in the certificate and associate's degree programs, providing the student with the opportunity to gain real-world experience while training.

Most psychiatric aides, however, learn their skills on the job from experienced workers before they can work without direct supervision. Some employers provide classroom instruction for newly hired aides, while others rely exclusively on informal on-the-job instruction by a licensed practical nurse or an experienced aide. Such training may last from several days to a few months. Technicians and aides may also attend lectures, workshops, and in-service training.

Licensure and Certification

Five states require licenses to serve as a psychiatric technician: Arkansas, California, Colorado, Missouri, and Kansas.[3] Although specific requirements vary, these states usually require psychiatric technicians to complete an accredited education program, pass an exam, and pay a fee to be licensed. Psychiatric aides are not required to be licensed.

Psychiatric technicians are able to achieve certification through the American Association of Psychiatric Technicians.[4] Four certification levels are available, and the levels vary according to amount of education and work-level experience attained. The certifications allow the technician to add the initials NCPT after their name, meaning Nationally

Certified Psychiatric Technician. The certification shows an employer a high level of competency. For those technicians who possess the NCPT certification, they may receive better pay and promotional opportunities.

Other Qualifications

Technicians and aides must be in good health and possess physical stamina, allowing them to lift, move, and sometimes restrain patients. Applicants for these positions should be compassionate, patient, understanding, emotionally stable, and dependable with a desire to help people. They should also be able to work as a team, have good communication skills, and be willing to perform repetitive and routine tasks. They need good observational skills so that they can recognize signs of discomfort or changes in patient behavior.

Advancement

Additional training is required for significant advancement. Some become licensed in those states that license psychiatric technicians. Some become licensed practical nurses or registered nurses. Others may pursue college degrees in nursing, special education, social work, psychology, sociology, or related fields.

Employment Trends

Employment is expected to grow much faster than the national average for all occupations. Psychiatric technicians and aides will be needed in residential care facilities because the number of people with cognitive mental diseases, such as Alzheimer's disease, will increase as the nation's population ages and people live longer.

Employment Change

The employment of psychiatric technicians is expected to grow 5%, and employment of psychiatric aides is expected to grow 5%, about as fast as the national average. Psychiatric technicians and aides are a small occupation compared to nursing aides, orderlies, and attendants. Most psychiatric technicians and aides currently work in hospitals, but the industry most likely to see growth will be residential facilities for people with developmental disabilities, mental illness, and substance abuse problems. There is a long-term trend toward treating psychiatric patients outside hospitals because it is more cost-effective and allows patients greater independence. Demand for psychiatric technicians and aides in residential facilities will rise in response to increases in the number of older persons, many of whom will require mental health services. Demand for these workers will also grow as an increasing number of mentally disabled adults, formerly cared for by their aging parents, will need care.

Job growth also could be affected by changes in government funding of programs for the mentally ill. Federal

TABLE 34.3 Projections Data for Employment Trends of Psychiatric Technicians and Aides, 2019–2029				
Occupational Title	Employment, 2019	Projected Employment, 2029	Change, 2019–2029 Number	Percentage
Psychiatric technicians and aides	142,300	159,800	17,500	12%
Psychiatric technicians	82,800	93,800	11,000	13%
Psychiatric aides	59,500	66,000	6,500	11%

Data from Bureau of Labor Statistics, U.S. Department of Labor. Occupational Outlook Handbook. U.S. Department of Labor; 2020. https://www.bls.gov/ooh/healthcare/psychiatric-technicians-and-aides.htm?view_full#tab-6

health legislation has expanded the number of people who have access to health insurance. Coverage of mental health disorders will expand to more people due to federal health insurance reform.

Job Prospects

With the nation's population living longer and suffering from cognitive mental disorders, the need for psychiatric technicians and aides will increase. Correctional facilities will see an increase in the need for psychiatric technicians and aides because of the aging prison population. Those care centers offering assistance to those suffering from developmental disabilities, mental illness, and substance abuse will see the need to hire psychiatric technicians and aides. **TABLE 34.3** shows some projection data provided by the U.S. Department of Labor.

Earnings

Median annual wages of psychiatric technicians were $35,030 in May 2020. The lowest 10% earned less than $24,960, and the highest 10% earned more than $59,020. Median annual wages in the industries employing the largest number of psychiatric aides in May 2020 is shown in **TABLE 34.4**.

Median annual wages of psychiatric aides were $31,570 in May 2020. The lowest 10% earned less than $21,840, and the highest 10% earned more than $48,880. Median annual wages in the industries employing the largest numbers of psychiatric aides in May 2020 is shown in **TABLE 34.5**.

Related Occupations

Other occupations that help people who need routine care or treatment include childcare workers, home health aides and personal and home care aides, licensed practical and licensed vocational nurses, medical assistants, nursing assistants and orderlies, occupational therapist assistants and aides, registered nurses, and social and human service assistants.

TABLE 34.4 Median Annual Wages in the Industries Employing the Largest Numbers of Psychiatric Technicians, May 2020	
Psychiatric and substance abuse hospitals: state, local, and private	$35,250
General medical and surgical hospitals; private	$34,380
State government, excluding education and hospitals	$47,290
Outpatient mental health and substance abuse centers	$32,610
Residential mental health and substance abuse facilities	$31,520

Data from Bureau of Labor Statistics, U.S. Department of Labor. Occupational Outlook Handbook. U.S. Department of Labor; 2020. https://www.bls.gov/ooh/healthcare/psychiatric-technicians-and-aides.htm?view_full#tab-5

TABLE 34.5 Median Annual Wages in the Industries Employing the Largest Numbers of Psychiatric Aides, May 2020	
Psychiatric and substance abuse hospitals: state, local, and private	$33,520
State government, excluding education and hospitals	$32,580
Residential mental health and substance abuse facilities	$28,080

Data from Bureau of Labor Statistics, U.S. Department of Labor. Occupational Outlook Handbook. U.S. Department of Labor; 2020. https://www.bls.gov/ooh/healthcare/psychiatric-technicians-and-aides.htm?view_full#tab-5

Additional Information

For more information about a career and certification as a psychiatric technician, contact:

- American Association of Psychiatric Technicians, 1220 S St., Suite 100, Sacramento, CA 95811. https://psychtechs.org

LEARNING PORTFOLIO

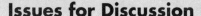

Issues for Discussion

1. Many individuals become home health, personal care, or psychiatric aides because they like to help people on a daily basis as a caregiver. While important, the desire to care for others is not all that is needed to be successful in these careers. Brainstorm and discuss with your classmates and instructor other attributes that are needed to make an individual successful in any of these careers.

2. Psychiatric technicians and aides sometimes work with prisoners housed in correctional facilities. Brainstorm and discuss with your classmates and instructor the challenges this setting poses to a psychiatric technician or aide and what actions a technician or aide can take to address these challenges.

Enrichment Activities

1. Develop a chart to compare and contrast the following factors among the professions discussed in this chapter: educational requirements, employment trends, opportunities for advancement, salary potential, and possible career ladders.

2. Use the internet to research your state's requirements for any of the professions discussed in this chapter. List these requirements if they exist. Compare and contrast licensing, certification, and registration for this career with any other career you have examined in this course.

CASE STUDY: DIRECT CARE DUTIES

Jillian is working as a home health aide. Her patient is a 70-year-old female who is recovering from a lengthy hospital stay and has a decubitus ulcer on her sacrum. She was recently providing care for her client when she noted a discrepancy in the documentation that was recorded in the chart. Jillian immediately reported the discrepancy to her supervisor.

Based on the information you have read about home health aides, answer the following questions.

1. True or false? As a home health aide, it is most likely that Jillian was performing medication administration and possibly dressing changes for this patient's wound.

2. True or false? It is likely that Jillian is at risk of exposure to infection and/or communicable disease while performing her duties as a home health aide.

3. True or false? As a home health aide, Jillian was not permitted to have access to documentation in the patient's record.

4. True or false? Jillian was correct in reporting the discrepancy to her supervisor as soon as she identified there was an issue.

5. True or false? Jillian's job duties can be physically demanding, and therefore she must guard herself and reduce the risk for back injury.

CASE STUDY: A DAY IN A PSYCHIATRIC TECHNICIAN'S LIFE

Izzy just arrived on the unit where she works as a psychiatric technician. She has been assigned to monitor vitals on the patients on her floor and administer medications during the morning rounds. Later in her shift, Izzy discovered a patient who was becoming agitated and belligerent with his roommate. Izzy immediately reported the behavior to her supervisor, who instructed Izzy to restrain the patient. Near the end of her shift, Izzy was told to help discharge a patient from the unit and then assist a patient with a craft activity.

Based on the information you have read about psychiatric aides, answer the following questions.

1. True or false? As a psychiatric technician, Izzy should not be responsible for patient vital signs and medication administration.

2. True or false? Izzy's work duties should be limited to bathing and grooming patients.

3. True or false? After discovering the agitated patient, Izzy was correct in reporting the incident to her supervisor because she works with a team of caregivers on the unit.

4. True or false? Applying restraints to a patient is not within the scope of practice for Izzy.

5. True or false? As a psychiatric technician, Izzy is permitted to assist with discharges and recreational activities.

LEARNING PORTFOLIO

References

1. Office of the Assistant Secretary for Planning and Evaluation, U.S. Department of Health & Human Services. *Evaluation Design Options for the Long-Term Care Registered Apprenticeship Program.* https://aspe.hhs.gov/reports/descriptive-analysis-us -department-labors-long-term-care-registered-apprenticeship -programs Accessed 09/02/2021

2. Ibid.

3. Institute of Justice. *License to Work.* https://ij.org/report /license-work-2/ltw-occupation-profiles/ltw2-psychiatric -technician/ Accessed 09/02/2021

4. American Association of Psychiatric Technicians. *The Certification Process.* https://psychtechs.org/the-certification -process/ Accessed 09/02/2021

PART FIVE

Health-Related Professions

Veterinarians and environmental scientists, specialists, and technicians impact the health of all Americans by ensuring a safe water and food supply, while occupational health and safety specialists and technicians ensure safe working conditions for employees.

OBJECTIVES

The following objectives are for chapters in Part V. After studying the chapters in this part, the student should be able to:

- Describe the responsibilities and work of each profession.
- Summarize the role of each profession in supporting human health.
- Classify the specialties in each profession.
- Discuss the environment in which the work takes place.
- Identify any healthcare personnel who assist the professionals with their work.
- Compare and contrast the following factors among the professions: educational requirements, employment trends, opportunities for advancement, salary potential, and career ladders.
- List other professionals who do similar tasks or have similar responsibilities.
- Discuss the advantages of the national organizations to which professionals belong.
- Explain the concept and process of interprofessional education (IPE) and interprofessional practice (IPP) in health care.

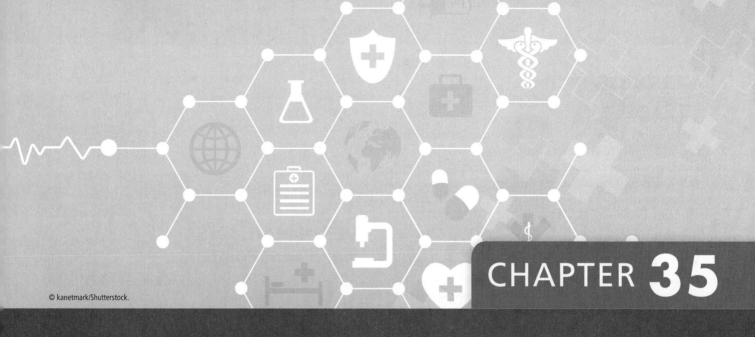

© kanetmark/Shutterstock.

CHAPTER **35**

Veterinary Medicine and Other Careers Working with Animals*

KEY TERMS

American Association for
 Laboratory Animal Science
 (AALAS)
Animal and human health
Animal and Plant Health
 Inspection Service (APHIS)
Animal trainer
Center for Veterinary Medicine
 (CVM)
Companion animal veterinarian
Doctor of Veterinary Medicine
 (DVM/VMD)
Euthanize
Food animal veterinarian

Food safety and inspection
 veterinarian
Groom
Groomer
Keeper
Kennel attendant
Livestock health
Manual dexterity
Nonfarm animal caretaker
Pet sitters
Public health
Research
Research veterinarian

Self-contained underwater
 breathing apparatus (SCUBA)
Standards for pure food from
 animal sources
Transmissible diseases
Veterinary College Admission
 Test (VCAT)
Veterinary Medical College
 Application Service (VMCAS)
Veterinary Technician National
 Examination (VTNE)
Veterinarians
Veterinary technologists and
 technicians

* All information in this chapter, unless otherwise indicated, was obtained from Bureau of Labor Statistics. *Occupational Outlook Handbook 2020–2021 Edition.* Washington, DC: U.S. Department of Labor; 2021.

463

WORKING WITH ANIMALS

For people who enjoy animals, many careers offer opportunities to spend all day caring for, training, or assisting with animals. Examples of occupations that involve working with animals are agricultural workers on farms and ranches; groomers and animal trainers in stables, pet stores, and zoos; and veterinarians, veterinary technologists, and technicians in clinics and hospitals.[1] One of the advantages for many animal workers is that they are self-employed and can set their work schedules. A disadvantage for farmers, ranchers, and veterinarians is that a large financial investment is required to set up a business. Another disadvantage for all animal workers is that the work can be emotionally and physically demanding with a high risk for physical injury.

Educational and experience requirements vary from a high school diploma for groomers to a two-year associate's degree for veterinary technicians to eight years of college for veterinarians. On-the-job training is common for animal workers who do not obtain a college degree; animal trainers and pet sitters can become certified to be more competitive for jobs.

Wages for workers caring for animals vary and are related to the educational requirements and job responsibilities. Median annual wages in May 2020 ranged from $26,080 for nonfarm animal caretakers and $36,260 for veterinary technologists and technicians to $99,250 for veterinarians. Expected growth from 2020 to 2030 is higher than average for careers that involve working with animals from 33% for animal caretakers to 17% for veterinarians and 15% for veterinary technologists and technicians.

This chapter will review careers for animal care and service workers, veterinary technologists and technicians, and veterinarians.

VETERINARY MEDICINE

Veterinary medicine is one of the oldest healing arts and involves both **animal and human health**. One of its main functions is the control of diseases transmissible from animals to humans and the discovery of new knowledge in comparative medicine.

Veterinarians contribute to human as well as animal health. Some veterinarians research ways to prevent and treat various human health problems. For example, veterinarians contributed greatly to conquering malaria and yellow fever, solved the mystery of botulism, produced an anticoagulant used to treat some people with heart disease, and defined and developed surgical techniques for humans, such as hip and knee joint replacements and limb and organ transplants.

Veterinary medicine has come to the rescue of a complex food supply. Doctors of Veterinary Medicine monitor the food supply. They guard the health of all domestic protein-producing animals and set and enforce **standards for pure food from animal sources**. Safeguarding our food supply by ensuring **livestock health** and wholesomeness is one of veterinary medicine's most important functions. Veterinarians involved in food security often work along the country's borders as animal and plant health inspectors, where they examine imports and exports of animal products to prevent disease here and in foreign countries. Through this work, the whole population is served indirectly (**FIGURE 35.1**).

VETERINARIANS
Significant Points

- Veterinarians should love animals and be able to get along with their owners.
- Graduation from an accredited college of veterinary medicine and a state license are required; admission to veterinary school is competitive.
- About 80% of veterinarians work in veterinary services.

Work Description

Veterinarians diagnose and treat diseases and injuries in animals. Specifically, they care for the health of pets, livestock, and animals in zoos, racetracks, and laboratories. Some veterinarians use their skills to protect humans against diseases carried by animals by working in **public health** or by conducting clinical **research** on human and animal health problems at universities. Others work in basic research, broadening our knowledge of animals and medical science, and in applied research, developing new ways to use knowledge. Most veterinarians diagnose animal health problems, vaccinate against diseases, medicate animals suffering from infections or illnesses, treat and dress wounds, set fractures, perform surgery, and advise owners about animal feeding, behavior, and breeding. They advise animal owners about general care, medical conditions, and treatments including prescription medications. When an animal is near the end of life because of a disease or injury, the veterinarian will **euthanize** the animal to reduce the suffering of both the animal and the owner. Veterinarians who treat animals use medical equipment such as stethoscopes, surgical instruments, and diagnostic equipment, including radiographic and ultrasound equipment. Veterinarians working in research use a full range of sophisticated laboratory equipment.

Companion animal veterinarians treat pets and generally work in private clinics and hospitals and animal shelters. According to the American Veterinary Medical Association (AVMA), more than 66% of veterinarians who work in private clinical practice work exclusively with companion animals.[2] They most often care for cats and dogs but also treat other pets, such as birds, ferrets, and rabbits. These veterinarians diagnose and provide treatment for animal health problems, consult with owners of animals about preventative health care, and carry out medical and

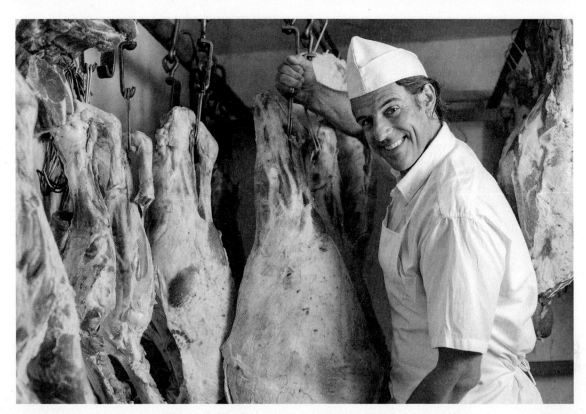

FIGURE 35.1 Some veterinarians work as food inspectors to ensure the food supply is safe.
© Tyler Olson/Shutterstock.

surgical procedures, such as vaccinations, dental work, and setting fractures.

Food animal veterinarians work with farm animals such as poultry, pigs, cattle, and sheep. Equine veterinarians work with horses and donkeys. In 2018, about 6% of private practice veterinarians diagnosed and treated horses.[2] Livestock or large animal veterinarians work with farm animals such as poultry, pigs, cattle, and sheep. There often is a certain amount of overlap between equine veterinarians and livestock veterinarians in some rural areas with limited veterinary coverage. In 2019, about 9% of private practice veterinarians had a practice that consisted primarily of food animals but may have included equine as well as companion animals, especially in rural areas.[2]

Farm animal veterinarians are comparable to a physician who is a general practitioner who cares for people of all ages from delivering a baby to visiting a patient in a nursing home. Veterinarians in general practice often work in rural areas with farmers and ranchers who own a variety of animals; they may assist cows in the delivery of a calf for a difficult birth to euthanizing animals near the end of life. They spend much of their time at farms and ranches treating illnesses and injuries and testing for and vaccinating against disease. Veterinarians check animals for **transmissible diseases** such as *Escherichia coli* and advise owners on the treatment of their animals. They may advise owners or managers about feeding, housing, and general health practices. Horses, poultry, fleece animals, and food animals represent enormous financial investments for their owners, and veterinarians are

vital in maintaining the health of the animals. Veterinarians who work with livestock or horses usually drive to farms or ranches to provide veterinary services for herds or individual animals.

Food safety and inspection veterinarians—employed by both the state and federal governments—inspect and test livestock and animal products for major animal diseases, provide vaccines to treat animals, enhance animal welfare, conduct research to improve animal health, and enforce government food safety regulations. They design and administer animal and public health programs for the prevention and control of diseases transmissible among animals and between animals and people.

Research veterinarians work in laboratories with physicians and other scientists, conducting clinical research on human and animal health problems. These veterinarians may perform tests on animals to identify the effects of drug therapies, test new surgical techniques, or advise pet food manufacturing companies. They may also research how to prevent, control, and eliminate food- and animal-borne illnesses and diseases.

Branches of the federal government that employ veterinarians are the United States Department of Agriculture (USDA), National Institutes of Health (NIH), Centers for Disease Control (CDC), and Food and Drug Administration (FDA). Veterinarians employed by the USDA's **Animal and Plant Health Inspection Service (APHIS)** are meat, poultry, or egg product inspectors who examine slaughtering and processing plants; they also check live animals and carcasses

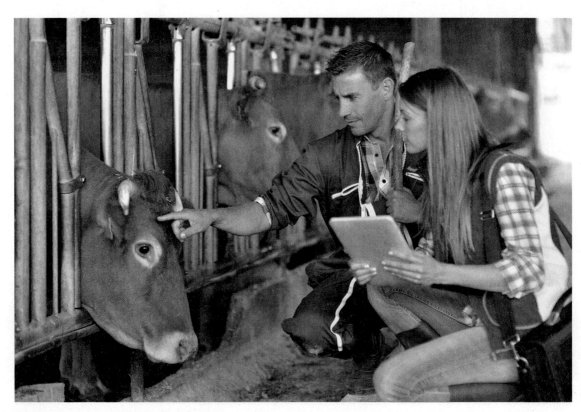

FIGURE 35.2 Veterinarians keep dairy cattle healthy for milk production.
© Goodluz/Shutterstock.

for disease, and enforce government regulations regarding food purity and sanitation (**FIGURE 35.2**).

The **Center for Veterinary Medicine (CVM)** in the FDA employs veterinarians who make recommendations for the safety of pet food as well as drug safety, such as antibiotics used in both humans and livestock. Veterinarians working for the CDC monitor food-borne illness, especially illnesses transmitted through meat and dairy products such as *Salmonella*, *E. coli*, and *Listeria*; for the NIH, veterinarians do research to improve the detection of the presence of bacteria that cause food- and animal-borne illness as well as the transmission of disease through food and water. In addition, U.S. Army Corps and U.S. Air Force veterinarians monitor the health and well-being of military working dogs and horses.

Work Environment

In 2020 about 80% of veterinarians worked in the veterinary services industry. Others held positions at colleges or universities; in private industry, such as in medical and research laboratories; and in federal, state, or local governments. About 11% of veterinarians were self-employed or had their own private practice.

Veterinarians working in nonclinical areas, such as public health and research; work in clean, well-lighted offices or laboratories; and have working conditions similar to those of other professionals who work in these environments. However, veterinarians who work in food safety and inspection

travel to farms, slaughterhouses, and food-processing plants to inspect the health of animals and to ensure that the facility follows safety protocols.

Veterinarians who work with livestock or horses spend time driving between their offices and farms or ranches. They work outdoors in all kinds of weather and may have to treat animals or perform surgery, often under unsanitary conditions, such as a stall or a shed. Veterinarians in private or clinical practice often work long hours in a noisy indoor environment. Those in group practices may take turns being on call for evening, night, or weekend work; solo practitioners may work extended hours—including weekend hours—responding to emergencies or squeezing in unexpected appointments. Veterinarians in private practice often work more than 40 hours per week. Sometimes they have to deal with emotional or demanding pet owners. When working with animals that are frightened or in pain, they risk being bitten, kicked, or scratched. The work can be emotionally stressful, as veterinarians care for abused animals, euthanize sick ones, and offer support to the animals' anxious owners. Working on farms and ranches, in slaughterhouses, or with wildlife can also be physically demanding.

Employment Opportunities

Veterinarians held about 86,800 jobs in 2020. The majority are employed in a solo or group practice. Most others were salaried employees of colleges or universities; medical schools; private industry, such as research laboratories and pharmaceutical companies; and federal, state, or local governments.

The federal government employs civilian veterinarians, chiefly in the Food Safety and Inspection Service (FSIS) within the USDA and the FDA Center for Veterinary Medicine. Veterinarians working for FSIS inspect poultry, beef, and swine processing plants to ensure that the plant is following food safety protocols. Those working for the FDA research the safety of commercial food and drugs used for companion animals and livestock. A few veterinarians work for zoos, but most veterinarians caring for zoo animals are private practitioners who contract with the zoos to provide services, usually on a part-time basis. In addition, many veterinarians hold veterinary faculty positions in colleges and universities and are classified as teachers.

Educational and Legal Requirements

Veterinarians must obtain a **Doctor of Veterinary Medicine (DVM)** degree and a state license. Admission to veterinary school is competitive.

Education and Training

Prospective veterinarians must graduate with a DVM degree (sometimes called VMD) from a four-year program at an accredited college of veterinary medicine that includes classroom, laboratory, and clinical components. In 2020, 33 colleges in the United States and five colleges in Canada met accreditation standards set by the Council on Education of the American Veterinary Medical Association (AVMA). Students can apply electronically to specific colleges through the **Veterinary Medical College Application Service (VMCAS)**, a centralized application program for participating veterinary medical colleges.[3] The webpage listed at the end of the chapter includes tips for completing an application.

The prerequisites for admission to veterinary programs vary. Although not required, most applicants to veterinary school have a bachelor's degree. Veterinary medical colleges typically require applicants to have taken many science classes, including biology, chemistry, anatomy, physiology, zoology, microbiology, and animal science. Most programs also require math, humanities, and social science courses. Applicants without a bachelor's degree face a difficult task in gaining admittance.

Pre-veterinary courses should emphasize the sciences. Veterinary medical colleges typically require applicants to have taken classes in organic and inorganic chemistry, physics, biochemistry, general biology, animal biology, animal nutrition, genetics, vertebrate embryology, cellular biology, microbiology, zoology, and systemic physiology. Some programs require calculus; some require only statistics, college algebra, and trigonometry or precalculus. Most veterinary medical colleges also require some courses in English or literature, other humanities, and the social sciences.

In addition to satisfying pre-veterinary course requirements, applicants must submit test scores from the Graduate Record Examination (GRE), the **Veterinary College Admission Test (VCAT)**, or the Medical College Admission Test (MCAT), depending on the preference of the college to which they are applying. Admission to veterinary school is competitive, especially for out-of-state students. In 2021, 46% of applicants were accepted. Admission rates were 20% to 66% for in-state students applying to veterinary schools across the U.S. compared to 3% to 10% for out-of-state students.[4] Since only 30 states have a school of veterinary medicine, cooperative arrangements in Western and Southern states make it possible for students in states without a veterinary school to be eligible for in-state tuition.[5] Students can strengthen their application by gaining volunteer or work experience with animals either on a farm, ranch, or animal shelter or by working with veterinarians in clinics or a research laboratory. Male students and those representing the ethnic and racial diversity of the U.S. may have a greater chance of being admitted since currently the majority of students in veterinary schools are female and white (80%) and the American Association of Veterinary Medical Colleges include a greater diversity of students in their strategic plan.[4]

Because of the length of training, the average loan debt for veterinarians for 83% of graduates from U.S. veterinary colleges in 2018 was $183,014.[6] Suggestions for limiting student debt are to develop a financial plan, take time between college graduation and attending veterinary school to work and save money, and establish residency to reduce the cost of out-of-state as well as increase the chances for admission.[7] The USDA sponsors a loan repayment program for veterinary medicine students to prepare veterinarians to practice in rural and other high-need areas in food animal production, food safety, and public health.[8] The USDA also funds a similar grant program that supports practice in rural areas as well as food animal production and food safety.[9]

In veterinary medicine programs, students take courses on normal animal anatomy and physiology as well as disease prevention, diagnosis, and treatment. Most programs include three years of classroom, laboratory, and clinical work. Students typically spend the final year of the four-year program doing clinical rotations in a veterinary medical center or hospital. In veterinary schools today, increasingly, courses include general business management and career development classes to help new veterinarians learn how to effectively run a practice.

New graduates with a DVM degree may begin to practice veterinary medicine once they receive their license, but many new graduates choose to enter a one-year internship. Interns receive a small salary but often find that their internship experience leads to better-paying opportunities later, relative to those of other veterinarians. Nearly all physicians complete a residency program before practicing as a physician. However, fewer graduates of veterinary medicine seek board certification, which requires the completion of a three- to four-year residency program that provides intensive training in one of the 41 AVMA-recognized veterinary specialties. Examples are anesthesia, dentistry, emergency and critical care, internal medicine, microbiology, nutrition, and zoological medicine.[10]

Licensure

All states and the District of Columbia require veterinarians to have a license. Requirements vary by state, but all states require prospective veterinarians to complete an accredited veterinary program and to pass the North American Veterinary Licensing Examination. Veterinarians working for the state or federal government may not be required to have a state license, because each agency has different requirements.

Most states not only require the national exam but also have a state exam that covers state laws and regulations. Few states accept licenses from other states, so veterinarians who want to be licensed in another state usually must take that state's exam. Nearly all states have continuing education requirements for licensed veterinarians.

Certification and Other Qualifications

The American Board of Veterinary Practitioners (AMVP) offers certification in 11 specialties, such as avian practice, beef cattle practice, canine and feline practice, food animal practice, and shelter medicine practice. Some veterinarians obtain certification after practicing several years instead of completing a residency program.[11] Although certification is not required for veterinarians, it can show exceptional skill and expertise in a particular field and is often required for veterinarians that work in teaching hospitals affiliated with colleges of veterinary medicine. To sit for the certification exam, veterinarians must have a certain number of years of experience in the field and complete additional education. Requirements vary by specialty.

Personal qualities to be successful as a veterinarian are compassion for both animals and their owners and excellent interpersonal skills necessary for communicating with owners about the condition of their animals and treatment options. Veterinarians should love animals and get along with their owners, especially pet owners, who usually have strong bonds with their pets. Management skills are important for veterinarians supervising technicians and other workers in clinics, hospitals, and laboratories or directing inspectors in the food industry. The ability to solve problems and make decisions is important when making a diagnosis and selecting the best treatment option for ill or injured animals as well as changing a treatment plan when necessary. In addition, **manual dexterity** is required for veterinarians because they must control their hand movements and be precise when treating injuries and performing surgery.

Advancement

DVMs who do an internship after graduation will have an advantage when applying for competitive or better-paying positions or in preparation for a residency program for a specialty area of practice such as surgery or ophthalmology. Veterinarians in private practice can expect to expand their practice by providing excellent care and customer service.

Employment Trends

The employment of veterinarians is expected to be greater than average through 2030.

Employment Change

Employment of veterinarians is projected to grow 17% from 2020 to 2030, above average for all occupations. Veterinary services are expected to be in greater demand as a result of pet owners' desire to prolong the life of their pets by treating chronic diseases (e.g., treatment for cancer or diabetes).

In private practice, demand for veterinarians will increase as more people are expected to take their pets for visits. Also, veterinary medicine has advanced considerably, and many of the veterinary services offered today are comparable to health care for humans, including cancer treatments and kidney transplants. Many pet owners consider their pets as members of the family and place a high value on their pets, an example of the human–animal bond. Pet owners are becoming more aware of the availability of advanced care and are more willing to pay for intensive veterinary care than owners in the past. Furthermore, the number of pet owners purchasing pet insurance is rising, increasing the likelihood that considerable money will be spent on veterinary care.

Although veterinary services are growing, the number of new graduates from veterinary schools has increased to roughly 4,000 per year, resulting in greater competition for jobs than in recent years.[4] Additionally, most veterinary graduates are attracted to companion animal care, so there will be fewer job opportunities in that field.

Job opportunities in farm animal care will be better because fewer veterinarians compete to work on large animals. Also, there will be some job opportunities available in the federal government in food safety, animal health, and public health. There also will be employment growth in fields related to food and animal safety, disease control, and public health. As the population grows, more veterinarians will be needed to inspect the food supply and to ensure animal and human health. Homeland security also may provide opportunities for veterinarians involved in efforts to maintain abundant food supplies and minimize animal diseases in the United States and in foreign countries.

Job Prospects

Candidates can expect very strong competition for most veterinarian positions. Job seekers with specializations and prior work experience should have the best job opportunities.

Occupational Title	Employment, 2020	Projected Employment, 2030	Change, 2020–2030	
			Number	Percentage
Veterinarians	86,800	101,300	14,500	17%

TABLE 35.1 Projections Data for Veterinarians, 2020–2030

Bureau of Labor Statistics, U.S. Department of Labor. Occupational Outlook Handbook 2014–2015 Edition. U.S. Department of Labor; 2014.

Given the training they receive from veterinary school, veterinarians are highly qualified for nontraditional industry positions in fields such as public health, disease control, corporate sales, and population studies. With potentially fewer opportunities in companion animal care, many graduating veterinarians will likely have better job prospects in these areas. **TABLE 35.1** shows projections data.

Earnings

Median annual wages of veterinarians were $99,250 in May 2020; the top 10% earned more than $164,490, and the bottom 10% earned less than $60,690.

Related Occupations

Related occupations include biological scientists, chiropractors, dentists, medical scientists, optometrists, physicians and surgeons, podiatrists, and veterinary technologists and technicians.

VETERINARY TECHNOLOGISTS AND TECHNICIANS
Significant Points

- Animal lovers get satisfaction from this occupation, but aspects of the work can be unpleasant, physically and emotionally demanding, and sometimes dangerous.
- There are primarily two levels of education and training for entry to this occupation: a two-year program for veterinary technicians and a four-year program for technologists.
- Employment is expected to grow much faster than average.
- Overall job opportunities should be excellent; however, keen competition is expected for jobs in zoos and aquariums.

Work Description

Owners of pets and other animals today expect superior veterinary care. To provide this service, veterinarians use the skills of **veterinary technologists and technicians**, who perform many of the same duties for a veterinarian that a nurse would for a physician. Although specific job duties vary by employer, there is often little difference between the tasks carried out by technicians and technologists despite differences in formal education and training. However, most technicians work in private clinical practice, while many technologists have the option to work in more advanced, research-related jobs at colleges and universities. Many veterinary technologists and technicians work in private clinics, animal hospitals, and veterinary testing laboratories (**FIGURE 35.3**).

Both conduct clinical work in a private practice under the supervision of a licensed veterinarian. They often perform various medical tests and treat and diagnose medical conditions and diseases in animals. For example, they may perform laboratory tests such as urinalysis and blood counts, assist with dental care, prepare tissue samples, take blood samples, and assist veterinarians in a variety of other diagnostic tests. Some technicians record case histories, develop X-rays, provide specialized nursing care, administer anesthesia, and assist with surgery. Some may sterilize laboratory and surgical equipment and provide routine postoperative care (**FIGURE 35.4**). Occasionally, veterinary technologists vaccinate newly admitted animals.

Experienced technicians may discuss a pet's condition with its owners and train new clinic personnel. Veterinary technologists and technicians assisting small-animal practitioners usually care for small pets, such as cats and dogs, but can perform a variety of duties with livestock and exotic animals. Very few veterinary technologists work in mixed-animal practices where they care for both small animals kept as pets and large animals such as horses or cattle.

Besides working in private clinics and animal hospitals, some technologists and technicians work in research facilities under the guidance of veterinarians or physicians. Even though educational levels are different, technologists and technicians who work in research-related jobs do similar work. For example, they are responsible for making sure that animals are handled carefully and humanely. They may administer medications, prepare samples for laboratory examinations, or record information on an animal's genealogy, diet, weight, medications, food intake, and clinical signs of pain and distress. They help veterinarians or scientists on research projects in areas such as biomedical research, disaster preparedness, and food safety.

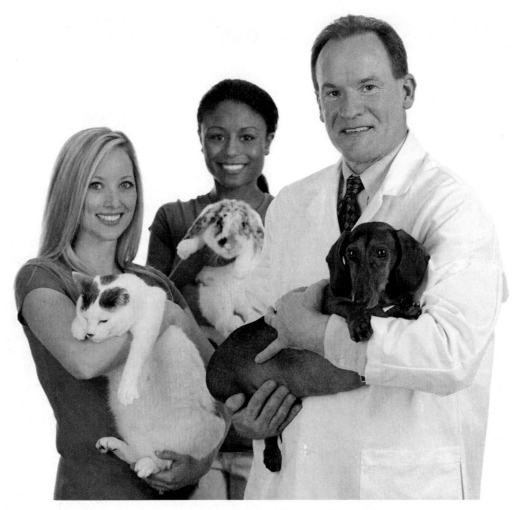

FIGURE 35.3 Veterinary technologists and technicians work in small animal clinics with veterinarians.
© Sean Locke Photography/Shutterstock.

Work Environment

Veterinary technologists and technicians typically work in private clinics, laboratories, and animal hospitals. They may also work in boarding kennels, animal shelters, and zoos. Some of the work may be unpleasant and physically and emotionally demanding. For example, they may witness abused animals or may need to help euthanize sick, injured, or unwanted animals. Those working for humane societies and animal shelters often deal with members of the public, some of whom might react with hostility to any implication that they as owners are neglecting or abusing their pets. Veterinary technologists and technicians have a higher rate of injuries and illnesses than the national average for all employees. When working with scared or aggressive animals, they may be bitten, scratched, or kicked, and such injuries can be very serious when the animal involved is large (e.g., a large dog or a horse) or potentially carries infection (e.g., cat scratch fever).

Many clinics and laboratories are staffed 24 hours a day, so technologists and technicians may work evenings, weekends, and holidays. Many have variable schedules, and some must work seven days a week.

Employment Opportunities

Veterinary technologists and technicians held about 114,400 jobs in 2020. About 90% worked in veterinary services. The remainder worked for colleges and universities, scientific and research services, and social advocacy organizations such as animal shelters.

Educational and Legal Requirements

There are primarily two levels of education and training for entry to this occupation: a two-year program for veterinary technicians and a four-year program for veterinary technologists. Typically, both technologists and technicians must pass a credentialing exam and must become registered, licensed, or certified, depending on the state in which they work.

Education and Training

Most entry-level veterinary technicians have a two-year associate's degree from an AVMA-accredited community college program in veterinary technology in which courses

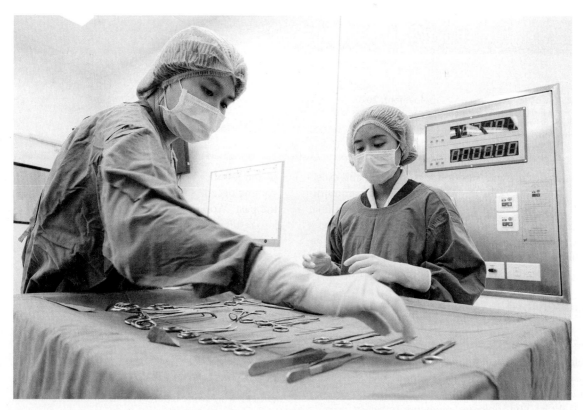

FIGURE 35.4 Veterinary technicians assist with surgery by maintaining sterile instruments.
© nimon/Shutterstock.

are taught in clinical and laboratory settings using live animals. In 2021 there were 213 veterinary technology programs in 48 states and Puerto Rico accredited by the AVMA; of these, 25 programs culminated in a four-year bachelor's degree in veterinary technology and the remainder offered an associate's degree in veterinary technology. Graduation from an AVMA-accredited program allows students to take the credentialing exam in any state in the country.[11]

Those interested in careers as veterinary technologists and technicians should take as many high school science, biology, and math courses as possible. Science courses taken beyond high school, in an associate's or bachelor's degree program, should emphasize practical skills in a clinical or laboratory setting.

Technologists and technicians usually begin work as trainees under the direct supervision of a veterinarian. Entry-level workers whose training or educational background encompasses extensive hands-on experience with diagnostic and medical equipment usually require a shorter period of on-the-job training.

Licensure

Each state regulates veterinary technicians and technologists differently; however, all states require successful completion of a credentialing exam following coursework. Most states use the **Veterinary Technician National Examination**

(VTNE). Candidates are tested for competency through an examination that is regulated by the State Board of Veterinary Examiners or the appropriate state agency. Passing the exam assures the public that the technician or technologist has sufficient knowledge to work in a veterinary clinic or hospital. Depending on the state, candidates may become registered, licensed, or certified. Candidates usually can have their passing scores transferred from one state to another if both states use the same exam.

Certification and Other Requirements

The **American Association for Laboratory Animal Science (AALAS)** certification is recommended for those seeking employment in a research facility. AALAS offers certification for three levels of technician competence, with a focus on three principal areas: animal husbandry, facility management, and animal health and welfare. Those who wish to become certified must satisfy a combination of education and experience requirements prior to taking one of the AALAS examinations. Work experience must be directly related to the maintenance, health, and well-being of laboratory animals and must be gained in a laboratory animal facility as defined by AALAS.[12] For more information about certification, go to the AALAS website listed under *Additional Information* at the end of the chapter.

Desirable personal characteristics of veterinary technologists and technicians are compassion for animals and their

TABLE 35.2 Projections Data for Veterinary Technologists and Technicians, 2020–2030

Occupational Title	Employment, 2020	Projected Employment, 2030	Change, 2020–2030	
			Number	Percentage
Veterinary technologists and technicians	114,400	131,500	18,300	15%

Data from Bureau of Labor Statistics, U.S. Department of Labor. Occupational Outlook Handbook. U.S. Department of Labor; 2020. https://www.bls.gov/ooh/healthcare/veterinary-technologists-and-technicians.htm#tab-6

owners when dealing with sick or injured animals and excellent communication skills in order to be able to communicate with supervisors and other staff members and animal owners. They also need to notice details about the animal's behavior to identify any illness and injury during testing or when giving medications. Manual dexterity is necessary in handling and treating animals and laboratory instruments.

Advancement

As they gain experience, technologists and technicians take on more responsibility and carry out more assignments with little veterinary supervision. Some eventually may become supervisors. They can specialize in a particular discipline. Specialties include dental technology, anesthesia, emergency and critical care, and zoological medicine.

Employment Trends

Employment is expected to grow much faster than average from the need to replace veterinary technologists and technicians who leave the occupation.

Employment Change

The employment of veterinary technologists and technicians is projected to grow 15% from 2020 to 2030, much faster than the average for all occupations. Pet owners are becoming more affluent and more willing to pay for advanced veterinary care. Because veterinarians perform specialized tasks, clinics and animal hospitals are increasingly using veterinary technologists and technicians to provide more general care and perform more laboratory work. Furthermore, veterinarians will continue to prefer higher-skilled veterinary technologists and technicians over veterinary assistants for more complex work.

Continued support for public health, food and animal safety, and national disease control programs, as well as biomedical research on human health problems, also will contribute to the demand for veterinary technologists, although the number of positions in these areas is lower than in private practice.

Job Prospects

Overall job opportunities are expected to be good, particularly in rural areas. However, the number of veterinary technology programs has been growing rapidly in recent years,

so the number of new graduates available for jobs over the coming decade should result in greater competition than in the past. Workers who leave the occupation each year will also result in job openings. **TABLE 35.2** shows projections data.

Earnings

The median annual wages of veterinary technologists and technicians were $36,260 in May 2020. Veterinary technologists in research jobs earned more than in other types of jobs.

Related Occupations

Others who work extensively with animals include animal care and service workers, veterinarians, veterinary assistants, and laboratory animal caretakers.

ANIMAL CARE AND SERVICE WORKERS
Significant Points

- Animal lovers get satisfaction in this occupation, but the work can be unpleasant, physically and emotionally demanding, and sometimes dangerous.
- Most workers are trained on the job, but employers generally prefer to hire people who have experience with animals and a high school diploma.
- Zookeepers and marine mammal trainers usually require a bachelor's degree.
- Most positions will present excellent employment opportunities; however, keen competition is expected for jobs as zookeepers and marine mammal trainers.
- Earnings are relatively low.

Work Description

Animal care and service workers provide care for animals. They feed, water, groom, bathe, and exercise pets and other nonfarm animals. Job tasks vary by position and place of work. Boarding kennels, pet stores, animal shelters, veterinary hospitals and clinics, stables, aquariums and natural aquatic habitats, zoological parks, and many laboratories house animals and employ animal care and service workers. They also clean, disinfect, and repair animal cages. They play with the animals, provide companionship, and observe behavioral changes that could indicate illness or injury. The following are examples of types of animal care and service workers.

Nonfarm animal caretakers often work with cats and dogs in animal shelters. All caretakers attend to the basic needs of animals, but experienced caretakers may have more responsibilities, such as helping vaccinate or euthanize animals that are seriously ill or injured under the direction of a veterinarian. Caretakers also may have administrative duties, such as keeping records, answering questions from the public, educating visitors about pet health, or screening people who want to adopt an animal.

Animal trainers train animals for riding, security, performance, obedience, or assisting people with disabilities. Most animal trainers work with dogs and horses, but some work with marine mammals, such as dolphins. They help animals become familiar with human contact as well as the human voice and teach animals to respond to commands. Trainers teach a variety of skills. For example, some may train dogs to guide people with disabilities such as blindness; others teach animals to cooperate with veterinarians or train animals for a competition or performance such as a circus. Training also can be a good tool for facilitating the relocation of animals from one habitat to another—for example, easing the process of loading horses onto trailers. Trainers work to display the talent and ability of an animal, such as a dolphin, through interactive programs to educate

and entertain the public. In kennels, veterinary clinics, or pet supply stores, **groomers** specialize in maintaining a pet's appearance. In addition to cutting, trimming, and styling pets' fur, groomers clip nails, clean ears, and bathe pets (**FIGURE 35.5**).

Groomers may operate their own business, work in a grooming salon, or run their own mobile grooming service that travels to clients' homes. Demand for mobile grooming services is growing because services are convenient for pet owners and allow the pet to stay in a familiar environment. Groomers typically groom dogs and cats, which may include cutting, trimming, shampooing, and styling fur; clipping nails; and cleaning ears. Groomers clean and sanitize equipment to prevent the spread of disease as well as maintain a clean and safe environment for the animals. Groomers also schedule appointments and collect general information on the pets' health and behavior. Groomers sometimes are the first to notice a medical problem, such as an ear or skin infection that requires veterinary care.

In stables, **grooms** are responsible for feeding, grooming, and exercising horses. They saddle and unsaddle horses, give them rubdowns, and cool them off after a ride. Grooms clean stalls, polish saddles, and organize the tack room (where the harness, saddle, and bridle are stored). They also take care of food and supplies for the horses. Experienced grooms sometimes help train horses.

In zoos, **keepers** care for animals in zoos where they plan diets, feed, and monitor the eating patterns of animals.

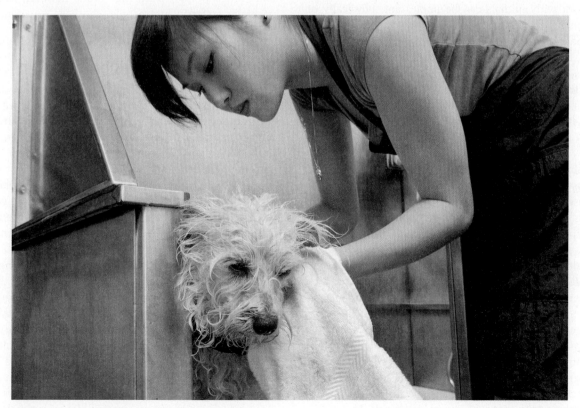

FIGURE 35.5 Animal groomers bathe and trim fur and nails of pets.
© bikeriderlondon/Shutterstock.

They also clean the animals' enclosures, monitor their behavior, and watch for signs of illness or injury. Depending on the size of the zoo, they may work with one species or multiple species of animals. Keepers may help raise young animals, and they often spend time answering questions from the public.

Kennel attendants care for pets while their owners are working or traveling. Basic attendant duties include cleaning cages and dog runs, and feeding, exercising, and playing with animals. Experienced attendants also may provide basic health care, bathe animals, and attend to other basic grooming needs or assist with obedience training.

In private homes, **pet sitters** look after animals while their owner is away. They go to the pet owner's home, allowing the pet to stay in familiar surroundings. Most pet sitters feed, walk, and play with pets daily. More experienced pet sitters also may bathe, groom, or train pets. Pet sitters typically care for dogs, cats, or other small pets. By caring for the pet in its normal surroundings, trauma is reduced, and the animal can maintain the usual diet and exercise pattern.

Work Environment

Many animal caretaker jobs require little or no training and have flexible work schedules, making them suitable for people seeking a first job or for temporary or part-time work; some have their own business.

Work with animals can be unpleasant, physically or emotionally demanding, and sometimes dangerous. Their work often involves kneeling, crawling, repeated bending, and occasionally lifting heavy supplies such as bales of hay or bags of feed. Animal caretakers must take precautions when treating animals with germicides or insecticides. They may work outdoors in all kinds of weather, and the work setting can be smelly and noisy. Caretakers of show and sports animals are often required to travel to competitions.

Animal care and service workers who witness abused animals or who assist in euthanizing unwanted, aged, or hopelessly injured animals may experience emotional distress. Those working for private humane societies and municipal animal shelters often deal with members of the public, some of whom may be hostile. Such workers must maintain a calm and professional demeanor while helping enforce the laws regarding animal care. Animal care and service workers have a higher rate of injuries and illnesses than the national average. Caretakers may be bitten, scratched, or kicked while holding, cleaning, or restraining an animal.

The advantages of working as an animal caretaker are that many jobs require little or no training and have flexible work schedules, making them suitable for people seeking a first job or for temporary or part-time work. About one-fourth of animal caretakers were self-employed in 2019.

Disadvantages are that animals need care around the clock, so many facilities, such as kennels, zoos, animal shelters, and stables, operate 24 hours a day. Therefore, caretakers often work irregular hours, including evenings, weekends, and holidays. Pet sitters often work weekends and holidays because that is when pet owners leave town. However, pet groomers and pet sitters have the flexibility of setting their schedule.

Employment Opportunities

Animal care and service workers held 272,400 jobs in 2020. About 32% worked in personal services, and 26% were self-employed. Animal trainers held 60,200 jobs in 2020; 44% were self-employed, while 22% worked in agriculture or forestry and 11% worked in animal production or aquaculture. Animal care and service workers are employed at kennels; others work at zoos, stables, animal shelters, pet stores, veterinary clinics, and aquariums. A significant number of caretakers worked for animal humane societies, racing stables, dog and horse racetrack operators, zoos, theme parks, circuses, and other amusement and recreation services.

Educational and Legal Requirements

On-the-job training is the most common way animal care and service workers learn their work; however, employers generally prefer to hire people who have experience with animals.

Education and Training

On-the-job training is the usual way that animal care and service workers learn their job, but many animal care facilities require at least a high school diploma, and many employers prefer to hire those who have experience with animals. Animal care and service workers begin by performing basic tasks and work up to positions that require more responsibility and experience. Some workers are trained before starting a position; for example, caretakers in shelters can attend training programs through the Humane Society of the United States and the American Humane Association.

Pet groomers often learn their trade by training under the guidance of an experienced groomer, although they can also attend one of 50 state-licensed grooming schools. The length of each program varies with the school and the number of advanced skills taught. Dog trainers and horse trainers typically qualify by taking courses at community colleges or vocational and private training schools. Most zoos require keepers to have a bachelor's degree in biology, animal science, or a related field, and marine mammal trainers usually need a bachelor's degree in marine biology, animal science, biology, or a related field.

Licensure

Licenses are not required to be employed as animal caretakers or trainers.

Certification and Other Qualifications

Although not required, certifications available in many animal service occupations may help workers establish their credentials and enhance their skills. For dog trainers, certification by a professional association or one of the hundreds of private vocational or state-approved trade schools can be advantageous. The National Dog Groomers Association of America offers certification for master status as a groomer. To earn certification, applicants must demonstrate their practical skills and pass two exams. The National Association of Professional Pet Sitters offers a home-study certification for those who wish to become pet care professionals. Topics include business management, animal care, and animal health issues, and applicants must pass a written exam to earn certification.

Desirable personal characteristics for animal care workers are compassion when working with animals and their owners and excellent customer service skills to satisfy pet owners. Other needed qualities are patience and problem-solving skills, especially for animal trainers who may need to change their approach for different animals. Often, four to five trainers work with a group of animals at one time; therefore, trainers should be able to work as part of a team. Physical stamina is important for animal care and service workers because their work often involves kneeling, crawling, bending, and occasionally lifting heavy supplies, such as bags of food.

Marine mammal trainers must also be good swimmers; certification in using a **self-contained underwater breathing apparatus (SCUBA)** is a plus.[14] Most horse-training jobs have maximum weight requirements for candidates due to the weight-bearing limits some horses may have because of prior injury or simply the animal's small size (e.g., ponies).

Advancement

With experience and additional training, caretakers in animal shelters may become adoption coordinators, animal control officers, emergency rescue drivers, assistant shelter managers, or shelter directors. Pet groomers who work in large retail establishments or kennels may, with experience, move into supervisory or managerial positions. Experienced groomers often choose to open their own salons or mobile grooming businesses.

Advancement for kennel caretakers takes the form of promotion to kennel supervisor, assistant manager, and manager; those with enough capital and experience may open up their own kennels. Zookeepers may advance to senior keeper, assistant head keeper, head keeper, and assistant curator, but very few openings occur, especially for the higher-level positions.

Employment Trends

Because many workers leave this occupation each year, there will be excellent job opportunities for most positions. However, keen competition is expected for jobs as zookeepers and marine mammal trainers.

Employment Change

Employment of animal care and service workers is expected to grow 33% over the 2020 to 2030 decade, faster than the average for all occupations. The companion pet population, which drives employment of animal caretakers in kennels, grooming shops, animal shelters, and veterinary clinics and hospitals, is anticipated to increase. Pet owners—including a large number of Baby Boomers, whose disposable income is expected to increase as they age—are expected to increasingly purchase grooming services, daily and overnight boarding services, training services, and veterinary services, resulting in more jobs for animal care and service workers. As more pet owners consider their pets part of the family, demand for luxury animal services and the willingness to spend greater amounts of money on pets should continue to grow. Demand for marine mammal trainers, on the other hand, is expected to grow slowly.

Demand for animal care and service workers in animal shelters is expected to grow as communities increasingly recognize the connection between animal abuse and abuse toward humans and continue to commit private funds to animal shelters, many of which are working hand in hand with social service agencies and law enforcement teams.

Animal care and service workers will continue to be needed as the variety and number of pet services increases. Employment in kennels, grooming shops, and pet stores is projected to increase to keep up with the growing demand for animal care. Job opportunities for animal care and service workers may vary from year to year because the strength of the economy affects demand for these workers. Pet owners tend to spend more on animal services when the economy is strong.

Job Prospects

Due to employment growth and the need to replace workers who leave the occupation, job opportunities for most positions should be excellent. Prospective groomers also will face excellent opportunities as the companion dog population is expected to grow and services such as mobile grooming continue to grow in popularity.

Candidates for positions as marine mammal trainers, horse trainers, and zookeepers, however, will face very strong competition, since there are relatively few positions and because of the popularity of these occupations. Furthermore, the cost of owning and riding horses is too high for many people, so employment of horse trainers is not expected to grow as fast as employment of those who train companion pets, such as dogs.

TABLE 35.3 Projections Data for Animal Care and Service Workers, Animal Trainers, and Nonfarm Animal Caretakers, 2020–2030

Occupational Title	Employment, 2020	Projected Employment, 2030	Change, 2020–2030	
			Number	Percentage
Animal care and service workers	332,700	443,400	110,800	33%
Animal trainers	60,200	77,400	17,200	28%
Animal caretakers	272,400	366,100	93,600	33%

Data from Bureau of Labor Statistics, U.S. Department of Labor. Occupational Outlook Handbook. U.S. Department of Labor; 2020. https://www.bls.gov/ooh/personal-care-and-service/animal-care-and-service-workers.htm#tab-6

TABLE 35.3 shows projections data from the National Employment Matrix.

Earnings

Wages are relatively low. Median annual wages were $26,080 for animal caretakers and $31,520 for animal trainers in May 2020. Median annual wages in the industries employing the largest numbers of animal caretakers in May 2020 are shown in **TABLE 35.4**.

Related Occupations

Others who work extensively with animals include agricultural workers, animal control workers, biological scientists, farmers, ranchers, agricultural managers, veterinarians, veterinary assistants and laboratory animal caretakers, and veterinary technologists and technicians.

Additional Information

For information on careers in veterinary medicine and a listing of AVMA-accredited veterinary medical colleges and veterinary technology programs, contact:

TABLE 35.4 Median Annual Wages in the Industries Employing the Largest Numbers of Animal Caretakers, May 2020

Industry	Salary
Other personal services	$25,910
Retail trade	$25,400
Social advocacy organizations	$25,080
Professional, scientific, and technical services	$25,050

Data from Bureau of Labor Statistics, U.S. Department of Labor. Occupational Outlook Handbook. U.S. Department of Labor; 2020. https://www.bls.gov/ooh/personal-care-and-service/animal-care-and-service-workers.htm#tab-5

- American Veterinary Medical Association, 1931 N. Meacham Rd., Suite 100, Schaumburg, IL 60173-4360. http://www.avma.org/

For information on veterinary education including applying to schools of veterinary medicine, loans, and scholarships, contact:

- Association of American Veterinary Medical Colleges, 655 K St. NW, Suite 725, Washington DC, 20001. http://www.aavmc.org
- VIN Foundation, 413 F St., Davis, CA 95616. https://vetschoolbound.org/applysmarter/

For information on board certification for specialties in veterinary practice, contact:

- American Board of Veterinary Practitioners, P.O. Box 1868, Mt. Juliet, TN 37121. https://abvp.com/veterinary-certification/

For veterinary licensing boards in the United States and Canada, contact:

- National Board of Veterinary Medical Examiners, P.O. Box 1356, Bismarck, ND 58502. http://www.nbvme.org/licensing-boards-list/

For information on the Veterinary Technician National Examination (VTNE) required for state licensure, contact:

- American Association of Veterinary State Boards, 380 W. 22nd St., Suite 101, Kansas City, MO 64108. https://www.aavsb.org/vtne/

For information on obtaining a veterinary position with the federal government, visit:

- Office of Personnel Management through USAJOBS. https://www.usajobs.gov/

For information on certification as a laboratory animal technician or technologist, contact:

- American Association for Laboratory Animal Science, 9190 Crestwyn Hills Dr., Memphis, TN 38125. http://www.aalas.org/

For information on jobs for veterinary technicians, contact:

- The National Association of Veterinary Technicians in America (NAVTA), P.O. Box 1227, Albert Lea, MN 56007. http://www.navta.net/

For career information and information on training, certification, and earnings of a related occupation—animal control officers—contact:

- National Animal Control Association, 40960 California Oaks Rd, #242, Murrieta, CA. http://www.nacanet .org

For information about internships in zoos and aquariums, contact:

- American Association of Zoos & Aquariums, 8403 Colesville Rd, Suite 710, Silver Spring, MD 20910. https://www.aza.org/careers-zoos-aquariums/

For general information on pet grooming careers, including workshops and certification information, contact:

- National Dog Groomers Association of America, P.O. Box 101, Clark, PA 16113. http://www.national doggroomers.com

For information on pet sitting, including certification information, contact:

- National Association of Professional Pet Sitters, P.O. Box 362, Huron, Ohio 44839. http://www.petsitters.org

LEARNING PORTFOLIO

Issues for Discussion

1. Go to the Association of American Veterinary Medical Colleges to learn more about becoming a veterinarian and review the brochure "Become a Veterinarian and Make a Difference." What are the course recommendations for high school and college students? List three other recommendations for gaining more knowledge and experience to strengthen an application to veterinary school. March 2014. https://www.aavmc.org/wp-content/uploads/2020/09/career-brochure-web.pdf

2. View the 2½-minute video from CareerOneStop that explains the role of a veterinary technician at https://youtu.be/CHuStDPc2pM. List some of the duties of the technician in a veterinary clinic.

3. View the 18-minute video "Day in the Life of a Veterinarian" to learn what a veterinarian does and her path to being accepted at a veterinarian school at https://youtu.be/VMaejf0EStU. Discuss the role of the veterinarian in communicating with the animal's owner about the necessary diagnostic procedures and surgical treatments.

Enrichment Activities

1. View the 12-minute video "VetVidEpisode1EquineVeterinarianFinalDraft" as a student interviews a practicing veterinarian to learn how college students can prepare to apply to veterinarian school as well as experiences in veterinarian school. https://www.youtube.com/watch?v=j5IyO4DIhTc

2. View the 2½-minute video "The Voices of our Profession: My Passion, My Profession" from the American Veterinary Medical Association, in which veterinarians describe how they became interested in the profession. https://www.youtube.com/watch?v=w9s3b5dG_bI

3. View the four-minute video "What You Need to Know about Paying for Veterinary School" from the American Veterinary Medical Association to learn how to fund a veterinary education. https://www.youtube.com/watch?v=s43eQ_xa51c

4. Read books about the life of a country veterinarian in the United Kingdom written by James Herriot in *All Creatures Great and Small* or view the series by the same name as part of *Masterpiece* produced by the Public Broadcasting System (PBS).

CASE STUDY: VETERINARY MEDICINE AND OTHER CAREERS WORKING WITH ANIMALS

Stephanie is a junior in high school and has been meeting with her guidance counselor to work on applications for college. She is considering a career working with animals but is not sure what careers are available other than being a veterinarian. Her family has always had a dog, which Stephanie helped select from the local animal shelter. Stephanie has often visited her grandfather who has a cattle ranch but also has a few alpacas that provide fiber that he sells to a local yarn shop.

Based on the information you have read about careers working with animals, answer the following questions.

1. The requirement to become a veterinarian is:
   A. bachelor's degree in animal science.
   B. Doctor of Veterinary Medicine.
   C. residency program in critical care.
   D. certification in one of 11 specialties.

2. Stephanie's guidance counselor recommends that she gain experience working or volunteering in settings where she will be working with animals during the summers or after school, now and during college. For which of the following positions could Stephanie qualify?
   A. Animal caretaker at a no-kill shelter
   B. Animal trainer at the local aquarium
   C. Veterinary technician at the local veterinarian practice
   D. Technologist in an animal research lab

3. Stephanie is concerned about the cost of veterinary school. What options does she have to reduce the amount of money needed for school loans?
   A. Establish state residency before applying
   B. Apply for a loan through a repayment program
   C. Work and save money before applying
   D. All of the above

4. True or false? Students in veterinary schools lack diversity by sex, race, and ethnicity.

LEARNING PORTFOLIO

References

1. Royster S. Working with animals. *Career Outlook*. April 2015. http://www.bls.gov/careeroutlook/2015/article/working-with-animals.htm Accessed September 8, 2021.

2. American Veterinary Medical Association. *Market Research Statistics: U.S. Veterinarians 2018.* https://www.avma.org/resources-tools/reports-statistics/market-research-statistics-us-veterinarians-2018 Accessed September 8, 2021.

3. Association of American Veterinary Medical Colleges. *Veterinary Medical School Admission Requirements (VMSAR).* https://applytovetschool.org/ Accessed September 8, 2021.

4. Annual Data Report 2020-2021. Washington, DC: American Association of Veterinary Medical Colleges; May 2021, p. 1-65. https://www.aavmc.org/wp-content/uploads/2021/05/2021-AAVMC-Annual-Data-Report.pdf Accessed September 8, 2021,

5. VIN Foundation. *What are my Chances of Getting into Veterinary School?* https://vetschoolbound.org/what-are-my-chances-of-getting-into-veterinary-school/ Accessed September 8, 2021.

6. American Veterinary Medical Association. *Student Debt Advocacy.* https://www.avma.org/advocacy/national-advocacy/student-debt Accessed September 8, 2021.

7. American Veterinary Medical Association. *What You Need to Know about Paying for Veterinary School.* https://www.youtube.com/watch?v=s43eQ_xa51c Accessed September 8, 2021.

8. U.S. Department of Agriculture. *The Veterinary Medicine Loan Repayment Program.* https://nifa.usda.gov/program/veterinary-medicine-loan-repayment-program Accessed September 8, 2021.

9. United States Department of Agriculture. *Veterinary Services Grant Program.* https://nifa.usda.gov/program/veterinary-services-grant-program Accessed September 8, 2021.

10. American Veterinary Medical Association. *What Do Board-Certified Veterinary Specialists Do?* https://www.avma.org/education/veterinary-specialties/what-board-certified-veterinary-specialists-do Accessed September 8, 2021.

11. American Board of Veterinary Practitioners. *Recognized Veterinary Specialties.* https://abvp.com/veterinary-certification/recognized-veterinary-specialties/ Accessed September 8, 2021.

12. American Veterinary Medicine Association. *Programs Accredited by the AVMA Committee on Veterinary Technician Education and Activities (CVTEA).* https://www.avma.org/education/accreditation/programs/accredited-programs-cvtea Accessed September 8, 2021.

13. American Association for Laboratory Animal Science. *Technician Certification.* https://www.aalas.org/certification/technician-certification Accessed September 8, 2021.

14. International Marine Animal Trainers' Association. *How to Become a Trainer: Careers with Marine Mammals.* https://www.imata.org/become_a_trainer Accessed September 8, 2021.

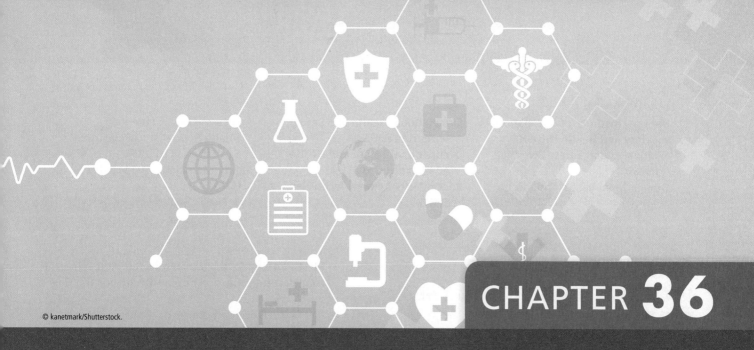

© kanetmark/Shutterstock.

CHAPTER 36

Occupational Health and Environmental Science*

KEY TERMS

American Board of Industrial
    Hygiene (ABIH)
Board of Certified Safety
    Professionals (BCSP)
Centers for Disease Control and
    Prevention (CDC)
Certified Hazardous Materials
    Manager
Certified Industrial Hygienist
    (CIH)
Certified Safety Professional
    (CSP)
Climate change analyst
Compliance

Construction Health and Safety
    Technician (CHST)
Environmental chemist
Environmental health specialist
Environmental Protection
    Agency (EPA)
Environmental restoration
    planner
Ergonomist
Hazardous Materials Manager
Health physics technicians
Health physicist
Industrial or occupational
    hygiene technicians

Industrial or occupational
    hygienist
Industrial ecologist
Institute of Hazardous Materials
    Management (IHMM)
Junior Commissioned Officer
    Student Training and Extern
    Program (JRCOSTEP)
Mine examiner
National Environmental Health
    Association (NEHA)
National Environmental
    Health Science & Protection
    Accreditation Council (EHAC)

* All information in this chapter, unless otherwise indicated, was obtained from Bureau of Labor Statistics. *Occupational Outlook Handbook 2020–2021 Edition*. Washington, DC: U.S. Department of Labor; 2021.

National Institute of Occupational Safety and Health (NIOSH)

National Radon Safety Board (NRSB)

Occupational health and safety specialist

Occupational Health and Safety Technician (OHST)

Occupational Safety and Health Administration (OSHA)

Radon Measurement Technician (RMT)

Registered Environmental Health Specialist or Registered Sanitarian (REHS/RS)

Safety Management Specialist (SMS)

U.S. Public Health Service (USPHS)

PROTECTING THE WORKER—PROTECTING THE ENVIRONMENT

Occupational health and safety specialists protect workers from accidents and injuries by monitoring **compliance** to safety laws and regulations in the workplace. Environmental scientists and specialists ensure the health of the population by protecting the air, water, soil, and food supply from toxins and pathogenic organisms.

Occupational health and safety professionals inspect worksites for compliance to safety regulations that protect workers from physical, chemical, or biological harm. The most common industries employing occupational health and safety specialists are pipeline transportation of crude oil and natural gas, oil and gas extraction, and mining. Safety measures include providing rest periods to avoid physical injury and wearing protective gear to prevent exposure to chemicals and pathogenic organisms.

Environmental scientists and specialists monitor air, soil, and water for toxins and pathogens harmful to the health of humans, plants, and animals. Many are employed as consultants for management, scientific, and technical services; others are employed by waste management services, architectural and engineering firms, and social advocacy organizations. These specialists are first responders after a natural disaster such as a flood or an oil spill; they take samples of the water and locally grown foods to detect toxic chemicals or pathogens such as bacteria. If the water supply is contaminated, the public is advised to use bottled water until the water supply is safe to use.

For students interested in worker safety or the environment, there are opportunities to work for the federal, state, or local government; for hospitals; or for consulting firms.

OCCUPATIONAL HEALTH AND SAFETY SPECIALISTS
Significant Points

- The major employers are local, state, and federal governments.
- The demand for occupational health and safety specialists is expected to grow as fast as other occupations.
- Most jobs require a bachelor's degree, although some regulators learn the skill through on-the-job training.

Work Description

Occupational health and safety specialists analyze many types of work environments and work procedures. Specialists inspect workplaces for compliance to regulations on safety, health, and the environment. They also design programs to prevent disease or injury to workers and damage to the environment.

Occupational health and safety specialists examine lighting, equipment, ventilation, and other conditions and materials in the workplace that could affect employee health, safety, comfort, and performance. Specialists seek to increase worker productivity by reducing absenteeism and equipment downtime. They also seek to save money by lowering insurance premiums and workers' compensation payments and by preventing government fines.

Some specialists develop and conduct employee safety and training programs. These programs cover a range of topics, such as how to use safety equipment correctly and how to respond in an emergency. In addition to protecting workers, specialists also work to prevent harm to property, the environment, and the public by inspecting workplaces for chemical, physical, radiological, and biological hazards. Specialists who work for governments conduct safety inspections of industry for compliance with government health and safety standards and regulations; when standards and regulations are not followed, specialists can impose a fine ranging from several thousand to millions of dollars.

Occupational health and safety specialists work with engineers and physicians to control or fix potentially hazardous conditions or equipment and to design and implement procedures to prevent potentially hazardous work conditions. Specialists investigate accidents and incidents to identify causes and to determine how they might be prevented in the future. They also work closely with occupational health and safety technicians to collect and analyze data in the workplace.

The tasks of occupational health and safety specialists vary by industry, workplace, and types of hazards affecting employees. The following are examples of types of occupational health and safety specialists. **Ergonomists** consider the

TABLE 36.1 Distribution of Occupational Health and Safety Specialists by Industry, 2020

Industry	Percentage
Government	22%
Manufacturing	17%
Construction	12%
Management, scientific, and technical consulting services	8%
Hospitals	4%

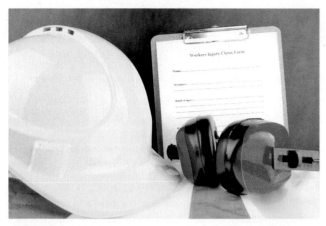

FIGURE 36.1 Occupational health and safety professionals promote the use of safety equipment to prevent injury of workers.
© simez78/Shutterstock.

design of industrial, office, and other equipment to maximize workers' comfort, safety, and productivity. **Health physicists** work in locations that use radiation and radioactive material. They help protect people and the environment from hazardous radiation used in research and medical treatment or from nuclear power plants, among other sources. **Industrial or occupational hygienists** identify workplace health hazards, such as lead, asbestos, noise, pesticides, and communicable diseases.

Work Environment

Occupational health and safety specialists work in a variety of settings, such as offices, factories, construction sites, hospitals, gas and oil fields, and mines. Their jobs often involve considerable fieldwork and travel. They may be exposed to strenuous, dangerous, or stressful conditions. Specialists use gloves, helmets, respirators, and other personal protective and safety equipment to minimize illness and injury (**FIGURE 36.1**).

In the federal government, specialists are employed by various agencies, including the **National Institute for Occupational Safety and Health (NIOSH)** and the **Occupational Safety and Health Administration (OSHA)**. Most large government agencies employ specialists to protect agency employees. In addition to working for governments, occupational health and safety specialists work in management, scientific, and technical consulting services; education services; hospitals; and manufacturing. Most occupational health and safety specialists work full time. Some specialists may work weekends or irregular hours in emergency situations.

Employment Opportunities

Occupational health and safety specialists held about 98,000 jobs in 2020 (**TABLE 36.1**).

Educational and Legal Requirements

Occupational health and safety specialists typically need a bachelor's degree. Specialists usually receive on-the-job training in inspection procedures and regulations. Some states may require licensure for specific specialties.

Education and Training

Occupational health and safety specialists typically need a bachelor's degree in occupational health, safety, or a related scientific or technical field, such as engineering, biology, or chemistry.

For some positions, a master's degree is required in industrial hygiene, health physics, or a related subject. Typical courses include radiation science, hazardous materials management and control, risk communications, and respiratory protection. These courses may vary, depending on the specialty in which a student wants to work. For example, courses in health physics focus on topics that differ from those in industrial hygiene.

The **Board of Certified Safety Professionals (BCSP)** website lists qualified bachelor's and master's level programs in safety, health, and environmental practices.[1] Internships are not required, but employers may prefer to hire candidates who have participated in one. High school students interested in becoming occupational health and safety specialists should take courses in English, math, chemistry, biology, and physics.

Although occupational health and safety specialists learn standard laws and procedures in their formal education, they also need some on-the-job training for specific work environments. For example, a specialist who will inspect offices needs different on-the-job training than a specialist inspecting factories.

Licensure

Licensure is generally not required for occupational health and safety specialists, although requirements vary by state and specialty.

TABLE 36.2 **Projections Data for Occupational Health and Safety Specialists, 2020–2030**

Occupational Title	Employment, 2020	Projected Employment, 2030	Change, 2020–2030	
			Number	Percentage
Occupational health and safety specialists	98,000	104,800	6,800	7%

Data from Bureau of Labor Statistics, U.S. Department of Labor. Occupational Outlook Handbook. U.S. Department of Labor; 2020. https://www.bls.gov/ooh/healthcare/occupational-health-and-safety-specialists-and-technicians.htm#tab-6

Certification and Other Qualifications

Although certification is voluntary, many employers encourage it. Certification is available through several organizations, depending on the field in which the specialists work. Specialists must have graduated from an accredited educational program and have work experience to be eligible to take most certification exams. A **Certified Safety Professional (CSP)** is a safety professional who has met education and experience standards, has successfully completed the certification exam, and is authorized by the BCSP to use the CSP designation. Educational requirements are a bachelor's degree in any field or an associate's degree in safety and health plus experience. Applicants for the CSP designation are also required to have four years of relevant work experience. To keep their certification, specialists are usually required to complete periodic continuing education.[2] The **American Board of Industrial Hygiene (ABIH)** offers certification as a **Certified Industrial Hygienist (CIH).** Those applying for CIH status typically have a bachelor's degree in biology, chemistry, engineering, or physics.[3] Desirable qualities and skills for specialists are the ability to use advanced technology for testing toxic chemicals. Specialists need to be detail oriented, knowledgeable about safety standards and regulations, and able to recognize when standards are not being met. Problem-solving and communication skills are necessary to find solutions to unsafe working conditions and to communicate safety instructions and concerns to employees and managers. Physical stamina is also important because specialists often stand for long periods of time or work in settings which can be uncomfortable, such as underground mines or outdoor work sites in all kinds of weather.

Advancement

Specialists with advanced degrees and certification can expect to advance in the profession.

Employment Trends

Demand for occupational health and safety specialists is projected to be about average for all occupations.

Employment Change

Employment is projected to grow 7% from 2020 to 2030, above average for all occupations. For example, technological advances that allow manufacturing workers to use new machinery will require specialists to create and enforce procedures to ensure the safe use of the machinery. The increased adoption of nuclear power as a source of energy may lead to job growth for specialists in that field. These specialists will be needed to maintain the safety of both the power plant workers and the surrounding environment.

Also, specialists will be necessary because insurance and workers' compensation costs have become a concern for many employers and insurance companies. An aging population is remaining in the workforce longer than past generations, and older workers usually have a greater proportion of workers' compensation claims.

Job Prospects

Job opportunities for individuals with advanced degrees are expected to be good. Candidates with certification may enjoy more job opportunities. Projected needs for occupational health and safety specialists are shown in TABLE 36.2.

Earnings

The median annual wage for occupational health and safety specialists was $76,340 in May 2020 TABLE 36.3 lists median salaries by industry.

Related Occupations

Occupations with similar educational requirements and job responsibilities are health and safety engineers,

TABLE 36.3 **Median Annual Salaries for Occupational Health and Safety Specialists, 2020**

Manufacturing	$77,370
Hospitals, state, local, private	$77,160
Government	$74,720
Construction	$74,550
Management, scientific, and technical consulting	$73,740

Data from Bureau of Labor Statistics, U.S. Department of Labor. Occupational Outlook Handbook. U.S. Department of Labor; 2020. https://www.bls.gov/ooh/healthcare/occupational-health-and-safety-specialists-and-technicians.htm#tab-5

environmental scientists and specialists, and occupational health and safety technicians.

OCCUPATIONAL HEALTH AND SAFETY TECHNICIANS
Significant Points

- Major employers are government, construction, and manufacturing firms.
- Some jobs require an associate's degree; others provide on-the-job training.
- Demand for employees is above average.

Work Description

Technicians work closely with and often under the supervision of occupational health and safety specialists to conduct tests and collect samples and measurements as part of workplace inspections. For example, they may collect and handle samples of dust, mold, gases, vapors, or other potentially hazardous materials. They also work with specialists to increase worker productivity by reducing worker absences and equipment downtime, which saves companies money by lowering insurance premiums and workers' compensation payments, and preventing government fines.

Technicians test and identify work areas for potential health and safety hazards. They may examine and test machinery and equipment such as scaffolding and lifting devices at construction sites to be sure that they meet appropriate safety regulations. They may check that workers are using required protective gear, such as masks and hardhats. Technicians also check that hazardous materials are stored correctly (**FIGURE 36.2**).

Although all occupational health and safety technicians work to maintain the health of workers and the environment, their responsibilities vary by industry, workplace, and types of hazards affecting employees. For example, a technician may do testing at a waste-processing plant or may inspect the lighting and ventilation in an office setting. Both of these inspections are focused on maintaining the health of the workers and the environment.

The following are examples of types of occupational health and safety technicians. **Health physics technicians** work in industries that use radiation and radioactive material by monitoring exposure to hazardous radiation and appropriate removal of waste. **Industrial or occupational hygiene technicians** examine the workplace for health hazards, such as exposure to lead, asbestos, pesticides, or infectious disease. **Mine examiners** inspect mines for proper air flow and potential health hazards such as the buildup of methane or other harmful gases.

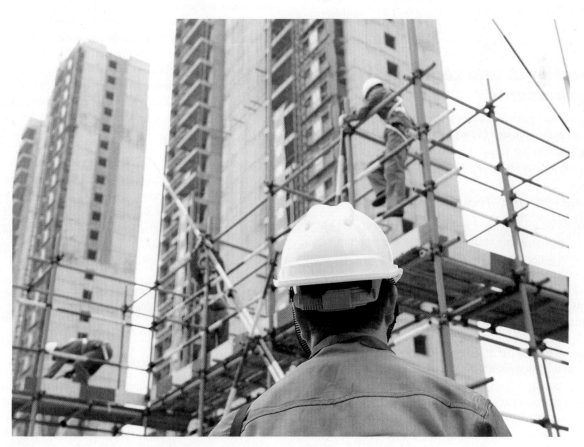

FIGURE 36.2 Occupational health and safety technicians monitor the safety at worksites.
© hxdbzxy/Shutterstock.

TABLE 36.4 Distribution of Occupational Health and Safety Technicians by Industry, 2020

Industry	Percentage
Manufacturing	23%
Government	13%
Construction	17%
Management, scientific, and technical consulting	10%

Data from Bureau of Labor Statistics, U.S. Department of Labor. Occupational Outlook Handbook. U.S. Department of Labor; 2020. https://www.bls.gov/ooh/healthcare/occupational-health-and-safety-specialists-and-technicians.htm#tab-3

Work Environment

Occupational health and safety technicians work in a variety of settings, such as offices, factories, construction sites, and mines. Their jobs often involve considerable fieldwork in all kinds of weather and travel. Most work full time but may work irregular hours when there is an emergency such as extreme weather or a chemical spill.

Employment Opportunities

There were 21,300 employed occupational health and safety technicians in 2020. The majority work for local manufacturing and consulting firms (**TABLE 36.4**).

Educational and Legal Requirements

Occupational health and safety technicians typically enter the occupation through one of two paths: Some technicians learn through on-the-job training, and others enter with postsecondary education such as an associate's degree or certificate.

Education and Training

Employers typically require technicians to have at least a high school diploma. Some employers may prefer to hire technicians who have earned an associate's degree or certificate from a community college or vocational school. These programs typically take two years or less. They include courses in respiratory protection, hazard communication, and material handling and storage procedures. Postsecondary programs include instruction on standards, laws, and procedures; however, some on-the-job training is usually required to familiarize the technician with specific work environments.

On-the-job training covers specific laws, inspection and testing procedures, and recognizing hazards. The length of training varies with the employee's level of experience and education and the industry in which he or she works. Some technicians enter the occupation through a combination of related work experience and training. They may take

on health and safety tasks at the company where they are employed at the time. For example, an employee may volunteer to complete annual workstation inspections for an office where he or she already works.

Licensure

Licensure is not required for occupational health and safety technicians; however, certification may be required by employers.

Certification and Other Qualifications

Certification is not required to become an occupational health and safety technician; however, many employers encourage it. To apply for certification, technicians must have a high school diploma and related on-the-job experience and pass a standardized health and safety exam. The BCSP offers three certifications at the technician level. **Construction Health and Safety Technician (CHST)** certification requires the applicant to have experience in construction safety. **Occupational Health and Safety Technician (OHST)** certification is designed for workers who perform occupational health and safety tasks as part of their job duties. **Safety Management Specialist (SMS)** certification requires 10 years of experience in management safety–related programs.[4]

Desirable qualities and skills for occupational health and safety technicians are the ability to use computers and complex testing equipment. Attention to detail and problem-solving skills are important to recognize when standards and regulations are not being met and to make the necessary changes to meet these standards. Good communication skills are necessary when working with specialists and other employees when collecting samples of possible toxins.

Advancement

Occupational health and safety technicians can become occupational health and safety specialists by earning a bachelor's or advanced degree. Technicians with knowledge in more than one area of health and safety along with knowledge of general business functions will have the best prospects for advancement

Employment Trends

Employment is projected to grow faster than average for all occupations.

Employment Change

Employment of occupational health and safety technicians is projected to grow 9% from 2020 to 2030, faster than average for all occupations. Increased adoption of nuclear power as a source of energy may lead to job growth as new regulations and precautions need to be enforced. Technicians will be needed to collect and test data to maintain the safety of both the workers and the environment. Insurance and workers' compensation costs have become a concern for many employers and insurance companies. Occupational health and safety technicians will be needed to work with occupational health and safety specialists in maintaining safety for all workers.

Job Prospects

Technicians with knowledge in more than one area of health and safety as well as general business functions will have better job prospects. Technicians can complete many routine tasks with little or no supervision. As a result, some employers may operate with more technicians because they are more cost effective than specialists. **TABLE 36.5** lists employment projections for occupational health and safety technicians.

Earnings

The median annual wage for occupational health and safety technicians was $53,340 in May 2020. **TABLE 36.6** lists median salaries for industries that employ technicians.

Similar Occupations

Occupations with similar education and experience requirements and job responsibilities are construction and building inspectors, environmental science and protection technicians, fire inspectors and investigators, and occupational health and safety specialists.

ENVIRONMENTAL SCIENTISTS AND SPECIALISTS
Significant Points

- Local, state, and federal governments, consulting firms, and engineering firms are the major employers.
- Most jobs require a bachelor's degree in environmental science or other science.
- Demand for jobs will be greater than average.

Work Description

Environmental health is a branch of public health concerned with all aspects of the natural and built environment that may affect human health. An environmental health specialist inspects environmental health systems to make sure they are in compliance with local, state, and federal regulations established to keep citizens safe and healthy. They use their knowledge of the natural sciences to protect the environment and human health. They may clean up polluted areas, advise policy makers, or work with industry to reduce waste.

These specialists analyze environmental problems and develop solutions. For example, many specialists work to reclaim lands and waters that have been contaminated by pollution. Others assess the risks that new construction projects pose to the environment and make recommendations to governments and businesses on how to minimize the environmental impact of these projects. Some specialize in food safety and do inspections of food processing plants or restaurants. Others may do research and provide advice on manufacturing practices, such as advising against the use of chemicals that are known to harm the environment (**FIGURE 36.3**).

The federal government and many state and local governments have regulations to ensure that there is clean air to breathe, safe water to drink, safe food to eat, and no hazardous materials in the soil. The regulations also place limits on development, particularly near sensitive ecosystems such as wetlands. Many environmental scientists and specialists work for the government to ensure that these regulations are followed. Others work for consulting firms that help companies comply with regulations and policies. Some environmental scientists and specialists focus on environmental regulations that are designed to protect people's health, while others focus on regulations designed to minimize society's impact on the ecosystem. The following are examples of types of specialists:

TABLE 36.6 Median Annual Salaries for Occupational Health and Safety Technicians, 2020

Construction	$58,370
Manufacturing	$52,230
Government	$52,210
Management, scientific, and technical consulting	$47,890
Hospitals	$44,140

Data from Bureau of Labor Statistics, U.S. Department of Labor. Occupational Outlook Handbook. U.S. Department of Labor; 2020. https://www.bls.gov/ooh/healthcare/occupational-health-and-safety-specialists-and-technicians.htm#tab-5

TABLE 36.5 Projections Data for Occupational Health and Safety Technicians, 2020–2030

Occupational Title	Employment, 2020	Projected Employment, 2030	Change, 2020–2030	
			Number	Percentage
Occupational health and safety technicians	21,300	23,200	1,900	9%

Data from Bureau of Labor Statistics, U.S. Department of Labor. Occupational Outlook Handbook. U.S. Department of Labor; 2020. https://www.bls.gov/ooh/healthcare/occupational-health-and-safety-specialists-and-technicians.htm#tab-6

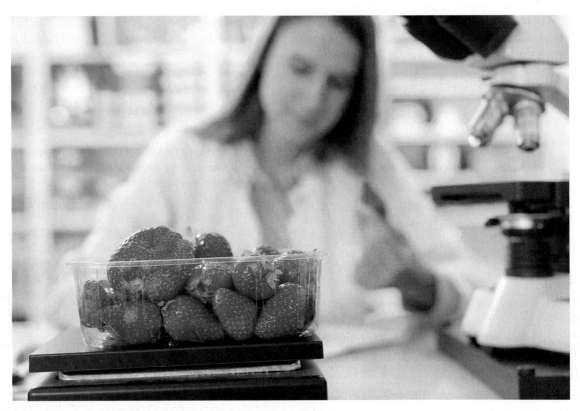

FIGURE 36.3 Environmental scientists monitor the safety of the food supply.
© science photo/Shutterstock.

Climate change analysts study effects on ecosystems caused by the changing climate. They may do outreach education activities and grant writing typical of scientists. **Environmental restoration planners** assess polluted sites and determine the cost and activities necessary to clean up the area (**FIGURE 36.4**).

Environmental health specialists study how environmental factors impact human health. They investigate potential environmental health risks, such as soil and water contamination caused by nuclear weapons manufacturing. **Industrial ecologists** work with industry to increase the efficiency of their operations and thereby limit the impacts these activities have on the environment. They analyze costs and benefits of various programs, as well as their impacts on ecosystems.

Other environmental scientists do work and receive training that is similar to that of other physical or life scientists but focus on environmental issues. **Environmental chemists** are an example; they study the effects that various chemicals have on ecosystems. For example, they look at how acids affect plants, animals, and people and work in waste management and remediation of contaminated soils, water, and air.

Work Environment

Environmental scientists and specialists work in offices and laboratories. Some may spend time in the field gathering data and monitoring environmental conditions firsthand, but this work is much more likely to be done by environmental science and protection technicians.

Fieldwork can be physically demanding, and environmental scientists and specialists may work in all types of weather. Specialists may need to travel to meet with clients or present research at conferences. Most environmental scientists and specialists work full time. They may have to work long or irregular hours when working in the field.

Employment Opportunities

Environmental scientists and specialists held about 87,100 jobs in 2020. Most environmental scientists and specialists work for private consulting firms, engineering firms, or local, state, or federal governments (**TABLE 36.7**). Many work in laboratories although they also work in the field to inspect sites. Federal agencies that employ environmental scientists and specialists include the **Environmental Protection Agency (EPA)**, **U.S. Public Health Services (USPHS)**, and **Centers for Disease Control and Prevention (CDC)**.

Education and Legal Requirements

Most jobs for environmental scientists and specialists require a bachelor's degree in environmental science or another science field such as biology, chemistry, or engineering.

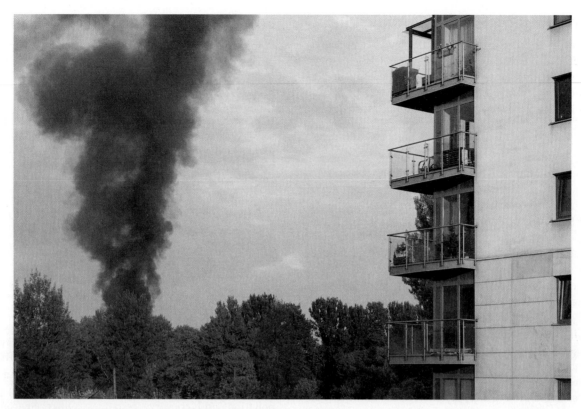

FIGURE 36.4 Environmental scientists work with industry to reduce air pollution.
© Eunika Sopotnicka/Shutterstock.

TABLE 36.7 Distribution of Environmental Scientists and Specialists by Industry, 2020

Industry	Percentage
Management, scientific, and technical consulting services	25%
State government	24%
Local government	12%
Engineering services	10%
Federal government	6%

Education and Training

For most entry-level jobs, environmental scientists and specialists must have a bachelor's degree in environmental science or a science-related field, such as biology, chemistry, physics, geosciences, or engineering. However, a master's degree may be needed for advancement. Environmental scientists and specialists who have a doctoral degree make up a small percentage of the occupation, and this level of training is typically needed only for the relatively few postsecondary teaching and basic research positions.

A bachelor's degree in environmental science offers a broad approach to the natural sciences. Students typically take courses in biology, chemistry, geology, and physics.

Students often take specialized courses in hydrology, waste management, and fluid mechanics as part of their degree as well. Classes in environmental policy and regulation are also beneficial. Students who want to reach the doctoral level and have a career in academia or as an environmental scientist doing basic research may find it advantageous to major in a more specific natural science such as chemistry, biology, physics, or geology rather than the broader environmental science degrees. The **National Environmental Health Science & Protection Accreditation Council (EHAC)** is the accrediting agency for environmental health degree programs. As of 2020, there were 28 accredited undergraduate and nine graduate programs in the United States.[5,6] Students should look for opportunities, such as classes and internships, that allow for work with computer modeling, data analysis, and geographic information systems. Students with experience in these programs will be the best prepared to enter the job market.

Licensure

Many states recognize graduation from an EHAC-accredited program as the standard needed to become a registered environmental health specialist or sanitarian. Registration is required for some positions with the federal government. For example, only students from accredited programs are eligible to participate in the **Junior Commissioned Officer Student Extern Training Program (JRCOSTEP)**; graduation from an accredited program is a requirement to enter the U.S. Public Health Service.[7]

Certification and Other Qualifications

Registration and certification in different areas of environmental health are available for those wishing to be more competitive in the job market. The **Institute of Hazardous Materials Management (IHMM)** offers the credential **Certified Hazardous Materials Manager** for those with experience evaluating sites for hazardous contaminants in the air, soil, and water and designing remediation programs.

The **National Environmental Health Association (NEHA)** offers certification for workers in environmental health. The most common is the **Registered Environmental Health Specialist or Registered Sanitarian (REHS/RS)** credential. Workers with this credential have the skills to manage an emergency response, sewage, hazardous materials, and vector control (managing mammals, birds, and insects that transmit disease pathogens).[8] The **Ecological Society of America (ESA)** offers certification as an Associate Ecologist, Ecologist, and Senior Ecologist based on the number of years of experience in the field.[9]

Desirable qualities and skills for specialists are analytical and problem-solving skills to evaluate data and find solutions to environmental pollution. Excellent communication skills are necessary to present data, explain results, and write technical reports. Interpersonal skills are also important, since specialists work with teams of other scientists, engineers, and technicians; also, results are presented to business owners or plant managers, who can be defensive. Scientists spend a lot of time alone analyzing data and preparing reports, so self-discipline is important.

Advancement

Environmental scientists and specialists often begin their careers as field analysts, research assistants, or technicians in laboratories and offices. As they gain experience, they earn more responsibilities and autonomy and may supervise the work of technicians or other scientists. Eventually, they may be promoted to project leader, program manager, or other management or research position. Some environmental scientists and specialists begin their careers as scientists in related occupations, such as hydrology or engineering, and then move into the more interdisciplinary field of environmental science. Others work as researchers or faculty at colleges and universities.

Employment Trends

Employment of environmental scientists and specialists is projected to grow faster than the average for all occupations.

Employment Change

Employment of environmental scientists and specialists is projected to grow 8% from 2020 to 2030, faster than the average for all occupations. Heightened public interest in the hazards facing the environment, as well as the increasing demands placed on the environment by population growth, is projected to spur demand for environmental scientists and specialists.

Most employment growth for environmental scientists and specialists is projected to be in private consulting firms that help clients monitor and manage environmental concerns and comply with regulations. However, most jobs will remain concentrated in the various levels of government and closely related industries, such as publicly funded universities, hospitals, and national research facilities.

More businesses are expected to consult with environmental scientists and specialists in the future to help them minimize the impact their operations have on the environment. For example, environmental consultants help businesses develop practices that minimize waste, prevent pollution, and conserve resources. Other environmental scientists and specialists are expected to be needed to help planners develop and construct buildings, utilities, and transportation systems that protect natural resources and limit damage to the land.

Job Prospects

Environmental scientists and specialists should have good job opportunities. In addition to growth, many job openings will be created by scientists who retire, advance to management positions, or change careers. TABLE 36.8 shows some job projections data from the U.S. Department of Labor.

Earnings

The median annual wage for environmental scientists and specialists was $73,230 in May 2020. TABLE 36.9 shows salaries for the major employers, including the government and consulting services.

TABLE 36.8 Projections Data for Environmental Scientists and Specialists, 2020–2030

Occupational Title	Employment, 2020	Projected Employment, 2030	Change, 2020–2030	
			Number	Percentage
Environmental scientists and specialists	87,100	94,400	7,300	8%

Data from Bureau of Labor Statistics, U.S. Department of Labor. Occupational Outlook Handbook. U.S. Department of Labor; 2020. https://www.bls.gov/ooh/life-physical-and-social-science/environmental-scientists-and-specialists.htm#tab-6

TABLE 36.9 Median Annual Salaries for Environmental Scientists and Specialists, 2020	
Federal government	$103,180
Engineering services	$75,780
Management, scientific, and technical consulting	$71,690
Local government	$69,840
State government	$67,700

Data from Bureau of Labor Statistics, U.S. Department of Labor. Occupational Outlook Handbook. U.S. Department of Labor; 2020. https://www.bls.gov/ooh/life-physical-and-social-science/environmental-scientists-and-specialists.htm#tab-5

Related Occupations

Some occupations that have similar educational requirements and job responsibilities are agricultural and food scientists, atmospheric scientists, geoscientists, occupational health and safety specialists, chemists, environmental engineers, and zoologists and wildlife biologists.

ENVIRONMENTAL SCIENCE AND PROTECTION TECHNICIANS
Significant Points

- Major employers are state and local governments, consulting firms, testing laboratories, and engineering firms.
- Most jobs require an associate's degree.
- Demand for these technicians is expected to be higher than average.

Work Description

Environmental science and protection technicians monitor the environment and investigate sources of pollution and contamination, including those affecting health. Many environmental science and protection technicians work under the supervision of environmental scientists and specialists, who direct the technicians' work and evaluate their results. They often work on teams with scientists, engineers, and technicians in other fields to solve complex problems related to environmental degradation and public health. For example, they may work on teams with geoscientists and hydrologists to manage the cleanup of contaminated soils and groundwater around an abandoned bomb manufacturing site.

Most environmental science and protection technicians work for state or local governments, testing laboratories, or consulting firms. In state and local governments, environmental science and protection technicians spend a lot of time inspecting businesses and public places and investigating complaints related to air quality, water quality, and food

safety. Sometimes they may be involved with enforcement of environmental regulations. They may protect the environment and people's health by performing environmental impact studies of new construction or by evaluating the environmental health of sites that may contaminate the environment, such as abandoned industrial sites.

Environmental science and protection technicians work in testing laboratories collecting and tracking samples and performing tests that are often similar to what is done by chemical technicians, biological technicians, or microbiologists. However, the work done by environmental science and protection technicians focuses on topics that are directly related to the environment and how it affects human health.

In consulting firms, environmental science and protection technicians help clients monitor and manage the environment and comply with regulations. For example, they help businesses develop cleanup plans for contaminated sites, and they recommend ways to reduce, control, or eliminate pollution. Also, environmental science and protection technicians conduct feasibility studies for and monitor the environmental impact of new construction projects. Environmental science and protection technicians typically specialize in either laboratory testing or fieldwork and sample collection. However, it is common for laboratory technicians to occasionally collect samples from the field and for fieldworkers to do some work in a laboratory.

Work Environment

Technicians work in laboratories, offices, and the field. Fieldwork offers a variety of settings. For example, a technician may investigate an abandoned manufacturing plant or work outdoors testing the water quality of lakes and rivers. Technicians may work around streams and rivers monitoring the levels of pollution caused by runoff from agricultural fields, cities, and landfills, or they may have to use the crawl spaces under a house to neutralize natural health risks such as radon. While working outdoors, they may be exposed to adverse weather conditions (**FIGURE 36.5**).

In the field, environmental science and protection technicians spend most of their time on their feet, which can be physically demanding. They also may need to carry and set up testing equipment, which can involve some heavy lifting and frequent bending and crouching.

Environmental science and protection technicians typically work full time. In some cold climates, the ground may freeze, thus limiting the ability to take samples. This may cause some workers to work seasonally. They may also need to travel to meet with clients or to perform fieldwork. This may occasionally require technicians to work long or irregular hours.

Employment Opportunities

Environmental science and protection technicians held about 34,200 jobs in 2020. Most worked for state or local

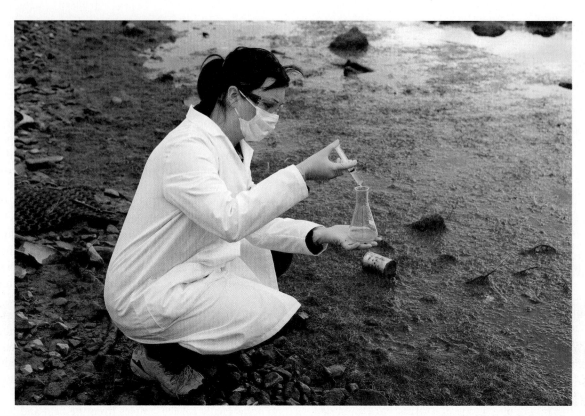

FIGURE 36.5 Environmental science and protection technicians sample and test water for toxins.
© cubephoto/Shutterstock.

governments (25%), consulting firms (25%), testing laboratories (11%), or engineering firms (7%).

Education and Legal Requirements

Environmental science and protection technicians typically need an associate's degree or two years of postsecondary education, though some positions may require a bachelor's degree.

Education and Training

Environmental science and protection technicians typically need an associate's degree in environmental science, environmental health, public health, or a related degree. Because of the wide range of tasks, environments, and industries in which these technicians work, there are jobs that do not require postsecondary education and others that require a bachelor's degree.

A background in natural sciences is important for environmental science and protection technicians. Students should take courses in chemistry, biology, geology, and physics. Coursework in mathematics, statistics, and computer science also is useful because technicians routinely do data analysis and modeling.

Many schools offer internships and cooperative-education programs, which help students gain valuable experience while attending school. Internships and cooperative-education experience can enhance the students'

employment prospects. Many technical and community colleges offer programs in environmental studies or a related technology, such as remote sensing or geographic information systems (GIS). Associate's degree programs at community colleges traditionally are designed to provide easy transfer to bachelor's degree programs at colleges and universities.

Technicians whose jobs involve handling hazardous waste typically need to complete training per OSHA standards. The length of training depends on the type of hazardous material that workers handle. The training covers health hazards, personal protective equipment and clothing, site safety, recognizing and identifying hazards, and decontamination.

Licensure

In some states, environmental science and protection technicians need a license to do certain types of environmental and health inspections. For example, some states require licensing for technicians who test buildings for radon. Licensure requirements vary by state but typically include minimum levels of education and experience and a passing score on an exam.

Certification and Other Qualifications

The **National Radon Safety Board (NRSB)** offers **Radon Measurement Technician (RMT)** certification in radon measurement of buildings. Requirements are

TABLE 36.10 Median Annual Salaries for Environmental Science and Protection Technicians, 2020

Local government	$51,510
Engineering services	$49,360
State government	$47,970
Management, scientific, and technical consulting	$43,890
Testing laboratories	$40,560

Data from Bureau of Labor Statistics, U.S. Department of Labor. Occupational Outlook Handbook. U.S. Department of Labor; 2020. https://www.bls.gov/ooh/life-physical-and-social-science/environmental -science-and-protection-technicians.htm#tab-5

completing training courses and an exam and to submit radon measurements.[10]

Desirable qualities and skills for environmental science and protection technicians are the ability to carry out a wide variety of laboratory and field tests with accuracy. Critical thinking skills are necessary to determine the best way to address environmental hazards. Good communication skills are necessary to work with specialists and other employees when collecting samples of possible toxins. Excellent listening and writing skills are necessary to follow instructions and communicate results in written reports. Interpersonal skills are needed to work with scientists and other technicians and managers and others at the worksite.

Advancement

Job candidates with an associate's degree and laboratory experience should have the best job opportunities.

Employment Trends

Public interest in the environment is expected to increase demand for careers in environmental science.

Employment Change

Employment of environmental science and protection technicians is projected to grow 11% from 2020 to 2030, faster than the average for all occupations. Heightened public interest in the hazards facing the environment, as well as the increasing demands placed on the environment by population growth, is expected to spur demand for environmental science and protection technicians. Most employment growth for environmental science and protection technicians is projected to be in consulting firms. More businesses and governments are expected to use these firms in the future to help them monitor and manage the environment and comply with regulations.

Job Prospects

Environmental science and protection technicians should have good opportunities for employment. Job candidates with an associate's degree and laboratory experience should have the best opportunities.

Earnings

The median annual wage for environmental science and protection technicians was $46,850 in May 2020; the median annual wages in the top five industries employing these technicians are shown in **TABLE 36.10**.

Additional Information

For more information about occupations in safety, a list of safety and related academic programs, and credentialing, visit:

- BCSP Foundation, 8645 Guion Rd, Indianapolis, IN 46268; https://www.bcspfoundation.org/ and https:// www.bcsp.org/Get-Involved/Career-Paths-in-Safety

For more information about becoming a Certified Safety Professional:

- Board of Certified Safety Professionals. *Certified Safety Professional.* https://www.bcsp.org/CSP

For information about undergraduate and graduate degree programs in environmental health science and scholarship opportunities, contact:

- Association of Environmental Health Academic Programs (AEHAP), P.O. Box 66057, Burien, WA 98166. https://www.aehap.org/member-programs.html
- National Environmental Health Science & Protection Accreditation Council (EHAC), P.O. Box 66057, Burien, WA 98166. https://www.nehspac.org/about-ehac/

For information about certification and credentialing options and requirements for environmental health scientists, contact:

- National Environmental Health Association, 720 S. Colorado Blvd., Suite 1000-N, Denver, CO 80246-1926. http://www.neha.org/professional-development /credentials

For information on student internships or becoming a commissioned officer in the U.S. Public Health Service in Environmental Health or Occupational Health, contact:

- Commissioned Corps of the U.S. Public Health Service. *Explore Opportunities.* https://www.usphs.gov /professions/environmental-health/

Information on obtaining an internship or job with the federal government can be obtained by visiting:

- USAJOBS. Students & recent graduates. https://www .usajobs.gov/Help/working-in-government/unique -hiring-paths/students/

LEARNING PORTFOLIO

Issues for Discussion

1. Watch the one-minute video "Workers' Safety and Health Rights on the Job" from the U.S. Department of Labor. List the industries represented in the video and worker safety concerns for that industry. https://www.youtube.com/watch?v=MjnWMQeufI0

2. Go to the National Institute for Occupational Safety and Health (NIOSH) website and review the list of industries and occupations. Choose one industry/occupation from the list and review the sources of worker injury or illness for that particular industry/occupation. Are there specific recommendations for the industry to protect the worker? https://www.cdc.gov/niosh/index.htm

3. Watch the two-minute video "Environmental Health Careers" from the Association of Environmental Health Academic Programs (AEHAP). Summarize the components of the environment that are monitored by environmental health specialists to protect the health of all humans. https://vimeo.com/50335987

4. Go to the Environmental Protection Agency website and link to "Compliance and Enforcement and then to Civil Cases and Settlements." Choose one case to review. What industry was involved in the case? What standard or regulation was not followed? What was the penalty? http://cfpub.epa.gov/enforcement/cases/

Enrichment Activities

1. Review information about the NIH Summer Internship Program and the NIEHS Scholars Connect Program, opportunities to work in a research laboratory, attend seminars, and present results at a poster session. https://www.niehs.nih.gov/careers/research/

2. Watch the two-minute video "Preventing Mercury Exposure in Florida" from the CDC Environmental Public Health Tracking Program. Who is most susceptible to negative health effects of mercury? http://ephtracking.cdc.gov/showTrackingInAction.action

3. Watch the two-minute video "Environmental Health Careers" from the Association of Environmental Health Academic Programs (AEHAP). Summarize the components of the environment that are monitored by environmental health specialists to protect the health of all humans. https://www.youtube.com/watch?v=qVc38zRk9M8

4. Go to the Environmental Protection Agency (EPA) website to learn more about climate change and programs of the EPA to address this problem. https://www.epa.gov/climate-indicators

CASE STUDY: OCCUPATIONAL HEALTH AND ENVIRONMENTAL SCIENCE

Hunter has been completing research for his environmental science class. Hunter reviewed some of the requirements for becoming an occupational health and safety specialist. He was very interested to learn about the educational requirements as well as the projected job growth in this area.

Hunter has been studying biology and will graduate in May with his bachelor's degree. He plans on searching for a job within the local, state, or federal government after graduation. Because of Hunter's anticipated degree completion, he will be eligible for Graduate Safety Practitioner (GSP) designation. GSP designation is one pathway to sit for the Certified Safety Professional (CSP) exam.

The following questions relate to occupational health and environmental science. Please help Hunter answer them based on what you have learned from this chapter.

1. Hunter is meeting the basic educational requirement for an occupation health and safety specialist by:
   A. graduating in May.
   B. studying environment science.
   C. receiving his bachelor's degree.
   D. researching job opportunities.

2. Hunter's best chance of employment with the government is based on the fact that _____ of specialists work for a government agency.
   A. 70%
   B. 60%
   C. 45%
   D. 20%

3. Once Hunter completes his CSP exam, he will need to complete which of the following in order to keep his certification?
   A. Yearly community service hours
   B. Periodic continuing education
   C. Exam completion every two years
   D. Thirty additional internship hours

LEARNING PORTFOLIO

References

1. Board of Certified Safety Professionals. *Academic Database.* https://www.bcsp.org/resources/academic-database Accessed September 8, 2021

2. Board of Certified Professionals. *Certifications.* https://www.bcsp.org/ Accessed September 8, 2021.

3. ABET-American Board of Industrial Hygiene. *Accredited IH Programs.* http://www.abih.org/become-certified/abet-accredited-ih-programs Accessed September 8, 2021.

4. Board of Certified Safety Professionals. *BCSP. A Complete Guide to Safety Certification.* 2nd ed. August 2021. https://online.fliphtml5.com/pbcyp/ijfs/#p=3 Accessed September 2021.

5. National Environmental Health Science & Protection Accreditation. *EHAC Undergraduate Accredited Programs.* https://www.nehspac.org/about-ehac/accredited-programs-ehac-undergraduate-programs/ Accessed September 8, 2021.

6. National Environmental Health Science & Protection Accreditation. *EHAC Graduate Accredited Programs* https://www.nehspac.org/about-ehac/accredited-programs-ehac-graduate-programs/ Accessed September 8, 2021.

7. Commissioned Corps of the U.S. Public Health Service. *Students.* https://www.usphs.gov/students/ Accessed September 8, 2021

8. National Environmental Health Association. *REHS/RS Credential.* https://www.neha.org/professional-development/credentials/rehsrs-credential Accessed September 8, 2021

9. Ecological Society of America. *Certification Requirements.* https://www.esa.org/certification/certification-requirements-checklist/ Accessed September 8, 2021

10. National Radon Safety Board. *How to Become Certified.* https://www.nrsb.org/for-professionals/how-to-get-certified/ Accessed September 8, 2021.

APPENDIX A

Salaries for Health Professionals

PROFESSION	MEDIAN YEARLY SALARY
Animal care and service worker	$26,080
Athletic trainer	$49,860
Audiologist	$81,030
Cardiovascular technologist and technician	$59,100
Chiropractor	$70,720
Community health worker	$42,000
Dental assistant	$41,180
Dental hygienist	$77,090
Dental laboratory technician	$38,620
Dentist	$164,010
Dietetic technician	$30,110
Dietitian/nutritionist	$63,090
Environmental science and protection technician	$46,850
Environmental scientist and specialist	$73,230
Emergency medical technician (paramedic)	$36,650
Exercise physiologist	$50,280
Genetic counselor	$85,700
Health Education Specialist	$56,500
Health information specialist	$44,090

All information in this chapter, unless otherwise indicated, was obtained from Bureau of Labor Statistics. *Occupational Outlook Handbook 2020–2021 Edition*. Washington, DC: U.S. Department of Labor; 2021.

PROFESSION	MEDIAN YEARLY SALARY
Home health and personal care aide	$27,080
Magnetic resonance imaging technologists	$74,690
Massage therapist	$43,620
Medical assistant	$35,850
Medical and clinical laboratory technician	$49,213*
Medical and clinical laboratory technologist	$65,333*
Medical and health service manager	$104,280
Medical equipment repairer	$51,610
Medical transcriptionist	$35,270
Mental health counselor	$47,660
Nuclear medicine technologist	$79,590
Nursing assistant	$30,850
Nurse, practical/vocational (LPN/LVN)	$48,820
Nurse, registered	$75,330
Occupational health and safety specialist	$76,340
Occupational health and safety technician	$53,340
Occupational therapist	$86,280
Occupational therapy aide	$30,180
Occupational therapy assistant	$62,940
Ophthalmic laboratory technician	$38,620
Optician, dispensing	$38,530
Optometrist	$118,050
Orthotists and prosthetists	$70,190
Pharmacist	$128,710
Pharmacy technician	$35,100
Phlebotomist	$36,320
Physical therapist	$91,010
Physical therapy aide	$28,450
Physical therapy assistant	$59,770
Physician assistant	$115,390
Physician/surgeon	$208,000
Podiatrist	$134,300
Psychiatric technician	$35,030
Psychologist	$82,180
Radiation therapist	$86,850
Radiologic technologists and technicians	$61,900
Recreational therapist	$47,710

PROFESSION	MEDIAN YEARLY SALARY
Respiratory therapist	$62,810
Social and human service assistant	$35,960
Social worker	$51,760
Sonographers, diagnostic, medical	$75,920
Speech-language pathologist	$80,480
Surgical technologist	$49,710
Veterinarian	$99,250
Veterinarian technologist or technician	$36,260

Notes: (1) Only salaries of major health professions are shown. Space limitation does not permit the listing of all health and health-related jobs. (2) Earnings vary with education, experience, level of responsibility, performance, industry, amount of unionization, geographic area, specialized services rendered, and whether the practitioner is self-employed or part time. (3) No attempt is made to show variance by specialties. (4) Salaries shown are income averages and change rapidly over time. (5) For details, updates, and data on unlisted health professions, consult the *Additional Information* section for each profession in the chapters.

Use the resources and internet websites where applicable.

Am J Clin Pathol. 2021; 155 (5): 649–673. https://doi.org/10.1093/ajcp/aqaa197 Salary Survey, 2019.

Data from Bureau of Labor Statistics, U.S. Department of Labor. Occupational Outlook Handbook. U.S. Department of Labor; 2020.

APPENDIX B

Sources of Career Information

This appendix is provided for student use from the Bureau of Labor Statistics/U.S. Department of Labor online publications *Occupational Outlook Handbook* and the newsletter *Career Outlook,* also available from the Bureau of Labor Statistics website. Following are several places to begin collecting information on careers and job opportunities.

Like any major decision, selecting a career involves a lot of fact finding. Fortunately, some of the best informational resources are easily accessible. You should assess career guidance materials carefully. Information that seems out of date or that glamorizes an occupation—overstates its earnings or exaggerates the demand for workers, for example—should be evaluated with skepticism. Gathering as much information as possible will help you make a more informed decision. Use many different sources of information including some of the following.

PEOPLE YOU KNOW

One of the best resources can be your friends and family. They may answer some questions about a particular occupation or put you in touch with someone who has experience in the field. This personal networking can be invaluable in evaluating an occupation or an employer. These people will be able to tell you about their specific duties and training as well as what they did or did not like about a job. Your contacts who have worked in an occupation locally also may be able to give you a recommendation and get you in touch with specific employers.

EMPLOYERS

This is the primary source of information on specific jobs. Employers often post lists of job openings and application requirements, including the exact training and experience required, starting wages and benefits, and advancement opportunities and career paths.

INFORMATIONAL INTERVIEWS

People already working in a particular field often are willing to speak with people interested in their field. An informational interview will allow you to get good information from experts in a specific career without the pressure of a job interview. These interviews allow you to determine how a certain career may appeal to you while helping you build a network of personal contacts. Another way to learn more about different careers and work settings is to volunteer in a hospital, clinic, diagnostic or research laboratory, or community agency.

PROFESSIONAL SOCIETIES, TRADE GROUPS, AND LABOR UNIONS

These groups have information on an occupation or various related occupations with which they are associated or actively represent, such as training requirements, earnings, and listings of local employers. These groups may train members, or they may be able to put you in contact with organizations or individuals who perform such training. One valuable source for finding organizations associated with occupations is the *Encyclopedia of Associations*, a publication that lists trade associations, professional societies, labor unions, and other organizations. Professional organizations are also listed at the end of each chapter in this text for each health profession.

GUIDANCE AND CAREER COUNSELORS

Counselors can help you make choices about which careers might suit you best. They can help you establish what occupations suit your skills by testing your aptitude for various types of work and determining your strengths and interests. Counselors can help you evaluate your options and search for a job in your field, or help you select a new field altogether. They can also help you determine which educational or training institutions best fit your goals and then assist you in finding ways to finance them. Some counselors offer other services such as interview coaching, résumé building, and help in filling out various forms. Counselors in secondary schools and postsecondary institutions may arrange guest speakers, field trips, or job fairs.

You can find guidance and career counselors at many institutions, including:

- High school guidance offices
- College career planning and placement offices
- Placement offices in private vocational or technical schools and institutions
- Vocational rehabilitation agencies
- Counseling services offered by community organizations
- Private counseling agencies and private practices
- State employment service offices

When using a private counselor, check to see that the counselor is experienced. One way to do so is to ask people who have used the counselor's services in the past. Counselors affiliated with high schools, colleges, and state employment services usually do not charge for services. However, private counseling agencies and counselors in private practice typically charge a fee. The National Board of Certified Counselors and Affiliates is an institution that accredits career counselors. To verify the credentials of a career counselor and to find a career counselor in your area, contact:

- National Board for Certified Counselor and Affiliates, 3 Terrace Way, Greensboro, NC 27403. https://www.nbcc.org/

POSTSECONDARY INSTITUTIONS

Colleges, universities, and other postsecondary institutions typically put a lot of effort into helping place their graduates in good jobs because the success of their graduates may indicate the quality of their institution and may affect the institution's ability to attract new students. Postsecondary institutions commonly have career centers with libraries of information on different careers, listings of related jobs, and alumni contacts in various professions. Career centers frequently employ career counselors who generally provide their services only to their students and alumni. Career centers can help you build your résumé, find internships that can lead to full-time positions, and tailor your course selection or program to make you a more attractive job applicant.

LOCAL LIBRARIES

Libraries can be an invaluable source of information. Because most areas have libraries, they can be a convenient place to look for information. Also, many libraries provide free access to the internet and e-mail, although many libraries require registering for a time slot for using the internet. Libraries may have information on local and national job openings, potential contacts within occupations or industries, colleges and financial aid, vocational training, individual businesses or careers, and writing résumés. Libraries frequently have subscriptions to various trade magazines that can provide information on occupations and industries. Your local library also may have video materials. These sources often have references to organizations that can provide additional information about training and employment opportunities. Some libraries offer programs to aid in the job search. If you need help getting started or finding a resource, ask your librarian for assistance.

INTERNET RESOURCES

A wide variety of career information is easily accessible on the internet. Many online resources include job listings, résumé posting services, and information on job fairs, training, and local wages. Many employment services offer free, unlimited internet use. Many of the resources listed elsewhere in this section list internet sites that include valuable information on potential careers. No single source contains all information on an occupation, field, or employer; therefore, you will likely need to use a variety of sources.

The website ExploreHealthCareers.org is designed for students interested in health careers. The site provides many resources, for example, exploring career interests with self-administered surveys, applying for college, and financing college. The Career Search section describes numerous health careers with the expected salary and the years of education and/or training required. The website is listed https://explorehealthcareers.org/

Company Websites

Many companies also list job openings on their sites, so search for positions that fit your skills, interests, and experience. Even if there are no current openings that fit your needs, some companies accept résumés or applications to keep on file for when a position does become available.

Job Boards

The internet abounds with sites that host job listings. Many of these sites allow you to upload and submit your résumé to employers electronically. You can also set up an account and include other kinds of information about yourself, such as any certifications. Employers can then search your résumé and contact you when there are job opportunities. Some sites also allow you to set up a list of keywords that describe the types of jobs in which you are interested. These sites will generate an email when there are positions that match your keywords. Some job boards require a paid membership before you can apply for jobs or search all of their listings; however, since many job boards are free, weigh the costs against the benefits of paying for a job board's services.

Social Networking

Keep your social networking profiles current, and be sure that your social media profiles contain only appropriate content that you want prospective employers to see. Use privacy settings to prevent other users from identifying you in photos or tagging your comments. Monitor social networking sites and remove anything that could appear unprofessional. Use these sites to connect with friends, family, and current, former, and potential colleagues who might be helpful to you in your job search.

Also use social networking sites to connect with companies that interest you. Reach out to employees and ask them if they'd be willing to talk to you about their work. Many companies post job listings on their social networking pages. In addition, you may want to join discussion groups related to the industries that interest you, but remember to stay professional in everything you post.

Online Sources from the U.S. Department of Labor

The Bureau of Labor Statistics within the U.S. Department of Labor website includes the *Occupational Outlook Handbook* with information about hundreds of occupations, including what the work is like, educational and training requirements, salaries, and professional organizations (http://www.bls.gov/ooh/). *Career Outlook*, a newsletter found on the Bureau of Labor Statistics website, has a variety of articles about occupations and career planning (http://www.bls.gov/careeroutlook/). The U.S. Department of Labor has a number of other resources, including the following:

- **CareerOneStop** centers offer employment and training opportunities, skills assessments, and job seeking help. http://www.careeronestop.org/
- **mySkills myFuture,** maintained by CareerOneStop, can help you match your past skills and experience with occupations. http://www.myskillsmyfuture.org/
- **Employment and Training Administration** features information about employment and training opportunities, including for veterans. https://www.doleta.gov/
- The **Office of Disability Employment Policy** offers a return-to-work toolkit for employers and for people with a disability. http://www.dol.gov/odep/

- **O*NET** has a database with information about hundreds of occupations. The database is searchable by skills, education level, job outlook, and other keywords. https://www.onetonline.org/
- Your **State Labor Market Information** may have career tools and data specific to your area. http://www.bls.gov/bls/ofolist.htm

RESOURCES FOR SPECIFIC GROUPS

The U.S. Equal Employment Opportunity Commission (EEOC) is responsible for enforcing federal laws that make it illegal to discriminate against a job applicant or an employee because of the person's race, color, religion, sex (including pregnancy), national origin, age (40 or older), disability, or genetic information. The laws apply to all types of work situations, including hiring, firing, promotions, harassment, training, wages, and benefits (http://www.eeoc.gov).

Organizations described in this section provide information designed to help specific groups of people. Consult directories in your library's reference center or a career guidance office for information on additional organizations.

Workers with Disabilities

Information on employment opportunities, transportation, and other considerations for people with a wide variety of disabilities is available from:

- National Organization on Disability, 77 Water Street, 13th Floor, New York, NY 10005. http://www.nod.org/

For information on workplace accommodations for people with disabilities, contact:

- Job Accommodation Network (JAN), P.O. Box 6080, Morgantown, WV 26506. http://www.jan.wvu.edu

Workers Who Are Blind

Information on employment services for the visually impaired can be obtained by contacting:

- American Foundation for the Blind. 1401 South Clark St., Suite 730, Arlington, VA 22202. 1-202-502-7600 https://www.afb.org/research-and-initiatives/employment
- American Printing House for the Blind. Career Connect. 1-800-232-5463 https://aphcareerconnect.org/about/

Older Workers

Internet sites that specialize in supporting the older worker include the following:

- Senior Community Service Employment Program. U.S. Department of Labor. Employment and Training Administration. https://www.dol.gov/agencies/eta/seniors

- AARP. https://www.aarp.org/work/job-search/employer-pledge-companies/?cmp=RDRCT-03ec1060-20200401
- National Council on the Aging, 251 18th St. South, Suite 500, Arlington, VA 22202. http://www.ncoa.org
- Retirement Jobs.com. http://retirementjobs.com/search/
- National Caucus and Center on Black Aging, Inc., 1220 L St. NW, Suite 800, Washington, DC 20005. http://www.ncba-aged.org

Veterans

Contact the nearest regional office of the U.S. Department of Labor's Veterans Employment and Training Service.

- http://www.dol.gov/agencies/vets/

Contact the U.S. Veterans Administration for programs to transition to civilian employment.

- http://www.benefits.va.gov/benefits/
- My Next Move for Veterans. https://www.mynextmove.org/vets/

Women

- Department of Labor, Women's Bureau, 200 Constitution Ave. NW, Room S-3002, Washington, DC 20210. http://www.dol.gov/agencies/wb

OBTAINING JOBS WITH THE FEDERAL GOVERNMENT

Many jobs for healthcare workers and health-related professions are available with the federal government.

Office of Personnel Management

Information on obtaining civilian positions within the federal government is available from the U.S. Office of Personnel Management through USA Jobs, the federal government's official employment information system. Use this resource for locating and applying for job opportunities with the federal government including the Department of Veteran Affairs.

- USA Jobs. https://www.usajobs.gov

The Office of Personnel Management offers programs for students and new graduates to prepare for government positions:

- Pathways for Students and Recent Graduates to Federal Careers. https://www.opm.gov/policy-data-oversight/hiring-information/students-recent-graduates/

Military

The military employs and has information on hundreds of occupations as either an enlisted service member or officer. Information is available on tuition assistance programs, which provide money for school and educational debt repayments. Your local military recruiting office can provide information on military service. Also read "Military Careers" in the *Occupational Outlook Handbook* to learn more about job opportunities in the Armed Forces. You can also find more information on careers in the military at Today's Military: https://www.todaysmilitary.com

APPENDIX C

How to Create an Effective Résumé

Information in this appendix was modified from "Tips for Writing a Federal Resume," U.S. Department of Labor, available at https://www.dol.gov. This discussion offers examples of résumé preparation. The final version of any individual résumé will depend on the job seeker's career plans and choices.

PURPOSE OF A RÉSUMÉ

- Marketing tool—sells YOU!
- Summarizes how your skills and abilities can contribute to the work of a company or other employer.
- Helps you land a job interview.
- Serves as an employer screening tool.

To write the most effective résumé, you need to determine the career field that interests you and research the following:

- The career field you would like to pursue
- Where the jobs are and who is hiring
- What qualifications and credentials you need to attain
- How best to market your qualifications

Tips for an Effective Résumé

- Tailor your résumé to the position to which you apply by customizing the résumé to speak to the position advertised.
- Review the job announcement for key words and use those words and language in your résumé.
- Make your résumé appealable and readable by using a straightforward format, spell checking, and avoiding tables and text-based graphics.

- Highlight job-related skills that fall into any of these categories: self-management (e.g., dependable, resourceful, etc.); functional (e.g., operate equipment, analysis, etc.); or technical (e.g., sales, computer programming, etc.).
- Highlight your accomplishments, your achievements, and results you have met, as long as you are truthful.
- Translate your experiences to align with the mission of the organization to which you are applying.
- Minimize use of technical jargon unless it is addressed in the job announcement.
- Keep to one page until you have 8 to 10 years of experience to place on the résumé.

Helpful Hint

Remember that employers frequently use digital tracking systems to sort job applications and these systems depend on keywords. You should understand how to find these keywords and use them to your advantage in your résumé. Look to the job description itself for guidance on the keywords contained in it. You can create a word cloud from the job description, using free software such as Wordle.net. Once the keywords are known, employ them in your résumé and cover letter as appropriate.

Chronological Format

- Focuses on your work history with most recent position first.
- Allows potential employers to follow your career history and career progression easily.

- Applies well in situations where you plan to continue in the same line of work.

Functional Format

- Focuses on your skills and experience; skills are grouped into functional areas.
- Used most often when changing careers, to address employment gaps, or when you don't have a lengthy work history.

Combination Format

- Combines the chronological and functional résumé formats.
- Highlights skills while providing the chronological work history that some employers prefer.
- Offers the most comprehensive view of your career to date.

Targeted Format

- Customized to a specific job.
- Written specifically to the employer's needs.

The résumé's objective statement is important and must refer specifically to the position sought. The résumé will then be directed to the appropriate company personnel. There are other, more specialized résumé formats, but they will not be discussed here.

RÉSUMÉ COMPARISON

One can evaluate the appropriateness of each of the four types of résumé formats by studying the comparison chart in **FIGURE C.4**. Only a few of the many aspects of preparing a suitable résumé are discussed here. For more details, major reference sources are:

- The original U.S. Department of Labor document mentioned at the beginning of this appendix.
- The career development centers located in most educational institutions, including high schools, colleges, and universities.
- Public library resources devoted to jobs and careers.

RÉSUMÉ FORMATS

The four major résumé formats to choose from are:

1. Chronological (see **FIGURE C.1**)
2. Functional (see **FIGURE C.2**)
3. Combination (see **FIGURE C.3**)
4. Targeted (see **FIGURE C.4**)

Joe Dough
2345 Brook Avenue, Englewood, Colorado 12345
(123) 456-7890
Joe.Dough@email.com

OBJECTIVE: Seeking a position as an armed security guard for Pinkerton Services

KEY QUALIFICATIONS

• Top Secret Clearance	• Security	• Instruction
• Bilingual English/Spanish	• Conflict Resolution	• Leadership
• Management	• Operations	• Procurement

EXPERIENCE

20XX–present Security Specialist U.S. Marine Corps

- Supervised security for $100 million of highly sensitive equipment resulting in zero loss in a 3-year period.
- Implemented new system security plan that led to increased lockdown protection for incarcerated personnel.
- Provided leadership of 25 personnel ensuring in a 30% decrease in staff turnover and a 10% increase in promotions.
- Expertly managed development of investigative reports – recognized as Supervisor of the Quarter for efficiency and accuracy of written instructions and documents.
- Communicated effectively with diverse populations; efficiently managed a diverse workforce and inmate population resulting in a 10% decrease in inmate violence.

20XX–20XX Warehouse Supervisor Micro Chemical, Inc., Denver, CO

- Supervised a crew of 15 in daily operations, including evaluation and discipline resulting in a company-record promotion rate for staff.
- Monitored complex cataloging and ordering systems by implementing a fast-track procurement system decreasing supply turnaround by 20%.
- Proficient at using Windows 7, Microsoft Office, and PeopleSoft Databases.

20XX–20XX Security Guard Mayfield Mall, Denver, CO

- Coordinated work assignments for a four member security team by boosting morale and encouraging an innovative and safe working environment.

EDUCATION

- U.S. Marine Corps Security Specialist
- Metro State College – 42 Semester Units in Administration of Justice, Denver, CO

FIGURE C.1 Chronological.

Joe Dough
2345 Brook Avenue, Englewood, Colorado 12345
(123) 456-7890
Joe.Dough@email.com

SUMMARY

Provides leadership, instruction, and supervision of 25 personnel. Decreased staff turnover by 30% and increased staff promotions by 10%. Consistently recognized for excellent leadership.

KEY QUALIFICATIONS

- Top Secret Clearance
- Bilingual English/Spanish
- Management

- Security
- Conflict Resolution
- Operations

- Instruction
- Leadership
- Procurement

EXPERIENCE

Security

- Supervised security for $100 million of highly sensitive equipment resulting in zero loss in a 3-year period.
- Implemented new system security plan that led to increased lockdown protection for incarcerated personnel.

Investigation

- Investigated security and safety violations and wrote detailed incident reports – led to Mayfield Mall being recognized as the "Safest Shopping Facility in the Mountain States."
- Expertly managed development of investigative reports – recognized as Supervisor of the Quarter for efficiency and accuracy of written instructions and documents.

Communication

- Communicated effectively with diverse populations; efficiently managed a diverse workforce and inmate population resulting in a 10% decrease in inmate violence.
- Proficient at using Windows 7, Microsoft Office, and PeopleSoft Databases.

Supervision

- Provided leadership of 25 personnel ensuring in a 30% decrease in staff turnover and a 10% increase in promotions.

EDUCATION

- U.S. Marine Corps Security Specialist
- Metro State College – 42 Semester Units in Administration of Justice, Denver, CO

FIGURE C.2 Functional.

Joe Dough
2345 Brook Avenue, Englewood, Colorado 12345
(123) 456-7890
Joe.Dough@email.com

SUMMARY

Provides leadership, instruction, and supervision of 25 personnel. Decreased staff turnover by 30% and increased staff promotions by 10%. Consistently recognized for excellent leadership.

KEY QUALIFICATIONS

- Top Secret Clearance
- Bilingual English/Spanish
- Management

- Security
- Conflict Resolution
- Operations

- Instruction
- Leadership
- Procurement

EXPERIENCE

Security

- Supervised security for $100 million of highly sensitive equipment resulting in zero loss in a 3-year period.
- Implemented new system security plan that led to increased lockdown protection for incarcerated personnel.

Investigation

- Investigated security and safety violations and wrote detailed incident reports – led to Mayfield Mall being recognized as the "Safest Shopping Facility in the Mountain States."
- Expertly managed development of investigative reports – recognized as Supervisor of the Quarter for efficiency and accuracy of written instructions and documents.

Communication

- Communicated effectively with diverse populations; efficiently managed a diverse workforce and inmate population resulting in a 10% decrease in inmate violence.
- Proficient at using Windows 7, Microsoft Office, and PeopleSoft Databases.

Supervision

- Provided leadership of 25 personnel ensuring in a 30% decrease in staff turnover and a 10% increase in promotions.

EMPLOYMENT HISTORY

- 20XX-20XX Security Specialist U.S. Marine Corps
- 20XX-20XX Warehouseman Supervisor Micro Chemical, Inc., Denver, CO

EDUCATION

- U.S. Marine Corps Security Specialist
- Metro State College – 42 Semester Units in Administration of Justice, Denver, CO

FIGURE C.3 Combination.

Targeted	Advantages	Disadvantages	Best Used By
Chronological	–Widely used format –Logical flow, easy to read –Showcases growth in skills and responsibility –Easy to prepare	–Emphasizes gaps in employment –Not suitable if you have no work history –Highlights frequent job changes –Emphasizes employment but not skill development –Emphasizes lack of related experience and career changes	–Individuals with steady work record
Functional	–Emphasizes skills rather than employment –Organizes a variety of experience (paid and unpaid work, other activities) –Disguises gaps in work record or a series of short–term jobs	–Viewed with suspicion by employers due to lack of information about specific employers and dates	–Individuals who have developed skills from other than documented employment and who may be changing careers –Individuals with no previous employment –Individuals with gaps in employment –Frequent job changers
Combination	–Highlights most relevant skills and accomplish-ments –De–emphasizes employment history in less relevant jobs –Combines skills developed in a variety of jobs or other activities –Minimizes drawbacks such as employment gaps and absence of directly related experience	–Confusing if not well organized –De–emphasizes job tasks, responsibilities –Requires more effort and creativity to prepare	–Career changers or those in transition –Individuals reentering the job market after some absence –Individuals who have grown in skills and responsibility –Individuals pursuing the same or similar work as they've had in the past

FIGURE C.4 Targeted Résumé Comparison Chart.

APPENDIX D

Infection Control

OVERVIEW OF INFECTION CONTROL

Students in the health professions are expected to be familiar with infection control practices during their clinical rotations. A review of this appendix plus orientation at the clinical site will prepare students to follow infection control procedures. Also, a poster with specific infection control procedures is usually posted on the patient's or resident's door in hospitals and skilled nursing facilities. In addition, many educational programs require that students receive the same immunizations that are required by state law for healthcare workers before beginning clinical rotations. These include vaccinations for hepatitis B; influenza; chickenpox; measles, mumps, and Rubella (MMR), tetanus, diphtheria, and pertussis or whooping cough (Tdap).

Infection control practices are necessary for all who work in health care regardless of the setting: doctor's office, dentist's office, outpatient clinic, hospital, surgical suite, home care, or skilled nursing facility. Consistent infection control practices prevent the spread of infection between healthcare workers and patients and among patients. The term **universal precautions** has been used in the past to prevent contact with infectious agents present in the blood of asymptomatic patients with bloodborne infections—for example, human immunodeficiency virus (HIV) or hepatitis B or C virus. The Centers for Disease Control and Prevention (CDC) now recommends using a more universal term, **standard precautions**, to include all body fluids that may contain transmissible infectious agents—for example, secretions from the respiratory tract and excretions from the urinary and digestive tracts.

Staff from the environmental services/housekeeping department in hospitals, skilled nursing facilities, and outpatient clinics are responsible for thoroughly **cleaning and sanitizing** patient/resident rooms and examination and treatment rooms as well as common areas including the inside of elevators and the lobby. **Environmental services** staff are also responsible for cleaning a room after a patient or resident is discharged from the facility. However, staff providing direct patient care including nursing staff are responsible for **cleaning and sanitizing** patient care equipment such as a blood pressure cuff and tray tables or countertops after dressing a wound or inserting a urinary catheter. Hospitals, surgery centers, dental clinics, and outpatient clinics also use special ovens to **sterilize** surgical instruments after each use.

Each healthcare facility has designated staff members responsible for developing infection control policies and procedures, educating employees, and monitoring practices within the facility. Hospitals typically have an infection control committee represented by staff from various departments within the hospital. Nursing homes and other long-term care facilities should also have a working committee represented by environmental services, nursing, and other departments within the facility. In order to track infectious outbreaks in institutions and communities, hospitals and nursing homes monitor infectious outbreaks and report to the city and state health departments, who report individual cases to the CDC. Physicians are also responsible for reporting individual cases to the city and state health departments.

In addition to standard precautions, there are specific precautions for preventing infections from microorganisms transmitted by (1) direct or indirect contact with body fluids, (2) respiratory droplets, and (3) respiratory droplets that are airborne. The designated terms for these precautions are contact precautions, droplet precautions, and airborne precautions. This appendix summarizes common infectious diseases that can be transmitted by each method and precautions to prevent the transmission of these diseases.

Additional resources and a glossary with definitions and/or further explanations to facilitate understanding infection control terms are included in this appendix.

STANDARD PRECAUTIONS FOR ALL PATIENT CARE

1. Perform **hand hygiene** (**FIGURE D.1**).[1]
2. Use **personal protective equipment (PPE)** whenever there is an expectation of possible exposure to infectious material.[1]
3. Follow **respiratory hygiene**/cough etiquette principles (**FIGURE D.2**).[1]
4. Properly handle and properly **clean and disinfect** patient care equipment and instruments/devices.[1]
5. Follow safe injection practices.[1]
6. Ensure healthcare worker safety including proper handling of needles and other sharps.[1]

HOW INFECTIONS SPREAD

Germs are a part of everyday life and are found in our air, soil, and water and in and on our bodies. Some germs are helpful; others are harmful. Many germs live in and on our bodies without causing harm, and some even help us stay healthy. Only a small portion of germs are known to cause infection.

HOW DO INFECTIONS OCCUR?

An infection occurs when pathogenic organisms or germs enter the body, increase in number, and cause a response or infection in the body. An infectious agent or germ refers to a virus, bacteria, fungus, or protozoa that can cause an illness.[2] The most common infectious agents in healthcare settings are viruses and bacteria. Three things are necessary for an infection to occur:

- Source: places and persons where infectious agents (germs) live (e.g., sinks, surfaces, human skin, and digestive tract[2])

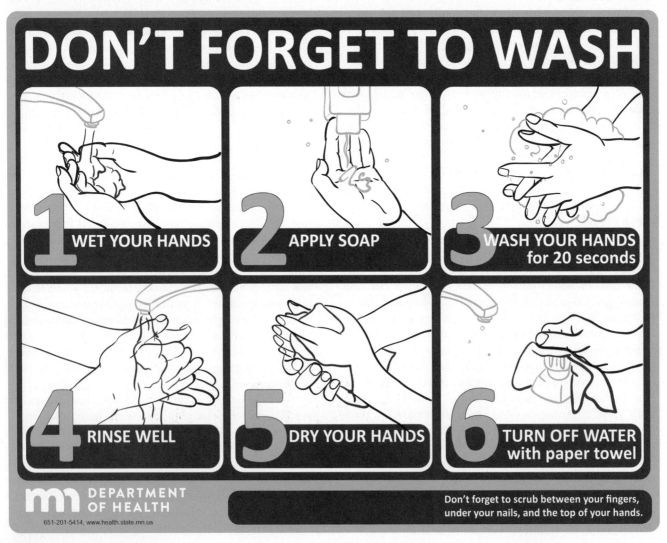

FIGURE D.1 Proper hand hygiene.
Reproduced from Minnesota Department of Health. Don't Forget to Wash. m Department of Health; n.d. https://www.health.state.mn.us/people/handhygiene/wash/dontforget.html

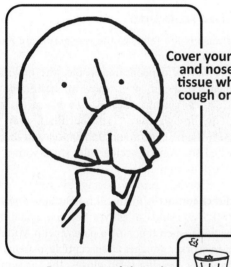
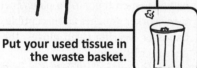
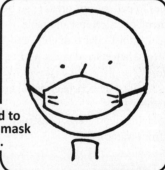
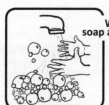
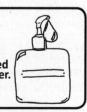

FIGURE D.2 Respiratory hygiene.

Reproduced from Minnesota Department of Health. Cover Your Cough. m Department of Health; n.d. https://www.health.state.mn.us/people/cyc/hcpposter.html

- Susceptible: a person at risk for developing an infection if exposed to a cold virus or bacterial pneumonia because of age, disease, or medical treatment[2]
- Transmission: a way germs are moved to the susceptible person[2]

Sources

A source is an infectious agent or germ and refers to a virus, bacteria, or another microbe such as a fungus that causes illness.

People

In healthcare settings, germs are found in many places. People are one source of germs including:

- Patients
- Healthcare workers
- Visitors and household members

People can be sick with symptoms of an infection or **colonized** with germs (not have symptoms of an infection but able to pass the germs to others).[2] For example, the respiratory tract of a person may be colonized several days before the person shows any symptoms (fever, cough, sore throat), and the disease can be transmitted to a coworker, who also becomes ill.[2]

Environmental Source

Germs are also found in the healthcare environment. Examples of environmental sources of germs include:

- Dry surfaces in patient care areas (e.g., bed rails, medical equipment, countertops, and tables)[2]
- Wet surfaces, moist environments, and biofilms (e.g., cooling towers, faucets and sinks, and equipment such as ventilators)[2]
- Indwelling medical devices [e.g., catheters and intravenous (IV) lines][2]
- Dust or decaying debris (e.g., construction dust or wet materials from water leaks)[2]

Susceptible Person

A **susceptible** person is someone who is not vaccinated or otherwise immune or a person with a weakened immune system at high risk of becoming infected. For an infection to occur, germs must enter a susceptible person's body and invade tissues, multiply, and cause a response. Individuals are susceptible under the following conditions:

- When patients are sick and receive medical treatment in healthcare facilities, the following factors can increase their susceptibility to infection:
  - Underlying medical conditions: Patients in health care who have underlying medical conditions such as diabetes, cancer, or HIV are **immunocompromised** and at increased risk for infection because these illnesses decrease the immune system's ability to fight infection.[2]

  - Certain medications used to treat medical conditions, such as antibiotics, steroids, and certain cancer medications, and drugs used to prevent rejection of a transplanted organ (kidney, liver) increase the risk of some types of infections. Patients receiving these medications are considered **immunosuppressed** because the medications suppress normal functioning of the immune system.[2]
  - Common devices and procedures used in health care such as urinary catheters, IV tubes, and surgery provide a way for germs to enter the body and increase the risk of infection.[2]

Recognizing the factors that increase patients' susceptibility to infection allows healthcare workers to recognize risks and perform basic infection prevention measures to prevent infection from occurring.

Transmission

Transmission refers to the way germs are moved to the susceptible person.

Germs depend on people, the environment, and/or medical equipment to move in healthcare settings. There are a few general ways that germs travel in healthcare settings: through contact (i.e., touching), sprays and splashes of body fluids or secretions, inhalation, and sharps injuries (i.e., when someone is accidentally stuck with a used needle or sharp instrument).[2]

Contact moves germs by touch. An example of **direct contact** is methicillin-resistant *Staphylococcus aureus* (MRSA). Hands or gloves become contaminated with the bacteria when touching a patient with MRSA; if the healthcare worker touches a susceptible patient before washing hands or wearing clean gloves, the susceptible patient can develop MRSA.[2]

In an example of **indirect contact**, the healthcare provider's hands become contaminated by touching germs present on medical equipment or high-touch surfaces, and the provider then carries the germs on their hands and spreads them to a susceptible person when proper **hand hygiene** is not performed before touching the susceptible person.

Sprays and splashes occur when an infected person coughs or sneezes, creating droplets that carry germs short distances (within approximately 6 feet), although the germs do not survive in the air for extended periods of time. These germs can land on a susceptible person's eyes, nose, or mouth and can cause infection—for example, pertussis (whooping cough) or meningitis. Using proper **respiratory hygiene** can prevent droplet infections.[2]

Inhalation occurs when germs are aerosolized in tiny particles that survive on air currents over great distances and time and reach a susceptible person. Airborne transmission can occur when infected patients cough, talk, or sneeze germs into the air—for example, tuberculosis (TB) or measles—or when germs are aerosolized by medical equipment or by dust from a construction zone—for example, nontuberculous mycobacteria (fungus found in soil) or aspergillus (fungus found in mold). The bacteria that cause TB can travel more than 6 feet and remain in the air for several hours after someone infected with the disease coughs or sneezes. If a healthcare worker forgets to wear an N-95 mask when caring for a patient with active TB, they can become exposed to the bacteria that cause TB (*Mycobacterium tuberculosis*) and become infected with TB.[2]

Sharps injuries can lead to infections—for example, Human Immunodeficiency Virus (HIV), hepatitis B virus (HBV), and hepatitis C virus (HCV). Infection can occur when bloodborne pathogens enter a healthcare worker through a skin punctured by a used needle or sharp instrument used on a patient.[2]

CONTACT PRECAUTIONS

Use **contact precautions** (FIGURE D.3) for patients with known or suspected infections that represent an increased

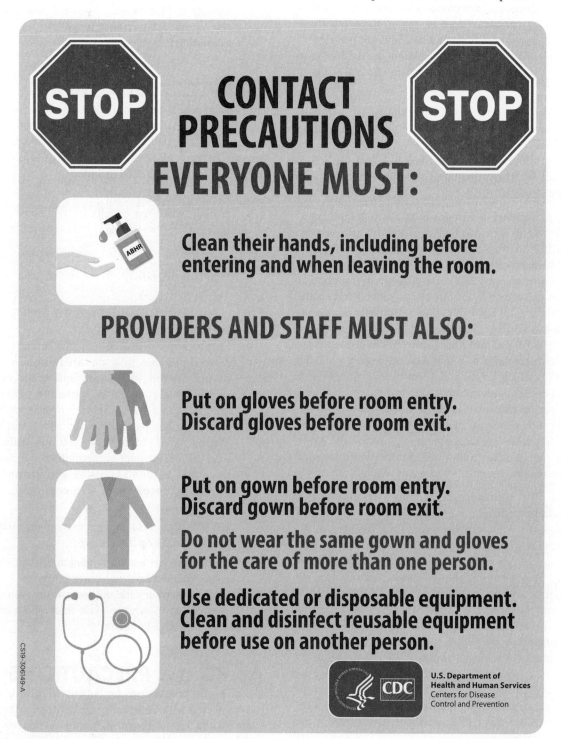

FIGURE D.3 Contact precautions.

Reproduced from Centers for Disease Control and Prevention, U.S. Department of Health and Human Services. Contact Precautions. Centers for Disease Control and Prevention; n.d. https://www.cdc.gov/infectioncontrol/pdf/contact-precautions-sign-P.pdf

risk for contact transmission. Contact precautions are used when germs (virus or bacteria) are spread by directly touching the patient or touching items that have been in contact with the patient.[3]

Direct contact involves body-surface to body-surface contact and physical transfer of microorganisms between a susceptible person (host) and an infected or colonized person.

Contact precautions are indicated for persons with gastrointestinal illness with symptoms of vomiting and diarrhea and incontinent persons (stool or urine), including those who use incontinent products such as diapers or pads.

Examples of when contact precautions are used:

- Stool incontinence
- Draining wounds
- Uncontrolled secretions (nasal or oral)
- Pressure ulcers
- Generalized skin rash
- Patient with **bowel ostomy** tubes
- Patient with bags draining body fluids—for example, urine

Examples of bacterial infections spread through direct contact are someone with methicillin-resistant *Staphylococcus aureus* (MRSA) of the skin or a wound or contact with stool, urine, or urinary catheter for someone with vancomycin-resistant *Enterococcus* (VRE). Overuse of the antibiotics methicillin and vancomycin can cause bacteria to become resistant to the antibiotics, requiring substituting an alternative antibiotic.[3]

Examples of viral infections caused by direct contact are nasal or oral secretions as a source of respiratory syncytial virus (RSV), which causes a mild respiratory illness with symptoms of the common cold.[3]

Indirect contact involves contact of a susceptible person (host) with a contaminated intermediate object such as bed rails, tray tables, medical equipment, needles, dressings, gloves, or contaminated (unwashed) hands.[3] Recommended precautions to prevent infections through contact are:

1. Use PPE appropriately as shown in **FIGURE D.4**, including gloves and gowns. Wear a gown and gloves for all interactions that may involve contact with the patient or the patient's environment. Donning PPE upon room entry and properly discarding before exiting the patient room are done to contain or prevent the spread of pathogens.[3]
2. Limit transport and movement of patients outside the room for medically necessary purposes. When transport or movement is necessary, cover, contain, or prevent drainage from the infected or colonized areas of the patient's body. Remove and dispose of contaminated PPE and perform hand hygiene before transporting patients on contact precautions. Don clean PPE to handle the patient at the transport location.[3]

3. Use disposable or dedicated patient-care equipment (e.g., blood pressure cuffs). If common use of equipment for multiple patients is unavoidable, clean and disinfect such equipment before use on another patient.[3]
4. Prioritize cleaning and disinfection of the rooms of patients on contact precautions, ensuring rooms are frequently cleaned and disinfected (e.g., at least daily or before use by another patient if in an outpatient setting) and focusing on frequently touched surfaces and equipment such as tray tables, countertops, and examining tables.

DROPLET PRECAUTIONS

Use **droplet precautions** for patients known or suspected to be infected with pathogens transmitted by respiratory droplets that are generated by a patient who is coughing, sneezing, or talking (**FIGURE D.5**). Examples of infections when droplet precautions are used include:

- COVID-19 (coronavirus)
- Pertussis (whooping cough)
- Influenza
- Diphtheria
- Pneumonia
- Meningitis (bacterial)[3]

1. Source control: Put a mask on the patient when providing care.[3]
2. Ensure appropriate patient placement in a single room if possible. In acute care hospitals, use single rooms. In long-term care and other residential settings, make decisions regarding patient placement on a case-by-case basis, considering infection risks to other patients in the room and available alternatives. In ambulatory settings, place patients who require droplet precautions in an exam room or cubicle as soon as possible and instruct patients to follow **respiratory hygiene**/cough etiquette recommendations.[3]
3. Use PPE appropriately. Don mask upon entry into the patient room or patient space.[3]
4. Limit transport and movement of patients outside the room for medically necessary purposes. If transport or movement outside the room is necessary, instruct the patient to wear a mask and follow respiratory hygiene/cough etiquette.[3]

AIRBORNE PRECAUTIONS

Use **airborne precautions** for patients known or suspected to be infected with pathogens transmitted by the airborne route (**FIGURE D.6**). Airborne germs are carried in very small droplets through the air when an infected person coughs,

SEQUENCE FOR PUTTING ON
PERSONAL PROTECTIVE EQUIPMENT (PPE)

The type of PPE used will vary based on the level of precautions required, such as standard and contact, droplet or airborne infection isolation precautions. The procedure for putting on and removing PPE should be tailored to the specific type of PPE.

1. GOWN

- Fully cover torso from neck to knees, arms to end of wrists, and wrap around the back
- Fasten in back of neck and waist

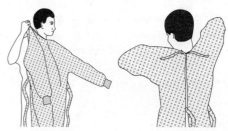

2. MASK OR RESPIRATOR

- Secure ties or elastic bands at middle of head and neck
- Fit flexible band to nose bridge
- Fit snug to face and below chin
- Fit-check respirator

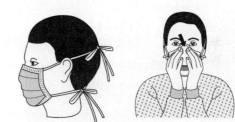

3. GOGGLES OR FACE SHIELD

- Place over face and eyes and adjust to fit

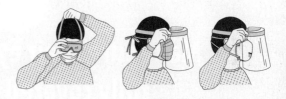

4. GLOVES

- Extend to cover wrist of isolation gown

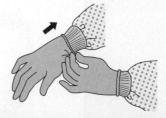

USE SAFE WORK PRACTICES TO PROTECT YOURSELF
AND LIMIT THE SPREAD OF CONTAMINATION

- Keep hands away from face
- Limit surfaces touched
- Change gloves when torn or heavily contaminated
- Perform hand hygiene

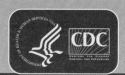

CS250672-E

FIGURE D.4 The proper sequence of putting on personal protective equipment (PPE).

Reproduced from Centers for Disease Control and Prevention. Sequence for Putting on Personal Protective Equipment (PPE). Centers for Disease Control and Prevention; n.d. https://www.cdc.gov/niosh/npptl/pdfs/PPE-Sequence-508.pdf

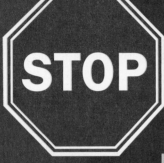
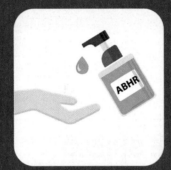
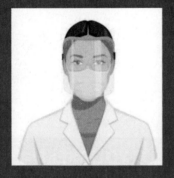
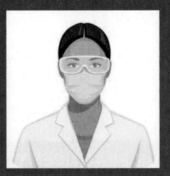
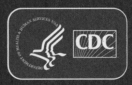

FIGURE D.5 Droplet precautions.

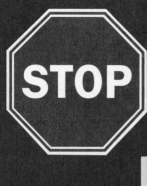
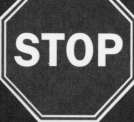
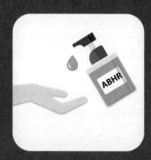
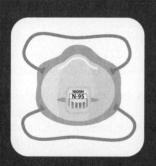
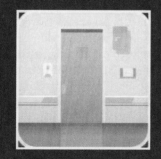
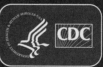

AIRBORNE PRECAUTIONS

STOP **STOP**

EVERYONE MUST:

Clean their hands, including before entering and when leaving the room.

Put on a fit-tested N-95 or higher level respirator before room entry.

Remove respirator after exiting the room and closing the door.

Door to room must remain closed.

U.S. Department of
Health and Human Services
Centers for Disease
Control and Prevention

CS19-306149-A

FIGURE D.6 Airborne precautions.

Reproduced from Centers for Disease Control and Prevention, U.S. Department of Health and Human Services. Airborne Precautions. Centers for Disease Control and Prevention; n.d. https://www.cdc.gov/infectioncontrol/pdf/airborne-precautions-sign-P.pdf

sneezes, or talks. The droplets can remain suspended in the air for several hours and travel more than 6 feet in distance.[3] Examples of when airborne precautions are used:

- Tuberculosis
- Measles
- Chickenpox
- Disseminated or widespread herpes zoster (shingles)

Recommended precautions for preventing airborne infections are:

1. Source control: Put a mask on the patient when providing care.[3]

2. Ensure appropriate patient placement in an **airborne infection isolation room (AIIR)** constructed according to the guideline for isolation precautions. Air pressure in the AIIR is lower than the air pressure outside the AIIR, which prevents movement of contaminated air from the AIIR to other parts of the hospital.[3]

3. In settings where airborne precautions cannot be implemented due to limited engineering resources, masking the patient and placing the patient in a private room with the door closed will reduce the likelihood of airborne transmission until the patient is either transferred to a facility with an AIIR or returned home.

4. Restrict susceptible healthcare personnel from entering the room of patients known or suspected to have tuberculosis, measles, chickenpox, or disseminated zoster (shingles) if other immune healthcare personnel are available.[3]

5. Use personal PPE appropriately, including a **National Institute for Occupational Safety and Health (NIOSH)-approved N95 respirator** (face mask) that filters out 95% of airborne particles. The mask should be fitted to the individual to prevent gaps that would allow airborne particles to enter around the mask.

6. Limit transport and movement of patients outside the room for medically necessary purposes. If transport or movement outside an AIIR is necessary, instruct patients to wear a surgical mask, if possible, and observe respiratory hygiene/cough etiquette. Healthcare personnel transporting patients who are on airborne precautions do not need to wear a mask or respirator during transport if the patient is wearing a mask and infectious skin lesions are covered.[3]

7. Immunize susceptible persons as soon as possible following unprotected contact with vaccine-preventable infections (e.g., measles or chickenpox).[3]

Glossary

Airborne precautions Precautions followed to prevent transmission of infectious disease when the germ causing the disease is spread primarily through the air. Germs that can spread through the air cause tuberculosis, chickenpox, measles, and herpes zoster. Precautions for the healthcare worker are to wear personal protective equipment (PPE) (N-95 mask, gown, and gloves) and to ask the patient to wear a mask when providing care. Vaccinating individuals exposed to the germs previously listed will prevent the disease. Childhood immunizations for chickenpox and measles and adult immunizations for herpes zoster are public health programs in the United States to prevent these infectious diseases.

Airborne infection isolation room (AIIR) Rooms designed to prevent the spread of droplets expelled by a patient with tuberculosis or other diseases transmitted by germs that travel through the air. The room has negative pressure (compared to the rest of the hospital), which prevents contaminated air from moving into the hallway or other rooms.

Bowel ostomy An opening on the outside surface of the abdomen from the intestinal tract. The ostomy is formed when part of the small bowel or large bowel is surgically removed because of disease. The ostomy allows stool to empty into a bag attached to the ostomy site.

Cleaning Removing soiled material from countertops, examining tables, medical equipment and tools, patient rooms and examining rooms, and common areas in a hospital or nursing home facility with soap and water to remove any visible material.

Colonization The presence of microorganisms (virus or bacteria) on the skin or in the respiratory, digestive, or urinary tract of a person who has no symptoms of a disease; however, someone who is colonized can transmit the microorganism to a susceptible person who then develops an infectious disease.

Contact precautions Precautions used when germs (virus or bacteria) are spread by directly touching the patient or touching items that have been in contact with the patient. Precautions are used in patients with gastrointestinal illness, incontinent persons (stool or urine), or those with a skin rash or open wounds. Precautions include wearing personal protective equipment (PPE), including a mask, gown, and gloves.

Direct contact Contact between the gloved hands of the healthcare worker and contaminated skin or wound, contaminated stool or urine, colostomy bag, urinary catheter, or used continence products. Transmission of infectious disease by contact can be prevented by wearing gloves when caring for patients and disposing of dirty gloves properly to prevent the transfer of germs from the infected patient to equipment, solid surfaces, or other patients or healthcare workers.

Droplet precautions Precautions used for patients known or suspected to be infected with pathogens transmitted by respiratory droplets that are generated by a patient who is coughing, sneezing, or talking. Droplets are a source of viral infection—for example, coronavirus, whooping cough, influenza, bacterial diphtheria, meningitis, and viral or bacterial pneumonia. Immunizations are available to prevent all of these diseases.

Environmental cleaning Cleaning areas in healthcare settings to prevent healthcare-acquired infections; cleaning and sanitizing equipment and surface areas after each use, before and after surgical, dental, or treatment procedures, and in the hospital or clinic rooms between patients.

Hand hygiene Washing hands with soap and water before and after treating a patient and after removing gloves to prevent the transmission of germs that cause infection between patients and between healthcare workers and patients. Also, the use of an alcohol-based sanitizer before touching a patient, before performing a procedure—for example, pulling a tooth—or after moving from a soiled patient site (open wound) to a clean patient site (inserting a urinary catheter).

Healthcare-associated infections (HAI) Infections that occur as a result of providing health care to a patient—for example, catheter-associated urinary tract infections, surgical site infections, bloodstream infections, pneumonia, and gastrointestinal infections.

Immunocompromised Individuals with weakened immune systems that are therefore unable to fight infections. Caused by disease—for example, HIV/AIDs, diabetes, or cancer.

Immunosuppressed Caused by medications used to treat medical conditions including antibiotics, steroids, certain cancer medications, and those prescribed after an organ transplant (kidney, liver, heart) or stem cell transplant. These medications/treatments suppress the immune system and increase the risk for infection.

Indirect contact Making contact with hospital equipment or surfaces such as tray tables, doorknobs, or hospital equipment that has been touched by a healthcare worker who has first touched an open wound or contaminated stool, urine, colostomy bag, or urinary catheter.

Infectious disease Diseases caused by germs (viruses, bacteria, fungi, parasites) that are transmitted from someone who has an infection to a healthy individual. Germs can also be transmitted from insects or animals to people to cause an illness.

National Institute for Occupational Safety and Health (NIOSH)-approved N95 Mask worn by healthcare professionals when caring for someone with an infection requiring airborne precautions—for example, tuberculosis (TB). The mask blocks entry of 95% of particles when worn correctly.

Personal protective equipment (PPE) Worn by healthcare workers when providing care for a patient with infectious disease; includes a mask, gown, gloves, and sometimes goggles.

Respiratory hygiene Procedures used in the community or a healthcare setting to prevent the transmission of all respiratory infections (common cold, influenza, coronavirus). Procedures are (1) covering the mouth and nose with a tissue when coughing or sneezing, (2) disposing of used tissue after each use in a waste container, and (3) washing hands with soap and water or alcohol-based solution after

disposing of tissue. In a healthcare setting patients with respiratory symptoms may be asked to wear a mask during clinic visits.

Sanitize Using approved disinfecting solutions and procedures to sanitize medical equipment and tools, patient or resident rooms, or examining rooms after use, especially by patients or residents with a known infection. Sanitizing will destroy nearly all pathogenic organisms that can cause infections transmitted between healthcare workers and patients.

Sterilize The final step after cleaning medical equipment and tools used for medical or dental treatment or surgery before the equipment or tools are reused. An example is an autoclave or special oven that uses steam heat under high pressure to destroy all pathogenic organisms (viruses, bacteria, fungus).

Susceptible Individuals at risk for developing an infectious disease because of a weakened immune system. Those over 65 years of age, those with chronic diseases (diabetes or cancer), or those taking medications to suppress the immune system—for example, after an organ transplant—are at risk for developing an infectious disease if exposed to the germ that causes the disease.

INTERNET RESOURCES ON INFECTION CONTROL

Many resources on infection control are available from the Centers for Disease Control and Prevention (CDC) within the U.S. Department of Health and Human Services. Many can be used for self-study.

For information about state laws requiring vaccination for healthcare workers:

- U.S. Department of Health and Human Services. Center for State, Tribal, Local, and Territorial Support. Public Health Law Program. *Vaccination Laws.* https://www.cdc.gov/phlp/publications/topic/vaccinationlaws.html

For a list of videos on infection control from the Centers for Disease Control and Prevention:

- Centers for Disease Control and Prevention, National Center for Emerging and Zoonotic Infectious Diseases (NCEZID), Division of Healthcare Quality Promotion (DHQP). *Project Firstline Videos.* https://www.cdc.gov/infectioncontrol/projectfirstline/resources/videos.html

Three- to six-minute YouTube videos from the Centers for Disease Control and Prevention:

These videos cover precautions for COVID-19 but can be applied to many other sources of infection.

- *Episode 1: What's the Goal of Infection Control?* https://www.youtube.com/watch?v=atLgq4fsVvo, May 25, 2021.
- *Episode 3: What's a Virus?* https://www.youtube.com/watch?v=iKfG15U8nVo, May 25, 2021.

- *Episode 6: How Do Viruses Spread from Surfaces to People?* https://www.youtube.com/watch?v=KmyxsnuREGs May 25, 2021.
- *Episode 9: What is Personal Protective Equipment (PPE)?* https://www.youtube.com/watch?v=e-t2yZsEo70 April 26, 2021.
- *Episode 10: Why is Eye Protection Recommended for COVID-19?* https://www.youtube.com/watch?v=kkruNHsMbMY April 26, 2021.
- *Episode 12: Why are Gowns Recommended for COVID-19?* https://www.youtube.com/watch?v=qG70h5MOADM April 26, 2021.
- *Episode 16: Cleaning? Disinfection? What is the Difference?* https://www.youtube.com/watch?v=dIuRI9OpjnY May 25, 2021.
- *Episode 21: Do We Really Have to Talk About Hand Hygiene? Again?* Yes!https://www.youtube.com/watch?v=n1oqVM-N3j8 May 25, 2021

- *Episode 22: Why Does Contact Time Matter for Disinfection?* https://www.youtube.com/watch?v=TCa7Gg1NUD4&t=24s April 16, 2021.
- *Episode 23: What is Source Control?* https://www.youtube.com/watch?v=9C2wwGm_Su4 April 16, 2021.

For a summary of infection control procedures for patients with cancer:

- National Center for Emerging and Zoonotic Infectious Diseases. Division of Healthcare Quality Promotion. *Preventing Infections in Cancer Patients. My Pocket Guide. A Quick Guide to CDC's Basic Infection Control and Prevention Plan for Outpatient Oncology Settings and Patient Education Resources.* https://www.cdc.gov/hai/pdfs/bicapp/cdc_pocketguide_final_508compliant.pdf

References

1. Centers for Disease Control and Prevention. *Standard Precautions for All Patient Care.* https://www.cdc.gov/infectioncontrol/basics/standard-precautions.html Reviewed January 26, 2016. Accessed April 7, 2021.
2. Centers for Disease Control and Prevention. *How Infections Spread.* https://www.cdc.gov/infectioncontrol/spread/index.html Last reviewed January 7, 2016. Accessed March 24, 2021.
3. Centers for Disease Control and Prevention. *Transmission Based Precautions.* https://www.cdc.gov/infectioncontrol/basics/transmission-based-precautions.html Reviewed January 7, 2016. Accessed April 7, 2021.

GLOSSARY

3D printing A manufacturing method whereby three-dimensional objects are quickly made on a machine connected to a computer containing blueprints for the object.

abdominal sonographer Ultrasound technician who specializes in inspecting a patient's abdominal cavity to help diagnose and treat conditions.

abuse A pattern of practices or customs that are unsound or inconsistent with ethical business, fiscal, or healthcare practices or customs.

Academy of Nutrition and Dietetics (AND) A professional organization committed to improving the nation's health and advancing the profession of dietetics through research, education, and advocacy.

Academy for Certification of Vision Rehabilitation (ACVREP) Agency that certifies orientation and mobility specialists and vision rehabilitation therapists.

accountable care organization (ACOs) Healthcare delivery model that ties provider reimbursement payment to the quality and cost of care for a patient population—for example, patients on kidney dialysis.

accreditation The process by which an external entity reviews an organization or program of study to determine if the organization or program meets certain predetermined standards.

Accreditation Council for Education in Nutrition and Dietetics (ACEND) A professional organization that offers accreditation for programs in nutrition and dietetics.

Accreditation Council for Genetic Counseling (ACGC) Agency that accredits academic programs in genetic counseling.

ACSM-Certified Clinical Exercise Physiologist (ACSM-CEP) Certified by the American College of Sports Medicine; requires a minimum of a bachelor's degree, 1,200 clinical hours, and completion of an exam.

ACSM-Certified Personal Trainer (CPT) Personal trainer certified by the American College of Sports Medicine.

activities of daily living (ADLs) Set of key capabilities used to evaluate need for personal care assistance for older adults

or disabled persons; includes bathing, dressing, toileting, and self-feeding.

acute infectious disease An illness with sudden onset that has an intense but short effect on the body.

ADA See American Dental Association.

adaptive equipment Special equipment designed to facilitate everyday functioning for patients.

administrative medical assistant A medical assistant who specializes in administrative tasks.

ADN See associate's degree in nursing.

ADN-to-BSN Educational program that allows nurses with an associate's degree in nursing (ADN) to complete a bachelor's degree in nursing (BSN).

ADN-to-MSN Educational program that allows nurses with an associate's degree in nursing (ADN) to enter and complete a master's degree in nursing (MSN).

adult day care services Program for the disabled or elderly who require health and/or support services; used to supplement home care services or a less costly option to being institutionalized.

advance premium tax credit Tax credit that can be used to reduce the cost of health insurance premiums for policies purchased from the Marketplace.

advanced airway devices Devices used to open or maintain a patient's obstructed or injured airway to maintain breathing.

advanced emergency medical technician The third level of a four-tier category of emergency medical technician who provides basic and limited advanced emergency medical care and transportation for critical and emergent patients who access the emergency medical system.

advanced practice registered nurse (APRN) Registered nurse with master's degree training who can serve as a primary care provider; includes nurse anesthetists, nurse midwives, nurse practitioner, and clinical nurse specialists.

aerosol Medications suspended in a gas that forms a mist the patient inhales.

Affordable Care Act (ACA) Healthcare reform legislation signed into law by President Barack Obama in March 2010 with a goal of increasing access to health insurance while controlling healthcare costs.

Aging Network System of federal, state, and local agencies committed to having older Americans live independently in their homes and communities.

alignment The proper form of a body part, such as a spine.

allopathic physician A physician offering medical care using pharmacologically active agents or surgical interventions to treat or suppress symptoms of diseases or injuries.

almshouses Facilities that provided care for the disabled or ill in the 1700s, before hospitals were established.

Alzheimer's disease A degenerative brain disease and the most common form of dementia; early symptoms are a decline in cognitive function that affects memory, language, and problem solving. Later stages require complete care.

ambulatory care Health care provided outside of institutional settings.

American Academy of Family Physicians (AAFP) Professional organization of primary care physicians who provide medical care for all ages. The academy supports family physicians through networking and continuing education and serves as an advocate through state and federal legislation.

American Academy of Nurse Practitioners Certification Program (AANPCB) Agency within the academy that offers specialty certification for nurse practitioners.

American Art Therapy Association (AATA) Professional and educational organization that advocates for the art therapy profession and provides continuing education programming and networking opportunities.

American Association of Colleges of Nursing (AACN) Represents all college and university programs in nursing education. Establishes quality standards and provides assistance in implementation. Promotes public support for professional nursing education, research, and practice.

American Association of Community Colleges (AACC) Advocates for community colleges that confer 2-year, associate degrees in the United States.

American Association for Laboratory Animal Science (AALAS) Agency that offers certification for veterinary technicians who work in animal research laboratories.

American Association of Cardiovascular and Cardiopulmonary Rehabilitation (AACVPR) Multidisciplinary professional association of health professionals in the field of cardiac and pulmonary rehabilitation.

American Board of Clinical Social Work (ABCSW) Administers advanced credentials for clinical social workers as a generalist, clinical supervisor, children/families practitioner, and psychoanalyst.

American Board of Examiners (ABE) Organization that promotes uniform practice standards for education and training and credentialing for clinical social workers.

American Board of Foot and Ankle Surgery (ABFAS) Agency that certifies podiatrists in the field of surgery.

American Board of Genetic Counseling (ABGC) Agency that administers qualifying exams for genetic counselors to become certified.

American Board of Hospice and Palliative Medicine Certifies physicians to practice in hospice and palliative care.

American Board of Industrial Hygiene (ABIH) Administers credentialing of Certified Industrial Hygienists to ensure the safety of workers in the field of industrial hygiene and the families of the workers.

American Board of Medical Specialties (ABMS) Agency that administers qualifying exams to practice in medical specialties—for example, surgery.

American Board of Podiatric Medicine Agency that certifies podiatrists in the field of medicine.

American Board of Veterinary Practitioners (AMVP) Professional organization that promotes excellence in veterinary care; offers certification in 11 specialties within veterinary practice, including beef cattle practice and feline practice.

American College of Nurse-Midwives (ACNM) Agency that accredits graduate programs for nurse-midwives.

American College of Sports Medicine (ACSM) Professional organization that promotes the advancement and integration of scientific research into educational and practical applications of exercise science and sports medicine.

American Dance Therapy Association (ADTA) Professional organization dedicated to the profession of dance/movement therapy.

American Dental Association (ADA) A professional organization that represents dentists nationwide and seeks to address the most important professional and public health issues.

American Hospital Association (AHA) A national industry trade group that supports hospitals, healthcare systems, and health networks as well the communities served.

American Kinesiotherapy Association (AKTA) Professional organization of registered kinesiotherapists that supports and advances the professional standards of kinesiotherapists.

American Medical Association (AMA) A professional medical organization that represents physicians nationwide and seeks to address the most important professional and public health issues.

American Midwifery Certification Board (AMCB) Organization that provides certification for midwives and nurse-midwives. (See certified midwives, certified nurse-midwives.)

American Music Therapy Association (AMTA) Professional organization with a mission to advocate for music therapy as a profession; promotes high quality educational programming, professional standards, credentialing, and research to support music therapy as a profession.

American Nursing Credentialing Center (ANCC) Organization that offers specialty certification for nurses; for example, informatics and cardiac rehabilitation.

American Osteopathic Association (AOA) Accrediting agency for graduates of osteopathic physicians; also administers certifying exams for specialty physicians.

American Physical Therapy Association (APTA) A national professional organization whose goal is to foster advancements in physical therapy practice, research, and education.

American Podiatric Medical Licensing Exam (APMLE) Exam required for graduates of podiatric medicine to practice podiatric medicine.

American Society of Exercise Physiologists (ASEP) Professional organization of exercise physiologists that promotes the profession and sets educational standards.

American Speech-Language-Hearing Association (ASHA) Agency that certifies speech-language pathologists and audiologists.

American Therapeutic Recreation Association (ATRA) Professional organization that represents the interests and needs of therapeutic recreation specialists.

American Veterinary Medical Association (AVMA) Professional organization that advocates for members, accredits educational programs and offers continuing education programs.

Americans with Disabilities Act of 1990 Civil rights law that prohibits discrimination against individuals with disabilities in all areas of public life: jobs, schools, transportation, and all public and private spaces open to the general public.

anatomy The study of the structure of organisms and their parts.

animal and human health Control of diseases transmissible from animals to humans.

Animal and Plant Health Inspection Service (APHIS) Division of the U.S. Department of Agriculture that protects and promotes U.S. agricultural health, including exports.

animal trainer Animal workers who train animals for riding, security, performance, obedience, or assisting people with disabilities.

anorexia nervosa An eating disorder involving a refusal to eat.

applied behavior analysis (ABA) Application of behavioral sciences in schools and clinics to improve behavioral problems and facilitate learning; part of treatment for autism spectrum disorder.

apprenticeship program Combination of on-the-job training and related instruction where workers learn the aspects of a specific occupation.

App Software program ("application") developed to run on a computer or mobile device to accomplish a specific purpose.

Area Agency on Aging (AAA) One of 622 agencies nationwide with the purpose of providing resources and supports for older adults; established in 1973.

Art Therapist (AT) Mental health professional that combines artistic, creative, and psychotherapeutic skills to encourage clients to express emotions through an art medium to promote physical, mental, and emotional health.

Art Therapist Registered-Board Certified (ATR-BC) The highest level of art therapy credential achieved by successfully passing a national examination; completion of graduate-level education in art therapy and clinical experience are required to sit for the exam.

Art Therapy Credentials Board (ATCB) Professional board responsible for ensuring educational and professional standards of registered and board-certified art therapists.

arterial blood sample A blood sample taken from an artery instead of a vein.

artificial intelligence (AI) The use of computers and technology to simulate intelligent behavior and critical thinking; one example of AI is predicting the spread of infectious diseases in a population.

assessment Taking steps to determine the needs of a specific population.

assistant administrator Administrator who manages the day-to-day responsibilities in large companies or facilities.

assisted-living facility Living facility primarily for seniors that provides meals, housekeeping, medication management, and other assistance with daily living activities as needed.

assistive devices Medical equipment designed to help patients with disabilities perform everyday tasks and activities. Also known as protective or preventive devices, including tape, bandages, and braces that athletes or their trainers use to protective, prevent, or avoid injuries during a sport or other form of training that involves the human body.

associate administrator Administrator who manages the day-to-day responsibilities in large companies or facilities.

Associate's Degree in Nursing (ADN) A two-year degree for individuals seeking to become a registered nurse.

Association for Education and Rehabilitation of the Blind and Visually Impaired (AER) Professional organization that provides support for professionals who work with those who are visually impaired.

Association of Nutrition and Foodservice Professionals (ANFP) Nonprofit organization that serves members through advocacy, education, and research; offers credentials for Certified Dietary Managers (CDMs) and Certified Food Protection Professional (CFPP).

Association of Social Work Boards (ASWB) Agency that offers the licensing exam required to practice social work.

athletic trainer A professional who instructs athletes on correct technique and appropriate conditioning to maximize athletic performance while minimizing risk of injury.

Audiologist Professional that works with people who have hearing, balance, and related ear problems.

audiology assistant Provides technical support for audiologists and extends services by completing routine tasks such as setting up and cleaning equipment and completing screening exams.

autism spectrum disorders (ASD) Group of developmental disabilities that can cause significant social, communication, and behavioral challenges.

automated analyzer Laboratory equipment that automatically prepares, measures, and reports content of body fluids or cells.

automated external defibrillator (AED) Portable device that checks the heart rhythm and restores a normal heart rhythm by sending an electric shock to the heart when the heart suddenly stops beating.

avian (bird) influenza Strains of influenza virus that normally infect birds, including poultry but can sometimes pass to humans.

Bachelor of Science in Nursing (BSN) A four-year degree obtained in order to become a registered nurse.

Bachelor's Degree in Social Work (BSW) Entry-level degree that prepares graduates to work as caseworkers, health educators, and social and human services assistants.

bar coding technology The use of an optical scanner to electronically capture information encoded on a product.

beam modification devices Devices that when kept in the path of a beam produce a desirable modification in the special distribution of the beam.

behavior analyst Specialist in the assessment and treatment of clients with skill deficits in language, motor, social, and reasoning skills.

behavioral disorder counselor A psychotherapist who helps clients modify their behavior in a specific aspect of their life (e.g., compulsive behavior or eating disorders).

behavioral health disorder Includes mental illness and substance use disorders.

behavioral health services Services for those with mental illness or substance use disorders; providers include psychiatrists, psychologists, clinical social workers, behavioral disorder counselors, and psychiatric nurses.

Behavioral Risk Factor Surveillance System (BRFSS) A public health program in which states collect data on behaviors that increase risk for chronic disease. Statistics are reported to the National Center for Health Statistics, a division of the Centers for Disease Control and Prevention (CDC).

Behavior Analysis Certification Board (BACB) Agency that certifies behavior analysts, assistant behavior analysts, and behavior technicians.

behavior therapist Professional who helps individuals to modify their behavior in an aspect of their life. As an example, a behavior therapist may be asked to modify the eating behavior of an obese person.

billing process The method of submitting and following up with claims made to government payers, insurance companies, and patients.

binge-eating disorder An eating disorder involving periods of binge eating that, unlike bulimia, are not followed by compensatory behaviors, such as purging, exercise, or fasting.

biological sciences The study of the branch of knowledge that deals with living organisms and vital processes.

biomedical engineer Person who uses their knowledge of biology, medicine, technology, and mechanical engineering to research and develop new equipment.

birth defects Structural changes in organs or other body parts in infants at birth; surgery may be required to improve function. Common birth defects are structural changes of the heart.

blood bank technologist Identifies blood types, antibodies, and antigens, and tests blood for viruses that could be transmitted during blood transfusions—for example, the human immune deficiency virus (HIV).

blood pH A measure of the acidity or alkalinity level of the blood.

Blue Cross and Blue Shield Private health insurance that covers both inpatient and outpatient services; first insurance plan to cover the cost of physician services in 1939.

Board Certified Specialist in Audiology (BCS-A) Audiologist who has met education and experience requirements and successfully completed the certification exam.

Board Certified Specialist in Child Language and Language Disorders (BCS-CL) Specialized certification for speech therapists in treating children with language differences and disorders.

Board Certified Specialist in Fluency (BCS-F) Specialized certification for speech therapists in treating speech disorders such as stuttering.

Board Certified Specialist in Interoperative Monitoring (BCS-IOM) Advanced specialized training plus the completion of an exam that trains audiologists to monitor the auditory nerve when there is a risk of damage during surgery.

Board Certified Specialist in Swallowing and Swallowing Disorders (BCS-S) Specialty certification for speech therapists who work with individuals with neurological diseases that affect swallowing.

Board Certified Dance/Movement Therapist (BC-DMT) Credential reflects the attainment of an advanced level of dance/movement therapy, including preparation for supervising and training others in the field and engaging in a private practice.

Board-Certified Assistant Behavior Analyst (BCABA) Certification as an assistant behavior analyst with bachelor's-level education who works under the supervision of a certified behavior analyst.

Board-Certified Behavior Analyst (BCBA) Certification as a board analyst with graduate-level education who is qualified to work independently and supervise the work of assistant behavior analysts and registered behavior technicians.

Board-Certified Diplomate in Clinical Social Work (BCD) Advanced generalist certification for clinical social workers.

Board of Certification, Inc. (BOC) Certification program for entry-level athletic trainers.

Board of Certified Safety Professionals (BCSP) Agency that certifies occupational health specialists and technicians.

bone injuries Damage to bone; many bone injuries are most common among athletes in certain sports—for example, injury to wrist bones among tennis players.

breast sonographer Ultrasound technician who specializes in studying diseases of the breast.

BSN See Bachelor of Science in Nursing.

BSW See Bachelor's Degree in Social Work (BSW).

budget The amount of money that is available for, required for, or assigned to a particular purpose.

bulimia nervosa An eating disorder characterized by cyclical binging and purging episodes.

bundling payments Method of controlling healthcare costs by reimbursing Medicare for all services for a procedure—for example, hip replacement surgery and home care after discharge from the hospital.

Bureau of Labor Statistics (BLS) Source of the *Occupational Outlook Handbook* that provides information about broad range of occupations with details about educational requirements, projected need, places of employment, and salaries.

Burwell v. Hobby Lobby, Inc. Supreme court case ruled that closely affiliated corporations opposed to contraceptives are exempt from insurance coverage for contraceptives for female employees.

business dietitian nutritionist Works as a professional resource for corporations in product development, as a sales professional, or as a food and nutrition marketing expert.

cancer registrar Individual who maintains a hospital-based registry of cancer patients.

capitation Paying a fixed amount per person for health services without regard to the volume of services provided.

cardiac rehabilitation program Individualized instruction on physical activity, nutrition, and stress management, especially after a heart attack or open heart surgery.

cardiographic technician Professional who specialize in vascular technology and perform noninvasive tests such as echocardiograms.

cardiology technologist Professional who assists physicians in diagnosing and treating heart and blood vessel ailments.

cardiopulmonary disorders Disease of the heart and /or lungs.

cardiac pulmonary resuscitation (CPR) Training in emergency treatment when someone's heart has stopped beating or someone has stopped breathing; treatment includes clearing of the airway, chest compressions, and rescue breathing.

cardiopulmonary technologist Professional who assists the physician in diagnosing and treating both heart and lung ailments.

cardiovascular invasive specialist Professional who assists physicians in diagnosing and treating heart and blood vessel ailments through the use of invasive procedures.

cardiovascular technician Professional who focuses on performing noninvasive tests such as echocardiograms.

cardiovascular technologist Professional who assists physicians by performing complex medical tests involving the heart and pulmonary system.

career development An organized planning method used to form an individual's work identity.

caregiving The process of providing personal care services for a senior friend or family member who is physically or mentally disabled or is experiencing dementia.

carrier testing Tests used to identify people who "carry" changes in DNA that are linked to disease.

cell counter Automated device used to count cells—for example before and after drug treatment to evaluate the effectiveness of treating an infectious disease.

Center for Medicare and Medicaid Innovation Division of CMS that tests various payment and service delivery models to achieve better health care while lowering costs by improving healthcare systems.

Center for Veterinary Medicine (CVM) Agency within the U.S. Food and Drug Administration (FDA) responsible for drug safety testing for drugs used by food and companion animals.

Centers for Disease Control and Prevention (CDC) Branch of the federal government that tracks the health of the nation and provides support to identify causes of epidemics and foodborne illnesses.

Centers for Medicare and Medicaid Services (CMS) Agency of the U.S. Department of Health and Human Services (HHS) that manages Medicare and Medicaid and strives to ensure effective, up-to-date healthcare coverage and to promote quality care for beneficiaries.

Certificate of Clinical Competence in Audiology (CCC-A) Issued to individuals who present evidence of their ability to provide independent clinical services to patients diagnosed with auditory disorders.

Certificate of Clinical Competence in Speech-Language Pathology (CCC-SLP) Issued to individuals who present evidence of their ability to provide independent clinical services to patients diagnosed with speech or language disorders.

certification The process or action of providing an individual with an official document attesting to their status or level of achievement.

certified athletic trainer Healthcare provider who specialize in prevention, treatment, and rehabilitation of injuries and illnesses in athletes and the physically active.

Certified Audiology Assistant (C-AA) Relatively new profession to support audiologists; postsecondary certification programs are available.

certified cardiac rehabilitation professional (CCRP) A professional who demonstrates knowledge and skills in exercise testing and counseling in nutrition, exercise training, and smoking cessation as well as management of weight, diabetes, blood pressure, and blood lipids.

certified clinical exercise specialist (CES) A professional who demonstrates knowledge and skills in conducting health screening and exercise testing, and evaluating strength and flexibility in healthy clients and those with cardiovascular, pulmonary, and metabolic diseases.

Certified Community Behavioral Health Clinics (CCBHCs) Clinics funded by the U.S. Congress in 2014 to meet the demand for behavioral health services in communities impacted by the opioid crisis and need for more comprehensive services for mental health and substance abuse disorders.

Certified Diabetes Care and Education Specialist (CDCES) Specialty certification for health professionals counseling patients with diabetes; requires experience and exam.

Certified Dietary Manager (CDM) Professional who has received the training and certification to manage a foodservice operation that meet the standards of local, state, and federal regulators.

Certified Hazardous Materials Manager Professional with experience evaluating sites for hazardous contaminants in the air, soil, and water and designing remediation programs.

Certified Health Education Specialist (CHES) Certification for entry-level health educators; eligibility for the certifying exam is a bachelor's degree in public health or health promotion.

Certified Industrial Hygienist (CIH) Certification that recognizes the competency of employees in evaluating health risks to workers in industrial settings.

certified midwife (CM) Practitioners who provide the same services as CNMs but who lack the training and certification of a registered nurse.

certified nurse-midwife (CNM) APRN who provides primary care to women, including gynecological exams, family planning advice, prenatal care, assistance in labor and delivery, and neonatal care.

certified nutrition specialist (CNS) Conferred by Board for Certification of Nutrition Specialists (BCNS); requirements are a graduate degree, clinical experience, and passing of exam.

certified nutrition support clinician (CNSC) Specialty certification conferred by the National Board of Nutrition Support Certification of the American Society for Enteral and Parenteral Nutrition (ASPEN) for health professionals.

Certified Orientation and Mobility Specialist (COMS) Has met education and experience standards and successfully completed the certification exam.

certified personal trainer (CPT) A certificate awarded by the American College of Sports Medicine to those who have successfully completed training in cardiopulmonary resuscitation (CPR) and automated external defibrillation (AED) and passed the certifying exam.

certified registered nurse anesthetist (CRNA) Provides anesthetics to patients in every practice setting, and for every type of surgery or procedure.

Certified Respiratory Therapist (CRT) Credential given to those who graduate from entry-level or advanced programs accredited by CoARC and pass a certifying exam.

Certified Safety Professional (CSP) Occupational health specialist or technician who has met education and/or experience requirements and successfully passed the certification exam.

Certified Speech-Language Pathology Assistant (C-SLPA) Professionals that provide support for speech language pathologists. A relatively new profession since training programs for certified speech language assistants were established in the early 2000s.

Certified Therapeutic Recreation Specialist (CTRS) Health professional qualified to use recreational activities (sports, arts, crafts, dance, music) to reduce stress and improve functioning in those with an illness, injury, or disability.

certified tumor registrar Individual who has met external requirements to maintain a registry of cancer patients.

Certified Vision Rehabilitation Therapist (CVRT) Health professional who has met education and experience requirements and successfully passed the certifying exam.

chest physiotherapy Treatment prescribed after surgery to help return the patient's lungs to their normal level of functioning and prevent the lungs from becoming congested.

chief executive officer (CEO) Professional who provides overall management direction to an organization.

child and family social worker Social worker who provides assistance to improve the social and psychological functioning of children and families.

child or adult protective services social worker Social worker who investigates reports of abuse and neglect and intervenes if necessary.

child welfare social worker Social worker who assesses the well-being of at-risk children and obtains services to protect them if necessary.

Children's Health Insurance Program (CHIP) Health insurance for children from families with incomes too high for Medicaid but too low to afford the cost of premiums for private health insurance.

Chiropractor Primary care professionals who focus on patients' overall health and work to relieve pain, increase mobility, and improve performance. They are sometimes referred to as Doctors of Chiropractic or chiropractic physicians.

chromosomes Contain DNA and unique characteristic passed from parents to offspring.

chronic disease A disease that is long in duration, reoccurs frequently, and progresses slowly.

Civilian Health and Medical Program of the Department of Veterans Affairs (CHAMPVA) Program that provides health care for family members of disabled or deceased member of the military services.

climate change analysts Researchers who analyze policies related to renewable energy and efficiency and make recommendations for legislation.

clinical care Service provided to an individual, group, or community to benefit their health status.

clinical chemistry specialist Technician who specializes in the chemical analysis of body fluids.

clinical decision support systems (CDSS) The variety of technologies that provide healthcare providers with diagnostic and treatment recommendations.

clinical dietitian nutritionist Provides nutritional services for patients in hospitals, nursing homes, clinics, or doctors' offices.

clinical documentation improvement (CDI) specialist Individual responsible for review of the patient's electronic health record and serves as the liaison to the clinical treatment team in documenting clinical care.

Clinical Exercise Physiology Association (CEPA) Affiliate Society of the American College of Sports Medicine (ACSM); promotes the profession of exercise physiologists to employers and supports the application of clinical exercise physiology for individuals at high risk or living with a chronic disease.

Clinical Laboratory Improvement Amendment (CLIA) Federal law to ensure quality standards for laboratory testing of human specimens (blood, body fluid, and tissue); used to diagnose, prevent, or treat disease.

clinical laboratory scientist See clinical laboratory technologist.

clinical laboratory technician Laboratory personnel trained at the associate's degree level; performs laboratory testing in conjunction with clinical laboratory technologists.

clinical laboratory technologist Often have supervisory responsibilities who generally have a bachelor's degree and perform a range of routine tests and laboratory procedures; work in cooperation with pathologists and other physicians.

clinical medical assistant A medical assistant who specializes in providing clinical care to patients.

clinical nurse specialist (CNS) Nurse who provides direct patient care and expert consultations in one of many nursing specialties; master's degree training required.

clinical preventive services Guidelines for primary care providers to use in screening and counseling patients to prevent or reduce the risk of heart disease, cancer, and infectious disease.

clinical psychologist Specializes in the assessment and treatment of persons with mental and emotional problems and illnesses.

clinical social worker (CSW) Provides counseling for clients with behavioral health problems (mental health and substance use disorders).

closely held corporations Companies in which more than 50% of stock in the corporation is owned by five or fewer individuals.

cloud computing The virtualization of servers.

Cochlear Implant Specialty Certification (CISC) American Board of Audiologists certification offered for audiologists with competency in cochlear implant surgery and rehabilitation after surgery.

code of ethics A written list of a profession's values and standards of conduct.

coder An individual who uses various classification systems to code, categorize, and report patient information for multiple purposes.

cognitive skills Competent use of one's intellectual activity (as thinking, reasoning, remembering, imagining, or learning words).

coinsurance The percentage of the cost of medical services paid by the consumer of the total cost of the service. For example, coinsurance for those enrolled in Medicare is 20%.

Commission on Accreditation of Athletic Training Education (CAATE) Accrediting agency for academic programs for athletic trainers.

Commission on Dietetic Registration (CDR) Agency that administers registration of dietitians.

Commissioned Corps Health professionals who work for federal public health services in different agencies within HHS.

Committee on Accreditation for the Exercise Sciences (CoAES) Accrediting agency for academic programs that prepare students for positions in the health, fitness, and exercise industry.

Commission on Accreditation for Respiratory Care (CoARC) Promotes quality respiratory therapy education through accreditation services.

Commission on Accreditation of Allied Health Education Programs (CAAHEP) Largest accrediting body for health science professions; accredits over 2,000 educational programs in 28 health science occupations.

Commission on Massage Therapy Accreditation (CMTA) Accredits both educational institutions and programs offering instruction in massage therapy and bodywork; recognized by the U.S. Department of Education.

communication The sharing of information between two or more people as a way to convey meaning.

communication disorder Disruption in the regular or normal functions of communication.

communication skills A set of skills that enables a person to convey information so it is received and understood.

Community and Social Service Occupations Professionals who work with individuals to assist them in obtaining needed care or services.

community dietitian nutritionist Individual that counsels on sound nutrition practices in settings outside of hospitals or long-term care facilities.

community engagement initiative The Centers for Medicare and Medicaid (CMS) allowed states to target Medicaid recipients to complete work or "work-equivalent" activities such as caregiving or being enrolled as a student as a condition of eligibility for Medicaid.

community health worker (CHW) Provides link between the community and health educators; implements strategies to improve health of individuals and communities.

community hospital Short-term general and specialty hospitals.

Community Mental Health Act Law passed in 1963 to establish Comprehensive Mental Health Centers throughout the United States.

Community Mental Health Centers (CMHC) Established in 1963 to serve the mental health needs in the United States as a result of a movement to deinstitutionalize those with mental illness. However, over time these centers were not adequately funded to meet mental health needs.

companion animal veterinarian Veterinarians who specialize in the care of animals that are considered pets—primarily cats and dogs—but also birds, ferrets, and rabbits.

complementary and alternative medicine (CAM) Medical treatments used to complement standard medical treatment—for example, the use of acupuncture to treat side effects of cancer treatment; alternative treatment is used instead of standard medical treatment—for example, following a special diet instead of using anticancer drugs prescribed by a physician.

compliance Adherence to regulations or rules.

compounding The actual mixing of ingredients to form powders, tablets, capsules, ointments, and solutions.

Comprehensive Osteopathic Medical Licensing Examination (COMLEX-USA) Exam required of graduates of osteopathic medicine to obtain a license to practice medicine.

computed tomography (CT) Radiography in which a three-dimensional image of a body structure is constructed by computer from a series of plane cross-sectional images made along an axis.

computerized physician order entry (CPOE) system A medication order and fulfillment system.

confidentiality The obligation of healthcare providers to not disseminate patient information beyond proper channels.

conflict of interest A clash between an individual's selfish interests and his or her obligations to an organization, group, or persons.

conflict resolution Finding a peaceful way for two or more parties to resolve a disagreement.

conflicts Serious disagreements or arguments.

congenital malformation A physical defect of an organ or body part that is present in the infant at birth.

Consensus Model for APRN Regulation Model to ensure consistency for the education, licensure, and certification of advanced practice registered nurses.

Construction Health and Safety Technician (CHST) certification Certification is available to technicians with experience in construction safety.

consultant dietitian nutritionist Nutritionist who works under contract with facilities or have private practices.

consultant pharmacist Pharmacists who travel to nursing homes or other facilities to monitor patients' drug therapy.

continuing care community Community or campus that allow residents to move from independent living to assisted living or to a skilled nursing facility as their needs change.

continuing education The process by which a professional seeks recurrent learning activities and training beyond the initial license or certificate.

coordinate To work with different groups or individuals to execute a plan.

Coordinated Program in Dietetics (CP) Undergraduate or graduate program in dietetics that includes clinical experience; graduates are eligible to take the registration exam.

copayment The share of the cost for healthcare services (for example, a doctor's visit) not covered by health insurance.

Coronavirus (COVID-19) One of a group of viruses that causes respiratory illness in animals and humans. Beginning in 2019 the virus resulted in a worldwide pandemic and many deaths.

corrective lenses Lenses worn in front of the eye to correct problems with vision; these can either be contact lenses or glasses.

cost sharing reduction Costs for out-of-pocket deductibles, coinsurance, and copayments are reduced for those obtaining health insurance through the Marketplace.

cost-sharing subsidy A provision of the Affordable Care Act includes subsidies for those enrolling in the Silver Health Plan; these subsidies can be used to pay for healthcare expenses not covered by health insurance such as deductibles and copayments for clinic visits or prescription drugs.

Council for Standards in Human Service Education (CSHSE) Agency that accredits educational programs in human services.

Council on Accreditation of Nurse Anesthesia Education Programs Accrediting agency for the institutions and programs of nurse anesthesia at the post-master's certificate, master's, or doctoral degree levels in the United States.

Council on Education for Public Health Agency that accredits schools and programs of public health.

Council on Podiatric Medical Education (CPME) Accrediting agency for schools of podiatric medicine.

Council on Professional Standards for Kinesiology (COPSKT) Administers accreditation standards for kinesiology education programs, and registration and continuing education programs for kinesiotherapists.

Council on Social Work Education Agency that accredits schools or programs of social work.

counseling psychologist A therapist who helps normal or moderately maladjusted persons, either individually or in groups, to gain self-understanding, recognize problems, and develop methods of coping with their difficulties.

coverage gap Refers to health insurance; for example, individuals who do not qualify for Medicaid because their income is too high yet are unable to purchase health insurance through the Marketplace because the cost of premiums is unaffordable.

CT technologist A radiographer who specializes in computed tomography.

cultural difference The customary beliefs, values, and traits of a racial, religious, or social group that distinguishes one from another.

cytotechnologist Technologist who screens human cell samples under a microscope for early signs of cancer.

dance movement therapy (DMT) Combining movement and psychotherapy to integrate emotional, cognitive, physical, and social aspects of an individual.

Data Service Hub Federally managed data services for consumers applying for health insurance through the Health Exchanges/Marketplace that link to Medicaid and the Children's Health Insurance Program (CHIP) and verifies income and citizenship status.

deductible The dollar amount paid out of pocket for healthcare services before health insurance will cover the cost.

deep tissue massage A form of massage therapy that targets large muscle groups to relieve pain and tension.

defibrillator An electronic device used to restore a heart by applying an electric shock to it.

dementia Decline in cognitive function that affects memory, language, and problem-solving skills. Causes are poor heart health, smoking, brain injury, and some diseases of the brain, including Alzheimer's disease and vascular dementia. Typical symptoms are getting lost in a familiar neighborhood, forgetting names of family members, or forgetting common words.

demographic Related to characteristics of the population: age, gender, race, and ethnicity.

dental assistant A professional who assists dentists by performing a variety of patient care, office, and laboratory duties.

dental ceramist A technician who makes porcelain and acrylic restorations.

dental hygienist A professional who cleans teeth, provides other preventive dental care, and teaches patients how to practice good oral hygiene.

dental laboratory technician A specialist who creates dental appliances according to a dentist's prescription. Dental laboratory technicians who create porcelain and acrylic restorations are often called dental ceramicists.

dental public health specialist A dentist who promotes good dental health and disease prevention within the community.

dentist A trained practitioner who diagnoses and treats problems with teeth and tissues in the mouth, along with giving advice and administering care to help prevent future problems.

developmental disability A term used in the United States and Canada to describe lifelong disabilities attributable to mental and/or physical impairments manifested prior to age 18.

developmental psychologists Psychiatric specialists in investigating the development of individuals from prenatal origins through old age.

diagnosis and treatment of illness Identifying and treating injury or disease.

diagnosis and treatment plan Identification of a disease and the detailed program of action for treating the patient.

diagnosis-related groups (DRGs) A set of payment categories that are used to classify patients for the purpose of hospital reimbursement with a fixed fee regardless of the actual cost and that are based on the diagnosis, surgical procedure used, age of patient, and expected length of stay.

diagnostic imaging The use of an image of a part of the body created by radiographic techniques to aid in a diagnosis.

diagnostic medical sonography Use of sound waves to generate an image for the assessment and diagnosis of various medical conditions.

Didactic Program in Dietetics (DPD) Undergraduate or graduate program that prepares college students to apply for a dietetic internship.

dietetic educator Health professional that specializes in the education of dietitian nutritionists and dietetic technicians.

dietetic internship (DI) Training program that includes clinical experience; graduates are eligible to take the registration exam.

diploma nurse A nurse who has received a diploma administered in a hospital.

direct support professional Aide who works with individuals who are developmentally or intellectually disabled.

discrimination Discrimination in health care refers to the marginalized—those of low income, racial and ethnic minorities, and those who identify as LGBTQ—who often experience obstacles in obtaining health care.

disease prevention services Public health programs designed to reduce the risk of injury or illness in the workplace or for the general public.

disparagement The action of belittling or criticizing the skills, knowledge, or qualifications of another professional.

disparities Wide differences in access to health care or quality of health care based on where one lives as well as income, educational level, race, ethnicity, gender expression, or sexual orientation.

dispensing optician A professional trained to fit and adjust eyeglasses, who may in some states also fit contact lenses according to prescriptions written by ophthalmologists or optometrists, but who does not examine eyes or prescribe treatment.

distributive health care A healthcare system in which delivery of services is not localized in one place, but instead is available in a variety of venues.

DO See Doctor of Osteopathy.

Doctorate in Clinical Social Work (DSW) Prepares graduates to administer educational programs including conducting research, providing supervision, and policy analysis in the field of social work.

Doctor of Audiology (AuD) Academic degree in audiology practice; required to become a licensed audiologist.

Doctor of Optometry Degree that requires the completion of a four-year program at an accredited optometry school, preceded by at least three years of pre-optometric study at an accredited college or university.

Doctor of Osteopathy (DO) A degree conferred by an osteopathic medical school. Osteopathic physicians have the same privileges and use similar techniques as allopathic physicians (MDs) but tend to emphasize a more hands-on approach, particularly with musculoskeletal injuries and disorders.

Doctor of Podiatric Medicine (DPM) Profession similar to MDs and Dos but trained in the medical and surgical care of the foot, ankle, and lower leg.

Doctor of Veterinary Medicine (DVM/VMD) Animal physician who is trained to treat diseases of companion and food animals.

documentation The process of entering a description of a patient's history, condition, diagnostic and therapeutic treatment, and results of treatment.

dosimetrist A technician who calculates the dose of radiation that will be used for treatment.

doulas Individual who provides emotional and physical support for women during pregnancy and childbirth and after the birth of the infant to promote the health and well-being of the mother and infant.

DRG validator One who performs quality review of records and data coded by the coding staff.

drug addiction A form of mental illness described as a chronic, relapsing brain disorder. Characteristics are compulsive drug seeking and continued use despite harmful consequences such as loss of a job or broken relationships. Addictive drugs include alcohol, cocaine, and opium related pain killers such as heroin, morphine, and synthetic opioids (fentanyl, oxycodone).

dual eligible Individual who is eligible for both Medicare and Medicaid services based on age and/or disability and income.

Early and Periodic Screening, Diagnostic, and Treatment (EPSDT) Services for infants, children, and adolescents under age 21 who are enrolled in Medicaid to identify and treat physical and developmental conditions and mental illness.

Ebola virus Causes rare and deadly infection endemic to Africa; the largest Ebola epidemic in history occurred in West Africa in 2014.

echocardiographer Technologist who uses ultrasound to examine the heart chambers, valves, and vessels.

economic effectiveness Ability of an individual to be financially self-sustaining within the parameters of an emotional or mental disability.

educational psychologist Designs, develops, and evaluates materials and procedures to resolve problems in educational and training programs.

electrical stimulation Use of a low-voltage electrical current to stimulate nerves for relief of pain.

electrocardiogram (ECG) An instrument for recording the changes of electrical potential occurring during the heartbeat that is used to diagnosis abnormalities of the heart.

electrocardiograph (ECG) technician Cardiovascular technician who specializes in ECGs, stress testing, and Holter monitor procedures.

electroencephalography (EEG) Procedure that measures the electrical activity of the brain.

electroneurodiagnostic technologist (EEG technologist) A technician who operates electroencephalographs to measure the electrical activity of the brain.

electronic health record (EHR) Individual patient health record stored in a computer database for easy access by physicians and other healthcare workers regardless of the setting—clinic, hospital, nursing home, or emergency care center.

electronic health record support specialist One who provides ongoing end-user support, maintenance, training, and customization of the EHR.

electronic materials management The tracking and managing of inventory of medical supplies, drugs, and other materials.

emergency equipment Equipment such as heart defibrillator, intravenous accessory, oxygen supply, and so on, intended for use in patients experiencing a medical emergency outside a hospital or similar facility.

emergency medical responder The first level of a four-tier category of emergency medical technician who is prepared to care for patients at the scene of an accident and while transporting patients by ambulance to the hospital under medical direction.

emergency medical services (EMS) A network of services coordinated to provide aid and medical assistance from primary response to definitive care, involving personnel trained in the rescue, stabilization, transportation, and advanced treatment of traumatic or medical emergencies.

emergency medical technician (EMT) The second level of a four-tier category of emergency medical technician who has more advanced training and can provide the most extensive prehospital care; however, what they are permitted to do varies by state.

emergency medicine A medical specialty in which physicians care for patients with acute illnesses or injuries that require immediate medical attention.

emergency skills Applicable to a medical emergency including, but not limited to, emergency care (health care at the basic life support level)—for example, spinal immobilization, administration of oxygen, and control of bleeding.

emotional disorders Difficulty in competent use of one's intellectual activity (as thinking, reasoning, remembering, imagining, or learning words).

emotional disturbance Inability to learn, build, or maintain interpersonal relationships, display of inappropriate behaviors, and tendency to develop physical symptoms or fears associated with personal or school problems that adversely affect a child's educational performance.

emotional stress Feeling of being suddenly overwhelmed by the tasks of everyday life.

employee assistance program (EAP) Mental health programs provided by employers to help employees deal with personal problems.

employer shared responsibility payment The Affordable Care Act requires employers with at least 100 full-time employees to either offer minimum essential health insurance coverage or make an employer shared responsibility payment to the Internal Revenue Service for each employee.

endodontist A dentist who performs root-canal surgery and therapy.

endotracheal intubation A procedure in which a tube is inserted into the trachea in order to facilitate breathing in a person with severe respiratory distress or obstruction.

engineering psychologist Deals with the design and use of the systems and environments in which people live and work.

environmental chemist Evaluates the impact of industrial chemical waste on the natural environment—plants, animals, and humans.

environmental factor Determinant of disease found in the surroundings of individuals and groups.

environmental health specialist Assesses air, water, and soil contamination from industrial waste or natural disasters.

Environmental Protection Agency (EPA) Branch of U.S. government that develops policies to protect the safety of air, soil, and water; monitors compliance by industry; and provides technical assistance in times of weather and other emergencies.

environmental restoration planner Assesses polluted land or water sites and determines cost of restoration.

epidemic An outbreak of disease in a certain geographic area in greater numbers than usual; the most common cause of an epidemic in the United States is influenza (flu).

e-prescribing The use of a computerized physician order entry system solely for medications.

equality Providing the same healthcare opportunities for everyone—for example, universal immunization for infants and children.

equity Removing obstacles to health care—for example, providing high quality health care regardless of income and providing transportation or child care to remove obstacles for prenatal care for women.

ergonomist Ensures comfort and safety of workers to prevent injury or illness in the workplace.

essential health benefits Comprehensive health services that the Affordable Care Act requires health insurance plans to offer through the Health Exchanges/Marketplace.

essential hospitals and health systems Facilities that provide health care to vulnerable populations with limited or no access to health care because of finances, insurance status, or health condition.

ethics The formal study of moral choices that conform to standards of conduct.

euthanize Veterinarians put animals to sleep when the animal is close to the end of life to reduce suffering. Some animal shelters euthanize animals when the animal has not been adopted by a family.

evidence-based practice Use of scientific evidence to guide practice decisions.

exclusive provider organization (EPO) Health plan that only covers the cost of providers inside the network.

executive order The president of the United States issues a directive or law instead of the usual process in which laws are passed by the House of Representatives and the Senate and then signed into law by the president. For example, short-term, limited-duration health insurance policies were allowed by states as the result of executive order in 2018.

expansion of Medicaid One of the components of the Affordable Care Act was to provide federal funds to expand the availability of Medicaid for low-income adults with incomes at 138% of the federal poverty level.

experimental or research psychologist Designs, conducts, and analyzes experiments to develop knowledge regarding human and animal behavior. Also referred to as research psychologist.

family practice A medical practice that provides health care regardless of age or sex while placing emphasis on the family unit.

family services social worker A social worker within either a government and/or nonprofit organization designed to better the well-being of individuals who come from unfortunate situations, whether environmental or biological.

federal poverty level (FPL) A measure of income level issued yearly by HHS used to determine eligibility for Medicaid, the Children's Health Insurance Program, and the cost of premiums for health insurance purchased through Health Exchanges.

Federally Facilitated Marketplace (FFM) Options for state governments to provide a Marketplace for consumers to purchase health insurance under the Affordable Care Act.

Federally Qualified Health Center (FQHC) Provides preventive, medical, dental, and mental health services to low-income, minority, and homeless individuals in both urban and rural underserved areas. Centers are qualified to receive reimbursement by Medicare and Medicaid.

Federation of State Massage Therapy Boards (FSMTB) Organization of state boards of message therapy that administer a common licensing exam for massage therapists regardless of state of residence.

fee-for-service payment Payment to a healthcare provider for each medical service rendered to a patient.

FFM-P State-Based Marketplace that operates in partnership with the federal government (FFM-P).

financial viability Ability to work, function, and develop on a financial level.

first responder Refers to the first "certified" person—for example, an emergency medical technician, a police officer, or a firefighter—who arrives at the scene of a disaster, accident, or life-threatening medical situation. The first responder's duties include providing medical assistance and calling other emergency caregivers to the scene.

fissure sealants In dentistry, one method of preventing cavities from developing in the pits and fissures identified in or near teeth is to seal them off with a special varnish called a pit and fissure sealant.

fluoroscopy An instrument used in medical diagnosis for observing the internal structure of opaque objects by casting a shadow of the object upon a fluorescent screen.

food animal veterinarian Specializes in the health care of cattle, poultry, swine, fish, and sheep.

foodborne illness Illness caused by food contaminated with a microscopic organism (virus, bacteria, or fungus) or toxins released by these organisms; can be caused by improper storage temperatures or inadequate cooking temperatures. Symptoms are typically vomiting and diarrhea.

Food Safety and Inspection Service (FSIS) A branch of the U.S. Department of Agriculture (USDA) responsible for ensuring the safety of meat, poultry and egg products. Inspectors work in meat and poultry processing plants.

food safety and inspection veterinarian Employed by both the state and federal government to inspect and test livestock and animal products for major animal diseases, provide vaccines to treat animals, enhance animal welfare, conduct research to improve animal health, and enforce government food safety regulations.

forensic psychologist A professional who works in the criminal justice and legal fields, often serving as an expert witness to explain the psychological aspects of a particular case.

frail elderly Physically weak patients of advanced age.

franchise Licensing granted to an individual or group to market a company's goods or services.

fraud The intentional deception of another person to that person's detriment.

free medical clinics (FMCs) Nonprofit, community-based or faith-based organizations that provide health care with little or no charge to low-income individuals who are uninsured or underinsured and are residents in the county where the clinic is located. Many who use free clinics are the homeless, those with a diagnosis of drug addiction or HIV/AIDS, and immigrants.

fringe benefit An employment benefit that has a monetary value but does not affect basic wage rates (e.g., health insurance or disability insurance).

functional magnetic resonance imaging (fMRI) A method of tracing the work of brain cells by tracking changes in oxygen levels and blood flow to the brain.

gamma scintillation camera Scanner used to take pictures of the radioisotopes as they pass through the patient's body.

genetic counselor A professional who gives information and advice regarding the risk of inherited conditions.

geriatrics Branch of medicine that deals with the problems and diseases of old age and aging people.

geriatric social worker Social worker who specializes in services to older adults.

geriatricians Primary care physicians who specialize in the care of those 65 years of age and older and focus on common health and social issues related to the aging process.

geropsychologist A psychologist who deals with the special problems faced by older adults.

globalization Ease of access to travel and transportation of food products. Increases exposure to communicable diseases and foodborne illness and adds to challenges in tracking the origin of disease or foodborne illness.

grammatical pattern Proper use of words and their meanings.

grooms Animal worker who is responsible for feeding, grooming, and exercising horses.

groomer Animal worker who specializes in maintaining a pet's appearance. In addition to cutting, trimming, and styling the pet's' fur, groomers clip nails, clean ears, and bathe pets.

gross domestic product (GDP) The standard measure of the value of the goods and services produced by a country minus the value of imports during a specified period of time.

group practice Physicians who often work as part of a team, coordinating care for a population of patients, providing backup coverage, and allowing for more time off.

gynecology A field of specialization that focuses on women's health.

health and visual sciences Course of study for a student in an optometry program; courses in pharmacology, optics, vision science, biochemistry, and systemic diseases are included.

health behaviors Actions of individuals that can promote health such as eating a healthy diet and participating in regular physical activity. Also, actions that can increase the risk for disease—for example, eating a less healthy diet, having infrequent physical activity, smoking, excessive use of alcohol or illicit drugs, and risky sexual behavior.

Health Care and Education Reconciliation Act of 2010 Modification of the original Patient Protection and Affordable Care Act with the addition of student loan reform.

healthcare administrator Individual who directs and controls the activities of a healthcare facility or division.

healthcare administrator An individual who plans, directs, coordinates, and supervises the delivery of health care. Sometimes referred to as a healthcare executive.

healthcare executive Leading manager or officer of a healthcare facility or organization.

healthcare facility One of a variety of settings where a patient can receive care.

HealthCare.gov Website operated by HHS that provides information for Americans seeking to obtain health insurance.

Healthcare Practitioners and Technical Occupations Professionals who work directly with patients or with patient laboratory samples to identify health status.

Healthcare Social Worker A social worker who helps patients and their families cope with chronic, acute, or terminal illness.

Healthcare Support Occupation Occupation with lower educational requirements and shorter training periods. For example, nursing assistants, medical assistants, dental assistants, and physical therapy assistants and aides.

health data analyst One who acquires, manages, analyzes, interprets, and transforms patient data into accurate, consistent, and timely information.

health disparities Differences in health outcomes (infant mortality or longevity) because of differences in race, ethnicity, immigration status, income, education, or employment.

Health Education Specialist Teach people about behaviors that promote wellness; develop and implement strategies to improve the health of both individuals and communities.

health educator Person who teaches healthy behaviors—e.g., diet, exercise—to improve the health of communities.

health equity When everyone has the same opportunity to be as healthy as possible because the obstacles (income, employment, education, gender expression, sexual orientation, race, ethnicity, immigration status, age) that prevent discrimination and lack of healthcare access are addressed.

Health Exchange (Marketplace) Site for selecting and purchasing health insurance as a result of the Affordable Care Act; can be online or at a physical site.

health informatics The science of how health information is technically captured, transmitted, and utilized.

health information Basic data (e.g., age, gender, height, weight), clinical conditions (e.g., diabetes, asthma), and many other health data about patients and their family health histories.

health information administrator Directs and controls the activities of the medical record department.

health information management (HIM) The body of knowledge required to acquire, analyze, and protect digital and traditional health information that is considered vital to the delivery of quality patient care.

health information personnel Administrators, technicians, transcriptionists, and medical librarians who work together to manage an information system that meets medical, administrative, ethical, and legal requirements.

health information technician Specialist who organizes and evaluates health records for completeness and accuracy.

health information technology (health IT) Broad concept that encompasses an array of technologies to record, store, retrieve, protect, share, and analyze health information.

Health Insurance Marketplace Also Health Exchange. Federally funded clearing house for enrolling in health insurance.

health literacy The ability of an individual to obtain, process, and understand health information and services needed to make appropriate health decisions.

health maintenance organization (HMO) Insurance provider that administers basic and supplemental health maintenance and treatment services to enrollees who pay a fixed fee.

health outcomes Health status of an individual or community as a result of preventive public health programs or medical intervention.

health physicist Profession that protects people and their environment from potential radiation hazards while ensuring the safe use of radiation in health care and research.

health physics technician Monitors industries that use radioactive materials to prevent exposure or harm to employees.

Health Professional Shortage Area (HPSA) Regions or zones identified by the Health Resources and Services Administration Shortage Designation branch of the HHS as medically underserved; lack of access to primary care, dental, or mental health providers; and groups who face economic, cultural, or linguistic barriers to health care.

health promotion services Education to help clients reduce the risk of illness, maintain optimal function, and follow healthy lifestyles through a wide variety of assistance and activities.

health psychologist Promotes good health through health maintenance counseling programs designed to help people achieve health-oriented goals, such as to stop smoking or lose weight.

health record An ordered set of documents or a collection of data that contains a complete and accurate description of a patient's history, condition, diagnostic and therapeutic treatment, and results of treatment.

Health Resources and Services Administration (HRSA) Agency of HHS with responsibility for improving access to health care for people who are geographically isolated or economically or medically vulnerable.

health savings account (HSA) A form of nontaxable savings that can be used to pay for medical care, often used by individuals in combination with high-deductible health plans (HDHPs).

health science librarian A person who provides essential health science information services to professional staff and personnel in medicine, dentistry, nursing, pharmacy, the allied health professions, and other related technologies.

health team A team of health personnel, each with a specialized function, brought together in accordance with the needs of the client and his or her family.

healthy behavior An action taken to attain, maintain, or regain good health and to prevent illness.

Healthy People 2020 The Office of Disease Prevention and Health Promotion within the U.S. Department of Health and Human Services establishes health goals every decade and compares health data with goals.

hearing aid dispenser Most states require that individuals who dispense hearing aids be licensed; some states may require that audiologists who fit hearing aids obtain a hearing aid dispenser license.

hearing impairment An inability to hear speech and other sounds clearly; an inability to understand and use speech in communication; or the inability to hear speech and other sounds at all.

hematology specialist and technologist Technician or technologist who specializes in the study of blood cells to identify diseases of the blood or to conduct blood type for blood transfusions.

high-deductible health plan with a Saving Option (HDHP/SO) A health insurance plan that requires individuals to pay a set amount of healthcare costs at the beginning of each calendar year before the health plan covers the costs. Usually premiums are lower than traditional health plans. Some plans have a savings account option.

high-frequency transducer Ultrasound transducer used exclusively for the study of breast tissue.

histotechnicians and histotechnologists Technician who cuts and stains tissue specimens for microscopic examination by pathologists.

Burwell v. Hobby Lobby, Inc. A U.S. Supreme Court ruling in favor of Hobby Lobby, a chain of craft stores owned by a Christian family that opposes the use of contraceptives. As a result of the ruling a closely held corporation can opt out of the requirements to cover the cost of contraceptives for female employees.

Holter monitoring A portable device that makes a continuous record of electrical activity of the heart in order to detect episodes of abnormal heart rhythms.

home and community based services (HCBS) Option for state Medicaid programs to cover the cost of providing health and personal care services for the elderly or disabled at home.

Home health agencies (HHAs) Agencies that provide nursing and medical care in the patient's home.

home health aide Direct care worker who works with patients needing long-term care and typically works for certified home health or hospice agencies that receive government funding.

home health care Supportive care provided in one's home.

hospice and palliative care medicine (HPM) Medical care to control pain and other symptoms in those with life-limiting or serious illness.

hospice and palliative care social worker Provides resources and emotional support for patients and their families when there is a serious illness or at the end of life.

Hospitalist Physician (or other primary care provider) who manages patients during the time of hospitalization, including admitting the patient, coordinating care during hospitalization, and following up after discharge.

hospital nurse Provides bedside care to patients admitted to a hospital.

Hospital Readmission Reduction Program (HRRP) A program under the Affordable Care Act to improve quality and reduce costs of care for patients readmitted to the hospital for pneumonia, congestive heart failure, or acute myocardial infarction. Medicare reduces prospective payments to hospitals that fail to meet the criteria for readmission for these three diagnoses.

hospital system Organization that includes more than one hospital or one hospital plus other healthcare organizations such as skilled nursing facilities.

Human Genome Project An international research project that sequenced and mapped all human genes and allows prediction of illness and adverse drug response.

Human Service Board-Certified Practitioner (HS-BCP) Recognized as having met educational and experience requirements to work in human services.

hygiene Personal behaviors that prevent the transmission of infectious disease by removing microorganisms that can cause infectious diseases of the skin, respiratory tract, or gastrointestinal tract. For example, frequent hand washing and bathing with soap and water.

immunizations Public health measures to immunize by vaccination to prevent the spread of infectious diseases within a population. For example, the flu vaccine in adults and measles, mumps, and hepatitis A and B vaccines in children.

immunology scientists and technologists Specialists with training in the study of the human immune system (white blood cells, antibodies) to diagnose the response of the body to infectious organisms or allergens or an abnormal response of the immune system for diseases such as rheumatoid arthritis.

independent activities of daily living (IADLs) See also Instrumental activities of daily living.

Indian Health Services (IHS) Agency within HHS that provides healthcare services for Native Americans and Alaskan Natives.

individual mandate Requirement of the ACA that all individuals are required to have health insurance or pay a tax penalty. The mandate was overturned by law effective January 1, 2019.

Individualized Supervised Practice Pathways (ISPPs) Option for Didactic Program in Dietetics to include supervised clinical experience needed to sit for the registration exam.

industrial ecologist Evaluates the impact of industry on the environment and the costs and benefits of specific programs/processes on the industry and the environment.

industrial or occupational hygienist Develops and monitors factors and stresses in the workplace that may cause injury, illness, or impaired health.

industrial or occupational hygiene technician Worker who monitors the workplace for health hazards to employees including air quality, noise emissions, and ionic radiation.

industrial psychologist Uses scientific techniques to deal with problems of motivation and morale in the work setting.

infant mortality The number of deaths in children less than one year of age per 1,000 live births; reflects the quality of health care.

infection control A discipline focusing on preventing the spread of healthcare-associated infections.

infectious disease Illness caused by pathogenic viruses, fungi, or bacteria and transmitted by person-to-person contact or through a vector such as an infected mosquito (e.g., malaria or West Nile virus).

informed consent Process of a patient giving permission to a healthcare provider to provide services in advance—for example before (1) an invasive procedure, (2) administering an experimental drug, or (3) enrolling in a research trial.

injury prevention Important part of school and community athletic programs insuring that appropriate equipment is worn when participating in team sports; common devices are helmets, elbow and knee pads, and wrist guards.

injury-prevention device Device used by athletes to prevent injury or to stabilize movement after injury to the feet, ankle, knee, wrist, or spine.

Institute of Hazardous Materials Management (IHMM) Professional organization that offers certification for workers in industries that expose workers to hazards including chemicals, noise, and radiation.

instrumental activities of daily living (IADLs) Complex self-care activities that are used to evaluate independence of disabled persons or older adults; examples are shopping, preparing meals, managing finances, and taking medications as prescribed.

insurance claim Form and documentation submitted to insurance companies to request compensation for medical expenses.

intermediate care facility for people with intellectual disability (ICF/ID) A facility that provides personal care and social services.

internal medicine The branch of medicine that deals with the diagnosis and (nonsurgical) treatment of diseases of the internal organs (especially in adults).

internship Supervised, practical experience to aid professional development.

interoperability The mechanism of electronic communication among organizations so that data can be incorporated from one system into another.

interprofessional education (IPE) Model for teaching students in the health professions about the roles and responsibilities of health professionals by functioning as a collaborative team during clinical training.

interprofessional practice (IPP) Process in which each team member participates in discussion and decision making to develop a plan of care for individual patients; improves quality of care and patient outcomes.

interventional X-ray machine High-resolution fixed X-ray equipment that allows physicians to diagnose and perform surgery in a minimally invasive manner.

invasive cardiology A heart specialty that requires the insertion of probes or other instruments into the patient's body.

ionizing radiation Any radiation, as a stream of alpha particles or X-rays, that produces ionization as it passes through a medium.

Junior Commissioned Officer Student Training and Extern Program (JRCOSTEP) Program in which college students are placed in federal government agencies for 31 to 120 days during school breaks. Students enrolled in a variety of programs are eligible to apply including those in environmental health, pharmacy, engineering, and nursing programs.

keeper Care for animals in zoos where they plan diets, feed, and monitor the eating patterns of animals.

kennel attendant Care for pets while their owners are working or traveling. Basic attendant duties include cleaning cages and dog runs, and feeding, exercising, and playing with animals.

Kinesiotherapist Formerly corrective therapist; uses rehabilitative exercise, reconditioning, and physical education to help clients unable to move because of injury or physical disability to become more mobile.

King v. Burwell The U.S. Supreme Court ruled in favor of the government on June 25, 2015, in a dispute over whether individuals who purchased health plans through a federal exchange (instead of a state exchange) would be eligible for premium subsidies.

language disorder An inability to use the symbols of language through appropriate grammatical patterns and the correct use of speech sounds.

laser surgery Surgery performed on the eyes using a laser tool, usually to correct a vision defect such as myopia (near-sightedness).

lensometer An instrument similar in shape to a microscope used by an ophthalmic laboratory technician to ensure the degree and placement of the curve are correct.

Liaison Committee on Medical Education (LCME) National accrediting agency for medical education programs in the United States and Canada.

licensed clinical social worker (LCSW) Clinical social worker who has met the requirement for supervised practice to become licensed to practice independently.

licensed practical nurse/licensed vocational nurse (LPN/LVN) Care for people who are sick, injured, convalescent, or disabled under the direction of physicians and registered nurses.

licensing A right conferred by a governmental body to practice an occupation or provide a service.

licensure The granting of a license by official or legal authority to perform medical acts and procedures not permitted by persons without such a license.

life expectancy Represents the average number of years of life that could be expected if current death rates were to remain constant; used as a gauge of the overall health of a population.

lifestyle Behaviors that impact the incidence and development of disease—for example, diet, physical activity, sexual activity, and the use of alcohol, illegal drugs, and cigarettes.

Little Sisters of the Poor v. Pennsylvania A U.S. Supreme Court ruling in favor of Little Sisters of the Poor allowing employers with moral or religious opposition to contraceptives to be exempt from contraceptive coverage in health plans.

livestock health General condition of animals kept or raised for meat, milk, eggs, or fiber.

Loan Repayment Program (LRP) The National Health Service Corps (NHSC) offers primary care medical, dental, and mental and behavioral healthcare providers the opportunity to have their student loans repaid while earning a competitive salary, in exchange for providing health care in urban, rural, or tribal communities with limited access to care.

longevity The length of human life; longevity usually refers to living past the estimated life expectancy or the average age of death.

long-term services and supports (LTSS) System of providing health and personal care support for the disabled, elderly, or others with chronic health problems in people's homes instead of an institution.

low birth weight Infants weighing less than 2,500 grams (5 pounds, 8 ounces) compared to the average birthweight of 8 pounds (3629 grams); more likely to occur in infants born before 37 weeks with complications requiring admission to a neonatal intensive care unit.

low-vision rehabilitation The restoration to normal or near-normal function in a patient with low vision.

LPN-to-BSN Training programs that allow licensed practice nurses (LPN) to obtain a bachelor's degree in nursing (BSN).

lung capacity The volume and flow of air during inhalation and exhalation.

MD See Doctor of Medicine.

magnetic resonance scanner/imaging (MRI) A noninvasive diagnostic technique based on nuclear magnetic resonance of atoms within the body induced by the application of radio waves to produce computerized images of internal body tissues.

maldistribution of health personnel A situation in which new health workers find it difficult to obtain jobs in their community, while other communities cannot find enough workers to fill the same type of healthcare jobs.

malpractice Professional misconduct.

mammography Use of X-rays to screen for cancer in breast tissue.

managed care organization (MCO) Healthcare plan with established cost controls and designed to improve quality of care.

management dietitian nutritionist Responsible for large-scale food services in hospitals, company cafeterias, prisons, schools, and colleges and universities.

manipulation A chiropractic technique used to adjust ("manipulate") a patient's spine or other parts of the patient's body so that the spine or other body part is in proper form.

manual dexterity The ability to quickly make coordinated movements of the hands and arms.

marketing Promoting, selling, and distributing a product or service.

marketplace subsidies The Affordable Care Act allows subsidies or tax credits for those who earn 400% or less of the federal poverty level; subsidies reduce the cost of health insurance premiums purchased through the federal market place.

Massage and Bodywork Licensing Examination (MBLEx) Licensing exam used by nearly all state licensing boards in the United States; licensure gives massage therapists the legal right to practice.

massage therapy Use of touch, pressure, and/or manipulation to ease pain or tension and reduce stress.

Master Certified Health Education Specialist (MCHES) An advanced credential for health educators with five years of experience in the field and successful completion of a competency exam.

master patient index A listing or database of all the patients treated by the healthcare provider, typically arranged according to an identification process.

Master of Science in Nursing (MSN) An advanced nursing degree that allows a nurse to obtain APRN status.

Master's Degree in Social Work (MSW) Advanced degree for social workers.

Meals on Wheels Service that supplies one hot meal a day to people who cannot or do not leave their homes.

Medicaid Healthcare program for low-income pregnant women, seniors at 100% and adults at 133% of the federal poverty level, and individuals with disabilities; jointly funded by federal and state governments.

Medicaid expansion See Expansion of Medicaid.

Medicaid spousal impoverishment provisions A program that allows for protection of a couple's financial resources so that a spouse can continue living in the community when his or her partner requires nursing home care.

Medicaid waiver A policy that allows individual states to test new ways to deliver and pay for healthcare services for Medicaid and the Children's Health Insurance Program (CHIP).

medical and clinical laboratory scientist (technologist) and technician Performs complex chemical, biological, hematological, immunological, and bacteriological tests of body fluids and tissue to assist physicians in making a medical diagnosis and to evaluate effectiveness of treatment.

medical and health services managers Executives who plan, direct, coordinate, and supervise the delivery of health care.

medical assistant Performs administrative and clinical tasks to keep the offices of physicians, podiatrists, chiropractors, and other health practitioners running smoothly.

medical billing The process of submitting and following up on claims to insurance companies in order to receive payment for services rendered by a healthcare provider.

Medical College Admission Test (MCAT) Exam required of students applying for schools of medicine, osteopathy, and veterinary medicine.

medical doctor (MD) A physician who has obtained a Doctor of Medicine (MD) degree at an accredited allopathic medical school.

medical equipment Devices used by health professionals to make a diagnosis, such as X-ray machines; to treat—for example, lasers used to repair detached retina; or for life support—for example, ventilators.

medical (health science) librarian Provides quick and efficient access to large volumes of information and materials to keep professional staff and personnel abreast of developments, new procedures and techniques, and other relevant data.

medical home The primary source of ongoing preventive care or disease management for an individual or family.

medical math The application of mathematical computations related to healthcare procedures.

medical nutrition therapy Application of the Nutrition Care Process in the management of disease that requires diet modification; the process begins with a nutrition assessment and followed by counseling of clients by a registered dietitian nutritionist (RDN).

medical reimbursement Payments made to healthcare providers in return for services.

medical social worker A social worker who usually works in a hospital setting to find resources for patients after being discharged from the hospital.

medical technology The procedures, equipment, and processes by which medical care is delivered.

medical terminology Specialized terminology used in medicine that allows healthcare providers to communicate specific details of a patient's condition in a precise manner.

medical transcriptionist (MT) An allied health professional that deals in the process of transcription or converting voice-recorded reports as dictated by physicians and/or other healthcare professionals into text format.

Medicare Provides health care to the disabled and those over 65 years of age.

Medicare Advantage Plan When a private health insurance company contracts with Medicare to provide all Part A (hospital) and Part B (outpatient) benefits including prescription drugs.

Medicare reimbursement Repayment from Medicare for out-of-pocket medical expenses.

Medicare Supplemental Health Insurance Health insurance purchased by Medicare beneficiaries to cover the cost of copayments for hospital and outpatient health services.

medication profile A computerized record of the customer's drug therapy.

Ménière's disease Disorder of the inner ear that causes dizziness (vertigo), hearing loss, and ringing in the ears.

mental health A state of emotional and psychological well-being.

mental health and substance abuse social worker Assesses and treats individuals with mental illness or substance abuse problems, including abuse of alcohol, tobacco, or other drugs.

Mental Health Parity and Addiction Equity Act of 2008 Federal law that requires that health insurance policies include coverage for mental illness, including outpatient counseling.

mental health services Diagnosis and treatment of patients with mental or emotional illnesses, including alcohol or substance abuse.

Methicillin-resistant *Staphylococcus aureus* (MRSA) A strain of the *S. aureus* bacteria that is resistant to many antibiotics. In community settings, MRSA is usually confined to the skin; in medical facilities, MRSA causes life-threatening bloodstream and surgical site infections and pneumonia.

microbiology specialist A specialist with training in the study of bacteria, viruses, and other microorganisms.

middle-level health worker Health professional with skills beyond those of a registered nurse and short of those of a licensed physician.

mine examiner A health and safety officer who inspects mines for compliance with federal and state safety regulations.

minimum essential coverage A standard set by the Affordable Care Act for the kind of coverage health insurance companies must provide in all policies.

mobile technology Equipment that can be carried or wheeled from place to place.

mortality Causes and rates of death in a population; monitoring mortality over time is used to develop policies to improve health outcomes.

MRI technologist Technologist radiographer who specializes in magnetic resonance imaging.

multidisciplinary team Medical group composed of several different specialties that evaluate the patient in terms of their individual specialties and work together to develop goals that meet the patient's needs.

muscle injuries Damage or injury to any of the muscles in the body. The various types of muscle injuries are categorized as strains, bruises (contusions), detachment injuries (avulsions), and exercise-induced injury or delayed-onset soreness. The thigh and back muscles are most commonly injured.

musculoskeletal system The body's bones (which make up the skeleton), muscles, tendons, ligaments, joints, cartilage, and other connective tissue which provide form, stability, and movement to the human body.

Music Therapist-Board Certified (MT-BC) Credential that identifies music therapists who have demonstrated knowledge, skills, and abilities necessary to practice music therapy.

Music Therapist (MT) Music is used within a therapeutic relationship to address the physical, psychological, cognitive, and social needs of individuals.

mutation Change in DNA sequence; may increase risk for birth defect or disease.

National Accrediting Agency for Clinical Laboratory Science (NAACLS) International accrediting agency that approves educational programs for clinical laboratory sciences.

National Association of Free & Charitable Clinics (NAFC) A nonprofit organization in the United States that supports local and regional organizations and volunteers who provide medical, dental, pharmacy, and behavioral health care to the economically disadvantaged who also are uninsured.

National Athletic Trainers' Association (NATA) A national association that distributes information about athletic trainers in education, services, and counseling and represents their interests in employment, accomplishments, and similar attributes.

National Board of Nutrition Support Certification (NBNSC) Independent board established by the American Society for Parenteral and Enteral Nutrition (ASPEN) that confers certification (CNSC) for dietitians specializing in nutrition support.

National Board of Certification and Recertification for Nurse Anesthetists (NBCRNA) Organization that offers a national certification exam for nurse anesthetists seeking to obtain or keep their certification and licensure.

National Board for Respiratory Care (NBRC) Administers exams for credentialing in respiratory care; credentials are used to qualify for licensure in most states.

National Center for Health Statistics (NCHS) A division within the CDC that collects data on factors contributing to health risks.

National Certification Board for Therapeutic Massage & Bodywork (NCBTMB) Certifies licensed massage therapists; certification is the highest voluntary credential for massage therapists.

National Coalition of Creative Arts Therapies Associations, Inc. (NCCATA) Coalition of six creative art therapies associations that promote the arts as primary therapeutic treatment. Included are art therapy, dance/movement therapy, drama therapy, music therapy, poetry therapy, and psychodrama.

National Collegiate Athletic Association (NCAA) An organization that represents the interests of college athletic programs and the students who participate in them.

National Commission for Health Education Credentialing, Inc. Agency that offers certification for the certified health educator specialist (CHES) or master certified health education specialist (MCHES).

National Commission on Certification of Physician Assistants (NCCPA) Agency that offers certification for physician assistants via the PANCE exam.

National Council Licensure Examination Either of two licensing exams required to become a registered nurse (NCLEX-RN) or a licensed practical or vocational nurse (NCLEX-PN).

National Council for Therapeutic Recreation Certification (NCTRC) Demonstrates knowledge, skill, and ability recognized as essential for therapeutic recreation practice.

National Council of State Boards of Nursing Nonprofit organization that provides support for nursing regulatory bodies in all states, the District of Columbia and four U.S. territories.

National Environmental Health Association (NEHA) Agency that offers certification for environmental health workers.

National Environmental Health Science and Protection Accreditation Council (EHAC) Agency that accredits educational programs in environmental health science.

National Federation of Independent Business v. Sebelius A June 2012 ruling by the U.S. Supreme Court that upheld the individual mandate—one of two provisions of the Affordable Care Act that were challenged in court—but rejected the other challenged provision and made it optional for states to expand Medicaid.

National Federation of Licensed Practical Nurses (NFLPN) Agency that offers specialty certification in IV therapy and gerontology.

National Health Expenditure (NHE) Estimates of total healthcare spending in the United States; includes measurement of expenditures for healthcare goods and services, public health activities, government administration, investment related to health care, and the net cost of health insurance.

National Health Services Corps (NHSC) An organization that negotiates agreements with primary care medical, dental, and mental health professionals to work in underserved areas with limited healthcare access in exchange for college loan repayments and scholarships.

National Institute of Mental Health (NIMH) Division within the National Institutes of Health that conducts research on mental disorders including anxiety, depression, schizophrenia, bipolar disorder, autism and others.

National Institute for Occupational Safety and Health (NIOSH) Division within the Centers for Disease Control (CDC); conducts research and makes recommendations to prevent worker injury and illness.

National Institutes of Health (NIH) Agency of the HHS that conducts research to discover causes and treatments for diseases.

National League for Nursing (NLN) Professional organization of nursing faculty.

National Radon Safety Board (NRSB) Provides training and certification for workers that test for radon or removing radon from homes and public buildings.

National Registry of Emergency Medical Technicians (NREMT) Certifies emergency medical service providers at five levels: first responder; EMT-Basic; EMT-Intermediate, which has two levels called 1985 and 1999; and paramedic.

National Society of Genetic Counselors (NSGC) Professional organization for genetic counselors.

navigator Individual mandated by the Affordable Care Act whose role is to assist consumers in applying for health insurance plans through the state or federal Health Exchange/Marketplace. Also called patient navigator.

NCLEX See National Council Licensure Examination.

negligence The failure to do something that a reasonably prudent person would do in the same or similar situation; alternatively, doing something that a reasonably prudent person would not do in the same or similar situation.

negotiation To work with another and arrive at a settlement.

nervous system A complex network of nerves and cells that carry messages to and from the brain and spinal cord to various parts of the body.

network Group of hospitals, physicians, and other healthcare providers as well as insurers and community agencies that deliver health services within a geographic area.

neuropsychologist Studies the relationship between the brain and behavior.

neurosonographer Ultrasound technician who focuses on the nervous system, including the brain.

newborn screening Testing of newborns to determine the presence of certain diseases that cause health or development problems.

nonfarm animal caretaker Often work with cats and dogs in animal shelters by feeding and watering the animals.

noninvasive procedure Technical care that does not require the insertion of probes or other instruments into the patient's body.

nuclear cardiology Nuclear imaging technique that involves using radioactive drugs to obtain images of the heart.

nuclear cardiology technologists Operates imaging devices to perform tests that require the use of radionuclides for diagnosis.

nuclear medicine Branch of radiology that uses radionuclides in the diagnosis and treatment of disease.

nuclear medicine computer tomography (CT) technologists Combines the use of radioisotopes with X-rays to create two-dimensional or three-dimensional images inside the human body.

nuclear pharmacist Pharmacist who prepares and dispenses radioactive pharmaceuticals.

nurse anesthetist Nurse who specializes in anesthesia and pain relief.

nurse-midwives Nurses who specializes in women's health and obstetrics, particularly labor and delivery.

nurse practitioners (NPs) Advanced practice registered nurses with a master's or a doctoral degree who have a dramatically expanded scope of practice beyond the registered nurse.

nursing assistant A trained professional who supports the nursing staff in hospitals, long-term care facilities, rehabilitation clinics, and doctor offices.

nutrition and dietetic technician, registered (NDTR) Professional trained at the associate's degree level to assist the registered dietitian nutritionist (RDN) in the delivery of food and nutrition services in hospitals, assisted living facilities, nursing homes, and schools.

nutrition support pharmacist Pharmacist that helps determine and prepare nutrition formulas given intravenously.

Obamacare A common term used to describe the Affordable Care Act; named after President Barack Obama, who signed the bill into law.

Obesity The condition of having a body mass index (BMI) that is higher than the BMI considered appropriate for a given height that occurs due to a complex combination of behavioral, genetic, metabolic, and environmental factors.

obstetric and gynecologic sonographer Ultrasound technician who specializes in the female reproductive system.

occupational health and safety specialist Bachelor's-trained professional that analyzes and inspects the work environment to identify practices with potential harm to employees; designs preventive programs and trains workers to respond to emergencies.

Occupational Health and Safety Technician (OHST) Entry level positions who receive on the job training, complete a certificate program, or associate's degree in the field. Identifies work areas for potential health and safety hazards.

Occupational Safety and Health Administration (OSHA) Division of the U.S. Department of Labor that monitors safety in the workplace.

occupational therapist Helps individuals with mental, physical, developmental, or emotional disabilities learn to perform the activities of daily living.

occupational therapist, registered (OTR) Credential awarded to those who graduate from an accredited educational program and pass a national certification examination.

occupational therapy Treatment for those recuperating from illness that encourages rehabilitation by performing the activities of daily life.

occupational therapy aide/assistant Helps patients develop, recover, and improve skills needed for activities of daily living and for being gainfully employed; works under the supervision of an occupational therapist.

ocular disease Eye disease that must be treated by an optometrist.

old-old Those over 85 years of age.

1973 Older Americans Act (OAA) An addition to a program established by the U.S. Congress in 1965 to provide resources and supports for the elderly, enacted primarily to create the Area Agency on Aging.

Omnibus Budget Reconciliation Act of 1987 (OBRA 87) A law passed by Congress that required Medicare and Medicaid standards and certification procedures for long-term care facilities to merge; ICF/ID standards were upgraded to be the same as skilled care facilities.

ophthalmic laboratory technicians Professional that grinds and creates lenses for glasses based on orders from dispensing opticians.

ophthalmic medical assistant A medical assistant who helps an ophthalmologist provide eye care.

Ophthalmologist A medical doctor specializing in treating diseases or injuries of the eye. Like optometrists, they also provide basic vision care, but they are also able to perform more advanced treatments such as surgery.

opioid use disorder A mental illness and brain disorder caused by addiction to drugs used to relieve pain such as morphine or synthetic opioids.

optics Coursework that must be completed by those who wish to work in the field of optometry.

optometric medical assistant A medical assistant who helps an optometrist provide eye care.

optometrist A medical professional that provides vision care to patients.

Optometry Admissions Test (OAT) A standardized exam that measures academic ability and scientific comprehension.

oral and maxillofacial surgeon A dentist who operates on mouths, jaws, teeth, gums, neck, and head.

oral pathologist A dentist who diagnoses diseases of the mouth.

oral surgeon A dentist who operates on the mouth and jaws.

orderly Attendant in a hospital responsible for the non-medical care of patients and the maintenance of order and cleanliness.

orientation and mobility (O&M) specialist Teaches people with blindness or visual impairments to move about effectively, efficiently, and safely in familiar and unfamiliar environments.

orthodontist The largest group of dental specialists, work to straighten teeth.

orthotic and prosthetic technician One who provides technical support to a certified individual in creating, repairing, and maintaining orthoses and prostheses.

orthotics and prosthetics (O&P) The evaluation, fabrication, and custom fitting of artificial limbs and orthopedic braces.

orthotist One who designs and fits corrective braces, inserts, and supports for body parts that need straightening or other curative functions.

osteopathic manipulative medicine (OMM) Use of hands to manipulate muscles and joints to diagnose and treat common symptoms such as headache, backache, or muscle strain.

osteopathic physician Physician with a Doctor of Osteopathy who places special emphasis on the body's musculoskeletal system, preventive medicine, and holistic patient care.

outcomes assessment The use of standardized, objective measures to gauge a patient's functionality at various stages of treatment.

out-of-pocket Cost of healthcare services not covered by private health insurance, Medicaid or Medicare, or Children's Health Insurance Program. Includes copayments for hospital and outpatient care and may include full payment for eye glasses, hearing aids, and dental work.

oxygen/oxygen mixture Treatment of gases to help patients suffering from breathing disorders.

palliative Intended to reduce or alleviate, but not cure.

palliative care Treatment of symptoms associated with a life-limiting or serious illness, including pain and inability to swallow.

pandemic When an infectious disease affects large numbers of people and spreads around the world. The COVID-19 virus increased in numbers in China (epidemic) but when the virus and illness caused by the virus spread around the world causing many deaths, the outbreak was considered a pandemic.

paraffin bath A form of pain relief that uses heated wax for medical purposes.

paramedic The fourth level of a four-tier emergency medical technician category who perform lifesaving interventions with both basic and advanced equipment typically found in an ambulance.

Patient Care Partnership Expectations for care of hospitalized patients by hospital staff; developed by the American Hospital Association in 2003.

Patient-Centered Medical Home (PCMH) Model for delivering health care in which a primary care provider (physician or advanced practice registered nurse) coordinates health care for individual patients.

patient navigator See navigator.

patient portal An online application that allow patients to interact and communicate with their healthcare providers.

Patient Protection and Affordable Care Act See Affordable Care Act (ACA).

patient registration The process of obtaining pertinent personal, financial, and social information from the patient about their medical history, contact information, and insurance billing data.

patient registration process An activity involving obtaining pertinent personal, financial, and social information from the patient about their medical history, contact information, and insurance billing data.

Pediatric Audiology Specialty Certification (PASC) Certification that signifies expertise in pediatric audiology and is the best option for treating children with hearing and balance disorders and hearing loss.

pediatric dentist A dentist whose work focuses on children and special-needs patients.

Pediatric Nursing Certification Board (NPCB) Agency that certifies nurses as pediatric specialists.

pediatric oncology Medical care of children with cancer.

pediatrics Medical care of infants, children, and young adults.

pedigree Family tree of health conditions, including cause and age of death of biological family members.

pedodontics Dentistry for children (see also pediatric dentist).

pedorthists One who selects, modifies, or creates footwear to address conditions of the foot and ankle.

perceptual skills Awareness of the elements of environment through physical sensation.

periodontist Specialize in treating the gums.

personal and home care aide Direct care worker who works with patients needing long-term care and is employed by public and private agencies that provide home care services.

personal care and service occupations Professionals who provide direct care services to individuals unable to care for themselves (e.g., disabled persons or older adults).

personal protective equipment (PPE) Refers to wearing face masks, gowns, and gloves in a healthcare setting to prevent the transmission of infectious disease.

personnel psychologist A psychologist who applies professional knowledge and skills to the hiring, assignment, and promotion of employees to increase productivity and job satisfaction.

pet sitters Most pet sitters feed, walk, and play with pets daily while the pet owner is away or unable to care for their pet.

pharmaceutical chemistry Physical and chemical properties of drugs and dosage forms. Also known as pharmaceutics.

pharmaceutical fees Established as part of the Affordable Care Act and monitored by the Internal Revenue Service. An annual fee imposed on businesses that manufacture or import branded prescription drugs.

pharmaceutical industry pharmacist Pharmacist that works the sales, research and development, or marketing divisions of pharmaceutical companies.

pharmaceuticals Medicinal drugs.

pharmaceutics The branch of pharmacology concerned with the preparation, use, or sale of medicinal drugs.

pharmacoeconomics The analysis of the costs and benefits of different drug therapies.

pharmacology The study of the effect drugs have on the human and animal bodies.

pharmacotherapist Health professional that specializes in drug therapy and works closely with physicians.

pharmacy administration The study of business aspects of pharmacy use and management.

pharmacy aide/assistant Often a clerk or cashier who primarily answers telephones, handles money, stocks shelves, and performs other clerical duties.

pharmacy informatics The application of information technology to the use of medications to improve patient care.

pharmacy technician Technician who helps licensed pharmacists provide medication and other healthcare products to patients.

philosophy Most basic beliefs, concepts, and attitudes of an individual or group.

phlebotomist Individual trained to draw blood from a patient for clinical or medical testing, transfusions, blood donations, or research.

photosensitivity Sensitivity to light from the sun.

physical disability A limitation on a person's physical functioning, mobility, dexterity, or stamina. Its definition can vary, depending on whether it is a medical, legal, cultural, or other issue.

physical therapist Professional trained to provide services that help restore function, improve mobility, relieve pain, and prevent or limit permanent physical disabilities.

physical therapist aide A professional who helps make therapy sessions productive, under the direct supervision of a physical therapist or physical therapist assistant.

physical therapist assistant Under the direction and supervision of physical therapists, he or she provides part of a patient's treatment.

physical therapy The treatment of disease, injury, or deformity by physical methods such as massage, heat treatment, and exercise rather than by drugs or surgery.

physician assistant (PA) A medical professional who may practice preventive, diagnostic, and therapeutic medicine under the supervision of a physician or surgeon. Responsibilities may include taking a medical history, conducting a physical exam, and ordering and interpreting lab tests and X-rays required for making a diagnosis.

Physician Assistant National Certifying Examination (PANCE) Examination that graduates of physician assistant training programs must pass to be certified and licensed in their profession.

physiology The study of how organisms and their body parts carry out the normal physical functions that allow them to exist.

picture archiving and communication system (PACS) Technology that captures and integrates diagnostic and radiological images from various devices, stores them, and disseminates them to a health record, a clinical repository, or other points of care.

pit and fissure sealants Sealants applied to the tooth to fill pits and fissures and provide a physical barrier on the tooth surface.

podiatric medical assistant A medical assistant who works closely with foot doctors.

policies Acceptable procedures of a governmental, corporate, or nonprofit body.

polysomnography The testing of multiple sleep parameters to diagnose sleep disorders.

positron emission scanners/tomography (PET) Nuclear medicine imaging technique that produces a three-dimensional image of body processes.

positron emission tomography (PET) technologists An imaging specialist who prepares and delivers to patients radioactive drugs for diagnosis and medical research.

Preadmission Screening and Resident Review (PASRR) Screening for mental illness or intellectual disability required for all admissions to Medicaid-certified nursing homes.

predictive genetic counseling Counseling provided when DNA changes are present that increase a person's chances of developing disease—for example, Alzheimer's disease.

preexisting condition Medical diagnosis present at the time health insurance is purchased.

preferred provider organization (PPO) Health insurance plan that covers the cost of providers within a network and outside of the network although copayments by the patient are higher for out-of-network providers.

premium The cost of health insurance covered by an employer, shared with the employee or purchased through a Health Exchange.

premium subsidy See premium tax credit.

premium tax credit Also premium subsidies; allowed by the Affordable Care Act for those who earn 400 % or less of the federal poverty level. The tax credit reduce the cost of health insurance premiums purchased through the federal market place.

prenatal screening Testing done of amniotic fluid during pregnancy to identify fetus with certain genetic diseases.

prescribed drug regimen Medications prescribed by one's healthcare provider to manage an acute or chronic illness.

preterm birth Birth that occurs before 37 weeks' gestation; can be caused by lack of prenatal care, underlying disease in the mother or multiple births. Preterm infants often need additional support, including care in a neonatal intensive nursery because of immature organ systems.

primary care Health care that focuses on prevention, early detection, and treatment and that takes general responsibility for individual patients.

primary care physicians, providers, or practitioners (PCPs) Healthcare practitioners who provide healthcare services for common injuries or illnesses; includes physicians, advanced practice registered nurses, and physician assistants.

privacy officer An individual responsible for developing and implementing requisite privacy policies and procedures, receiving complaints, and disseminating information about an entity's privacy practices.

private health insurance Health insurance provided through an employer or purchased by an individual through another group such as a professional organization.

Professional An individual with specialized learning engaged in a specified activity as an occupation.

professional certification Granted by health professionals' national organizations to ensure health professionals meet established levels of competency.

Professionalism The conduct, character, skills, and judgment of a trained person.

professional registration The listing of certified health professionals on an official roster kept by a state agency or health professionals' organization; some health professionals' organizations use the term *registration* interchangeably with *certification*.

Program An organized set of activities intended to produce a desired outcome (e.g., educational programs improve education).

Program of All-Inclusive Care for the Elderly (PACE) Program that provides comprehensive preventive, primary, acute, and long-term care services so older individuals with chronic care needs can continue living in their local community.

prosthetist One who designs, measures, fits, and adjusts artificial limbs for amputees and devices for people with musculoskeletal or neurological conditions.

prosthodontist A dentist who replacing missing teeth with permanent fixtures, such as crowns and bridges, or with removable fixtures such as dentures.

Protecting Access to Medicare Act of 2014 Law in the U.S. to fund and establish comprehensive mental health and substance use disorder services, Certified Community Behavioral Health Clinics (CCBHCs).

psychiatric aide Individual who works as part of a team to care for mentally impaired or emotionally disturbed individuals.

psychiatric genetic counseling Used to determine the risk for mental illness for individuals who have family members with behavioral or psychiatric disorders.

psychiatric or mental health technician Works as part of a team to provide care and treatment of emotionally or mentally disabled patients.

psychiatry The branch of medicine that deals with the diagnosis, treatment, and prevention of mental and emotional disorders.

psychological treatment Treatment aimed at changing the patient's interpersonal environment to alleviate symptoms of mental or emotional disturbance.

psychological variables The collection of factors that can affect or alter a person's coping and mental health.

psychology A scientific approach to gathering, quantifying, analyzing, and interpreting data on why people act as they do; it provides insight into varied forms of human behavior and related mental and physical processes.

psychometric psychologist Health professional that directly measures human behavior, primarily through the use of tests.

public health Focuses on the protection of the environment, including air, food, and water and improvement of community health.

public health dentistry Community dental health.

qualified health plan (QHP) Under the Affordable Care Act, a QHP is certified by the Health Insurance Marketplace to include essential health benefits.

quality improvement analyst One who analyzes, reviews, forecasts, trends, and presents information directed at improving the quality of patient care.

radiation oncologist A physician who specializes in therapeutic radiology.

radiation physicist A worker who calibrates the linear accelerator simulator and checks that radiation output is accurate.

radiation therapy Treatment of disease by exposure of diseased tissue to radiation.

radiologic technician/radiographer/X-ray technician Specialist who takes X-rays and administers nonradioactive materials into patients' bloodstreams for diagnostic purposes.

radiologic technologist Specialist who performs complex imaging procedures.

radiologist Diagnoses and treats illness by the use of X-rays and radioactive materials.

radionuclides Unstable atoms that emit radiation spontaneously.

radiopharmaceutical Radioactive drug.

radiopharmacist Applies the principles and practices of pharmacy and radiochemistry to produce radioactive drugs that are used for diagnosis and therapy. (See also nuclear pharmacist.)

Radon Measurement Technician (RMT) Knowledgeable about the health risks associated with radon (radioactive gas that occurs in nature) and knowledgeable about measuring radon.

recreational sports Those activities where the primary purpose of the activity is participation, with the related goals of improved physical fitness, fun, and social involvement often prominent.

recreation therapy A form of therapy that uses medically approved activities such as sports, games, and field trips, to treat or maintain the physical, mental, and emotional well-being of patients.

recreation therapist (RT) Practitioners in the field of recreation therapy use activity-based interventions to address the needs of clients with illnesses or disabilities as a means to psychological and physical health and recovery.

registered art therapist (ATR) Credential that ensures that an art therapist has successfully completed a graduate-level program in art therapy and completed supervised postgraduate clinical experience.

Registered Behavior Technician (RBT) Paraprofessional with 40 hours of postsecondary training; works under the supervision of a certified behavior analyst to carry out treatment programs.

registered clinical exercise physiologist (RCEP) Credential offered by the Clinical Exercise Physiology Association to promote the field of exercise physiology; eligibility is based on education and work experience.

Registered Dance/Movement Therapist (R-DMT) A credential that represents a basic level of competence in dance/movement therapy and qualifies the therapist to be employed as a dance/movement therapist in a clinical or educational setting.

registered dietitian nutritionist (RDN) Dietetic professional that has passed the registration exam after completing academic coursework and supervised clinical practice.

Registered Environmental Health Specialist or Registered Sanitarian (REHS/RS) Ensures clean air and safe food and water; manages sewage and hazardous materials; responds to natural disasters.

registered nurses (RNs) Nursing professionals who deliver therapy and treatment to patients as prescribed, educate patients and the public about various medical conditions, and provide emotional support to both patients and family members.

Registered Respiratory Therapist (RRT) Credential awarded to CRTs who have graduated from advanced programs and passed two separate examinations.

registered kinesiotherapist (RKT) One who has graduated from an accredited educational program in kinesiotherapy or exercise science, completed the registered examination, and maintained continuing education hours to maintain registration.

registration The listing of certified health professionals on an official roster kept by a state agency or health professionals' organization.

Rehabilitation The restoration of a person to normal or near-normal function after a physical or mental illness, including chemical addiction.

rehabilitation center A facility for providing therapy and training for rehabilitation.

rehabilitation psychologist Works with disabled persons, either individually or in groups, to assess the degree of disability and develop ways to correct or compensate for these impairments.

reimbursement To make a return payment to.

Religious Freedom Restoration Act of 1993 Limits the ability of the federal government to restrict the exercise of religious beliefs without compelling justification; used in defense of the right of businesses to be exempt from covering the cost of contraceptives for women in Hobby Lobby v. Burwell.

repetitive stress injuries Injuries that happen when too much stress is placed on a part of the body, resulting in inflammation (pain and swelling), muscle strain, or tissue damage. This stress generally occurs from repeating the same movements over and over again.

reproductive technology Methods used to assist couples with infertility to conceive.

research Collecting of information about a particular subject.

research dietitian nutritionist Nutritionist employed in academic medical centers or educational institutions, although some work in community health programs.

research veterinarian Provides medical services to support animals participating in medical research studies; also faculty in schools of veterinary medicine who teach, conduct research, and supervise the care of animals by students in veterinary medicine.

residential care community See assisted-living facilities.

respiratory therapy technician Technician working under the supervision of physicians or respiratory therapists to evaluate and treat patients with breathing disorders.

RN-to-BSN A degree program that enables registered nurses who do not have a bachelor's degree to obtain a BSN more quickly than would be the case for those without an RN.

RN-to-MSN Allows someone with a bachelor's degree obtain RN status upon completing a master's of science in nursing.

Safety Management Specialist (SMS) Knowledgeable about the operation of an industry to preserve the safety and health of employees and the environment; establishes safety management systems in the workplace.

school health educator Professional who helps children and young people develop the knowledge, attitudes, and skills they need to live healthfully and safely.

school nutrition specialist (SNS) Option for certification for dietetic technicians working in school nutrition programs; conferred by School Nutrition Association.

school psychologist A psychologist concerned with developing effective programs for improving the intellectual, social, and emotional development of children in an educational system or school.

school social worker Social worker who serves as the link between students' families and the school, strives to ensure students reach their academic and personal potential.

self-contained underwater breathing apparatus (SCUBA) Equipment that allows first responders to breathe underwater during a water rescue.

senior centers Focal point for services and referrals to resources for the elderly; funded by the federal government as a result of the Older Americans Act.

sepsis An inflammatory response to a serious and widespread infection; the response causes damage to organ systems and can cause shock and death.

serious mental illness (SMI) Mental illness that is difficult to treat and frequently interferes with normal functioning and the ability to maintain interpersonal relationships or employment; most common are schizophrenia and bipolar disorder.

shared responsibility for coverage When health insurance is purchased through a Health Exchange/Marketplace to share the cost of premiums between the consumer and the federal government.

short-term, limited-duration health policy Modification to the ACA in 2018 by executive order that allowed states to offer health insurance policies that did not meet ACA requirements for essential coverage and eliminating coverage for those with pre-existing conditions.

side effects A secondary and usually adverse effect of a medication or treatment.

skilled nursing facility (SNF) A nursing home that provides the level of care closest to hospital care.

skin puncture A procedure in which a needle is inserted into the skin in order to infuse a medication.

Small Business Health Options Program (SHOP) Part of the 2010 healthcare reform legislation; small businesses with up to 100 employees can purchase qualified coverage for employees through SHOP exchanges established at the state or regional level.

social and economic factors Lack of access to stable housing, nutritious food, employment, education, personal safety, and personal or family support.

social and human service assistant Personnel who assists patients in obtaining services.

social determinants of health (SDOH) The conditions under which people are born, live, work, and age. Lack of access to stable housing, nutritious food, employment, education, reliable transportation, and personal safety influences access to quality health care.

social psychologist Studies the effects of groups and individuals on the thoughts, feelings, attitudes, and behavior of the individual.

Social Security Act of 1935 Federal funding of state health departments for maternal and child health services.

Social Security Act of 1965 Established Medicaid, health insurance for low-income individuals, and Medicare, health insurance for the disabled and those 65 years of age and older.

social work administrator An administrator who performs overall management tasks in hospital, clinic, or other setting that offers social worker services.

social work planner and policy maker Professional who develops programs to address such issues as child abuse, homelessness, substance abuse, poverty, and violence.

social and economic factors Factors that impact health outcomes are lack of access to stable housing, nutritious food, employment, education, personal safety, or personal and family support.

soft tissue mobilization A form of therapy that seeks to loosen tightness and minimize pain through application of pressure and manual manipulation.

solo practitioner Physician who works in an independent setting instead of a group practice.

sonographer/ultrasound technologist An individual who collects reflected echoes and forms an image that may be videotaped, transmitted, or photographed for interpretation and diagnosis by a physician.

Spanish Flu (1918 Flu) Pandemic caused by a deadly H1N1 influenza A virus that lasted two years, spread worldwide, and caused many deaths.

specialty board certification Areas of specialty for dietitian nutritionists in gerontology, pediatrics, renal nutrition, sports nutrition, oncology, or advanced clinical practice; certification requires experience and exam.

speech disorder Identified by an individual's difficulty in producing speech sounds, controlling voice production, and maintaining speech rhythm.

speech-language pathologist (SLP) Assesses, diagnoses, treats, and helps to prevent disorders related to speech, language, cognitive-communication, voice, swallowing, and fluency.

speech-language pathology assistants (SPLA) Trained to support Speech-Language Pathologists in providing services.

speech recognition software Computer programs that collect spoken words, analyze those words, and present the results as data.

spinal adjustment A chiropractic technique used by applying thrusts of varying speed and forces to spinal joints that are not in alignment and causing dysfunction and related pain.

sport centers Area or locations in a private (e.g., spa, fitness) or public (e.g., stadium, school) environment where specific sports take place—for example, a football stadium, a tennis court, or a spa center.

sports medicine Specialty concerned with the prevention and treatment of injuries and disorders that are related to participation in sports.

standards for pure food from animal sources Measure of quality established to ensure safe food production from animal sources.

State-Based Marketplace (SBM) A place where individuals can purchase health insurance; can be a physical location or available online.

State Loan Repayment Program Available in 30 states for students in a variety of healthcare training programs.

Statistics Analysis of quantitative data to identify patterns.

strategic planning A careful, well-thought method of establishing goals, policies, and procedures.

stress testing Monitors the heart's performance while the patient is walking on a treadmill, gradually increasing the treadmill's speed to observe the effect of increased exertion on the heart.

Student to Service Loan Repayment Program For students in the last year of school training as a physician, dentist, nurse practitioner, or certified nurse-midwife. Loan repayment is in exchange for serving three years in a designated health professional shortage area.

substance abuse counselor Helps individuals overcome addictions to intoxicants and cope with life's stresses.

sudden infant death syndrome (SIDS) Sudden unexplained death in an infant younger than one year of age, usually between 1 and 4 months of age.

surgery The branch of medicine that deals with the diagnosis and treatment of injury, deformity, and disease by making physical alterations to tissue; surgical treatments range from minor procedures such as inserting stitches into external wounds to aid the healing process to major, invasive procedures used to alter, repair, remove, or transplant internal organs.

surgical technologist A technologist who assists in surgical operations under the supervision of surgeons, registered nurses, or other surgical personnel.

symptoms and response Evidence of disease and the bodies reaction to a course of treatment.

teacher's certificate, license A certification required for teaching in K-12 schools; must meet educational requirements.

technology Tools and systems used to deliver health care, including computerized medical records, automated laboratory analysis, surgical robotics, and sophisticated diagnostic imaging—computerized axial tomography (CAT) and magnetic resonance imaging (MRI). Advances in technology contribute to the high cost of health care in the United States.

telehealth Healthcare appointments delivered by the clinician through telecommunication technologies. Also, communicating appointment reminders, visit summaries, and laboratory and diagnostic results through an electronic record.

telemedicine The use of electronic communications and information technologies to provide or support clinical care at a distance.

telepractice Use of telecommunication technology to deliver professional services at a distance; used by speech language pathologists and other health professionals.

tests and measurements Methods of evaluating physical capacity and health.

The Joint Commission Organization that provides oversight for hospitals and long-term care facilities and other healthcare organizations, including home care, behavioral health care, ambulatory care, and laboratory services.

therapeutic exercise Medically recommended physical activity designed to improve function, address an impairment, or improve quality of life.

therapeutic recreation (TR) The field of practice for recreation therapists who use different recreational activities to treat or restore to a level of functioning or independence in those with injury or illness.

third-party reimbursement Payment for services rendered by a provider to a person in which an entity other than the receiver of the service is responsible for the payment. For a doctor, a patient, and an insurance company in the healthcare system, the insurance company is the third-party reimbursing the doctor's fee on the patient's behalf.

tinnitus Ringing or other noises in the ear; caused by noise exposure, ear infection, and often unknown causes; often associated with hearing loss.

transesophageal echocardiography A form of testing that involves placing a tube in the patient's esophagus to obtain ultrasound images.

transmissible diseases Infections caused by viruses or bacteria that are easily carried from one animal to another, or from animals to humans.

trauma center A hospital unit specializing in the treatment of patients with acute and life-threatening traumatic injuries.

tumor registrar Individual that compiles and maintains records of patients who have cancer to provide information to physicians and for research studies.

ultrasound machine An electronic device that uses vibrations of the same physical nature as sound to form a two-dimensional image used for the examination and measurement of internal body structures.

uncompensated care Health care or services provided by hospitals or healthcare providers that do not get reimbursed; usually because patients don't have insurance or personal funds to pay for the cost of care.

universal vaccination Public health program to prevent communicable diseases through vaccination programs of children, adolescents, and adults. Immunization programs for children have eliminated most childhood infectious diseases such as measles, mumps, meningitis, hepatitis A and B, and polio. Adult immunizations prevent bacterial pneumonia, shingles, and influenza.

U.S. Administration on Aging (AOA) Division within HHS agency, Administration for Community Living; provides a variety of home- and community-based services for older adults and disabled persons.

U.S. Department of Health and Human Services (DHHS) The U.S. government's principal agency for protecting the health of all Americans and providing essential human services, especially for those who are least able to help themselves.

U.S. Medical Licensing Examination (USMLE) Exam required of medical school graduates to become licensed to practice medicine.

U.S. Public Health Service (USPHS) Group of agencies that focus on making laws, allocating funds, and doing investigative work to protect the health of all Americans.

value-based care Paying providers of health care based on the quality of care instead of the volume or number of patients treated or the number of treatment procedures.

vascular technologist Technologist who assists physicians in the diagnosis of disorders affecting the circulation.

vendor-neutral archive A single, consolidated archive platform used to host files from different PACS software.

venipuncture A procedure in which a needle is inserted into a patient's vein in order to draw blood or infuse medication.

ventilator A machine that pumps air into the lungs.

vertigo Balance disorder with symptoms of dizziness or spinning; caused by ear infection, head injury, or certain medications.

veterans A person who has been discharged from the military.

Veterinarian Cares for the health of pets, livestock, and animals in zoos, racetracks, and laboratories.

Veterinary College Admission Test (VCAT) Admission requirement for applicants to schools of veterinary medicine.

Veterinary Medical College Application Service (VMCAS) Agency that represents colleges of veterinary medicine and a central location for application to schools of veterinary medicine.

Veterinary Technician National Examination (VTNE) Used by most states for licensure of veterinary technicians.

veterinary technologist/technician Technician who assists in the diagnosis and treatment of animals, usually in an animal hospital or clinic.

viral gastroenteritis Infection of the digestive tract caused by a virus transmitted between individuals. The most common cause of viral gastroenteritis in humans is the norovirus with symptoms of vomiting and diarrhea.

vision rehabilitation therapist (VRT) Health professional who provides instruction for the visually impaired to use community resources and assistive technology.

vision therapy Treatment for those with vision issues.

vital statistics Information that chronicles certain life events, like birth and death.

VMD See Doctor of Veterinary Medicine.

volunteer EMT Depending on the legal requirements of a state, this term refers to "volunteer first aid, rescue, and ambulance squad," which provides emergency medical services without receiving payment for those services.

vulnerable populations Demographic groups that are at heightened risk of a disease or injury due to characteristics specific to that group.

wearable technology A small computer that can be worn on a person.

wellness and health promotion Wellness is a healthy balance of the mind, body, and spirit that results in an overall feeling of well-being. Health promotion refers to the improvement of health or wellness. For example, stopping smoking is one means to promote one's health and wellness.

work-related injuries Injuries that occur in the workplace, which are often covered by workers' compensation; includes physical, psychological, and stress-related injuries.

work requirement waiver Beginning in 2018 the Centers for Medicare and Medicaid Services (CMS) established a waiver to allow states to require that recipients of Medicaid be employed or enrolled as a student to qualify for health insurance through Medicaid.

World Health Organization (WHO) Agency of the United Nations that directs and coordinates international health within the United Nations' system.

zoonotic diseases The spread of harmful microorganisms (virus, bacteria, parasites, fungi) between animals and people. An example is avian flu that is spread between birds or poultry and humans.

INDEX

Note: Italicized numbers indicate a term found in a figure or table.

Opticians Association of America, 213
optics, 209
optometric assistants, 440
optometrists
    additional information, 210–211
    advancement, 210
    earnings, 210, *211*
    education, 209
    employment change, 210
    employment opportunities, 209
    employment trends, 210
    job prospects, 210, *210*
    licensure, 209–210
    other qualifications, 210
    related occupations, 210
    training, 209
    work description, 208–211
    work environment, 209
Optometry Admissions Test (OAT), 209
oral and maxillofacial surgeons, 168
oral pathologists, 168
orderlies, 444. *See also* nursing assistants
    and orderlies
orientation and mobility (O&M)
    additional information, 332
    advancement, 328
    certification and other qualifications, 328
    earnings, 328
    education, 327–328
    employment opportunities, 327
    job prospects, 328
    licensure, 328
    related occupations, 328
    specialists, 326–328
    training, 327–328
    work description, 326–327
    work environment, 327
orthodontists, 168
orthopedic surgery, 128
orthotic and prosthetic technician,
    243, 244
orthotics and prosthetics (O&P)
    additional information, 245
    certification and other qualifications, 244
    earnings, 245, *245*
    education, 244
    employment change, 245
    employment opportunities, 244
    employment trends, 245
    job prospects, 245, *245*
    licensure, 244
    related occupations, 245
    training, 244
    work description, 243, *243*
    work environment, 243–244
Orthotics and Prosthetics Residency
    Centralized Application Service
    (OPRESCAS), 244
orthotists, 104
Osteopathic Manipulative Medicine
    (OMM), 126

osteopathic physicians, 126
otolaryngology, 128
outcomes assessment, 238
out-of-pocket, 46
    costs, 42
outpatient cardiac rehabilitation
    centers, 21
outpatient clinics, 21, 26
    as employer, 103–104
outsourcing, transcription work, 432
oxygen or oxygen mixtures, 382

P

PACS. *See* picture archiving and
    communication system
PAHCOM. *See* Professional Association
    of Healthcare Office Management
palliative care, 129
pandemic, 8
paraffin baths, 240
paramedics, 346, 347. *See also* EMT-
    paramedics
Paraprofessional Healthcare Institute, 456
Parkinson's disease, 414
Patient Care Partnership, 27
patient care, standard precautions for, 512
Patient-Centered Medical Home
    (PCMH), 22
patient-centered teams, 117
patient information, confidentiality of, 91
patient navigators, 321
patient portal, 89
patient registration, 86
    process, 90
Patient's Bill of Rights, 27
payment reforms, 73
PCMH. *See* Patient-Centered Medical
    Home (PCMH)
Pediatric Audiology Specialty
    Certification (PASC), 227
pediatric dentists, 168
pediatricians, 128, *132*
Pediatric Nursing Certification Board
    (PNCB), 152, 163
pediatric oncology, *150*
pediatric otolaryngologist, 221
pediatric RDNs, 184
pediatrics
    optometrists and, 208
    PAs and, 140
pedigree, 313
pedorthists, 243
people, infection control, 514
perceptual skills, 250
periodontists, 168
personal and home care aide, 99, 100, 103
personal care aides. *See* home health and
    personal care aides
personal protective equipment (PPE), 8,
    512, 516, 517

personal trainers, 262
personnel psychologists, 287
PET. *See* positron emission tomography
pet groomers, 474, 475
pet sitters, 474
pharmaceutical chemistry, 200
Pharmaceutical industry pharmacist,
    199, 545
pharmaceuticals, 198
pharmaceutics, 200
pharmacists, 198
    additional information, 201–202
    advancement, 201
    consultant, 199
    earnings, 199
    education, 200
    employment change, 201
    employment opportunities, 199
    employment trends, 201
    job prospects, 201, *201*
    licensure, 200
    nuclear, 199
    nutrition support, 199
    other qualifications, 200
    radiopharmacists, 199
    related occupations, 201
    work description, *198,* 198–199
    work environment, 199, *199*
pharmacoeconomics, 201
pharmacology, 200
pharmacotherapists, 199
pharmacy administration, 200
Pharmacy College Admissions Test
    (PCAT), 200
pharmacy informatics, 201
pharmacy residencies, 200
Pharmacy Technician Certification Board
    (PTCB), 203, 204
pharmacy technicians and aides
    additional information, 204
    advancement, 203
    certification and other qualifications, 203
    earnings, 204
    education, 203
    employment change, 203–204
    employment opportunities, 202
    employment trends, 203–204
    job prospects, 204, *204*
    related occupations, 204
    training, 203
    work description, 202
    work environment, 202
phenylketonuria (PKU), 313
philosophy, 339
phlebotomists, 396
    additional information, 401
    advancement, 400
    certification and other qualifications,
        400
    earnings, 401
    education, 400